Mammotrophic Assayables of Cocted and Embalmed Ichthyic Victualia

Anastasios Anthropos

Mammotrophic Assayables of Cocted and Embalmed Ichthyic Victualia

First Edition December 2025

Written by Anastasios Anthropos

CONTENTS

Topic	Page No.

Chapter - 1

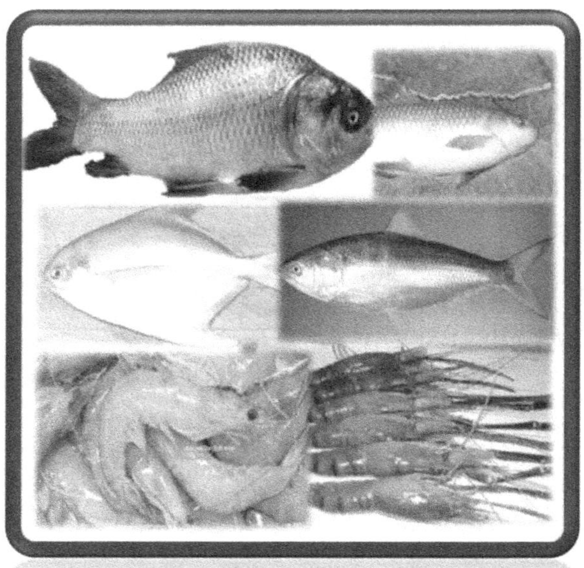

General Introduction

Fish are rich sources of high-quality protein and contain relatively low levels of cholesterol; therefore, they are often recommended for regular consumption. The major constituents of fish include moisture, protein, fat, minerals, and certain vitamins. Carbohydrate content in fish is generally negligible, while moisture content typically ranges from 60–80%. Protein content averages around 15–16%, and fat content varies widely, generally ranging from 2–13%, depending on the species. The nutritional composition of fish is influenced by several factors, including species, size, age, and seasonal variations. Since ancient times, fish has been recognized as an excellent source of animal protein in the human diet. Owing to its high-quality protein and low saturated fat content, fish is widely consumed across the world. It is also a rich source of omega-3 polyunsaturated fatty acids, which are known to reduce the risk of cardiovascular diseases in adults and play a crucial role in neural development in infants and young children, thereby supporting overall health.

In recent years, the lipid fraction of fish has gained significant nutritional importance due to its high content of polyunsaturated fatty acids. Fish are also considered a valuable source of essential minerals and vitamins. The total mineral content of raw fish flesh generally ranges from 0.6–1.5% of wet weight. Important minerals such as sodium, potassium, magnesium, calcium, iron, phosphorus, and iodine are present in fish and contribute significantly to human nutrition. The contents of sodium, potassium, calcium, magnesium, and phosphorus are approximately 1 mg per 100 g, while iron, zinc, and iodine are usually present in amounts less than 1 mg per 100 g. Different cooking methods can significantly affect the nutrient composition as well as the flavor profile of fish.

Several studies have reported the effects of various cooking techniques on the macro- and micronutrient content of different fish species. From a nutritional perspective, it has been observed that certain essential nutrients may be lost during the cooking process. Therefore, it is important to evaluate nutrient retention in cooked fish prepared using common domestic methods such as boiling, roasting, and frying. Fish is a highly perishable food commodity, and its preservation requires the application of appropriate techniques. Due to its high moisture and nutrient content, fish is highly susceptible to spoilage by microorganisms. Effective preservation methods are essential to prevent spoilage while maintaining the physical quality and nutritional value of fish. Spoilage primarily occurs due to rapid autolysis caused by endogenous enzymes, leading to changes in acidity that promote bacterial growth. Consequently, fish generally spoils more rapidly than other flesh foods and may begin to deteriorate within 12 hours of capture under the high temperatures typical of tropical regions. Common fish preservation methods include salting, drying, chilling, smoking, and freezing, which help extend shelf life and retain nutritional value.

Significance of the study

- Since fish is not usually consumed in the raw state, several different cooking methods are employed for the preparation for consumption. After cooking, the nutritive values of raw state fish are changed due to heat, temperature and the addition of water and oil. As the nutritive values of raw state and cooked fish differ from one another, this study can help to estimate the difference.
- Additionally, this study can also help to understand the best method of cooking for the retention of nutritive values and conclude which one is the most nutritious among the selected samples commonly consumed.
- Moreover preservation of the selected samples is carried out to estimate the nutritive value changes during preservation.
- The study is further compounded with the effect of different preservatives during preservation for 1, 2 days for estimating the immediate changes and for 14 and 15 days for estimating long-term changes of the samples, from the nutritional point of view.
- Mostly fish are preserved in the raw state and then cooked and consumed. So it is important to estimate their changes. Generally preservation for 2 days is very common in household level but those who have very little time to buy fish from the market daily, preserve fish for at least 2 weeks. This study basically helps to reveal the nutritional changes due to two different effects i.e. cooking and preservation with preservative and without preservative.

Samples of the study

Six most popular and abundant samples are selected for carrying out the study.

A. FRESH WATER SAMPLE

Fresh water fish can be defined as those fish, which spend their lives in fresh water bodies like lakes, rivers, where the salinity is less than 0.05%.

1. **CARP:** Carps are fishes of cyprinidiea family. They are highly cultured and domesticated in aquaculture for food. Fishes like *katla*, *rohu* and *mrigel* are the three major carps of India. Among these two major carps are chosen for the study -
   - *Rohu* (*Labeo rohita*) commonly known as *Rui*.
   - *Katla* (*Catla catla*) commonly known as *Katla*.
2. **CRUSTACEANS:** Crustaceans are a group of aquatic mandibulate arthropods, possessing calcareous and chitinous exoskeleton, a pair of modified appendages on each segment along with two pairs of antennae. These include shrimps, crabs, lobsters, wood lice and

many more. Among them two most popular and easily available samples are chosen for the study -

- Prawn (*Fenneropenaeus indicus*) commonly known as *bagda chingri.*
- Lobster (*Macrobrachium rosenbergii*) commonly known as *galda chingri.*

B. SALT WATER SAMPLE

Salt water fish are those which live in saline water or in basic environment i.e. 8.2 pH. India being surrounded by the Indian Ocean, Arabian sea, a variety of marine fish are found, such as salmon, tuna, cod, pomfret, *hilsa*, mackerel etc. Among them two most popular fish are chosen for the study-

- Pomfret (white variety) (*Pampus argenteus*) commonly known as Pomfret.
- *Hilsa* (*Tenualosa ilisha*) commonly known as *ilish.*

These species are commonly consumed in West Bengal especially in the Bengali community and there is no data regarding their nutritive values. Many researchers carried out different researches with marine fish and other edible aquatic species (as cited in chapter 2: Review of Literature) but the nutritional changes of these above samples are still unrevealed, hence these were chosen as the subject of the present study.

Information of the samples

a. Rohu (Labeo rohita):

Scientific classification:

Kingdom:	Animalia
Phylum:	Chordata
Class:	Actinopterygii
Order:	Cypriniformes
Family:	Cyprinidae
Genus:	*Labeo*
Species:	*L.rohita*

Fig.1.1 *Rohu*
Source: iucnredlist.org

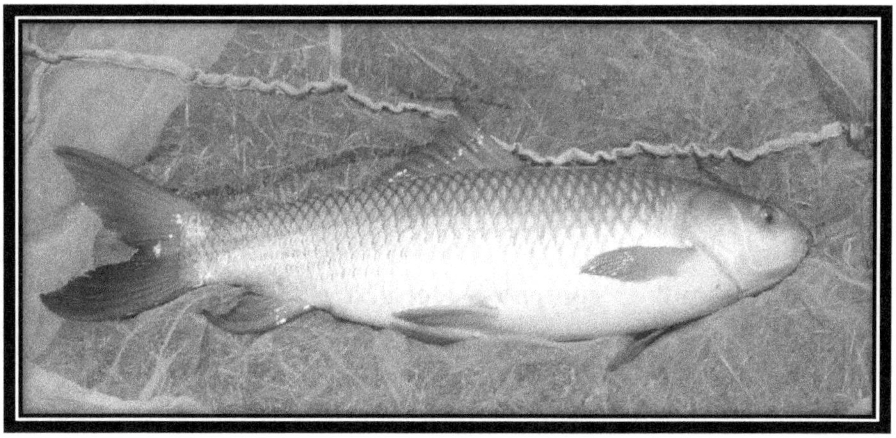

Fig.1.1.1 *Rohu*
Source: Rohu (*Labio rohita*) database

Rohu is one of the freshwater fishes of the carp family which is a very popular variety of fish in India and other parts of world especially south-east Asia. Among all carp species *rohu* is always popular due to its market demand and taste. This fish is generally collected from the pond by using the fishing nets when they attain at least 500 grams, but when they weigh 1 kg to 2 kg, the market demand is good[8].

Physical characteristics:

- *Rohu* has a thick body with narrow head and tail compared to *katla* and the weight of the head is less in *rohu* when compared with *katla.*
- The body is covered with scales except fins and head. Apart from this, the head is triangulated.
- Body surface and under body surface of *rohu* is brown in colour.
- The belly is silver-coloured and there is a total of 7 fins in the body.
- The maximum length is generally 1 meter.
- The body is slightly curved to upper side and it has two pairs of nostril.
- The scales are reddish in colour except the belly part[8].

Production areas of *Rohu*

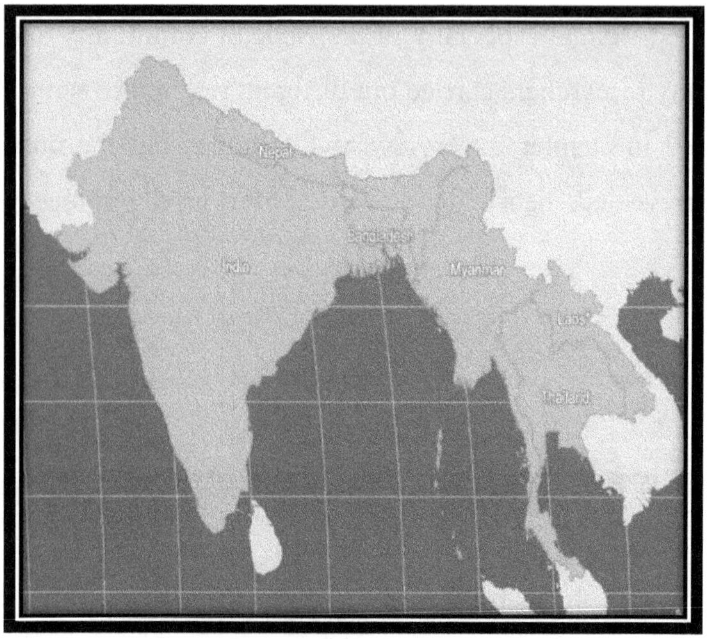

Fig.1.2 Habitat of *Rohu*
Source: FAO Fishery Statistics, 2006

Health benefits:

Although a diet consisting of fish is supposed to be healthy, it is not found on the plate so often. People prefer to have chicken and eggs over fish. For some, it is about personal preference, while for others, it becomes a matter of availability. But with improved transportation facilities, the problem of availability can be overcome to a great extent. But now there is an option of going for frozen fish in various types. The advantage of frozen fish is that it is well-cleaned and dressed, so it is easy for cooking readily.

- **Vitamin C content:** *Rohu* is a well known source of vitamin C, essential for maintaining good health. It keeps away diseases like common cold and cough and prevents other related diseases.
- **Protein rich:** Fish protein is one of the easily available forms of protein, which is needed for proper growth and development.
- **Low fat:** *Rohu* is low in fat being more beneficial for the body.
- **Booster of brain**: Consumption of this fish provides a lot of beneficial effects to the body,

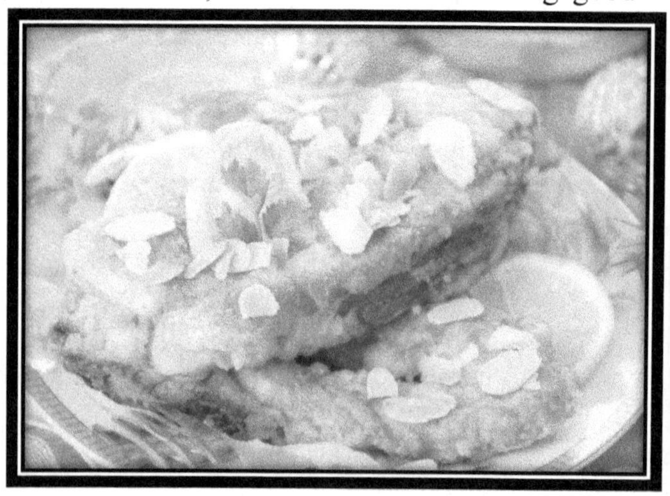

Fig.1.3 Recipe of *Rohu*
Source: Amazing Health Benefits of Rohu Fish

especially to the brains. It has been seen that a person consuming fish daily, has better memorising power and analysing skills along with
reduced level of emotional and behavioural problems.

- **Mineral source:** *Rohu* is the concentrated source of the minerals such as iron, zinc, iodine, potassium, calcium and selenium but the quantity may vary according to the type, age and size of the species, zone and season.
- **Reduction of Cancer:** Cancer is a deadly disease that affects people across the world. Antioxidants present in this fish are believed to be helpful in fighting against cancer to a great extent[9].

b. Katla (catla catla):

Scientific classification:

Kingdom:	Animalia
Phylum:	Chordata
Class:	Actinopterygii
Order:	Cypriniformes
Family:	Cyprinidae
Genus:	*Catla*
Species:	*C.catla*

Fig.1.4 ***Katla***
Source: iucnredlist.org

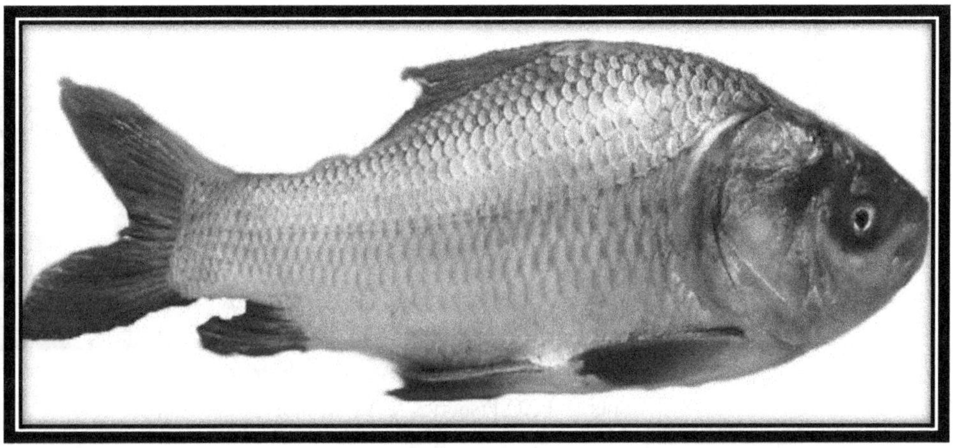

Fig.1.4.1 ***Katla***
Source: *Katla* fish farming

Katla is a fast growing and breeding for cultivating in the freshwater pond. It is very tasty as well as nutritious and very popular among the people throughout the south Asia. It is a carp species and its breeding rate in river, swamp and canal is very satisfactory. It is very hardy in nature and grows very faster comparatively to other fish. It contributes huge demand in the Asian market for providing economic growth of some Asian countries, such as Bangladesh and India.

Katla generally consumes small insects, leaves of plant, phyto-plankton and sometimes consumes zooplankton. They can be about 1m long and sexually matured at the age of 3-5 years. Usually a medium sized female *katla* contains about 1.5-3 millions of eggs. They lay eggs mainly in rainy season in the open water bodies [10].

Physical Characteristics:

- *Katla* is usually wide and flat in structure.
- It has big head compared to the body.
- It has wide and upwardly curved mouth usually.
- It has thin upper lip and the thick lower lip.

- It has more convex back than the belly.
- Upper side of the body is dark gray in colour and the side part of the body is silver in colour.
- It has blackish coloured fins[10].

Production areas of *Katla*:

Health benefits:

Katla is a concentrated source of fats and calories but the type of fat present is good for health. It also contains adequate amount of protein and some essential vitamins and minerals. It is greatly beneficial for the alimentary tract. Consuming 2-3 servings of fish in a week can reduce the risk starting from childhood asthma to prostate cancer. Healthy cooking practices such as baking, grilling, steaming can be applied to relish the fish.

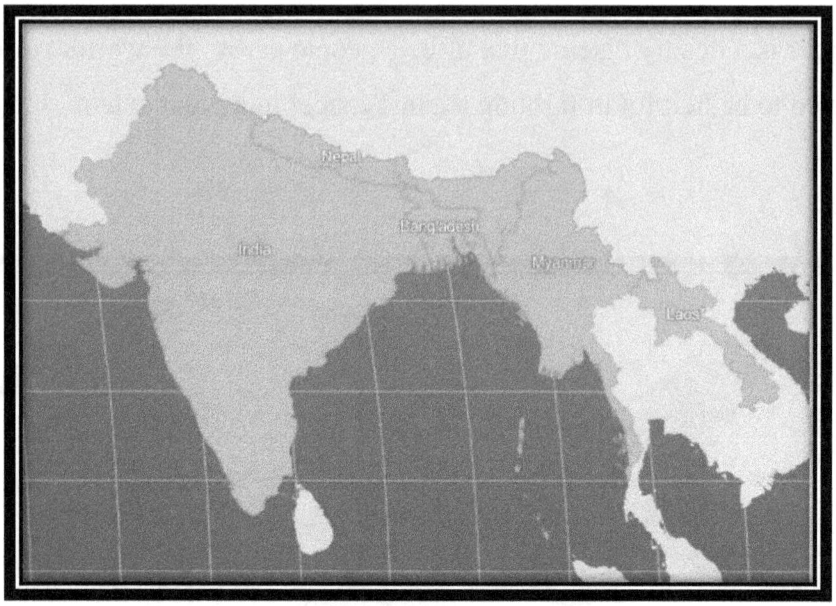

Fig.1.5. Habitat of *Katla*

Source: FAO Fisheries & Aquaculture *Catla catla*

- **Great for heart:** Due to the less content of saturated fat it can protect the heart and reduce the amount of cholesterol in the blood. It is recommended that having this fish regularly can lower the risk of heart disease.
- **Clearing the vessels:** Consumption of this fish can improve blood circulation and prevent the risk of thrombosis and inflammation.
- **Relief to joint pain:** It has been seen that eating this fish regularly as a part of a balanced diet helps to reduce the symptoms of swelling up of joints, rheumatoid arthritis.

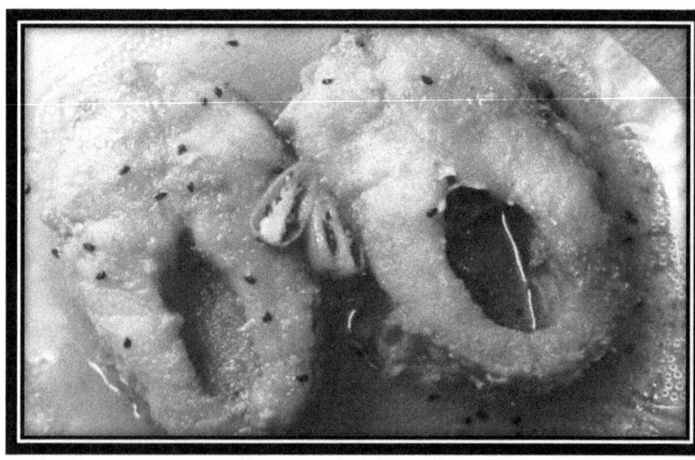

Fig.1.6. Recipe of *Katla*

Source: katla fish curry

- **Protection to eye health:** It helps to maintain the brightness of the eyes and can protect the eyesight from age-related macular degeneration (AMD), causing the retina to degenerate and the eyesight becomes blurred.
- **Essential micronutrients:** This fish is the good source of many essential nutrients such as iodine, selenium, zinc and potassium. Iodine is important for the thyroid gland, whereas selenium makes up

several important enzymes, having antioxidative properties that help to protect from oxidative damage[11].

c. Prawn (*Fenneropenaeus indicus*):

Scientific classification:

Kingdom:	Animalia
Phylum:	Arthropoda
Subphylum:	Crustacea
Class:	Malacostraca
Order:	Decapoda
Suborder:	Dendrobranchiata
Family:	Penaeidae
Genus:	Fenneropenaeus
Species:	*F. indicus*

Fig.1.7 Indian Prawn

Source: uniprot.org

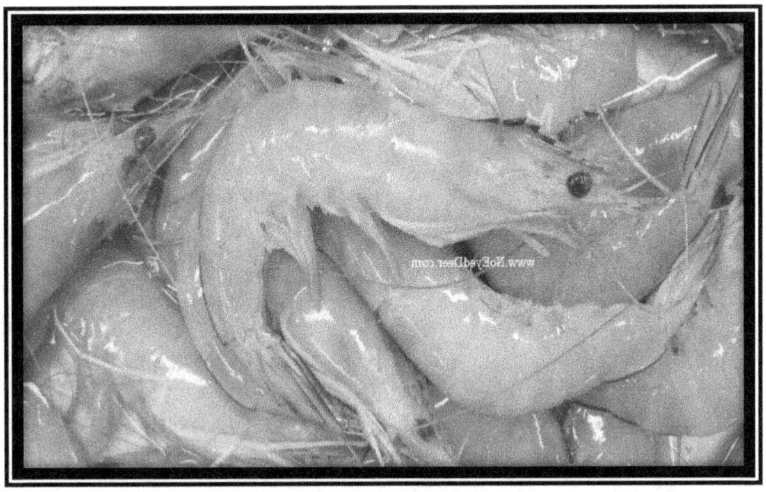

Fig.1.7.1 Indian Prawn

Source: Indian banana prawn, Malaysia

Brackish water aquaculture mainly exist in four states in India, namely Kerala, West Bengal, Goa and Karnataka. Shrimp farming is practiced traditionally in Kerala with one crop of salt tolerant paddy during the rainy season (June to September) and one crop of shrimp during the winter and spring season (November to April). These ponds are tidal; auto-stocking of mixed varieties of shrimp[12]. *F. indicus* is one of the major species in commercial fishery throughout south-east Asia. It is mostly caught off the east coast of Africa. This species is important for both offshore fishing and in pond culture mainly in the region of Bangladesh, Malaysia, Thailand, Indonesia and the Philippines[13].

Physical characteristics:

- Prawn has uniformly glabrous carapace and abdomen.
- It has hepatic and antennal spines on the carapace but no orbital spine present.
- It has sigmoidal curved rostrum armed with 7 or 8 dorsal and 5 or 6 ventral teeth. Telson is present with no lateral spine.
- It has shallow convexed rostral crest, adrostral carina reaches epigastric teeth along with well-defined gastro-orbital carina.
- It is slightly greyish or dull green in colour.
- It has antennal flagellum that is yellow or greenish yellow in colour.
- It has posterior half of uropods, which are yellowish in colour[14].

Production areas of Prawn:

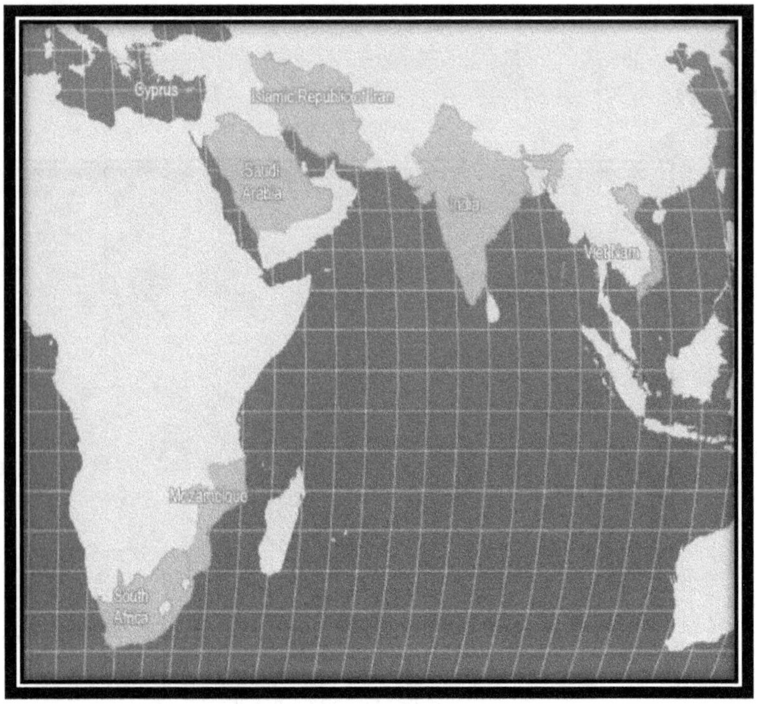

Fig. 1.8 Habitat of Prawn
Source: Fisheries and Aquaculture Department

Health benefits:

Though prawn may be small in size, they have good nutritional impact and health benefits. According to the U.S. Environmental Protection Agency and the Food and Drug Administration prawns contain relatively low level of mercury, Moreover the American Heart Association recommended that up to 6 ounces of cooked fish, shellfish and poultry can be consumed daily. Shrimps provide wide nutritional advantages due to the presence of adequate protein, vitamin and mineral contents[14].

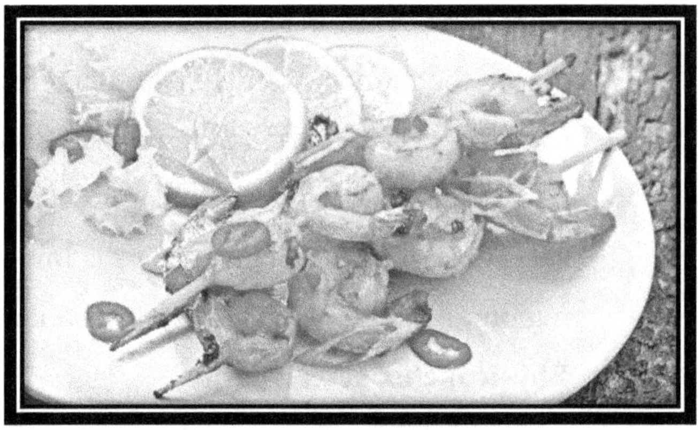

Fig.1.9 Recipe of Prawn
Source: food.ndtv.com

- **Glycemic Load:** Prawn contains low amount of carbohydrates, causing very low Glycemic Index rating.
- **Calorie content:** Calorie content of prawn is relatively low.
- **Macronutrients:** The flesh of prawn is composed of mainly protein and water, but some fat and cholesterol are also present.
- **Micronutrients:** Prawn is enriched with vitamin B_{12} and selenium. Moreover a fair amount of vitamin A, vitamin E, vitamin B_6, iron, magnesium, sodium, zinc and copper are also present in addition. Most importantly some amount of vitamin C is also present.
- **Vitamins for improving red blood cell health:** Vitamin A, present in prawn controls red blood cell development and activates genes that helps to develop functional red blood cells. It also helps the red blood cells to access the iron to transport oxygen throughout the body. Vitamin B_{12} also helps in the production of haem portion that is responsible for red blood cell for proper functioning[15].
- **Protein source:** Prawn is a healthy alternative source of protein. According to the U.S. Department of Agriculture, consumption of a minimum of 8 ounces of cooked prawn each week is beneficial for health. Other high saturated fat containing animal proteins, such as red meat can be replaced with

prawn, which can reduce the saturated fat intake but meet up the adequate protein requirements for being healthy[16].

d. Lobster *(Macrobrachium rosenbergii):*

Scientific classification:

Kingdom:	Animalia
Phylum:	Arthropoda
Subphylum:	Crustacea
Class:	Malacostraca
Order:	Decapoda
Infraorder:	Caridea
Family:	Palaemonidae
Genus:	*Macrobrachium*
Species:	***M. rosenbergii***

Fig 1.10 Lobster
Source: iucnredlist.org

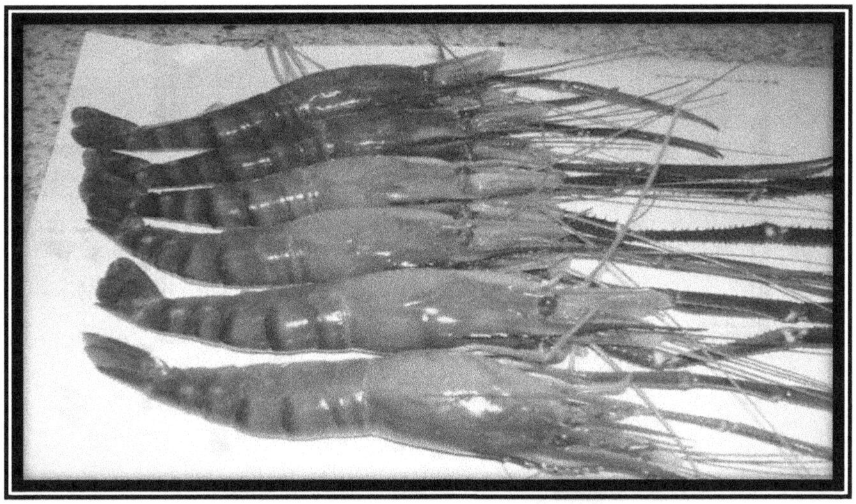

Fig 1.10.1 Lobster
Source: Penaeus Aquaculture

Macrobrachium rosenbergii, known as the giant river prawn is also commercially very important. It is found throughout the tropical and subtropical areas of the Indo-Pacific region, from India to southeastern Asia and northern Australia. It is one of the biggest freshwater prawns in the world and is widely cultivated in several countries. The larva stage of *M. rosenbergii* depends on brackish water but after becoming juvenile, the entire live spends in freshwater[17].

The cultivation of the giant prawns is found mostly in the lakes, rivers, swamps, irrigation ditches, canals and ponds. Most species need brackish water for the initial stages of life cycle, after that these are found in sea water, although some complete the life cycle in saline and fresh water lakes[18].

Physical characteristics:

- It has a very long rostrum, with 11-14 dorsal teeth and 8-10 ventral teeth.
- The tip of its telson reaches distinctly beyond the posterior spines of the telson.
- The adult male has very long second chelipeds in which all segments are elongate and have blunt spines.
- The movable finger of the second chelipeds of the adult male is covered by a dense velvet-like fur.
- The length of the adult male usually is about 33 cm long while adult females go up to 29 cm[19].

Production areas of Lobster:

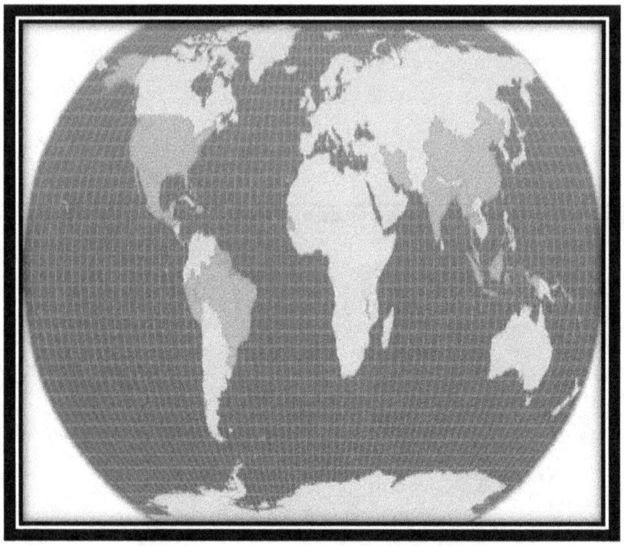

Fig.1.11. Habitat of Lobster
Source: FAO Fishery Statistics, 2006

Health benefits

Heart:

- The lobster contains a significant amount of sodium, which is beneficial for the heart.
- On the other hand beneficial fats are also found in the lobster which helps to prevent inflammation and atherosclerosis.
- The balanced ratio of omega-3 and omega-6 fatty acids found in lobster can help to maintain cholesterol balance in the human body.

Cognition:

- Adequate amount of unique vitamins and minerals are found in lobsters, especially Vitamin B_{12}, which helps to maintain nerve integrity and helps to keep the nervous system to function properly.
- Lobster contains adequate choline, which can increase the production of neurotransmitters which in turn maintain efficient functioning of brain and protect it from the effects of neurodegenerative diseases like Alzheimer's and Parkinson's.

Growth and Repair:

- One of the most important facts is the presence of high content of protein, which can give an energetic boost. Those who require high protein food lobster can be a good choice.

Reduction of Inflammation:

- As the lobster contains protein and "good" fat, inflammation can be reduced. Omega-3 fatty acids are important for the production of prostaglandins that can protect the body from arthritic conditions and even cardiovascular diseases.

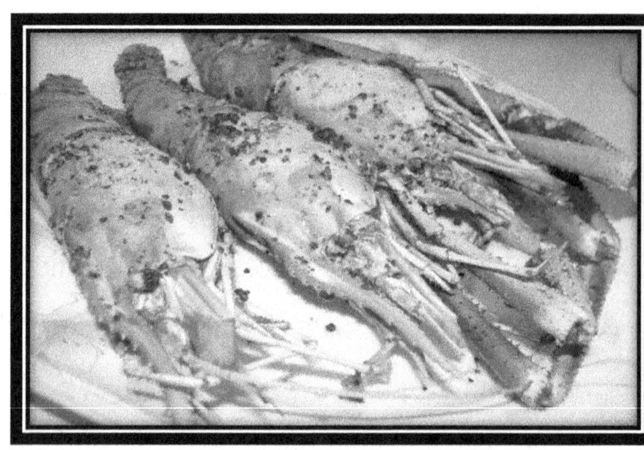

Fig.1.12 Recipe of Lobster
Source: Texas Fishing Forum

Strengthening bones:

- Lobster is not only delicious but also dense in some minerals such as calcium and phosphorus.

- These minerals are needed to increase the bone mineral density to prevent osteoporosis and other age-related bone disorders[20].

e. Pomfret (*Pampus argenteus)*:

Scientific classification:

Kingdom:	Animalia
Phylum:	Chordata
Class:	Actinopterygii
Order:	Perciformes
Family:	Stromateidae
Genus:	*Pampus*
Species:	*P. argenteus*

Fig. 1.13 White Pomfret
Source: iucnredlist.org

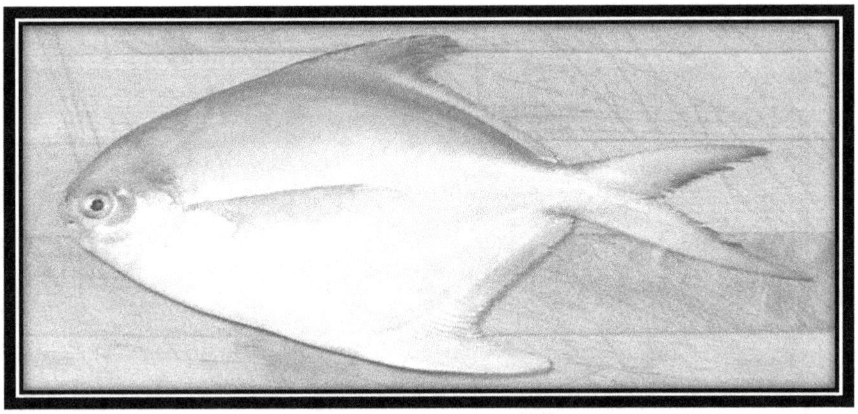

Fig. 1.13.1 White Pomfret
Source: Clovegarden.com

Pomfrets are commercially important fish in the Indo-Pacific region. Pomfret from Indian waters has long been considered to be *Pampus argenteus*. Silver pomfrets are usually silver or white in colour, with small scales. They can grow between the ranges of 4-6 kg[21].

They are pelagic fish, which live in the pelagic zone of ocean – being neither close to the bottom nor near the shore. They dwell generally near the bottom during the day and rise to the surface at night. They are usually found at 15- 40 m depth, generally over muddy bottoms. They feed on mostly zoo planktons[22].

Physical characteristics:

- The body of the pomfret is deep, compressed and oval in shape; dorsal and ventral parts of the body being equally convex.
- Dorsal and anal spines appear in a truncated form above skin. Anterior portion of soft dorsal are elevated.
- Moderately small mouth with weak jaws is observed.
- A nearly horizontal mouth is present, the maxillary enlarged to below anterior margin of eye.
- Teeth in jaws are present in single row and are closely set and fine. In adult, teeth are rudimentary.
- Eyes are with feeble adipose lids.
- Scales are small and deciduous in shape.
- Pelvic fins are absent, pectorals elongated and pointed. Caudal fins are forked with pointed lower lobe which is much larger than upper.
- Colour is generally white or silver. Upper surface of the body is neutral gray with a purplish shine[23].

Production areas of Pomfret:

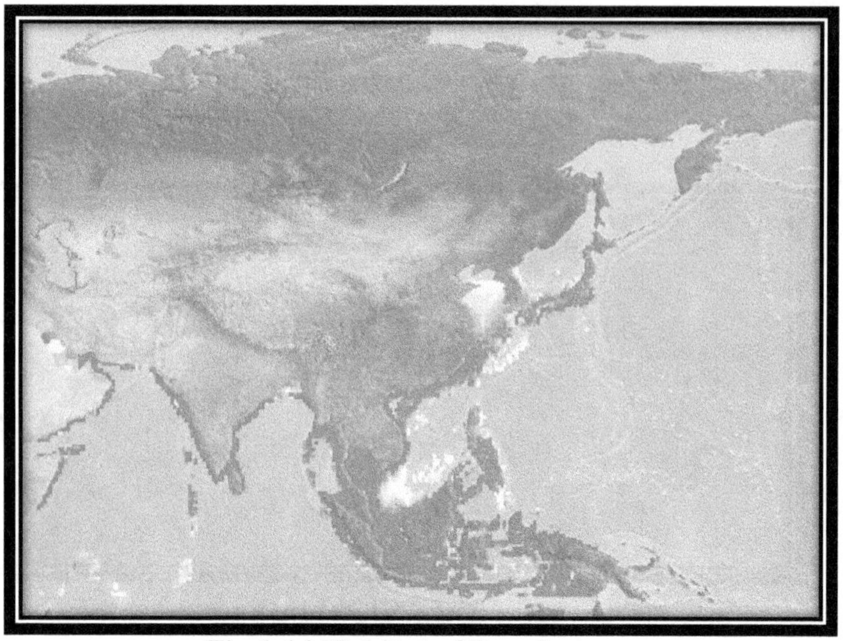

Fig.1.14 Habitat of Pomfret

Source: Fish Base

Health benefits:

- **Good for heart:** pomfret has less saturated fat and more omega-3 fatty acids that lower the amount of cholesterol in the blood and protect the heart from several degenerative diseases.
- **Clearing of the blood vessels:** Consumption of these fish can improve blood circulation and lower the risk of thrombosis. The EPA and DHA omega-3 oils in Pomfret help to prevent blood clots and inflammation.

- **Joint benefits:** It has been shown that consumption of this fish helps to remove the symptoms of rheumatoid arthritis. Recent studies have proved a relation between omega-3 fats and osteoarthritis, recommending that eating more sea fish could help to prevent the disease.
- **Effect on the eyes:** A previous study had suggested that omega-3 fatty acids are beneficial to protect the eyesight from age-related macular degeneration (AMD), causing the retina to degenerate and the eyesight becoming blurred. Pomfret contains retinol, which prevents nyctalopia.
- **Essential nutrients:** They contain essential minerals including iodine, selenium, zinc and potassium. They are also rich sources of many vitamins, including vitamins A and D.
- **Deep breath:** A number of researches have revealed that fish helps to protect the lungs; thus consumption of fish in a balanced meal makes the lungs stronger and healthier.
- **Emotional health:** Sea fish may also play a great inflence in preventing depression and help to avoid mood swing and post-natal depression.
- **Healthy skin:** Omega-3 fatty acids present in this fish helps to protect the skin from the harmful effects of the UV damage and also reduce the symptoms of skin disorders such as eczema and psoriasis.

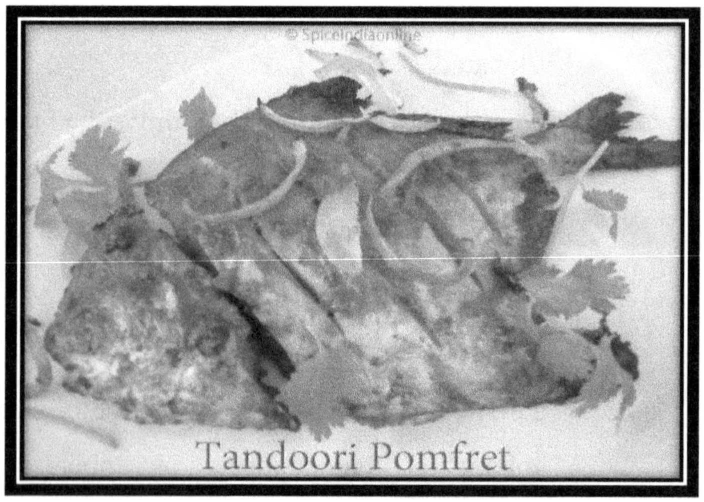

Fig.1.15 Recipe of Pomfret

Source: Seafood Recipes

- **Brain power:** Research has indicated that people who consume a plenty of sea fish have less chances to suffer from dementia and mental problems in later life. DHA is essential to improve the brain activity of children such as reading skills, behaviour and Attention Deficit Hyperactivity Disorder (ADHD) [24].

f. *Hilsa* (*Tenualosa Ilisha*):

Scientific classification:

Kingdom:	Animalia
Phylum:	Chordata
Class:	Actinopterygii
Order:	Clupeiformes
Family:	Clupeidae
Subfamily:	Alosinae
Genus:	Tenualosa(Hilsa)
Species:	*T. ilisha*

Fig.1.16 *Hilsa*
Source: iucnredlist.org

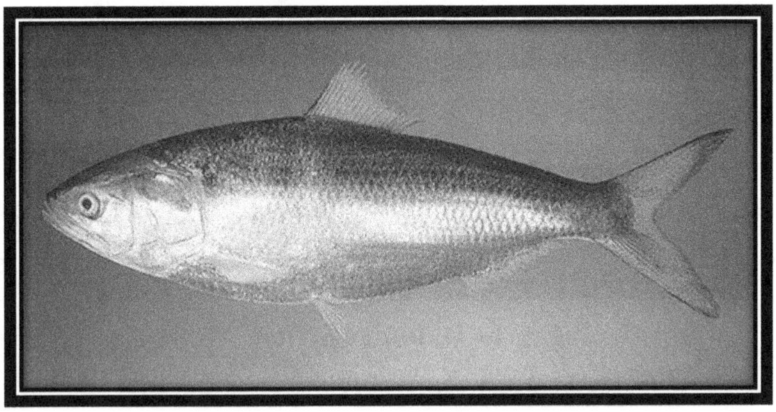

Fig.1.16.1. *Hilsa*
Source: Zipcodezo

Hilsa is a saltwater fish and live in a group in the coastal area of the sea. It is widely consumed in Bangladesh. Among the total fish production in Bangladesh about 30% is *hilsa.* A large number of the *hilsa* are caught from the rivers of Bangladesh like *Yamuna*, *Padma*, *Meghna*, and some others.

Though it is sea fish, but during breeding period it comes to the big rivers and lays eggs there and swims back to the sea after breeding. Fisherman also caught a large number of *hilsa* from the sea. But the river *hilsa* is tastier than sea *hilsa. Hilsa* generally consume different types of plankton, small plant, diatoms, protozoa, algae those are available under the water[25].

Physical characteristics:

- The body of the *hilsa* is covered with bright silver-coloured scales.
- Their backside is slightly green coloured and the body is flat from the both sides.
- The entire body of the fish is covered with big sized scales.
- Eyes are wide enough and the eye membranes are fatty.
- The head is rectangular and flat.
- They have dorsal fin, pelvic fin, caudal fin, pectoral fins and the anal fin is divided in two parts.
- The stomach of the fish is notched till pectoral fin.
- It has small mouth and there are no teeth in the jaw.
- It has about 18-19 cords in the dorsal fin[25].

Production area of *Hilsa*:

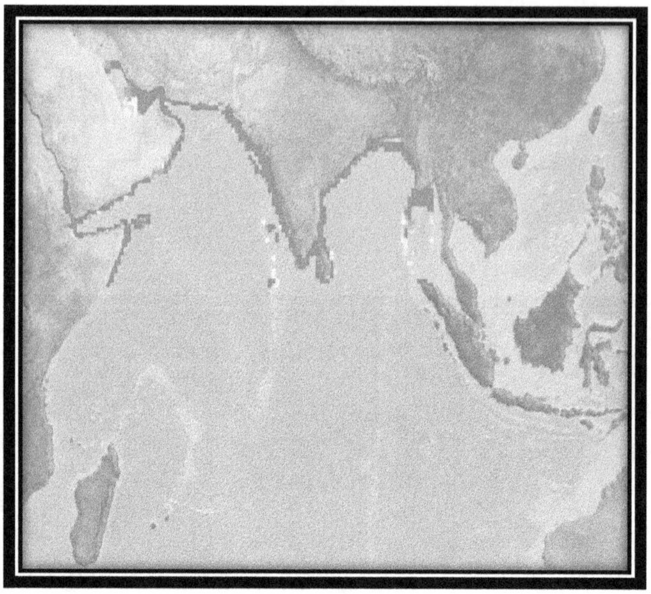

Fig. 1.17 Habitat of *Hilsa*
Source: *Tenualosa ilisha* (Hamilton, 1822), FishBase

Health benefit:

- They are good sources of omega 3 fatty acid. Studies showed that higher consumption of this fish help to protect skin from dermatitis.
- Nutritionist suggests that this fish can be consumed at least 2 to 3 times in a week. They claim to prevent a wide range of health problems from mental illness to blindness.
- This fish contains valuable fatty acid and lipid which play a vital role in providing pharmaceutical elements and physiological maintenance of body tissues.
- They contain high amount of omega 3 fatty acids such as EPA and DHA, which help to control several health problems such as hypertension, cardio vascular disease, obesity, stroke, diabetes, arthritis, cancer, depression etc.
- They are the good source of protein, fat, calcium and phosphorus along with some minerals. These minerals play a key role in metabolism as co-factors.
- The unique taste and flavour of *hilsa* is mainly due to the presence of certain fatty acids such as oleic acid, stearic acid and PUFA. They are also rich in vitamins A and D[26].

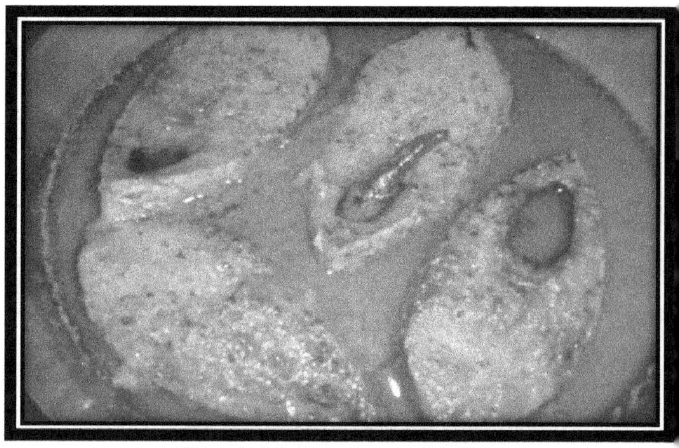

Fig.1.18 Recipe of *Hilsa*
Source: www.pinterest.com

Chapter – 2

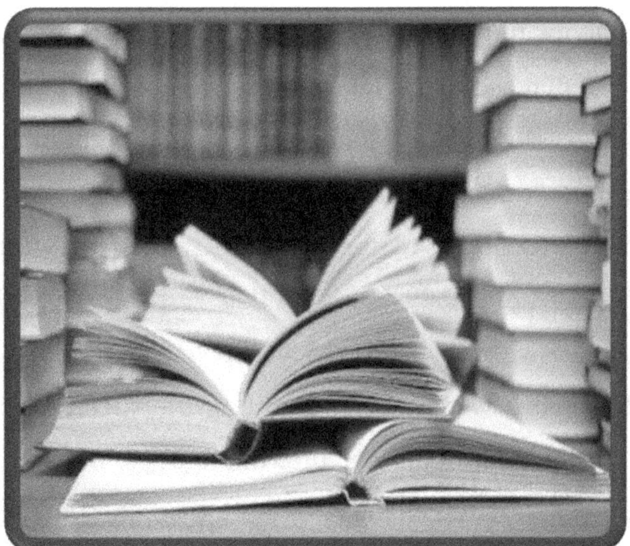

Review of Literature

In one study, three popular and easily available species of marine fish i.e. *Clupea harengus, Scomber scombrus* and *Trachurus trachurus* in Nigeria were subjected to several cooking methods such as boiling, frying and roasting and the effects of these cooking methods on the fish were observed. The protein content was reduced by frying for all the fish with very prominent effect on *Clupea harengus* and *Trachurus trachurus* and the spoilage was prevented. Fresh and fried *Clupea harengus* had 62.7 % and 10.6 % protein content respectively, while *Trachurus trachurus* had 57.3 % and 9.18 %. All the treatment methods reduced the ash content for all the fish species except for boiled *Scomber scombrus*. Boiling *Scomber scombrus* was the most nutritious among the three and due to the application of cooking methods the nutritive value was restored along with the flavour and texture. *Trachurus trachurus* was lowest in protein, whereas *Clupea harengus* was rich in protein but it was reduced with frying. Frying is better for long-time preservation but boiling was the better method for nutrient restoration. The results showed that the highest oil content present in *Scomber scombrus* that is (30.30%) followed by *Clupea harengus* (12.70%) while *Trachurus trachurus* had the lowest oil content (12.25%). This study also showed that the effect of treatment on a fish sample also depend on the type of fish species[27].

In yet another research in turkey, six commonly consumed marine fish in the raw state and cooked condition were subjected to analyses of amino acid and proximate compositions. All the fish samples showed significant changes in proximate content and amino acids composition for all cooking methods. Cooking significantly increases the essential, semi-essential, and other amino acids contents as compared to the fish species in the raw state. Grilled Atlantic bonito, anchovy, bluefish, fried mullet and hake appeared to be more valuable fish for obtaining the essential amino acids for humans. Moisture, fat, ash and carbohydrate contents of the raw fish ranged between 48.01% and 83.05%, 0.87% and 30.48%, 1.10% and 1.61%, and 0.09% and 8.70%, respectively. All the fresh fish experimented were high in protein ranges between 11.20-17.14 g/100 g and the content changed after treatment ranges between 18.11-25.65 g/100 g were observed among the species. Grilled and steamed fishes contained low fat as compared to the fried fish. The proximate contents, micro nutrient contents and amino acid composition showed the significant changes for all the cooking methods among all the fish species[28].

Another research showed that cooking methods were also applied to vegetable samples which could be a reference for the present study. Three cooking practices, i.e. boiling, steaming and stir-frying were used for 10 minutes to evaluate the effect on nutrient components, free amino acids, L-ascorbic acid, total phenol contents and antioxidant capacities of bamboo shoots (*Phyllostachys praecox*). Results indicated that boiling and stir-frying affect the nutrient composition by reducing the protein, soluble sugar, ash content. Total free amino acids content was 38.35% and 34.86%, respectively. Significant differences ($P<0.05$) were observed in free amino acids in the cooked samples. Due to the addition of edible oil the high fat content of stir-fried bamboo shoots increased by 52.85%. The L-ascorbic acid and total phenol contents were significantly reduced by boiling, while total phenol content was increased about 3.98% by steaming and stir-frying preserved 78.87% L-ascorbic acid. Results showed the antioxidant property of bamboo shoots could increase by stir frying. It could be concluded that stir-frying is more suitable for bamboo shoots as it helped to retain maximum antioxidant capacities[29].

In a recent study, the effect of using lemon juice and sun drying was investigated on the retention of vitamin C content of water-blanched and steamed *Amaranthus hybridus, Bidens pilosa* and *Cleome gynandra* indigenous vegetables preserved for six weeks. Results showed that the vitamin C retention was higher in lemon juice-treated samples as compared to the untreated samples, whereas steam-blanching was better than water-blanching for the retention of vitamin C. The percentages of vitamin C retention for the lemon juice treated steam and water-blanched vegetables after blanching were found to be 80% and 40% respectively, while for control steam- blanched vegetables, vitamin C retention ranged from 60-67.8% as compared to the retention of 20% for the control water-blanched vegetables. Results also revealed that six weeks stored vegetables had the higher vitamin C retention in lemon juice-treated blanched vegetables regardless to all the blanching types as compared to the control samples. Vegetable preservation with lemon juice as preservative and for the retention for vitamin C content is strongly effective. This study can also be the reference as it indicates the use of preservative for storage[30].

Another review revealed the effects of five common traditional cooking practices such as steaming, microwave cooking, boiling, stir-frying and stir-frying followed by boiling on the phyto chemicals and nutrient contents of broccoli. It had been seen that all the cooking methods except steaming caused significant losses of total soluble proteins, sugars and minerals. Steaming caused the lowest loss of total glucose, while stir-frying and stir-frying followed by boiling provided the highest loss. The two most popular methods for homemade dishes such as stir-frying and stir-frying followed by boiling caused huge losses of chlorophyll, vitamin C, soluble protein and sugar, whereas the steaming method was best to retain the nutrients of broccoli[31].

The effects of different cooking methods namely boiling, baking, frying and grilling were examined on the proximate and mineral composition of snakehead fish in a previous study. The protein and fat contents were significantly higher in frying and grilling. The moisture, protein, fat and ash contents of the fish in the raw state was 77.2 ± 2.39, 13.9 ± 2.89, 5.9 ± 0.45 and 0.77 ± 0.12% respectively. The ash content significantly increased, whereas the mineral contents such as Na, K, Ca, Mg, Fe, Zn and Mn were not affected by using the cooking methods. It was also observed that cu content increased and P content decreased in all the cooking methods except grilling. In this study, the grilling method is found to be the best choice for cooking[32].

Another study was carried out to investigate the changes in the macro and micro mineral components of common striped red mullet (*Mullus surmuletus*), sole (*Solea solea*) and whiting (*Merlangius merlangus*), indicating that concentrations of macro mineral in the edible parts of the fish species were found to be 444–1,559 mg/kg for sodium, 1,975–5,130 mg/kg for potassium, 228–658 mg/kg for magnesium, 187–1,105 mg/kg for calcium and 2,341–7,341mg/kg for phosphorus respectively [33].

Spoilage of fish occurs within 12 hours in the tropical regions due to the chemical and bacterial changes enhanced by high temperature. Spoilage begins soon after the death of the fish and processing should be carried out immediately to prevent the microbial growth and the reduction of nutrient contents. Salted and fermented *Labio* sp. was assessed to establish its nutritive value. It has been observed that the chemical composition of fermented species decreased. The magnitude of change between the fresh and treated materials significantly differed during storage [34].

Another study determined the nutrient composition and shelf life of dried *Clarias gariepinus* pre-treated with brine and vinegar. The fish were dried to average moisture content of 5.40 ±1.47% and stored differently at room temperature (26-30°C) for eight months. There were significant differences ($P<0.05$) between the nutrient compositions of the fish with the control having the highest values. Pre-treatment with salt and vinegar had no effect on the shelf life of dried *C. gariepinus*. Drying fish to an average moisture content of about 5% and storage in an airtight container may increase the shelf life of dried *C. Gariepinus*[35].

The review of the recent and classical literature revealed that loss of nutrients in fresh products during storage and cooking might be more substantial than commonly perceived. Canning and freezing processes might preserve nutritive value depending on the commodity. The initial thermal treatment of processed products caused loss of water-soluble and oxygen-labile nutrients. However, due to the lack of oxygen these nutrients were relatively stable during canning, whereas due to the short time of heating in blanching, frozen products initially lost some nutrients, but this loss was more during storage due to oxidation[36].

This study was carried out on Indian Mackerel (*Rastrelliger kanagurta*), Eel (*Monopterus albus*) and Cockle (*Anadara granosa*) to estimate the proximate composition and four micronutrients such as Cd, Cu, Mn and Zn. All the samples of each species were divided into two groups and each group was again divided into 3 sub-groups as replicates. The first group was kept uncooked, while the second group was fried. Both the raw state and fried samples were analyzed by using the standard methods to determine protein, lipid, ash, moisture and carbohydrate contents along with Cd, Cu, Mn and Zn contents. Results indicated Indian mackerel and eel had the higher protein content than cockle, whereas cockle had the higher Cd, Cu, Mn and Zn contents as compared to the Indian mackerel and eel. Hence the study concluded that from the nutritional aspect fish is better than shellfish[37].

A recent study was conducted on the fillets of *Platycephalus indicus* to analyze the effect of processing on proximate compositions. Results focused that frying significantly increased fat content in the fillet, whereas ash content was significantly reduced in boiling. Highest ash content of about 10.64% was recorded in baking method and the highest protein concentration 82.73% was obtained for boiled fillet. Lipid content of 17.27% was highest in fried fillet. *P. indicus* was rich in fat, protein and ash, thus its consumption should be encouraged[38].

The use of sulphiting agents is one of the oldest applications from Roman times to control the undesirable growth of microorganisms. Sulphur dioxide and the salts potassium bisulphite, potassium metabisulphite, sodium bisulphite, sodium metabisulphite and sodium sulphite are listed as GRAS in the US Code of Federal Regulations and it suggested that theses preservatives could not be used in foods containing adequate thiamine. Potassium metabisulphite is mainly used as an antimicrobial agent in soft fruit, fruit juices, wines, beverages, sausages, pickles and fresh shrimp. Sulphites are usually effective against moulds, yeasts and aerobic gram-negative bacilli. The microbial activity is produced by the undissociated sulphurous acid which enters the cell and reacts with thiol groups of proteins, enzymes and cofactors[39].

In a study, European sea bass (*Dicentrarchus labrax*) was used to analyze some metals such as Al, Ca, Cr, Cu, Fe, Mn, Ni, Pb, Se, Sr, Zn and P by comparing the concentration in the raw state and in the cooked fish. The European sea bass was cooked on pots made up of five different materials such as cast iron, aluminium, steel, teflon and ceramic. Results indicated that the micro element contents increased due to reduction of water content along with the release of the metals due to the surface contact of the pots. Cr, Se and Fe content decreased with cooking, whereas Pb content remains unchanged. The use of 2 model solutions, made of water and water and vinegar, demonstrates that the pots are not inert to the leaching of elements that could be found in the processed fish[40].

In this study, saturated brine, dry salt with 0.25 percent potassium sorbate and saturated brine with 0.3 percent sodium benzoate were applied separately on Bombay duck (*Harpodon nehereus*) and kept at ambient temperature for studying the storage period after sun drying. The primary objective of this study was to estimate the proximate composition and the changes in storage quality of dry fishes treated with chemical preservatives. The protein, fat, ash and moisture contents of dry fish treated by the three different preservatives were between the ranges of 53.91-56.33%, 5.94-11.77%, 14.78-21.96% and 6.9-7.42% respectively. The outcome of this study revealed that nutritive value of the chemically preserved dry fishes had a better storage life as compared to the saturated brine dry salt[41].

In one study, cooked fish balls were treated with salt solution and then vacuum packaged to determine the effectiveness for extending the shelf life. Freshly produced fish balls were divided into five groups - one group was air packaged, three groups dipped in salt solutions with concentration of 2.5, 5.0, 10.0%, and one group was vacuum packaged and preserved at 4^{0} C for 14 days. This study evaluated the changes in aerobic bacterial counts, pH, texture and sensory characteristics along with the shelf life depending on the bacterial counts and sensory evaluation. Vacuum packaged and 10% salt treated fish balls showed the shelf life extension of 6 days and 4 days respectively as compared to the shelf life of the control which is less than 3 days. Depending on sensory analysis, vacuum-packaging and 2.5% salt-immersed fish balls showed the shelf-life of fish balls by 6 days as compared to the control which is less than 9 days, but no significant ($P > 0.05$) differences present in the pH values for treated fish ball samples[42].

A study was carried out on the meat of male *Portunus pelagicus* to analyse fat, protein, ash and moisture contents. Water-soluble protein content along with the peptide-mapping of the fleshes of shark *Caracharhinus* spp. and *Thalapath Istiophorus* spp. was also determined. Moreover, fatty acid profile of the commercial fish oil and the crab meat were also determined by using gas chromatography. The results revealed the proximate composition of moisture, protein, ash and fat content found to be 89.4±0.072 %, 75.7±0.069%, 13.0±0.002% and 02.2±0.047% respectively in crab meat. Crab oil contained a high percentage of polyunsaturated fatty acids, representing 40.68 % of the total fatty acid content along with oleic acid (28.03%) and eicosapentaenoic acid (12.12%) as compared to the commercial fish oil. The study revealed that the meat of *P. Pelagicus* had high protein and low fat content. Thus, the consumption of crabs would be beneficial to prevent nutritional deficiencies[43].

In a study, New Zealand king salmon (*Oncorhynchus tshawytscha*) was subjected to common cooking procedures such as poached, steamed, micro-waved, pan fried and oven baked without oil and deep fried. The study aimed to investigate the fatty acid profile by gas chromatography to determine the optimal preparation techniques to achieve the nutritional and sensory qualities. Due to cooking in different methods moisture and lipid losses occurred. The fatty acid profile indicated minor differences between the methods, whereas deep fried salmon had increased in PUFA due to the uptake of linoleic acid present in the frying oil. All the cooking methods preserved the omega-3 fatty acids. However, deep-fried salmon showed the lowest amounts of omega-3 fatty acids. It is possible that an internal protection of omega-3 fatty acids in king salmon is present, but that needs further more researches[44].

In another study, cooked African catfish was used for the analyses of proximate composition, mineral and vitamin contents such as A, E, B_1, B_2, B_3 and B_6. Different cooking treatments like baking, grilling, microwave cooking and frying were used, resulting in the increased protein and ash contents in all the cooked fish. The fat content increased only in fried fillets, whereas the moisture content of cooked fish decreased. Mineral contents were also affected by cooking methods, except for Cu. Vitamin A content increased significantly in both grilled and fried fish, whereas vitamin E content increased in all the cooked fish. Vitamin B_1 content of the cooked fish significantly decreased but vitamin B_2 and B_3 contents of grilled fish significantly increased. Vitamin B_6 content of all the cooked fish significantly decreased except for the grilled fish. The study reveals that the vitamin and mineral contents were found to be high in grilled catfish[45].

In a research the sequential cooking–freezing–reheating (CFR) method was examined with sardine (*Sardina pilchardus*) fillets post cooking by the methods of frying, grilling, frozen, and then reheated using microwave ovens due to evaluate the changes in the fatty acid profile and proximate compositions. Both cooking and freezing–reheating affected ($P<0.001$) the proximate composition. Frying produced the highest moisture loss and fat gain, followed by grilling, and oven-baking. Microwave oven-reheating (MR) induced higher dehydration than conventional oven-reheating (OR), with grilled–frozen–MR samples also showing reduced fat and ash content. Frying significantly ($P<0.001$) affected the fatty acid composition of sardine, increasing oleic and linoleic acids and decreasing eicosapentaenoic and docosahexaenoic acids. Oven-baking and grilling affected the fatty acid content minimally. Freezing–reheating (FR) significantly affected ($P<0.001$) the fatty acid composition along with the increased oleic acid content and omega-3 fatty acids decreasing more in MR than in OR. However, the study revealed that OR should be used instead of MR when the CFR system is performed[46].

In a research, the effects of cooking, frying and smoking were studied on the chemical composition of two marine fish (*Sardinella sp., Dentex sp.*) and a freshwater fish (*Tilapia sp.*). The proximate compositions of the fish were similar to those of other fish reported in the previous literature. The fatty acid composition of the fish was not affected by smoking and cooking. The palm-kernel oil used in frying provided protection to the fatty acid pattern in the fried fish. High levels of omega 6 fatty acids were found in freshwater fish as well as in the marine fish. The fish contained appreciable amounts of Na, Ca, P and Mg along with the trace elements such as Fe, Cu, Zn and As. The study showed that B_1 is absent in sardine and tilapia, probably due to the thiaminase activity, whereas thiamine content was low in *Dentex sp* and vitamins B_2 and B_6 contents were very low in all the fish[47].

Another research investigated the impact of cooking on the fatty acid concentrations and the stability of long chain omega 3 fatty acids in three freshwater fish species such as rainbow trout, vendace and pike with different sizes and lipid contents. The domestic cooking practices used were boiling, baking, microwave oven cooking and frying with sunflower and rapeseed oils. Result disclosed that the long chain omega 3 fatty acids concentrations increased in fish flesh due to the elimination of moisture for subjecting to the cooking methods. Frying oils were absorbed by lean vendace and pike, and to some extent by medium fatty rainbow trout. *n*-6 fatty acids from cooking oils may interact with the biological activity of *n*-3 fatty acids[48].

In one study ground fillets of a low-fat fish which is frozen Alaska pollock (*Theragra chalcogramma*), and a high-fat fish which is Pacific mackerel (*Pneumataphorus japanicus*) were heated for 20 min at the intervals of temperature ranging from 40 - 115^{0}C, resulting in decrease of -SH groups and an increase of S-S bonds. The study revealed that the rapidity of reaction occurred at 95^{0}C and after 20 minutes it reached the equilibrium. This experiment indicated that temperatures higher than 50^{0}C caused oxidative changes of -SH groups to S-S bonds. cystine and cysteine lost due to the heating at 115^{0}C and S-S bonds to -SH groups formed at 95^{0}C, reducing the amino acid and protein content along with the increased digestibility when fed to rainbow trout (*Salmo gairdneri*) as compared to the raw fish protein. Freeze-drying did not affect digestibility and of S-S bond formation was not observed. The effect of heating on digestibility was found to be greater in the low-fat pollock as compared to the high-fat mackerel[49].

In a recent research the effects of baking, broiling, deep frying and microwave oven cooking on the proximate, mineral and fatty acid composition of grouper (*Epinephelus morio*), red snapper (*Lutjanus campechanus*), Florida pompano (*Trachinotus carolinus*) and Spanish mackerel (*Scomberomorus maculatus*) were determined. Cooking significantly changed the lipid content that was lost from fatty fillets. Baking, broiling or microwave cooking had no significant effect on the fatty acid composition of all the fillets. Major fatty acids were absorbed from the cooking medium by deep fried fillets, but the extent of fat absorption from the cooking medium decreased for fatty fillets due to the presence of excess lipid content. During the cooking of low fat species, sodium, potassium and magnesium levels were decreased, but these minerals were restored when high fat species were cooked[50].

Forty four samples of catfish (*Clarias gariepinus*) were found from a fish pond in NIFFR (NATIONAL INSTITUTE FOR FRESHWATER FISHERIES RESEARCH) and divided into 11 portions. Among these 5 portions were treated with increasing concentration of 1-5% potassium sorbate respectively, the next 5 portions were treated with increasing concentration of 1-5% sodium metabisulphite prior to smoking and the last portion was left untreated and served as control. After that they were smoked and preserved for 8 weeks at room temperature. Smoked samples were subjected to microbial, moisture contents and proximate analysis after 0, 2, 4, 6, and 8 weeks of storage. All the treated smoked samples were found to have Bacillus species but Streptococcus sp and E. coli were not found. Potassium sorbate (3%) reduced the Staphylococcus count to 0 throughout the 8th week of storage. Potassium sorbate found to be more efficient to control microbial quality and extension of the shelf life of smoked catfish[51].

In one research, the effects of individual extract of turmeric and shallot and the extract of the combination of turmeric and shallot on the storage quality of vacuum-packaged rainbow trout (*Oncorhynchus mykiss*) at 4^{0}C for 20 days. Fish samples were divided into 4 batches of which 3 batches were dipped in the aqueous solution of turmeric extract (1.5%), shallot extract (1.5%) and the combination of turmeric and shallot extract (1.5%+ 1.5%) for 30 minutes, while the 4th batch was served as the control sample and dipped in the distilled water. Microbiological (total plate count) as well as chemical evaluation (total volatile base nitrogen, peroxide value, and thio-barbituric acid value) along with sensory characteristics of the control and the treated samples were analysed at definite intervals. The results disclosed that the combination of two on the fish samples was effective to enable the good quality characteristics retention for longer period of time and to extend the shelf life during the refrigerated storage[52].

The effect of the salting on the storage quality of the smoked and non-smoked chub mackerel was studied over a period of 30 days. The result indicated that the applied preservation methods had a good effect on the fish samples. Total volatile basic nitrogen and tri-methylamine nitrogen values of salted and smoked samples remained constant during the 30 days of storage period. Salting had a good preservative effect but lower than the combined effect of salting and smoking. 2-Thiobarbituric acid (TBA)-reactive substances of salted and smoked samples increased during the storage period but remained at low levels after 30 days of storage as compared to TBA values of non-smoked samples. Salted and smoked samples showed constant Sensory characteristics during the storage period of 30 days, while slight textural differences between the two preservation methods were observed. The recoded sensory scores during storage had significant reduction for non-smoked samples, whereas it was higher for the salted samples[53].

One study focused on the effects of the application of 5% salt and cooking on the proximate composition, and the quality of various protein and lipid were measured at 30^0 C for the period of 30 days. Fermented fish silages were prepared from whole *tilapia* (*Oreochromis niloticus*), molasses and *Lactobacillus plantarum* starter culture. The silages were stable during fermentation and storage, and the nutrient contents remained constant. Increased degree of autolysis and ammonia production was noticed. Protein hydrolysis was prevented along with the decreased formation of total volatile bases by the addition of salt or cooking of substrate before fermentation due to the activity of endogenous auto-lysing enzymes. The energy content and the digestibility of the nitrogenous dry matter of silage-based diets for *tilapia* were higher in both the cooked and salted fish silages than in the raw state fish silage[54].

This study was designed to observe the performance of turmeric and salt treated product of *tengra* (*Mystus vittatus*). The salt and turmeric treated product included a combination of salting and drying process and addition of turmeric with salt as preservative. The other three treated products included turmeric, salted and unsalted products. Salted fish contained 2.0 to 3.0% salt, salt and turmeric treated fish contained 2.5 to 3.5% salt and 1 to 2% turmeric. Salt and turmeric treated products were preserved from 5-6 months and the other treated products varied from 3 to 5 months at refrigerated temperature. The sensory score of salt and turmeric treated product showed the highest average value of 7.63. The average total volatile nitrogen (TVN) of products and the turmeric treated salt were 5.45 and values of the product turmeric, salt and salt-treated were 5.91, 6.25 and 6.625 respectively. Thus it can be concluded that treatment with salt and turmeric was much more effective in preserving fish products, as it retained beneficial nutrients, higher sensory score and greater resistance to bacterial and enzymatic activity and longer period of time than other drying methods[55].

Another study examined the effects of different processing methods on the amino acid contents of four marine fishes commonly consumed in Nigeria: *Clupea harengus*, *Scomber scombrus*, *Trachurus trachurus* and *Urophycis tenuis*. The samples were boiled, roasted over hot charcoal and fried. The total amino acid contents ranged from 76.72 - 98.01 gm/100 gm protein and the total essential amino acids from 28.95 - 44.73 gm/100 gm protein for all the fish samples. Frying reduced the total amino acid contents, whereas boiling and roasting increased the content, but the values higher in roasted than boiled samples. Due to processing the essential amino acid contents were reduced in almost all the samples predominantly in the fried samples. Amino acid scores of the raw state, boiled and roasted samples had greater than 100%, while the fried samples had the limiting amino acids either leucine or threonine. The results revealed that roasting and boiling had the desirable effects on the amino acid contents of the fish samples[56].

An experiment was conducted where fillets cut from Atlantic cod, *Gadus morhua*, (post capture age 1, 3 and 5 days) were dipped in 2.5 to 5.0 percent fresh potassium sorbate, individually packaged in polyethylene pouches, iced and sensory evaluation was done at 2 to 3 days intervals until the end of acceptable shelf life. It was found that dipping fillets in 2.5 to 5.0 percent potassium sorbate and individually packaging them in plastic film, especially oxygen resistant polythene pouches, was definitely beneficial for extending the iced shelf life of the fillets. Dipping in potassium sorbate was effective in retarding trimethylamine (TMA) formation[57].

The effects of glaze, potassium metabisulphite and vacuum treatments were examined on physical (thawing loss, cooking loss, pH), chemical (TVB, TBA), microbiological (total mesophilic, physcrophilic bacteria) and sensory properties of anchovy stored at – 30^0 C for 180 days. During frozen storage period the number of total mesophilic and physcrophilic bacteria showed changes in the treated samples. Treatments with vacuum, glaze and meta- bisulphite had the positive effect on the protection of sensory properties of anchovy stored at -30^0 C for 180 days. All the sensory and chemical results indicated that the shelf life of anchovy stored at -30^0 C after normally packed, glazed and packed, dipped in metabisulphite solution and glazed and packed, and vacuumed were 90, 150, 90 and 180 days respectively[58].

Potassium metabisulphite was used to preserve crustaceans as well as to prevent melanosis. In this study, female species of shrimps *Aristèus antènnatus* were treated with 40% sodium metabisulphite at different concentrations, times and temperatures of immersion and subsequent freezing and storage were observed. Untreated shrimps showed the signs of melanosis post storage of 19 hours on crushed ice and their market value decreased at 27 hours, whereas shrimps treated with 2% solution for 5 minutes maintained their market value. Increasing the concentration reduced the appearance of spots but increased the residual SO_2 in the tissues. However < 10% of the sulphites penetrated into the edible part of the muscle and all the conditions experimented were safe from the legislation aspect. Melanosis had no effect on the test conditions by the duration of immersion in the metabisulphite solution. Quick freezing after immersion in sodium metabisulphite solution found to be a desirable method to prevent melanosis for three months without affecting the appearance of shrimps[59].

This study revealed the sensory, biochemical (Trimethylamine, hypoxanthine production) and microbiological characteristics during shelf-life at - 1^0C in shrimp (*Panaeus aztecus*), dipped in citric acid, ascorbic acid, potassium sorbate and 4-hexyl resorcinol solution. The lowest level of trimethylamine, hypoxanthine and the total psychrotrophic bacteria were found in samples dipped in all the solutions containing chemicals as compared to the control treatment. Sensory evaluation indicated that treatments did not alter the typical sensory characteristics of shrimp and were much effective to delay the bitter off-flavour formation within 26 days. This study contributed an alternative method other than conventional preservation of shrimp to extend the shelf-life[60].

A study was carried out on the composition of lipid of three fatty fishes (sardines, mackerel and salmon) to analyze the effect of deep-fat frying with sunflower oil. Results showed that total fat content was increased in sardines, whereas saturated fatty acids content decreased, especially in sardines and mackerel due to palmitic acid reduction. The raw state mackerel and sardines are the important source of omega 3 polyunsaturated fatty acids, which significantly decreased due to frying. In the raw state salmon contained low amount of eicosapentaenoic acid and docosahexaenoic acid which increased after frying. The ratio of omega 6 fatty acids and omega 3 fatty acids increased for all the fishes. Cholesterol content significantly increased in salmon and mackerel and decreased in sardine[61].

This study was done on the four silage type, prepared from the raw state and cooked whole herring and mackerel, by-products from the fillets of cod and saith. Each silage type was stored at 4, 20 and 50^0C for 48 days. The raw materials were analysed in fresh condition and after 2, 4, 8, 16, 32 and 48 days of preservation. Different storage temperatures and the length of the storage period did not affect crude protein, dry matter and total fat and amino acid content. Cooked and the raw state materials did not show any change in hydrolysis during storage[62].

A study was conducted on the proximate composition of male, female and berried females of freshwater prawn (*Macrobrachium rosenbergii*). The nutrient contents i.e. lipids, protein, carbohydrate, moisture, ash, free fatty acids, amino acids were analysed. They constituted one of the major sources of nutritive materials for humans. The organic constituents of Muscle tissue i.e. protein, carbohydrate, lipid, free amino acids and fatty acids revealed the nutritive nature of freshwater lobster. *M. rosenbergii* could be very widely used as food from the nutritional aspect and also a better choice for commercial culture[63].

This study was conducted to determine the nutritional analysis of *hilsa* from the six selected regions in Bangladesh. The protein, carbohydrate, moisture, fat, and energy value were determined. The pH and salt value were also estimated along with the vitamins A and C, whereas among the minerals calcium, iron, phosphorus, magnesium, manganese, copper and zinc. These values are useful references for the consumers to choose fish and shellfish based on their nutritional contents. These results suggested that the proximate composition of *hilsa* greatly varies due to physiological and environmental conditions, i.e. spawning, migration, and starvation or heavy feeding[64].

In yet another study with silver Pomfret (*Pampus argenteus*), evaluation of changes in the quality of frozen in the fresh condition as well as after holding in ice for 1, 2 and 4 days were carried out. Results showed that the shelf-life of the samples stored at-18^{0}C decreased rapidly if the pre-freezing iced storage was more than 1 day. The shelf-life of the iced frozen sample for 1, 2 and 4 days was 32, 20 and 16 weeks respectively. There was no correlation observed between the peroxide value and the organoleptic detection of rancid flavour. Free fatty acid levels were more in the samples frozen after iced storage for 1 day than the other samples[65].

Another study focused on the effect of both microwave and traditional cooking methods such as baking, grilling and frying on the nutrient composition of eels (*Anguilla anguilla*). Result indicated that moisture content was reduced by all the methods but the fat and protein contents were increased. The sodium and potassium content significantly decreased, whereas the calcium and magnesium contents increased and zinc content was not affected by cooking. Frying increased the manganese and iron contents, while grilling and microwave cooking increased the copper content. The ratio of saturated and monounsaturated fatty acids in cooked fish decreased, but Omega-3 polyunsaturated fatty acids were increased by all cooking methods. The grilling and microwave-cooking were the most desirable methods to restore the omega 3 and omega 6 ratio. The increased levels of docosahexaenoic acid in fried fish boost the nutritive value[66].

All the above literatures mainly disclose the changes of proximate composition, micronutrient content, fatty acid profile, amino acid profile and chemical parameters like peroxide value, total volatile base nitrogen, thio-barbituric acid value of different marine fish due to application of different cooking techniques along with the effects of preservation with different preservatives and other preservation techniques. These also reveal the sensory and microbiological evaluation post cooking and storage for longer period. But these reviews do not support the study of fish consumed in West Bengal mainly sweet water and salt water variations. So the present study focuses on the nutritional quality changes of those fish post cooking and preservation with both natural and synthetic preservatives.

Chapter – 3

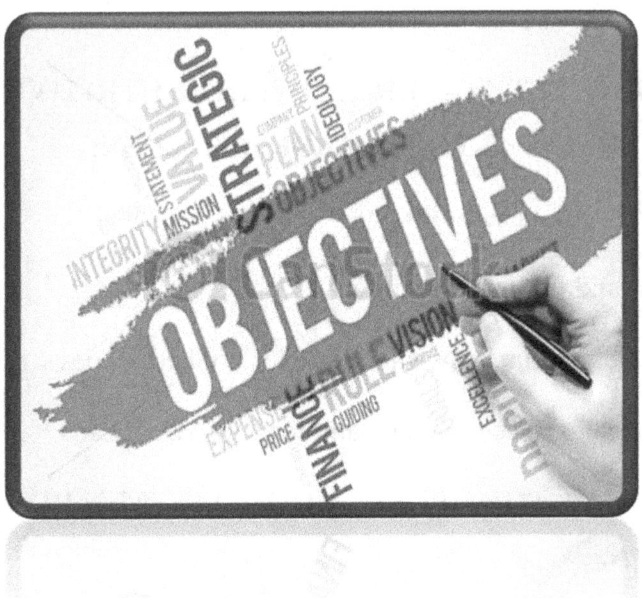

Aims & Objectives

The previous studies showed the nutritive values of different marine fish and their changes after cooking these fish. But there is no significant data of fish found in Bengal regarding the nutritive values and their changes during cooking. As fish is popularly consumed in West Bengal as a rich source of protein, the nutritive values and their changes during cooking is carried out in the present study.

A. IN CASE OF FRESH SAMPLES

- To estimate the nutritive values of selected samples in the raw state and cooked conditions.

B. IN CASE OF PRESERVED SAMPLES

- To estimate the nutritive values of the raw state samples after preservation on days 1, 2 and 14, 15.
- To estimate the nutritive values of the above samples after cooking on days 1, 2 and 14, 15.
- To estimate the nutritive values of the preserved raw state samples on days 1, 2 and 14, 15 in the raw condition (samples preserved with preservatives such as a combination of salt-turmeric and potassium metabisulphite).
- To estimate the nutritive values of the raw state samples preserved with selected preservatives on days 1, 2 and 14, 15 after cooking.

C. AFTER HAVING ESTIMATED ALL THE NUTRITIVE VALUES THE FOLLOWING COMPARISONS ARE TO BE MADE BETWEEN:

- Raw state and cooked samples
- samples with and without preservatives
- Preservatives containing raw state samples cooked on days 1, 2 and 14, 15
- Salt water samples, sweet water samples and crustaceans

D. TO ASCERTAIN THE BEST COOKING METHOD FOR NUTRITIVE VALUE RESTORATION.

E. EFFECT OF PRESERVATIVES ON THE NUTRITIVE VALUE OF THE SAMPLES AND IDENTIFICATION OF THE BEST ONE AMONG THE SELECTED PRESERVATIVES.

F. DETERMINATION OF THE BEST PRESERVATION DAY.

G. DETERMINATION OF THE BEST FISH FROM NUTRITIONAL ASPECT.

From the different reviews of literature the two preservatives are selected that is -

1. **Combination of salt & turmeric (Natural):** As this study focuses on the preservation and nutrient restoration of fish and other edible aquatic samples mainly consumed in West Bengal, salt and turmeric are the common household substances for preservation in this state.

2. **Potassium metabisulphite (Chemical):** Potassium metabisulphite is chosen as the chemical preservative to carry out this study. It has been used as an antifungal and antimicrobial agent in foods for many years, and has been generally recognized as safe (GRAS) by the U.S. Food and Drug Administration. It also helps to prevent melanosis or black spot, a dark discolouration, which is unattractive to consumers and reduces the market value of crustaceans. Literature showed that potassium metabisulphite was used to preserve crustaceans[57, 58] but its effect on fresh water and salt water fish is not observed still now. On the other hand its effect as preservative on nutrient retention of preserved fish has not yet been clearly established, this study helps to reveal this point of attention.

Chapter - 4

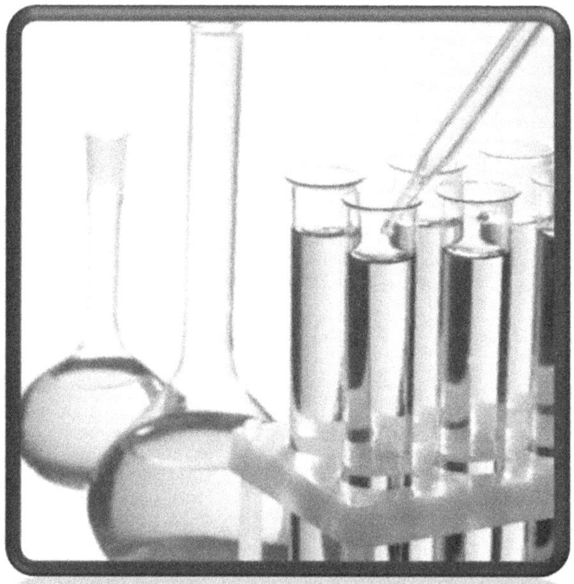

Materials and Methods

1. Sample preparation and cooking

Rohu (*Labeo rohita*), *katla* (*Catla catla*) and *hilsa* (*Hilsa ilisha*), each with a length of 25 – 30 cm and weight of 1 kg and pomfret (*Pampus argenteus*) with a length of 12cm and weight of 250–300 gm and prawn and lobster with a length of 10 cm, 25cm and weight of 50 gm and 90 gm respectively were obtained from the local fish market in Kolkata.

These were kept in a plastic container, transported to the laboratory and washed several times thoroughly under tap water to remove blood and excessive mucous. Subsequently, the fish sample was filleted into three sections. One section was divided into five groups and the other two divided into four groups.

In the first section, one group was used for immediate analysis in fresh condition and again divided into five sub-groups. One sub-group was left uncooked, while the other four were boiled, dry roasted in open pan, shallow fried and deep fried. Boiling was accomplished at 99–101^{0}C (temperature of water) for 10 minutes. Open pan dry roasting of fillets was done in a pan at 180^{0}C for 10 minutes. The fillets were fried in a household frying pan of 2 Litre of capacity at a temperature of approximately 180^{0}C for 10 minutes. Mustard oil was used as the medium for frying. 10 ml oil was used for shallow frying and 20 ml for deep frying.

The other two sections, each containing four groups was allowed to preserve up to 15 days in the refrigerator at -20^{0}C. One section was preserved with natural preservative - a combination of salt and turmeric (2% of the total weight of the sample) and another section was preserved with a chemical preservative KMS (Potassium metabisulphite) (2% of the total weight of the sample).

Each of these four groups was subdivided into five subgroups. One sub-group was left uncooked while the other four were then subjected to analysis post cooking on the day of preservation of 1st, 2nd, 14th and 15th.

1. b. Drip loss determination[67]

During storage of fish, drip loss (%) was determined by EZ drip loss method as the weight loss occurred during storage up to 15 days and thawing after freezing. The fillets were weighed before packaging and after each storage period. At each experimental storage period, the frozen fillets were thawed for at least 30 minutes and then drip loss was measured. Following this, fillets were subjected to cooking. The difference in weight (gm) was divided by the initial weight of the product (gm) and expressed as gm%.

Calculation

$$\text{Drip loss during storage (\%)} = \frac{W_l - W_c}{W_t - W_c} \times 100$$

Where,
W_c is the weight of the empty EZ-drip loss container alone.
W_t is the weight of EZ-drip loss container with sample and liquid.
W_l is the weight of the EZ-drip loss container with liquid.

1. c. Cooking yield determination[68]

Each fillet was cut into 5 pieces and 4 pieces were subjected to conventional cooking methods and weighed before and after cooking. They were allowed to each cooking method i.e. open pan dry roasting, boiling, shallow frying and deep frying for 10 minutes. After that they were left for 15 minutes at room temperature (20^0C) to cool down. The surface moisture and oil were dabbed dry with a paper towel before weighing for cooking yield determination. The cooking yield was calculated as the weight after cooking divided by weight before cooking and expressed as gm%.

Calculation

$$\text{Cooking yield percentage (\%)} = \frac{\text{Weight after cooking}}{\text{Weight before cooking}} \times 100$$

1. d. Preparation of the preservatives

Preservatives were taken at 2% of the amount of the weighed sample. At first they were prepared and then added to the sample for preservation.

i. Preparation of natural preservative

Table salt and turmeric were used in combination as natural preservative to preserve the sample. Both the preservatives are available in the market in powder form. So both the powders were taken in 1:1 ratio and mixed well and then were added to the sample at the dose of 2% of the total weight of the sample and spread uniformly so that each part of the samples were covered with the preservatives. After that they were packed in an air tight polythene container and stored in the refrigerator at -20^0C up to 15 days.

ii. Preparation of chemical preservative

Potassium metabisulphite (KMS) is a white crystalline powder. Its chemical formula is $K_2S_2O_5$. This salt (0.001gm) was taken in 100 ml distilled water to prepare a solution at the concentration of 0.001% level, or 10 ppm. From this 2 % (of the total weight of the sample) was added to the sample. 500 gm sample was taken and 10 ml of the prepared solution, containing 0.0001gm KMS was added to the sample and mixed well and preserved in an air tight polythene container and kept in the refrigerator at -20^0C up to 15 days. The permissible level of KMS for fish and shell fish is 100 ppm or 100 mg per litre[59]. In this study 1mg of KMS is actually used to preserve the fish and crustacean samples.

Maximum permitted level of KMS in food[67]

Food	Maximum permitted level (ppm/ mg per litre)
Fish and shell fish	**100**
Uncooked Crustaceans(Prawn, Shrimp, Lobster, Crab)	**30**
Cooked Crustaceans	**30**
Fully preserved fish including canned product	**1000**

- In this study, 10 ppm KMS solution was prepared and 10 ml of it was used in 500 gm of sample. 10 ml of the prepared KMS solution contains 0.0001gm KMS.
- Therefore 100ml of this solution will contain 0.001gm KMS and 1000 ml of solution will contain 0.01gm of KMS per 500 gm of sample and if 1 kg of sample is taken, the amount of KMS in the sample will be double, i.e. 0.02 gm or 20 mg or 20 ppm per kg which is quite below the maximum permissible level[67].

1. Nutrient contents analysis

Nutrient contents analyses for homogenized samples of cooked and raw state fish fillets were carried out in triplicate for the estimation of carbohydrate by anthrone method[68], protein by Lowry method[69], fat by Soxhlet extraction method[70], iron and calcium contents determined by AOAC method[71], moisture and ash by weight difference method[72] and determination of energy by energy conversion factor[73].

a. Estimation of carbohydrate by Anthrone Method [68]

Principle

Carbohydrates are dehydrated with concentrated H_2SO_4 to form furfuraldehyde, which condenses with anthrone to form a green coloured complex which can be measured by using the spectrophotometer. Anthrone reacts with monosaccharides, disaccharides, polysaccharides, dextrin, starch, gums and glycosides[74].

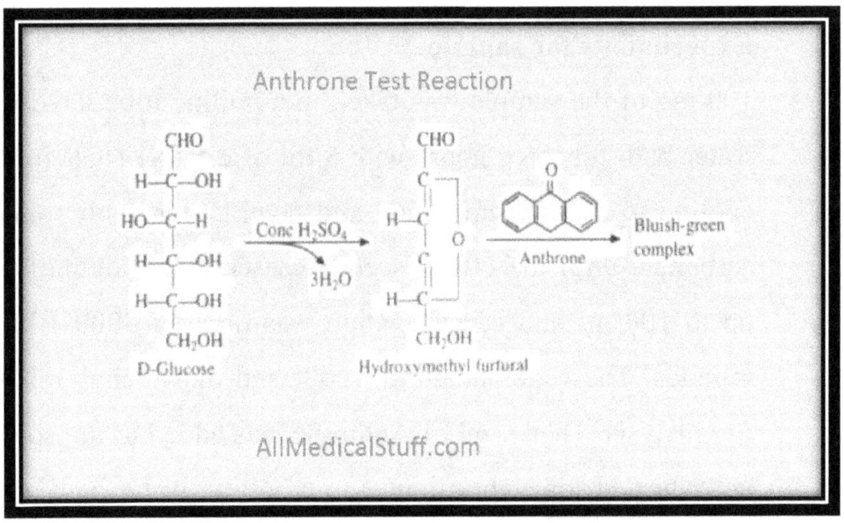

Fig.4.1 Anthrone reaction

Source: www. AllMedicalStuff.com

Materials

i. 2.5 (N) HCL

ii. Anthrone reagent

iii. Dextrose

iv. 95% H_2SO_4

v. Distilled water

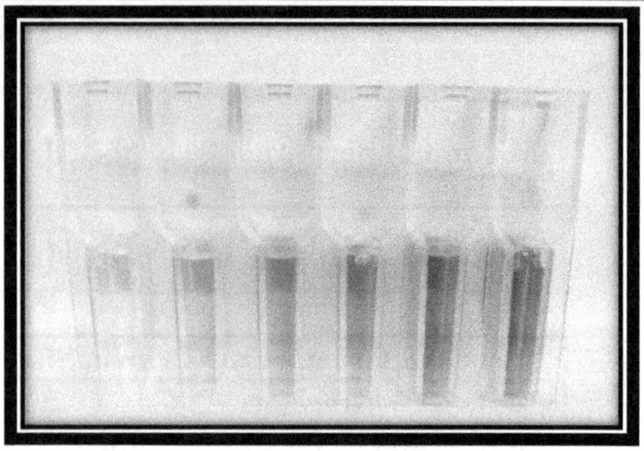

Fig.4.2 Standard of Anthrone
Source: slideplayer.com

Preparation of anthrone Reagent

200 mg of anthrone was added to 100 ml of ice cold 95% H_2SO_4 and kept for 30 minutes in ice box to dissolve the anthrone completely in ice. Then it was mixed well in acid and used for the experiments.

Preparation of standard curve by dextrose solution

100 mg of glucose was dissolved in100 ml of distilled water (stock solution). Then 10ml of stock solution was again mixed with 90 ml of distilled water.0, 0.2, 0.4, 0.6, 0.8 and1ml of working standards were taken in 6 test tubes from this solution. 0 served as blank. It only contained water. Then volume was made up to 1 ml by distilled water and 4 ml of anthrone reagent was added to all the test tubes. After that the test tubes were heated in water bath and cooled rapidly. After the appearance of dark green to green colour, the reading was taken at 630 nm in spectrophotometer (Perkin Elmer Lambda 25).

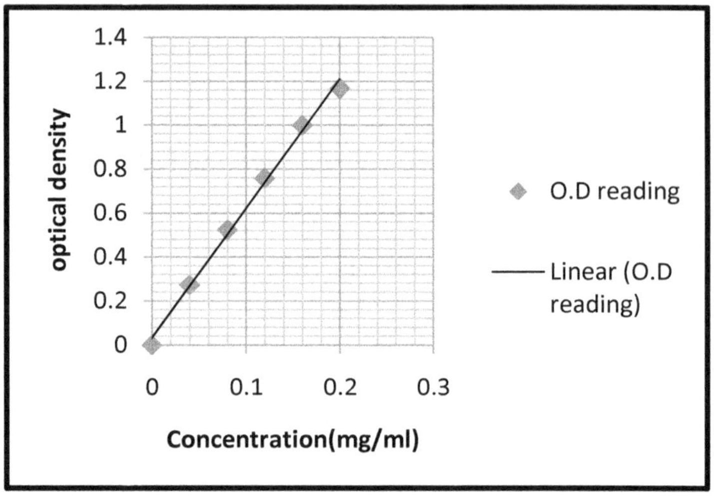

Fig 4.3 Standard curve of Carbohydrate

Experiments for sample

100 mg of the sample was taken in a boiling tube. Hydrolysis was carried out by keeping it in a boiling water bath for three hours with 5 ml of 2.5 (N) HCl followed by cooling to room temperature and neutralizing with solid sodium carbonate until the effervescence ceased. The volume was made up to 100 ml and centrifugation was done at 3000 RPM for 15 minutes. The supernatant was collected of which 1 ml was used for analysis. Then 4 ml of Anthrone was added to the solution, the latter heated for eight minutes in a boiling water bath and cooled rapidly. A green to dark green colour appeared. Then the reading was taken at 630 nm by a spectrophotometer (Perkin Elmer Lambda 25).

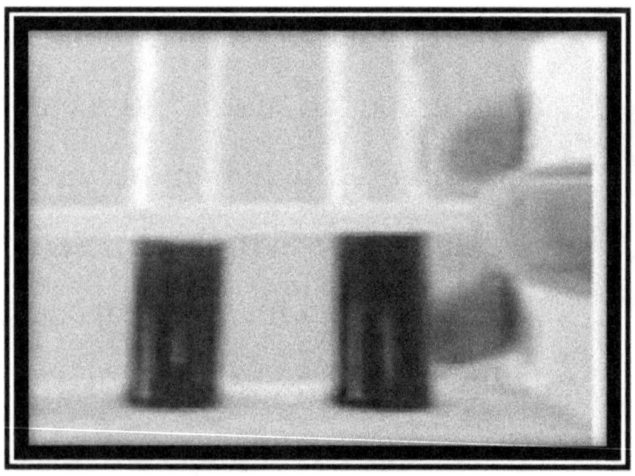

Fig.4.4 Anthrone test
Source: Open Science Publication

Calculation

The Optical Density (O.D.) reading from the standard curve results were plotted on the graph paper and the standard curve was drawn. Experimental results from the sample were plotted on the standard curve and the concentration of carbohydrate present in the measured sample was calculated from it. The amount of carbohydrate present in 100 mg of sample was calculated from the following formula -

$$\text{Total carbohydrate (mg/100 mg)} = \frac{\text{Mg of glucose}}{\text{Volume of test sample}} \times 100$$

This formula helps to calculate the amount of carbohydrate present in 100mg of sample and this result is used to convert the amount of carbohydrate in100 gm of sample by unitary method.

b. Estimation of Protein by Lowry Method [69]

Principle

Estimation of the total protein by Lowry method is one of the most commonly used colorimetric assays. This is a sensitive procedure due to the combination of two colour forming reactions i.e. Biuret reactions in which Cu_2^{++} reacts with a peptide bond of protein under alkaline conditions, resulting in reduction of cupric ions (Cu_2^{++}) to cuprous ions (Cu^+) and Lowry's reaction in which the Folin-Ciocaltaue reagent, containing phospho-molybdic complex which is a mixture of sodium tungstate, sodium molybdate and sodium phosphate, along with copper sulphate solution reacts with the protein producing a bluish-purple colour, which can be estimated by measuring the absorbance at 650-700nm in spectrophotometer.

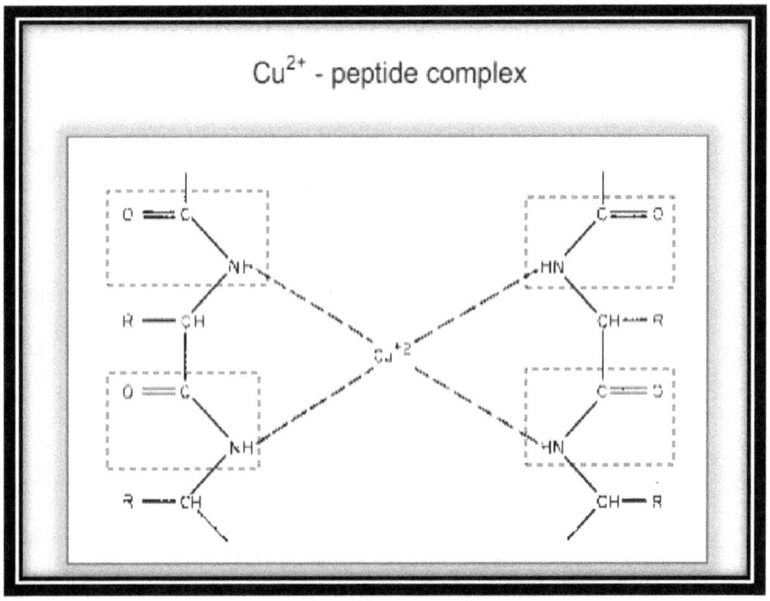

Fig.4.5 Lowry reaction

Source: shinaebiochem.blogspot

The bluish-purple colour is produced due to the reduction of phosphomolybdo tungstate to hetero-poly-molybdenum by the copper-catalysed oxidation of aromatic amino acids tryptophan and tyrosine. Thus the intensity of colour depends on the amount of these aromatic amino acids present and will thus vary for different protein samples. This method is advantageous as it can help to detect even a small quantity of protein present in the sample[75].

Materials

i. Sodium dihydrogen phosphate (NaH_2PO4)

ii. Di Sodium hydrogen phosphate (Na_2HPO4)

iii. Lowry reagent

iv. Folin-Ciocaltaue reagent

Reagent preparation

i. Lowry reagent:

a. Solution A: 2% sodium carbonate in 0.1(N) NaOH.

b. Solution B: 0.5% copper sulphate ($CuSO_4$) solution in 1% sodium potassium tartarate solution. These were prepared freshly.

50 ml of solution A with 1 ml of solution B were mixed well just prior to use.

ii. Folin-Ciocaltaue reagent: This is commercially available and was diluted with an equal volume of water just before use.

Preparation of standard Protein curve

Bovine Serum Albumin (BSA) was used as a standard protein due to its easy availability and low cost with improved purity. 50 mg of BSA was dissolved in 50 ml of saline solution (0.9 mg NaCl in 100 ml distilled water) in a volumetric flask (concentration-1mg/ml) to prepare the stock solution. 10 ml of standard stock solution was mixed with 40 ml of distilled water and 50 ml of working standard solution was made (concentration - 200μg/ml).

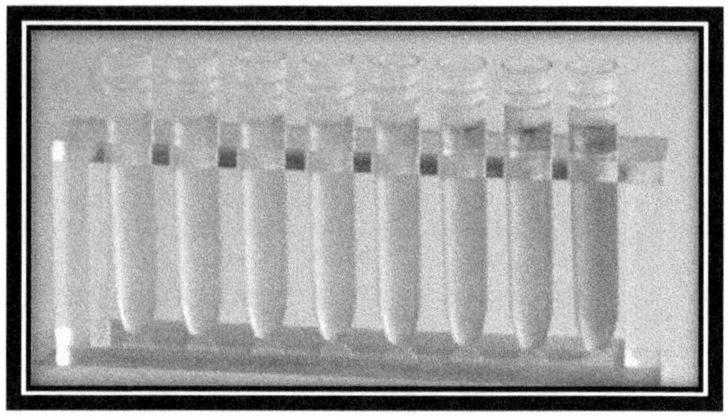

Fig.4.6 standard of Lowry assay

Source: G- Biosciences

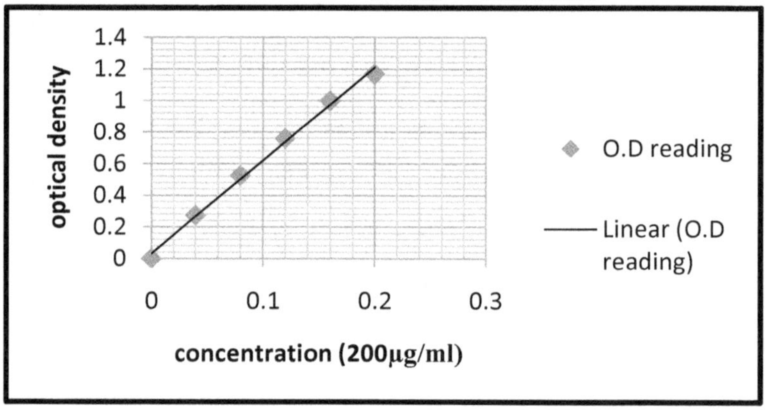

Fig. 4.7 Standard curve of Protein

0, 0.2, 0.4, 0.6, 0.8, and 1 ml of working standard were taken in test tubes. 0 contains only water. Then 5 ml of Lowry reagent was added to the test tubes and allowed to incubate for 10 minutes.

After that 0.5 ml of Folin-Ciocaltaue reagent was added and allowed to stand for 30 minutes. The optical density reading was taken at 660 nm with a spectrophotometer (Perkin Elmer Lambda 25) after the appearance of a dark blue colour.

Preparation of Phosphate Buffer Solution (PBS)

27.8 gm sodium dihydrogen phosphate (NaH_2PO4) was taken in a volumetric flask and 1000 ml of distilled water was added and mixed well. 53.6 gm disodium hydrogen phosphate (Na_2HPO4) was taken in another volumetric flask and again 1000 ml of distilled water was added and allowed to mix uniformly. After the preparation of two separate solution 16 ml of sodium dihydrogen phosphate solution and 84 ml of disodium hydrogen phosphate solution were added in another volumetric flask and the volume was made up to 200 ml with distilled water. The pH of this phosphate buffer solution was 7.6, measured by a pH meter (Labman LMPH -10).

Experiments for sample

200 mg of sample was taken and 20 ml of phosphate buffer solution was added and homogenized finely in a homogeniser (REMI Motors RQ-127 A/D, HP motor - 1/8, India), leaving it overnight. After that, it was cold – centrifuged (Cooling Centrifuge, REMI, India) at 5000 RPM for 20 minutes. The supernatant was collected and 1 ml was used for analysis. Then 5 ml of Lowry reagent was added to the supernatant and allowed to incubate for 10 minutes. After that 0.5 ml of Folin-Ciocaltaue reagent was added and incubated for 30 minutes until a dark blue colour appeared. The reading was taken at 660 nm with a spectrophotometer (Perkin Elmer Lambda 25).

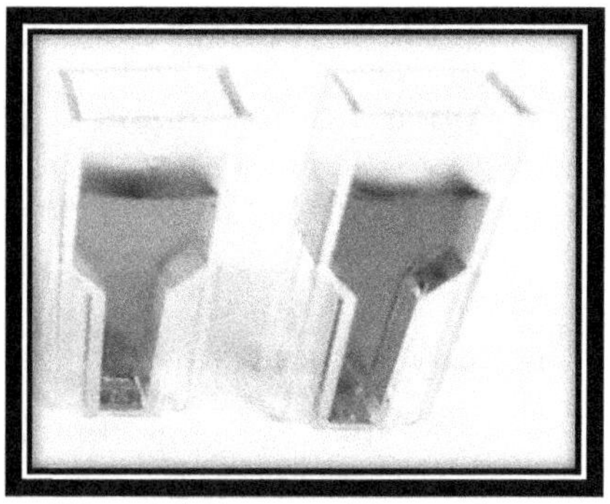

Fig. 4.8 Lowry Experiment
Source: En.wikipedia.org.

Calculation

The concentration of protein in the tested sample was obtained by plotting the O.D. reading from the experiment on the standard curve of BSA protein solution. This concentration was present in 1 ml of the tested sample and it was multiplied by 20 to calculate the amount of protein present in the 20 ml of buffer solution. This 20 ml buffer solution contained 200 mg of test sample. So the concentration of protein present in the 20 ml of buffer was equal to the concentration of 200 mg of sample. Thus this value of protein was converted to 100 gm of sample by unitary method.

c. Estimation of Fat by Soxhlet Extraction Method [70]

Principle

A Soxhlet extractor is a piece of laboratory apparatus invented in 1879 by Franz von Soxhlet. It was originally designed for the extraction of a lipid from a solid material. Typically, a Soxhlet extraction is used when the desired compound has a limited solubility in a solvent and the impurity is insoluble in that solvent. It allows for unmonitored and unmanaged operation while efficiently recycling a small amount of solvent to dissolve a larger amount of material[76].

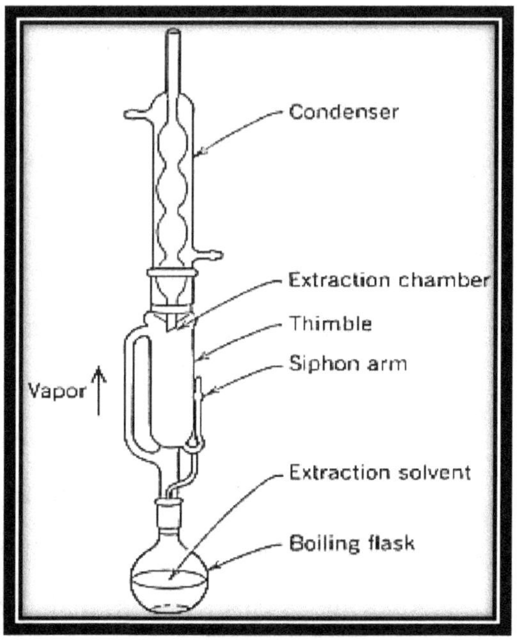

Fig.4.9 Soxhlet mechanism
Source: oleoresins.melbia.com

Experimental set up

- Soxhlet extractor
- Mantle heater
- Water condenser
- Flash evaporator

Experiment for sample

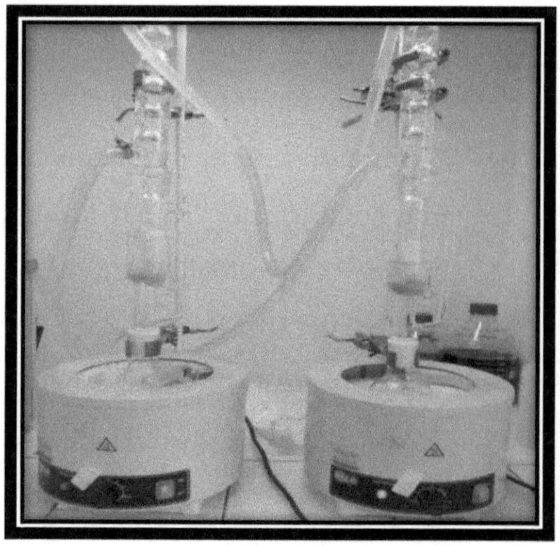

Fig. 4.10 Soxhlet Apparatus

5gm of dried sample wrapped in filter paper and the package was tied with crochet thread and placed inside the thimble of the apparatus. Then the extracting solvent petroleum ether of 60-80^{0}C boiling range was placed in a distillation flask placed on a heating mantel. The solvent was heated to reflux. The solvent vapour travelled up a distillation arm and flooded into the chamber housing the thimble. The condenser ensures that any solvent vapour that cooled, dripped back down into the chamber housing the solid material. The chamber containing the solid material slowly filled with warm solvent.

The fat present in the sample was dissolved in the solvent which was returned to the distillation flask. This cycle was allowed to continue for 12 hours. After complete extraction of the fat, the solvent was poured into a weighed petri dish, the solution evaporated and the final weight of the petri dish containing the fat was taken. From this, the amount of the fat was calculated.

Calculation

Amount of fat (gm/100 gm dried sample) =

$$\frac{\text{Final weight of Petri dish} - \text{Initial weight of Petri dish}}{\text{Weight of the dried sample}} \times 100$$

This formula helped to calculate the amount of fat present in 100 gm of dried sample. To determine the amount of fat in 100 gm of fresh fish, firstly, the unitary calculation was made to determine how much of fresh sample was equal to 100 gm of dried sample and the dried sample value was converted to fresh sample and the above formula was again used to calculate the amount of fat in 100 gm of fresh sample.

d. Estimation of Minerals by AOAC method after wet digestion [71]

Dried sample (500 mg) was taken in a 25 ml of volumetric flask and 10 ml of concentrated nitric acid was added to it and allowed to stand overnight. After that the volumetric flask was placed on a hot plate at temperature 200^{0}C and allowed to boil for 8 hours, when brown fumes were produced nitric acid was again added (about 20 to 30 ml) whenever the acid was about to be dry so that the sample does not get charred. Then 4 ml of perchloric ($HClO_4$) acid was added and boiled until brown fumes from the digestion ceased. After that the volume was made up to the mark by double distilled water and the solution was filtered. Aliquots of the solutions were transferred to polyethylene flasks and kept cool at 4^{0}C and this solution was used for the analysis of iron and calcium by atomic absorption spectrophotometer (Model No-iCE 3000 series of thermo scientific instrument).

Principle of atomic absorption spectrophotometer

Atomic absorption spectroscopy (AAS) is an analytical method, based on the absorption of UV-visible radiation by free atoms in the gaseous state. The food sample to be analysed is normally digested in acidic solution made aqueous and the aliquot is placed in the instrument, where it is heated to vaporise and atomise the minerals. A beam of radiation is passed through the atomised sample and the absorption of radiation is measured at specific wavelengths corresponding to the mineral that is to be analysed. The type and concentration of minerals present is obtained by measuring the location and intensity of the peaks in the absorption spectra. The reduction in intensity of an electromagnetic wave that travels through a sample is used to determine the absorbance. A (Absorbance) = -log (I/Io).

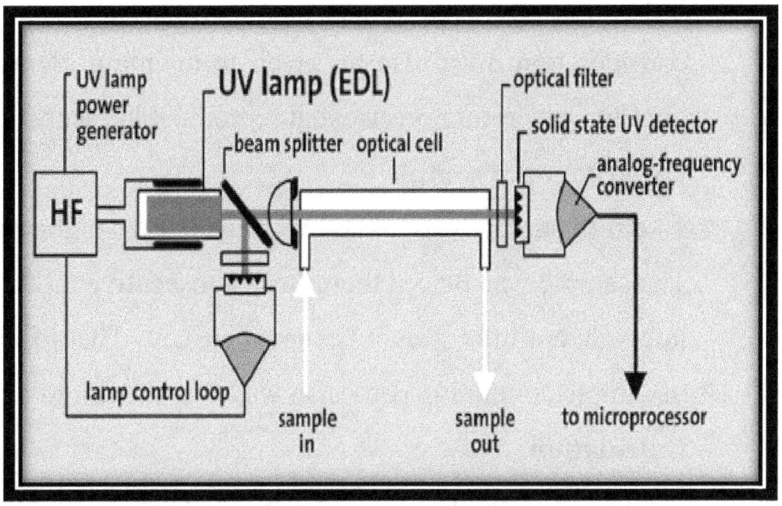

Fig.4.11 Atomic Absorption Spectroscopy (AAS)

Source: mercury-instrumentsusa.com

The Beer-Lambert law is used to relate the absorbance to the concentration of atoms in the sample: A = a.b.c, where A is absorbance, b is sample path length and c is concentration of absorbing species[77].

Calculation

Wet digested solution was fed to atomic absorption spectrophotometer and the concentration was given in mg/ml that is ppm (parts per million). The amount of minerals present in the sample was calculated by the following formula-

Amount of mineral (mg) =

$$\frac{\text{Concentration (ppm)} \times \text{Volume of Sample} \times \text{Dilution Factor}}{\text{Weight of the sample}} \times 100$$

e. Estimation of Moisture by weight difference method[72]

Principle

Moisture content influences the taste, texture, weight, appearance and shelf life of foodstuffs. Even a slight differentiation has adverse impact on the physical properties of food materials. The drying oven, commonly used for commercial purposes, is the established reference method for

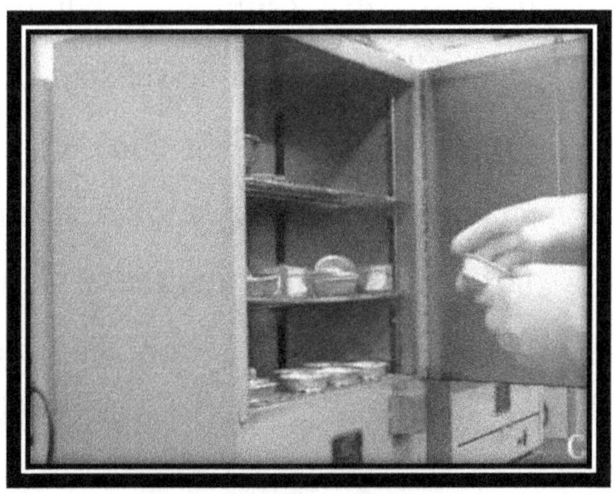

Fig.4.12 Hot Air Oven

loss by Thermo gravimetric analysis (TGA). In this procedure, a sample is weighed and subsequently heated to allow for the release of moisture. After this, the sample is cooled in the dessicator before re-weighing. Moisture content is calculated by the difference in wet and dry weights.

In this process, measuring accuracy and the resolution of the balance are extremely important. Careful consideration must also be given to maintain identical conditions, where temperature and duration are vital for generating precise and reproducible results[78].

Experiment of sample

10 gm of sample was taken in a previously weighed petri dish and placed in an oven, maintained at 60^0C. The sample was placed there for 7 consecutive days and the weight of the sample was checked at specific intervals until the weight became constant. The difference between the initial weight and the final weight of sample containing petri dish was converted into a percentage of moisture present in the sample.

Calculation

Moisture content of sample was calculated by the following formula -

$$\text{Moisture (\%)} = \frac{W_1 - W_2}{W_1} \times 100$$

W_1= weight (gm) of sample before drying

W_2 = weight (gm) of sample after drying

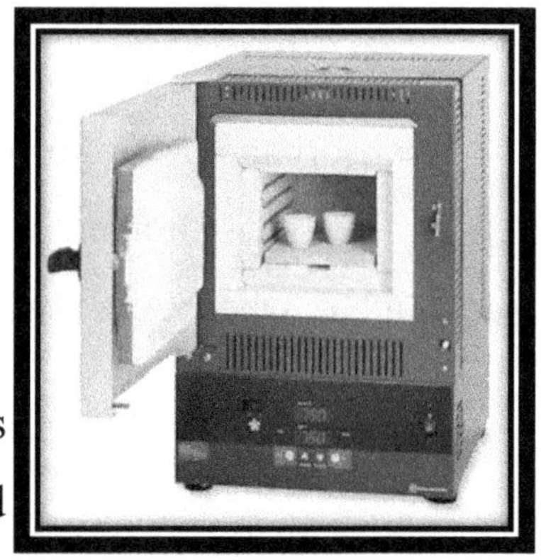

Fig. 4.13 Muffle furnace

f. Estimation of Ash by weight difference method[72]

Principle

The ash content of any substance is a measure of the total amount of minerals present in a food. Ash is the inorganic residue remaining after the water and organic matter have been removed by heating in the presence of oxidising agents, providing a measure of the total amount of minerals within a food. Ashing may also be used as the first step in preparing samples for analysis of specific minerals by atomic spectroscopy. Ash contents of fresh foods rarely exceed 5%, although some processed foods can have ash contents as high as 12%.

A high temperature muffle furnace capable of maintaining temperatures of between 500^0C - 600 ^{0}C is used for dry ashing procedure. Water and other volatile materials are vaporised and organic substances are burned in the presence of the oxygen in air to CO_2, H_2O and N_2. Most minerals are converted to oxides, sulphates, phosphates, chlorides or silicates. Although most minerals have fairly low volatility at these high temperatures, some are volatile and may be partially lost, e.g. iron, lead and mercury[79].

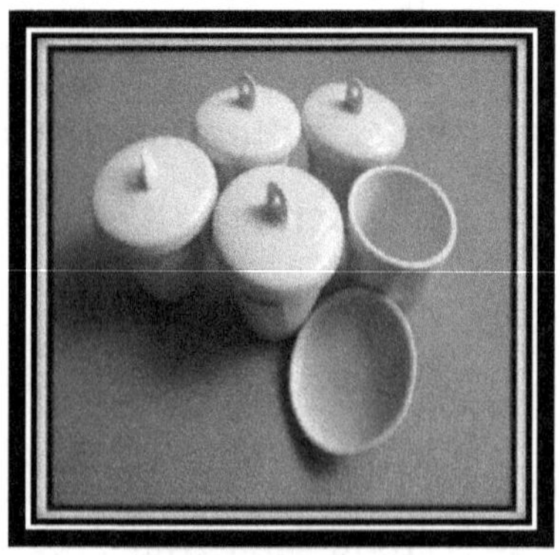

Fig. 4.14 Porcelain crucible

Experiment for sample

5 gm of dried sample was taken in a previously weighed crucible and placed in a muffle furnace (Bio Technics Muffle Furnace BTI-36) at temperature 600^0C for 8 hours. The weight was checked after that and the crucible was again placed in the furnace for at least 4 hours. The weight was checked again and the process was repeated until the weight became constant. The difference between the initial and the final weights of the sample containing crucible was the ash content of the sample.

Calculation

Ash content of the sample can be calculated by the following formula-

$$\text{Percentage of ash in dry weight (\%)} = \frac{\text{Amount of ash (gm)}}{\text{Dry weight of the sample}} \times 100$$

Amount of the ash can be calculated by the difference between the two weights of the crucible with the following formula-

Amount of ash (gm) = Initial weight of the crucible – Final weight of the crucible

g. Determination of Energy content by energy conversion factor[73]

Principle

The measurement of energy content of food is not technically difficult, but in practice such measurements are expensive, time-consuming and there are quite severe restrictions on the activities. In addition, knowledge of the energy content supplied by the dietary intake is often required in situations where its direct measurement is impossible or highly impractical. In these situations the only alternative method is to use a procedure for calculating the energy content of a food from its chemical composition.

The various systems of calorie conversion factors provide a method for performing this calculation. All the systems used at present have their origins in work carried out by different scientists such as Rubner, 1885; Atwater, 1903[80].

Experiment for sample

The energy content of the sample was determined by the summation of the amount of energy from carbohydrate, protein and fat. The carbohydrate and protein contents were multiplied by the conversion factor 4.1 and 4 respectively and the fat content was multiplied by 9.3 and the total calorie content was represented in Kcal per 100 gm of a sample.

2. Survey on fish consumption pattern

A survey was carried out to determine the fish consumption pattern and nutrition awareness among the adult women of Kolkata city. In total 100 samples were selected by snowball sampling technique from 4 zones of Kolkata city, *viz.* North, South, East and West. A structured questionnaire (Annexure-I) was prepared by consulting the experts. The questionnaire has 16 close-ended questions as follows:

- Demographic information of respondent

- Consumption pattern of fish and other edible aquatic animal
- The method of preparation of fish and other edible aquatic animal
- The method of preservation of fish and other edible aquatic animal

3. Statistical analysis

The effects of different cooking methods on the proximate composition and other nutrient contents of river fish, sea fish and crustaceans were analysed by using Mean and Standard Deviation. One way ANOVA was carried out for comparing the nutrient contents between the raw state and cooked samples along with the preservation days up to the 15th, preserved with and without natural and synthetic preservatives. Differences were considered to be significant when p value is < 0.05. Data was analysed by using SPSS package (Version 17). Correlation matrix was done to identify the correlations among the different variables of the different samples. Correlation of the variables is considered to be significant when the value is between $\pm$ 0.8-1.0. The values were checked at 0.05 and 0.01 levels of significance. Student t test and index number were also used to analyze some specific objectives of the study.

The significance of the survey study was analysed with the respect to certain variables by chi square test. Differences were considered to be significant when p value is < 0.05. Frequency distribution of the study variables were described by pie charts and bar diagrams.

Chapter - 5

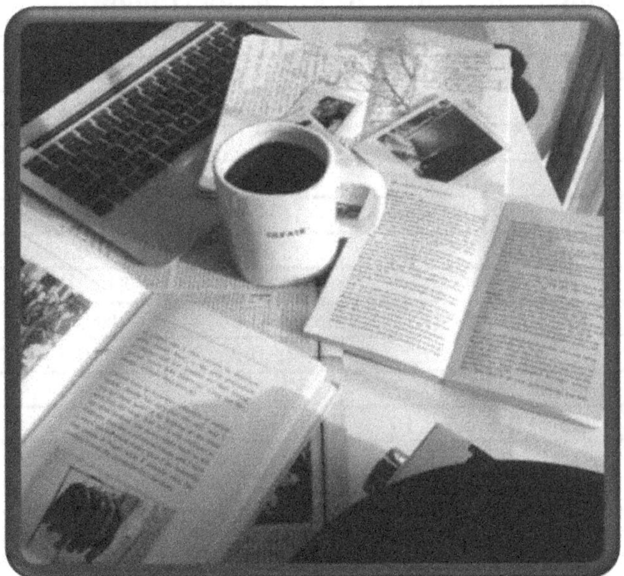

Results and Discussion

PART- A Experimental Results

In this study, percentage nutrient composition (carbohydrate, protein, fat, moisture, ash, iron, calcium and energy) has been analysed in three groups of fish and edible aquatic species, which includes Carp (*Rohu* and *Katla*), Crustaceans (Prawn and Lobster) and salt water fish (Pomfret and *Hilsa*). Differences in reported and observed values are due to the environmental conditions, type of breeding, size of the species, feed and nutrition of the species and other factors[83].

5.1 Carbohydrate content

Though fish contains very little amount of carbohydrate[1], this experiment is carried out to estimate the relative percentage of carbohydrate in different fish and edible aquatic species. Changes in carbohydrate content in different cooking methods and preservation conditions are also estimated. Carbohydrate estimation is carried out by Anthrone method[68].

5.1.1 *Rohu* (*Labeo rohita*)

It has been reported that *rohu* contains 4.4 gm of carbohydrate per 100 gm[84] in the raw condition. This value changes due to the application of different cooking methods and preservation conditions (vide Table no **5.1.1.1**).

Table no 5.1.1.1 Carbohydrate content of *Rohu* (gm/100gm)

Preservation	Duration	Raw state	Boiling	Dry roasting	Shallow frying	Deep frying
Control	Fresh	4.42±0.08	2.86±0.07	2.90±0.08	3.23±0.14	2.77±0.14
Control	24 hours	3.85±0.14	2.52±0.08	1.98±0.11	3.15±0.18	2.45±0.09
Control	48 hours	3.32±0.08	1.86±0.06	1.72±0.23	2.39±0.13	2.29±0.25
Control	14 days	2.06±0.20	1.44±0.22	1.50±0.36	1.71±0.38	1.51±0.36
Control	15 days	5.08±0.07	4.16±0.06	3.66±0.17	3.64±0.33	3.94±0.06
Salt & Turmeric	24 hours	4.78±0.09	2.52±0.07	1.68±0.03	3.88±0.03	4.64±0.18
Salt & Turmeric	48 hours	2.95±0.21	3.29±0.11	1.81±0.20	1.92±0.211	1.14±0.12
Salt & Turmeric	14 days	7.07±0.18	3.73±0.06	3.06±0.16	6.28±0.17	4.79±0.15
Salt &Turmeric	15 days	3.94±0.22	1.60±0.25	3.30±0.13	4.81±0.17	3.07±0.27
KMS	24 hours	3.86±0.12	1.83±0.16	1.35±0.21	1.20±0.18	1.66±0.12
KMS	48 hours	3.23±0.10	1.67±0.13	1.71±0.07	0.92±0.08	1.72±0.09
KMS	14 days	1.33±0.21	2.06±0.17	1.73±0.11	2.55±0.33	3.90±0.09
KMS	15 days	2.01±0.17	0.92±0.08	1.65±0.10	1.84±0.16	2.65±0.18

Values are expressed as mean±SD. Loss Restoration
Red digits represent the significant highest values from the raw state in different conditions.

In 14 days preservation without preservative, 15 days preservation with salt and turmeric and 14, 15 days preservation with KMS, carbohydrate losses mainly occur by boiling, whereas 24 hours and 48 hours preservation without preservative, 24 hours and 14 days preservation with salt and turmeric, losses occur by open pan dry roasting. In fresh condition and in 14 days preservation with salt and turmeric, nutrient loss occurs by deep frying.

Most of the retention occurs by shallow frying, but in 24 hours preservation with salt and turmeric, 48 hours, 14 days and 15 days preservation with KMS, retention occurs by deep frying and in 15 days control preservation without preservative and 24 hours preservation with KMS, retention occurs by boiling. 14 days preservation with KMS helps to increase the carbohydrate content in all the cooking methods more than the raw fish.

Boiling shows the increased carbohydrate content as compared to the raw value in 48 hours with salt and turmeric as well as 14 days KMS preservation. Open pan dry roasting and shallow frying show the increased carbohydrate content than the value of raw condition in 14 days KMS preservation, whereas deep frying shows the increased carbohydrate content as compared to the value of the raw state in 14 days and 15 days KMS preservation.

This is probably due to the loss of water from the fish for prolonged preservation with preservatives as well as the application of heat during cooking[48]. It is also possible that the molecular rearrangement occurs during cooking.

Fig. 5.1.1.2 Graphical representation of Carbohydrate content of *Rohu* with respect to different conditions

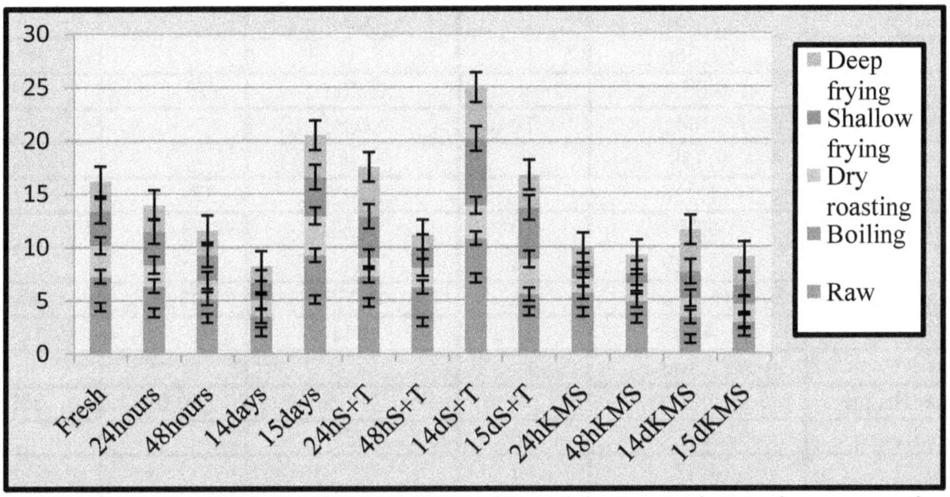

This graphical representation shows that among all the preservation conditions, **14 days preservation with salt and turmeric**[55] helps to increase the carbohydrate content in all the cooking methods except in open pan dry roasting. The possible reason for this may be the moisture loss due to prolonged preservation and the efficiency of salt and turmeric to inhibit the microbial growth and in turn the restoration of nutrient[34, 52].The graph also shows that salt and turmeric preservation increases the carbohydrate content as compared to the without preservative control preservation and KMS preservation.

Table no 5.1.1.3 ANOVA with regard to cooking conditions and preservation methods

Condition	Differences	Sum of Squares	df	Mean Square	F	Sig.
Fresh (control)	Between Groups	5.620	4	1.405	127.409	.000(S)
	Within Groups	.110	10	.011		
	Total	5.730	14			
24 hours (control)	Between Groups	6.347	4	1.587	100.044	.000(S)
	Within Groups	.159	10	.016		
	Total	6.505	14			
48 hours (control)	Between Groups	4.721	4	1.180	40.708	.000(S)
	Within Groups	.290	10	.029		
	Total	5.011	14			
14 days (control)	Between Groups	.775	4	.194	1.930	.182(NS)
	Within Groups	1.003	10	.100		
	Total	1.778	14			
15 days (control)	Between Groups	4.124	4	1.031	33.874	.000(S)
	Within Groups	.304	10	.030		
	Total	4.428	14			
24 hours (salt & turmeric)	Between Groups	21.229	4	5.307	1.455E3	.000(S)
	Within Groups	.036	10	.004		
	Total	21.266	14			
48 hours (salt & turmeric)	Between Groups	9.055	4	2.264	74.436	.000(S)
	Within Groups	.304	10	.030		
	Total	9.359	14			
14 days (salt & turmeric)	Between Groups	34.020	4	8.505	371.291	.000(S)
	Within Groups	.229	10	.023		
	Total	34.249	14			
15 days (salt & turmeric)	Between Groups	16.950	4	4.237	103.353	.000(S)
	Within Groups	.410	10	.041		
	Total	17.360	14			
24 hours (KMS)	Between Groups	14.060	4	3.515	129.035	.000(S)
	Within Groups	.272	10	.027		
	Total	14.332	14			
48 hours (KMS)	Between Groups	8.518	4	2.130	220.905	.000(S)
	Within Groups	.096	10	.010		
	Total	8.614	14			
14 days (KMS)	Between Groups	11.909	4	2.977	74.521	.000(S)
	Within Groups	.400	10	.040		
	Total	12.309	14			
15 days (KMS)	Between Groups	4.676	4	1.169	55.129	.000(S)
	Within Groups	.212	10	.021		
	Total	4.888	14			

$p<0.05$ S= Significant, NS= Non-significant. All abbreviations are on page so and so.

This statistical ANOVA table shows that all the values are significant, which means there is significant difference present in the values of carbohydrate content of *rohu* among different cooking methods and the raw state in respect to fresh condition along with different preservation methods.

Table no 5.1.1.4 Post hoc Duncan statistical analysis

Preservation	Duration	Raw state	Boiling	Dry roasting	Shallow frying	Deep frying
Control	Fresh	B,O,S,D^a	S, D^b	S, R^c	R,B,O,D^d	S, R^c
Control	24 hours	B,O,S,D^a	R,O,S^e	B,R,S,D^f	R,B,O,D^d	R,O,S^e
Control	48 hours	B,O,S,D^a	R,S,D^g	R,S,D^g	R,B,O^h	R,B,O^h
Control	14 days	B,O,S,D^a	-	-	-	-
Control	15 days	B,O,S,D^a	R,O,S^e	R,B^i	R,B^i	R,B^i
Salt & Turmeric	24 hours	B,O,S,D^a	R,O,S,D^j	B,R,S,D^f	R,B,O,D^d	R,B,O,S^k
Salt & Turmeric	48 hours	B,O,S,D^a	R,O,S,D^j	R,B,D^l	R,B,D^l	R,B,O,S^k
Salt & Turmeric	14 days	B,O,S,D^a	R,O,S,D^j	B,R,S,D^f	R,B,O,D^d	R,B,O,S,^{k}
Salt &Turmeric	15 days	B,O,S,D^a	R,O,S,D^j	R,B,S^m	R,B,O,D^d	R,B,S^m
KMS	24 hours	B,O,S,D^a	R,O,S^e	R,B,D^l	R,B,D^l	R,O,S^e
KMS	48 hours	B,O,S,D^a	S, R^c	S, R^c	R,B,O,D^d	S, R^c
KMS	14 days	B,O,S,D^a	R,S,D^g	R,S,D^g	R,B,O,D^d	R,B,O,S^k
KMS	15 days	B,O,S,D^a	R,O,S,D^j	R,B,D^l	R,B,D^l	R,B,O,S^k

R= Raw state, B= Boiling, O= Open pan dry roasting, S= Shallow frying, D= Deep frying. The same uppercase alphabets represent that there is no significant difference present among the variables.

This table shows the significant difference among the different variables such as cooking methods and preservation conditions. The raw state significantly differs from boiling, open pan dry roasting, shallow frying and deep frying in all the preservation methods and control conditions. In fresh condition, boiling significantly differs from shallow frying and deep frying. Both open pan dry roasting and deep frying in fresh condition and 48 hours preservation with KMS, significantly differ from shallow frying and the raw state. This pattern of difference is also found in boiling under 48 hours preservation with KMS, whereas shallow frying in fresh condition, 24 hours control preservation without preservative as well as salt and turmeric preservation, 14 days and 15 days salt and turmeric preservation, and 48 hours, 14 days KMS preservation, significantly differs from the raw state, boiling, open pan dry roasting and deep frying.

Boiling and deep frying in 24 hours control preservation without preservative and 24 hours KMS preservation and only boiling in 15 days control preservation, significantly differ from the raw state, open pan dry roasting and shallow frying. Open pan dry roasting in 24 hours control preservation without preservative, 24 hours, 14 days salt and turmeric preservation, significantly differs from the raw state, boiling, shallow frying and deep frying. Again boiling and open pan dry roasting in 24 hours control preservation without preservative and 14 days KMS preservation, significantly differ from the raw state, shallow frying and deep frying. Shallow frying and deep frying in 48 hours control preservation, significantly differ from the raw state, boiling and open pan dry roasting.

Open pan dry roasting, shallow frying and deep frying significantly differ from the raw state and boiling in 15 days control preservation without preservative. In 24 hours, 48 hours, 14 days, 15 days salt and turmeric preservation, boiling significantly differs from the raw state, open pan drying roasting, shallow frying and deep frying. Deep frying in 24 hours, 48 hours, 14 days salt and turmeric preservation and 14 days, 15 days KMS preservation, significantly differs from the raw state, boiling, open pan drying roasting and shallow frying.

Open pan dry roasting and shallow frying in 48 hours salt and turmeric preservation, 24 hours and 15 days KMS preservation, significantly differ from the raw state, boiling, open pan dry roasting and deep frying. Open pan dry roasting and deep frying in 15 days salt and turmeric preservation, significantly differ from the raw state, boiling, open pan dry roasting and shallow frying.

Table no 5.1.1.5 Gradation of cooking methods from higher to lower restoration with respect to preservation days

Preservation	Duration	Method 1	Method 2	Method 3	Method 4	Method 5
Control	Fresh	R	SF	OPDR	B	DF
Control	24 hours	R	SF	B	DF	OPDR
Control	48 hours	R	SF	DF	B	OPDR
Control	14 days	R	SF	DF	OPDR	B
Control	15 days	R	B	DF	OPDR	SF
Salt & Turmeric	24 hours	R	DF	SF	B	OPDR
Salt & Turmeric	48 hours	B	R	SF	OPDR	DF
Salt & Turmeric	14 days	R	SF	DF	B	OPDR
Salt &Turmeric	15 days	SF	R	OPDR	DF	B
KMS	24 hours	R	B	DF	OPDR	SF
KMS	48 hours	R	DF	OPDR	B	SF
KMS	14 days	DF	SF	B	OPDR	R
KMS	15 days	DF	R	SF	OPDR	B

R= Raw state, B= Boiling, OPDR= Open pan dry roasting, SF= Shallow frying, DF= Deep frying.

In all the preservation methods and fresh condition, carbohydrate retention occurs mainly in the raw state than the other cooking methods. In fresh condition, carbohydrate retention occurs firstly in the raw state then shallow frying, open pan dry roasting, boiling and deep frying. In 24 hours control preservation without preservative, the order changes from the raw state to shallow frying, boiling, deep frying and open pan dry roasting. In 48 hours control preservation without preservative, the order becomes the raw state, shallow frying, deep frying, boiling and open pan dry roasting. In 14 days control preservation without preservative, the order remains the raw condition, shallow frying, deep frying, open pan dry roasting and boiling. In 15 days control preservation without preservative, the order changes from the raw condition to boiling, deep frying, open pan dry roasting and then shallow frying.

In 24 hours salt and turmeric preservation, the order remains the raw state, deep frying, shallow frying, boiling and open pan dry roasting. In 48 hours salt and turmeric preservation, the order changes from boiling to the raw state, shallow frying, open pan dry roasting and then deep frying. In 14 days salt and turmeric preservation, the order remains the raw state, shallow frying, deep frying, boiling and open pan dry roasting. In 15 days salt and turmeric preservation, the order changes from shallow frying to the raw condition, open pan dry roasting, deep frying and then boiling.

In 24 hours KMS preservation, the order remains the raw state, boiling, deep frying, open pan dry roasting and shallow frying. In 48 hours KMS preservation, the order changes from the raw state to deep frying, open pan dry roasting, boiling and then shallow frying. In 14 days KMS preservation, the order is deep frying, shallow frying, boiling, open pan dry roasting and the raw condition. In 15 days KMS preservation, the order changes from deep frying to the raw condition, shallow frying, and open pan dry roasting and then boiling.

The overall analysis of carbohydrate content of *rohu* is mostly restored by the gradation of methods as the raw state>shallow frying> deep frying>open pan dry roasting>boiling.

Frying mainly restores[66] the nutrient as the oil can possibly create a protective layer, so that the carbohydrate cannot be leached out, but in boiling the soluble carbohydrates get dissolved and the content is reduced, and by throwing out the boiling water can also be the possible cause for the loss of carbohydrate. In open pan dry roasting the carbohydrates possibly get charred and hence the losses takes place. Thus among all the conventional studied cooking methods, **shallow frying** is the best method for cooking *rohu* to restore carbohydrate.

5.1.2 *Katla* (*Catla catla*)

It has been reported that *katla* contains 2.9 gm of carbohydrate per 100 gm[84] in the raw condition. This value changes due to the application of different cooking methods and preservation conditions (vide Table no **5.1.2.1**).

Table no 5.1.2.1 Carbohydrate content of *Katla* (gm/100gm)

Preservation	Duration	Raw state	Boiling	Dry roasting	Shallow frying	Deep frying
Control	Fresh	3.75±0.17	2.75±0.10	2.97±0.11	3.35±0.16	3.16±0.15
Control	24 hours	3.25±0.05	2.11±0.10	2.15±0.18	3.11±0.12	2.67±0.17
Control	48 hours	2.59±0.17	1.28±0.25	1.80±0.15	1.72±0.08	1.48±0.10
Control	14 days	5.65±0.15	1.36±0.10	2.72±0.25	2.12±0.11	3.02±0.08
Control	15 days	3.79±0.13	1.14±0.08	3.19±0.10	2.14±0.06	2.32±0.08
Salt & Turmeric	24 hours	5.45±0.40	1.98±0.07	2.65±0.15	3.42±0.15	3.69±0.16
Salt & Turmeric	48 hours	4.44±0.07	3.82±0.11	1.72±0.12	2.39±0.13	2.10±0.10
Salt & Turmeric	14 days	2.33±0.10	0.63±0.07	1.68±0.03	1.83±0.20	1.05±0.06
Salt & Turmeric	15 days	2.25±0.23	1.83±0.09	0.93±0.07	1.11±0.12	1.62±0.12
KMS	24 hours	3.01±0.18	2.23±0.13	1.94±0.08	2.14±0.09	2.41±0.06
KMS	48 hours	3.43±0.10	1.13±0.10	2.11±0.13	1.73±0.10	2.18±0.18
KMS	14 days	2.44±0.06	0.74±0.08	1.72±0.07	2.06±0.05	1.07±0.08
KMS	15 days	2.06±0.07	1.06±0.05	0.93±0.07	1.13±0.05	1.62±0.12

Values are expressed as mean±SD. ☐ Loss ☐ Restoration

In fresh condition, 24 hours, 48 hours, 14 days, 15 days control preservation without preservative and 24 hours, 14 days preservation with salt and turmeric as well as 48 hours, 14 days preservation with KMS, carbohydrate losses mainly occur by boiling, whereas in 48 hours and 15 days preservation with salt and turmeric as well as 24 hours and 15 days preservation with KMS, losses occur by open pan dry roasting. Most of the retention occurs by deep frying, but in fresh condition, 24 hours control preservation without preservative, 14 days preservation with salt and turmeric as well as with KMS, retention occurs by shallow frying, whereas in 48 hours and 15 days control preservation without preservative, retention occurs by open pan dry roasting, and 48 hours, 15 days preservation with salt and turmeric helps to retain carbohydrate by boiling.

14 days preservation with preservative shows the highest carbohydrate content in the raw state of *katla*, 24 hours preservation with salt and turmeric helps to increase the carbohydrate content in shallow frying and deep frying and 15 days preservation with salt and turmeric shows that the maximum retention occurs in open pan dry roasting, whereas 48 hours preservation with salt and turmeric indicates that highest retention occurs in boiling. This is probably due to the loss of water from the fish for the effect of prolonged preservation with preservative as well as the application of heat during cooking[48].

Fig. 5.1.2.2 Graphical representation of Carbohydrate content of *Katla* with respect to different conditions

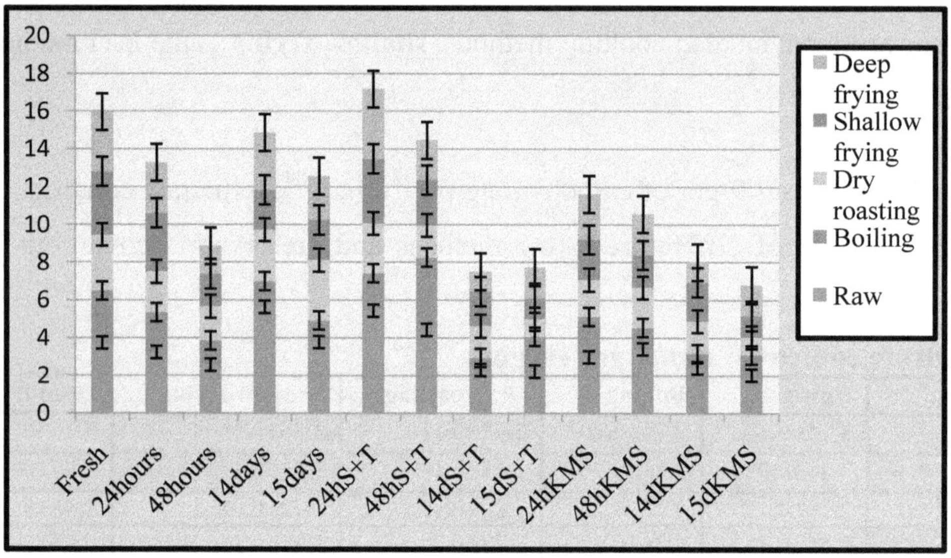

This graphical representation indicates that among all the preservation conditions, **24 hours preservation with salt and turmeric[55]** helps to increase the carbohydrate content in all the cooking methods except in boiling. The possible reason for this may be the moisture loss due to prolonged preservation that helps to concentrate the amount of carbohydrate and the efficiency of salt and turmeric to inhibit the microbial growth and in turn the preservation of nutrient[52].The graph also shows that salt and turmeric preservation comparatively increases the carbohydrate content more than that which is without preservative control preservation and KMS preservation.

Table no 5.1.2.3 ANOVA with regard to cooking conditions and preservation methods

Condition	Differences	Sum of Squares	df	Mean Square	F	Sig.
Fresh (control)	Between Groups	1.764	4	.441	21.565	.000(S)
	Within Groups	.204	10	.020		
	Total	1.968	14			
24 hours (control)	Between Groups	4.369	4	1.092	22.537	.000(S)
	Within Groups	.485	10	.048		
	Total	4.853	14			
48 hours (control)	Between Groups	2.984	4	.746	26.984	.000(S)
	Within Groups	.276	10	.028		
	Total	3.260	14			
14 days (control)	Between Groups	31.610	4	7.903	569.076	.000(S)
	Within Groups	.139	10	.014		
	Total	31.749	14			
15 days (control)	Between Groups	12.438	4	3.110	335.319	.000(S)
	Within Groups	.093	10	.009		
	Total	12.531	14			
24 hours (salt & turmeric)	Between Groups	20.546	4	5.137	103.241	.000(S)
	Within Groups	.498	10	.050		
	Total	21.044	14			
48 hours (salt & turmeric)	Between Groups	16.588	4	4.147	332.824	.000(S)
	Within Groups	.125	10	.012		
	Total	16.713	14			
14 days (salt & turmeric)	Between Groups	5.353	4	1.338	104.334	.000(S)
	Within Groups	.128	10	.013		
	Total	5.481	14			
15 days (salt & turmeric)	Between Groups	3.465	4	.866	43.674	.000(S)
	Within Groups	.198	10	.020		
	Total	3.663	14			
24 hours (KMS)	Between Groups	1.983	4	.496	35.557	.000(S)
	Within Groups	.139	10	.014		
	Total	2.122	14			
48 hours (KMS)	Between Groups	8.556	4	2.139	135.089	.000(S)
	Within Groups	.158	10	.016		
	Total	8.714	14			
14 days (KMS)	Between Groups	5.941	4	1.485	361.638	.000(S)
	Within Groups	.041	10	.004		
	Total	5.982	14			
15 days (KMS)	Between Groups	2.672	4	.668	102.025	.000(S)
	Within Groups	.065	10	.007		
	Total	2.737	14			

$p<0.05$ S= Significant, NS= Non-significant. All abbreviations are on page so and so.

This statistical ANOVA table shows that all the values are significant, which means there is significant difference present in the values of carbohydrate content of *katla* among different cooking methods and the raw state in respect to fresh condition along with different preservation methods.

Table no 5.1.2.4 Post hoc Duncan statistical analysis

Preservation	Duration	Raw state	Boiling	Dry roasting	Shallow frying	Deep frying
Control	Fresh	B,O,S,D^{a}	R,S,D^{b}	R,S,D^{b}	R,B,O^{c}	R,B,S^{d}
Control	24 hours	B,O,D ^{e}	R,S,D^{b}	R,S,D^{b}	B,O,D^{e}	R,B,O,S^{f}
Control	48 hours	B,O,S,D^{a}	R,O,S^{g}	R,B,D^{h}	R,B,D^{h}	R,B,O^{c}
Control	14 days	B,O,S,D^{a}	R,O,S,D^{i}	R,B,S,D^{i}	R,B,O,D^{k}	R,B,O,S^{f}
Control	15 days	B,O,S,D^{a}	R,O,S,D^{i}	R,B,S,D^{j}	R,B,O,D^{k}	R,B,O,S^{f}
Salt & Turmeric	24 hours	B,O,S,D^{a}	R,O,S,D^{i}	R,B,S,D^{j}	R,B,O^{c}	R,B,O^{c}
Salt & Turmeric	48 hours	B,O,S,D^{a}	R,O,S,D^{i}	R,B,S,D^{j}	R,B,O,D^{k}	R,B,O,S^{f}
Salt & Turmeric	14 days	B,O,S,D^{a}	R,O,S,D^{i}	R,B,D^{h}	R,B,D^{h}	R,B,O,S^{f}
Salt & Turmeric	15 days	B,O,S,D^{a}	R,O,S^{g}	R,B,D^{h}	R,B,D^{c}	R,O,S^{g}
KMS	24 hours	B,O,S,D^{a}	R,O^{l}	R,B,D^{h}	R,D^{m}	R,O,S^{g}
KMS	48 hours	B,O,S,D^{a}	R,O,S,D^{i}	R,B,D^{h}	R,B,O,D^{k}	R,B,S^{l}
KMS	14 days	B,O,S,D^{a}	R,O,S,D^{i}	R,B,S,D^{j}	R,B,O,D^{k}	R,B,O,S^{f}
KMS	15 days	B,O,S,D^{a}	R,D^{m}	R,S,D^{b}	R,O,D^{n}	R,B,O,S^{f}

R= Raw state, B= Boiling, O= Open pan dry roasting, S= Shallow frying, D= Deep frying. The same uppercase alphabets represent that there is no significant difference present among the variables.

This table shows the significant difference among the different variables such as cooking methods and preservation conditions. The raw state significantly differs from boiling, open pan dry roasting, shallow frying and deep frying in all of the preservation methods with preservatives and control conditions except in 24 hours control preservation without preservative. In fresh condition, 24 hours control preservation without preservative and 15 days KMS preservation, boiling significantly differs from the raw state, shallow frying and deep frying. Both shallow frying and deep frying in 24 hours preservation with salt and turmeric significantly differ from the raw state, boiling, open pan dry roasting and shallow frying in fresh condition. Deep frying in 48 hours control preservation without preservative significantly differs from the raw state, boiling and open pan dry roasting. Deep frying in fresh condition significantly differs from the raw state, boiling and shallow frying. The raw state and shallow frying in 24 hours control preservation without preservative, significantly differ from boiling, open pan dry roasting and deep frying.

Deep frying in 24 hours, 14 days, 15 days control preservation without preservative and 48 hours, 14 days salt and turmeric preservation along with 14 days KMS preservation, significantly differs from the raw state, boiling, open pan dry roasting and shallow frying. Boiling in 48 hours control preservation without preservative, 15 days salt and turmeric preservation, significantly differs from the raw state, open pan dry roasting and shallow frying, whereas deep frying significantly differs from the raw state, open pan dry roasting and shallow frying in 15 days salt and turmeric preservation and 24 hours KMS preservation. Open pan dry roasting in 48 hours control preservation without preservative and 14 days, 15 days salt and turmeric preservation, 24 hours, 48 hours KMS preservation, significantly differs from the raw state, boiling and deep frying, whereas shallow frying significantly differs from the raw state, boiling and deep frying in 48 hours control preservation without preservative as well as 14 days salt and turmeric preservation, and deep frying significantly differs from the raw state, boiling and shallow frying in 48 hours KMS preservation. Boiling in 14 days, 15 days control preservation without preservative, 24 hours, 48 hours, 14 days salt and turmeric preservation, and 48 hours, 14 days KMS preservation, significantly differs from the raw state, open pan dry roasting, shallow frying and deep frying.

Open pan dry roasting in 14 days and 15 days control preservation without preservative, 24 hours and 48 hours preservation with salt and turmeric and 14 days KMS preservation, significantly differs from the raw state, boiling, shallow frying and deep frying. Shallow frying in 14 days, 15 days control preservation without preservative, 48 hours salt and turmeric preservation, 48 hours and 14 days KMS preservation, significantly differs from the raw state, boiling, open pan drying roasting and deep frying. Boiling in 24 hours KMS preservation, significantly differs from the raw state and open pan dry roasting.

Shallow frying in 24 hours KMS preservation and boiling in 15 days KMS preservation, significantly differs from the raw state and deep frying. Again shallow frying in 15 days KMS preservation significantly differs from the raw state, open pan drying roasting and deep frying.

Table no 5.1.2.5 Gradation of cooking methods from higher to lower restoration with respect to preservation days

Preservation	Duration	Method 1	Method 2	Method 3	Method 4	Method 5
Control	Fresh	R	SF	DF	OPDR	B
Control	24 hours	R	SF	DF	OPDR	B
Control	48 hours	R	OPDR	SF	DF	B
Control	14 days	R	DF	OPDR	SF	B
Control	15 days	R	OPDR	DF	SF	B
Salt & Turmeric	24 hours	R	DF	SF	OPDR	B
Salt & Turmeric	48 hours	R	B	SF	DF	OPDR
Salt & Turmeric	14 days	R	SF	OPDR	DF	B
Salt &Turmeric	15 days	R	B	DF	SF	OPDR
KMS	24 hours	R	DF	B	SF	OPDR
KMS	48 hours	R	DF	OPDR	SF	B
KMS	14 days	R	SF	OPDR	DF	B
KMS	15 days	R	DF	SF	B	OPDR

R= Raw state, B= Boiling, OPDR= Open pan dry roasting, SF= Shallow frying, DF= Deep frying. Same colour represents the similar order.

In all the preservation procedures and fresh condition, carbohydrate retention occurs mainly in the raw state than the other cooking methods. In fresh condition and 24 hours control preservation without preservative, retention occurs firstly in shallow frying then deep frying, open pan dry roasting and boiling. In 48 hours control preservation without preservative, it changes in the order of open pan dry roasting followed by shallow frying, deep frying and boiling. In 14 days control preservation without preservative, the order is deep frying, open pan dry roasting, shallow frying and boiling. In 15 days control preservation without preservative, it remains in the order of open pan dry roasting, deep frying, shallow frying and boiling.

In 24 hours salt and turmeric preservation, the order changes from deep frying to shallow frying, open pan dry roasting and boiling. In 48 hours salt and turmeric preservation, the order of retention is boiling followed by shallow frying, deep frying and open pan dry roasting. In 14 days salt and turmeric preservation, the order becomes shallow frying, open pan dry roasting, deep frying and boiling. In 15 days salt and turmeric preservation, it remains in the order of boiling followed by deep frying, shallow frying and open pan dry roasting.

In 24 hours KMS preservation, the order changes to deep frying, boiling, shallow frying and open pan dry roasting. In 48 hours KMS preservation, it remains in the order of deep frying, open pan dry roasting, shallow frying and boiling. In 14 days KMS preservation, the order is shallow frying, open pan dry roasting, deep frying and boiling. In 15 days KMS preservation, the order becomes deep frying, shallow frying, boiling and open pan dry roasting.

The overall analysis of carbohydrate content of *katla* is mostly restored by the gradation of methods as the raw state>deep frying> shallow frying>open pan dry roasting>boiling.

Frying mainly restores[66] the nutrient as the oil can possibly create a protective layer, so that the carbohydrate cannot be leached out, but in boiling the soluble carbohydrates get dissolved and the content is reduced, and discarding this water can also be a possible cause for the loss of carbohydrate. In open pan dry roasting, the carbohydrates possibly get charred, causing reduction. Thus among all the studied conventional cooking methods, **deep frying** is the best method for cooking *katla* to restore carbohydrate. Additionally *katla* contains more fatty tissues as compared to *rohu* so the fat layers of this fish possibly also create a barrier to reduce the carbohydrate content in deep frying method.

5.1.3 Prawn (*Fenneropenaeus indicus*)

It has been reported that prawn contains 0.8 gm of carbohydrate per 100 gm[84] in the raw condition. This value changes due to the application of different cooking methods and preservation conditions (vide Table no **5.1.3.1**).

Table no 5.1.3.1 Carbohydrate content of Prawn (gm/100gm)

Preservation	Duration	Raw state	Boiling	Dry roasting	Shallow frying	Deep frying
Control	Fresh	1.06±0.20	0.71±0.07	0.98±0.12	0.85±0.06	0.50±0.09
Control	24 hours	0.88±0.10	0.41±0.09	0.55±0.13	0.88±0.10	0.51±0.17
Control	48 hours	1.03±0.20	0.52±0.02	1.01±0.07	0.71±0.09	0.95±0.04
Control	14 days	2.31±0.25	1.26±0.19	1.83±0.11	1.85±0.13	1.71±0.36
Control	15 days	2.25±0.05	0.63±0.079	0.62±0.06	1.61±0.07	1.87±0.19
Salt & Turmeric	24 hours	1.80±0.15	1.31±0.06	1.42±0.06	3.13±0.12	5.02±0.08
Salt & Turmeric	48 hours	3.13±0.12	2.11±0.10	3.74±0.08	2.35±0.11	3.91±0.10
Salt & Turmeric	14 days	1.94±0.11	1.11±0.10	0.91±0.07	1.93±0.11	1.54±0.08
Salt & Turmeric	15 days	3.14±0.06	1.63±0.14	2.93±0.07	4.30±0.11	4.15±0.14
KMS	24 hours	2.12±0.14	1.14±0.12	2.94±0.12	3.92±0.07	1.74±0.06
KMS	48 hours	1.11±0.12	0.83±0.07	0.73±0.07	1.62±0.07	2.74±0.06
KMS	14 days	1.01±0.07	0.56±0.07	1.65±0.11	0.93±0.07	1.36±0.12
KMS	15 days	1.06±0.05	0.45±0.05	1.55±0.06	1.27±0.07	2.30±0.11

Values are expressed as mean±SD. ☐ Loss ☐ Restoration
Red digits represent the significant highest values from the raw state in different conditions.

In 24 hours, 48 hours, 14 days control preservation without preservative and 24 hours, 48 hours, 15 days preservation with salt and turmeric as well as 24 hours, 14 days, 15 days preservation with KMS, carbohydrate losses mainly occur by boiling, whereas in 15 days control preservation without preservative, 14 days preservation with salt and turmeric as well as 48 hours preservation with KMS, losses occur by open pan dry roasting. In fresh condition, carbohydrate loss occurs by deep frying.

Most of the retention occurs by deep frying, but in 24 hours, 14 days control preservation without preservative, 14 days, 15 days preservation with salt and turmeric preservation and 24 hours preservation with KMS, carbohydrate retention occurs by shallow frying. In fresh condition, retention occurs by open pan dry roasting.

15 days preservation with salt and turmeric shows the highest carbohydrate content in the raw state and shallow fried prawn, whereas 48 hours preservation with salt and turmeric helps to increase the carbohydrate content in boiling and open pan dry roasting and 24 hours preservation with salt and turmeric indicates that highest retention occurs in deep frying.

Open pan dry roasting shows the increased carbohydrate content as compared to the raw state in 48 hours salt and turmeric preservation and 24 hours, 14 days, 15 days KMS preservation. Shallow frying shows the increased carbohydrate content in comparison to the raw state in 24 hours, 15 days salt and turmeric as well as 24 hours, 48 hours, 15 days KMS preservation, whereas deep frying shows the increased carbohydrate content as compared to the raw state in 24 hours, 48 hours, 15 days salt and turmeric preservation and 48 hours, 14 days, 15 days KMS preservation.

Here the effects of both the natural and artificial preservatives are prominent. They mostly help to increase the nutrient content. They probably prevent the growth of bacteria or help to modify the structural change of the carbohydrate, thus helping retention and the content becomes more than the raw state. The carbohydrate becomes concentrated due to the loss of moisture for the effect of prolonged preservation with preservatives as well as the application of heat during cooking[48].

Fig. 5.1.3.2 Graphical representation of Carbohydrate content of Prawn with respect to different conditions

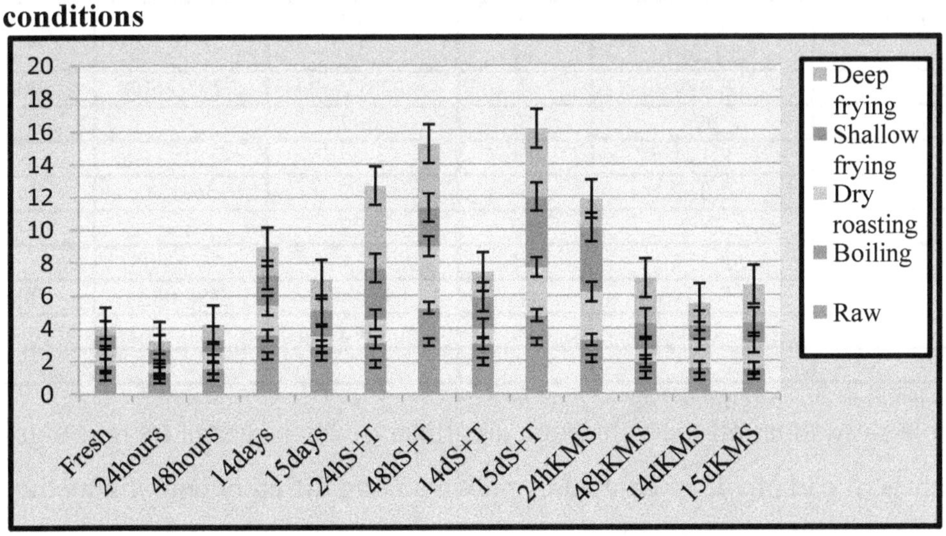

This graphical representation indicates that among all the preservation conditions, **15 days preservation with salt and turmeric**[55] helps to increase the carbohydrate content in all the cooking methods. The possible reason for this may be the moisture loss due to prolonged preservation that helps to concentrate the amount of carbohydrate and the efficiency of salt and turmeric to inhibit the microbial growth and in turn the preservation of carbohydrate[52]. The graph also shows that salt and turmeric preservation comparatively increased the carbohydrate content more than that which is without preservative control preservation and KMS preservation.

Table no 5.1.3.3 ANOVA with regard to cooking conditions and preservation methods

Conditions	Differences	Sum of Squares	df	Mean Square	F	Sig.
Fresh (control)	Between Groups	.597	4	.149	9.987	.002(S)
	Within Groups	.149	10	.015		
	Total	.747	14			
24 hours (control)	Between Groups	.583	4	.146	9.186	.002(S)
	Within Groups	.159	10	.016		
	Total	.741	14			
48 hours (control)	Between Groups	.594	4	.148	12.427	.001(S)
	Within Groups	.119	10	.012		
	Total	.713	14			
14 days (control)	Between Groups	1.709	4	.427	7.954	.004(S)
	Within Groups	.537	10	.054		
	Total	2.247	14			
15 days (control)	Between Groups	6.543	4	1.636	144.674	.000(S)
	Within Groups	.113	10	.011		
	Total	6.656	14			
24 hours (salt & turmeric)	Between Groups	29.312	4	7.328	503.756	.000(S)
	Within Groups	.145	10	.015		
	Total	29.457	14			
48 hours (salt & turmeric)	Between Groups	7.786	4	1.946	165.796	.000(S)
	Within Groups	.117	10	.012		
	Total	7.903	14			
14 days (salt & turmeric)	Between Groups	2.602	4	.651	63.406	.000(S)
	Within Groups	.103	10	.010		
	Total	2.705	14			
15 days (salt & turmeric)	Between Groups	13.964	4	3.491	287.712	.000(S)
	Within Groups	.121	10	.012		
	Total	14.085	14			
24 hours (KMS)	Between Groups	14.032	4	3.508	297.967	.000(S)
	Within Groups	.118	10	.012		
	Total	14.150	14			
48 hours (KMS)	Between Groups	8.099	4	2.025	275.360	.000(S)
	Within Groups	.074	10	.007		
	Total	8.173	14			
14 days (KMS)	Between Groups	2.067	4	.517	56.424	.000(S)
	Within Groups	.092	10	.009		
	Total	2.159	14			
15 days (KMS)	Between Groups	5.561	4	1.390	258.083	.000(S)
	Within Groups	.054	10	.005		
	Total	5.615	14			

$p<0.05$ S= Significant, NS= Non-significant. All abbreviations are on page so and so.

This statistical ANOVA table shows that all the values are significant, which means there is significant difference present in the values of carbohydrate content of prawn among different cooking methods and the raw state in respect to fresh condition along with different preservation methods.

Table no 5.1.3.4 Post hoc Duncan statistical analysis

Preservation	Duration	Raw state	Boiling	Dry roasting	Shallow frying	Deep frying
Control	Fresh	B,D^a	R,O^b	B,D^a	B,D^a	R,O,S^c
Control	24 hours	B,O,D^d	R,S^e	R,S^e	B,O,D^d	R,S^e
Control	48 hours	B,S^f	R,O,D^g	B,S^f	R,O,D^g	B,S^f
Control	14 days	B,O,S,D^h	R,O,S,D^i	R,B^k	R,B^k	R,B^k
Control	15 days	B,O,S,D^h	R,S,D^l	R,S,D^l	R,B,O,D^m	R,B,O,S^n
Salt & Turmeric	24 hours	B,O,S,D^h	R,S,D^l	R,S,D^l	R,B,O,D^m	R,B,O,S^n
Salt & Turmeric	48 hours	B,O,S,D^h	R,O,S,D^i	R,B,S^l	R,B,O,D^m	R,B,S^o
Salt & Turmeric	14 days	B,O,D^d	R,O,S,D^i	R,B,S,D^p	B,O,D^d	R,B,O,S^n
Salt & Turmeric	15 days	B,O,S,D^h	R,O,S,D^i	R,B,S,D^p	R,B,O^q	R,B,O^q
KMS	24 hours	B,O,S,D^h	R,O,S,D^i	R,B,S,D^p	R,B,O,D^m	R,B,O,S^n
KMS	48 hours	B,O,S,D^h	R,S,D^l	R,S,D^l	R,B,O,D^m	R,B,O,S^n
KMS	14 days	B,O,D^d	R,O,S,D^i	R,B,S,D^p	B,O,D^d	R,B,O,S^n
KMS	15 days	B,O,S,D^h	R,O,S,D^i	R,B,S,D^p	R,B,O,D^m	R,B,O,S^n

R= Raw state, B= Boiling, O= Open pan dry roasting, S= Shallow frying, D= Deep frying. The same uppercase alphabets represent that there is no significant difference present among the variables

This table shows the significant difference among the different variables such as cooking methods and preservation conditions. The raw state significantly differs from boiling and open pan dry roasting, shallow frying and deep frying in most of the preservation with preservatives and control conditions except fresh condition, 24 hours, 48 hours control preservation without preservative, 14 days preservation both by salt and turmeric as well as by KMS. In fresh condition, open pan dry roasting, raw state, and shallow frying significantly differ from boiling and deep frying, whereas boiling significantly differs from the raw state and open pan dry roasting.

Moreover, deep frying significantly differs from the raw state, open pan dry roasting and shallow frying in fresh condition, 24 hours control preservation without preservative and 14 days preservation by both the combination of salt and turmeric and by KMS, whereas the raw state and shallow frying significantly differ from boiling, open pan dry roasting and deep frying. In 24 hours control preservation without preservative, boiling, open pan dry roasting and deep frying significantly differ from the raw state and shallow frying. In 48 hours control preservation without preservative, the raw state, open pan dry roasting and deep frying significantly differ from boiling and shallow frying. In 14 days control preservation without preservative, boiling and shallow frying significantly differ from the raw state, open pan dry roasting and deep frying.

Boiling in 14 days control preservation without preservative and 48 hours, 14 days, 15 days salt and turmeric preservation along with 24 hours, 14 days, 15 days KMS preservation, significantly differs from the raw state, open pan dry roasting, shallow frying and deep frying. In 14 days control preservation without preservative, open pan dry roasting, shallow frying and deep frying significantly differ from the raw state and boiling, whereas boiling and open pan dry roasting significantly differ from the raw state, shallow frying and deep frying in 15 days control preservation without preservative, 24 hours salt and turmeric preservation and 48 hours KMS preservation.

Shallow frying significantly differs from the raw state, boiling, open pan dry roasting and deep frying in 15 days control preservation without preservative and 24 hours, 48 hours salt and turmeric preservation as well as in 24 hours, 48 hours, 15 days with KMS preservation. Deep frying significantly differs from the raw state, boiling, open pan dry roasting and shallow frying in 15 days control preservation without preservative, 24 hours, 14 days preservation with salt and turmeric preservation and 24 hours, 48 hours, 14 days, 15 days KMS preservation, whereas deep frying in 48 hours salt and turmeric preservation, significantly differs from the raw state, boiling and shallow frying.

Open pan dry roasting in 14 days, 15 days salt and turmeric preservation as well as 24 hours, 14 days, 15 days KMS preservation, significantly differs from the raw state, boiling, shallow frying and deep frying. Both shallow frying and deep frying in 15 days salt and turmeric preservation significantly differ from the raw state, boiling and open pan dry roasting.

Table no 5.1.3.5 Gradation of cooking methods from higher to lower restoration with respect to preservation days

Preservation	Duration	Method 1	Method 2	Method 3	Method 4	Method 5
Control	Fresh	R	OPDR	SF	B	DF
Control	24 hours	SF	R	OPDR	B	DF
Control	48 hours	R	OPDR	DF	SF	B
Control	14 days	R	SF	OPDR	B	DF
Control	15 days	R	DF	SF	B	OPDR
Salt & Turmeric	24 hours	DF	SF	R	OPDR	B
Salt & Turmeric	48 hours	DF	OPDR	R	SF	B
Salt & Turmeric	14 days	R	SF	DF	B	OPDR
Salt &Turmeric	15 days	SF	DF	R	OPDR	B
KMS	24 hours	SF	OPDR	R	DF	B
KMS	48 hours	DF	SF	R	B	OPDR
KMS	14 days	OPDR	DF	R	SF	B
KMS	15 days	DF	OPDR	SF	R	B

R= Raw state, B= Boiling, OPDR= Open pan dry roasting, SF= Shallow frying, DF= Deep frying.

In all the preservation techniques and fresh condition, carbohydrate retention occurs mainly in the raw state than the other cooking methods. In fresh condition, retention occurs firstly in the raw state then open pan dry roasting, shallow frying, boiling and deep frying. In 24 hours control preservation without preservative, the order changes to shallow frying, raw state, open pan dry roasting, boiling and deep frying. In 48 hours control preservation without preservative, the order is the raw state, open pan dry roasting, deep frying, shallow frying and boiling. In 14 days control preservation without preservative, the order becomes the raw state, shallow frying, open pan dry roasting, boiling and deep frying. In 15 days control preservation without preservative, it remains in the order of the raw state, deep frying, shallow frying, boiling and open pan dry roasting,

In 24 hours salt and turmeric preservation, the order changes to deep frying, shallow frying, raw state, open pan dry roasting and boiling. In 48 hours salt and turmeric preservation, the order is deep frying, open pan dry roasting, raw state, shallow frying and boiling. In 14 days salt and turmeric preservation, the order changes to the raw state, shallow frying, deep frying, boiling and open pan dry roasting. In 15 days salt and turmeric preservation, the order becomes shallow frying, deep frying, raw state, open pan dry roasting and boiling.

In 24 hours KMS preservation, the order changes to shallow frying, open pan dry roasting, raw state, deep frying and boiling. In 48 hours KMS preservation, the order is deep frying, shallow frying, raw state, boiling and open pan dry roasting. In 14 days KMS preservation, the order becomes open pan dry roasting, deep frying, raw state, shallow frying and boiling. In 15 days KMS preservation, the order becomes deep frying, open pan dry roasting, shallow frying, raw state and boiling.

The overall analysis of carbohydrate content of prawn is mostly restored by the gradation of methods as the raw state>deep frying> shallow frying>open pan dry roasting>boiling.

Frying mainly restores[66] the nutrients as the oil can possibly create a protective layer so that the carbohydrate cannot be leached out, but in boiling the soluble carbohydrates get dissolved and the content is reduced, and discarding this boiling water can also be the possible cause for the loss of carbohydrate. Losses occur in open pan dry roasting as the carbohydrate possibly gets charred. Thus among all the studied conventional cooking methods, **deep frying** is the best method for cooking prawn in order to restore carbohydrate though the amount of carbohydrate is very low in prawn.

5.1.4 Lobster (*Macrobrachium rosenbergii*)

It has been reported that lobster does not contain carbohydrate, [84] but this study shows the carbohydrate content in both the raw state as well as the changes due to the application of different cooking methods and preservation conditions (vide Table no **5.1.4.1**).

Table no 5.1.4.1 Carbohydrate content of Lobster (gm/100gm)

Preservation	Duration	Raw state	Boiling	Dry roasting	Shallow frying	Deep frying
Control	Fresh	2.65±0.13	2.15±0.13	1.51±0.14	2.47±0.13	1.51±0.10
Control	24 hours	1.65±0.13	1.51±0.09	1.11±0.10	1.63±0.11	1.29±0.06
Control	48 hours	1.15±0.13	0.95±0.15	0.78±0.11	1.16±0.00	0.19±0.05
Control	14 days	3.49±0.16	0.59±0.10	2.02±0.11	2.44±0.36	2.91±0.10
Control	15 days	3.22±0.20	0.54±0.10	1.17±0.21	2.19±0.17	2.21±0.19
Salt & Turmeric	24 hours	3.91±0.10	0.50±0.05	1.01±0.07	1.92±0.10	2.12±0.10
Salt & Turmeric	48 hours	3.91±0.10	0.92±0.10	1.92±0.10	1.66±0.07	2.61±0.07
Salt & Turmeric	14 days	3.85±0.05	0.45±0.50	0.73±0.10	1.11±0.12	1.86±0.07
Salt & Turmeric	15 days	3.95±0.13	0.43±0.07	1.10±0.10	2.68±0.07	3.18±0.07
KMS	24 hours	4.52±0.07	2.12±0.10	1.90±0.10	1.83±0.12	2.11±0.10
KMS	48 hours	3.26±0.05	1.31±0.10	1.56±0.05	1.25±0.05	1.86±0.07
KMS	14 days	3.25±0.05	0.40±0.05	0.66±0.07	1.25±0.05	1.15±0.05
KMS	15 days	3.25±0.08	0.86±0.07	1.66±0.07	2.25±0.05	3.75±0.05

Values are expressed as mean±SD. ☐ Loss ☐ Restoration

Red digit represents the significant highest values from the raw state in a single condition.

In fresh condition, 24 hours control preservation without preservative, carbohydrate losses mainly occur by open pan dry roasting, whereas in 48 hours control preservation without preservative losses occur by deep frying. But in 14 days, 15 days control preservation without preservative, 24 hours, 48 hours, 14 days, 15 days preservation with salt and turmeric as well as in 14 days and 15 days preservation with KMS, losses occur by boiling. In 24 hours and 48 hours KMS preservation, losses take place in shallow frying. In most of the cases significant losses occur by boiling. Most of the retention occurs by deep frying, but in fresh condition, 24 hours, 48 hours, 14 days and 15 days control preservation without preservative, retention occurs by shallow frying. All preservation conditions with salt-turmeric and KMS, retention occur in deep frying except in 24 hours preservation with KMS, where retention takes place in boiling.

24 hours preservation with KMS shows the highest carbohydrate content in the raw state and boiled lobster, whereas 14 days control preservation without preservative helps to increase the carbohydrate content in open pan dry roasting and shallow frying, and 15 days KMS preservation shows that the maximum retention occurs in deep frying. Moreover, deep frying increases the carbohydrate content as compared to the raw state probably due to the concentrated form of carbohydrate for extreme moisture loss with respect to the other cooking methods.

Here also the effects of both the natural and artificial preservatives are prominent as they help to increase the nutrient content. They probably help to modify the structural change of carbohydrate and it becomes concentrated due to the loss of moisture for the effect of prolonged preservation so that more retention occurs as compared to preservation without preservative.

Fig. 5.1.4.2 Graphical representation of Carbohydrate content of Lobster with respect to different conditions

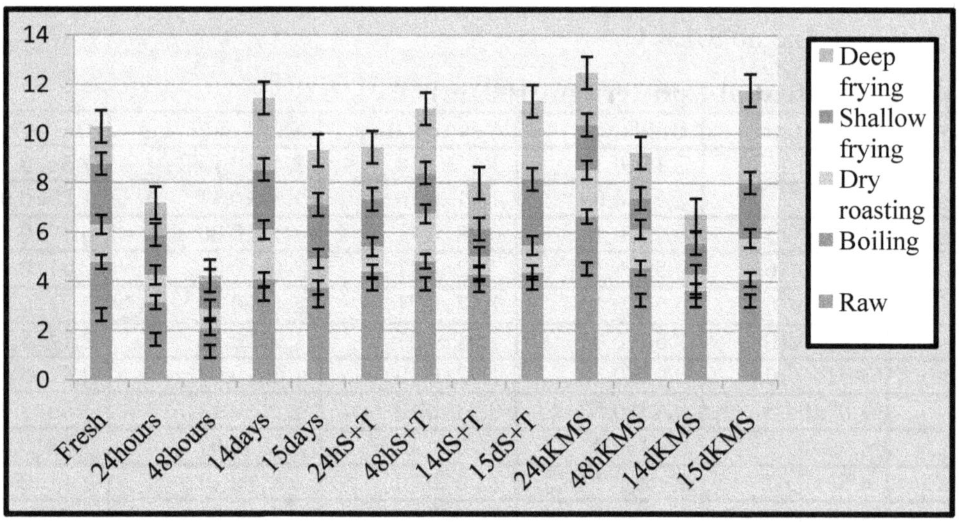

This graphical representation indicates that among all the preservation conditions, **24 hours preservation with KMS**[59] helps to increase the carbohydrate content amongst all the cooking methods. The possible reason for this may be the moisture loss due to prolonged preservation, that helps to concentrate the amount of carbohydrate and the efficiency of KMS to inhibit the microbial growth and in turn the preservation of carbohydrate in lobster[39]. The graph also shows that KMS preservation comparatively increases the carbohydrate content more than that which is without preservative control preservation and salt-turmeric preservation.

Table no 5.1.4.3 ANOVA with regard to cooking conditions and preservation methods

Condition	Differences	Sum of Squares	df	Mean Square	F	Sig.
Fresh (control)	Between Groups	3.387	4	.847	49.730	.000(S)
	Within Groups	.170	10	.017		
	Total	3.557	14			
24 hours (control)	Between Groups	.643	4	.161	14.357	.000(S)
	Within Groups	.112	10	.011		
	Total	.755	14			
48 hours (control)	Between Groups	1.899	4	.475	37.039	.000(S)
	Within Groups	.128	10	.013		
	Total	2.028	14			
14 days (control)	Between Groups	14.415	4	3.604	92.308	.000(S)
	Within Groups	.390	10	.039		
	Total	14.805	14			
15 days (control)	Between Groups	12.938	4	3.235	96.747	.000(S)
	Within Groups	.334	10	.033		
	Total	13.273	14			
24 hours (salt & turmeric)	Between Groups	20.563	4	5.141	629.469	.000(S)
	Within Groups	.082	10	.008		
	Total	20.644	14			
48 hours (salt & turmeric)	Between Groups	15.396	4	3.849	435.736	.000(S)
	Within Groups	.088	10	.009		
	Total	15.484	14			
14 days (salt & turmeric)	Between Groups	22.322	4	5.581	744.078	.000(S)
	Within Groups	.075	10	.007		
	Total	22.397	14			
15 days (salt & turmeric)	Between Groups	25.709	4	6.427	714.139	.000(S)
	Within Groups	.090	10	.009		
	Total	25.799	14			
24 hours (KMS)	Between Groups	15.496	4	3.874	363.180	.000(S)
	Within Groups	.107	10	.011		
	Total	15.602	14			
48 hours (KMS)	Between Groups	8.151	4	2.038	411.378	.000(S)
	Within Groups	.050	10	.005		
	Total	8.200	14			
14 days (KMS)	Between Groups	15.088	4	3.772	1.191E3	.000(S)
	Within Groups	.032	10	.003		
	Total	15.119	14			
15 days (KMS)	Between Groups	14.411	4	3.603	727.300	.000(S)
	Within Groups	.045	9	.005		
	Total	14.456	13			

$p<0.05$ S= Significant, NS= Non-significant. All abbreviations are on page so and so.

This statistical ANOVA table shows that all the values are significant, which means there is significant difference present in the values of carbohydrate content of lobster among different cooking methods and the raw state in respect to fresh condition along with different preservation methods.

Table no 5.1.4.4 Post hoc Duncan statistical analysis

Preservation	Duration	Raw state	Boiling	Dry roasting	Shallow frying	Deep frying
Control	Fresh	B,O,D^{a}	R,O,S,D^{b}	R,B,S^{c}	B,O,D^{a}	R,B,S^{c}
Control	24 hours	O,D^{d}	O,D^{d}	R,B,S^{c}	O, D^{d}	R,B,S^{c}
Control	48 hours	O,D^{d}	O,D^{d}	R,S,D^{e}	O,D^{d}	R,B,O,S^{f}
Control	14 days	B,O,S,D^{g}	R,O,S,D^{b}	R,B,S,D^{h}	R,B,O,D^{i}	R,B,O,S^{f}
Control	15 days	B,O,S,D^{g}	R,O,S,D^{b}	R,B,S,D^{h}	R,B,O^{j}	R,B,O^{j}
Salt & Turmeric	24 hours	B,O,S,D^{g}	R,O,S,D^{b}	R,B,S,D^{h}	R,B,O,D^{i}	R,B,O,S^{f}
Salt & Turmeric	48 hours	B,O,S,D^{g}	R,O,S,D^{b}	R,B,S,D^{h}	R,B,OS,D^{i}	R,B,O,S^{f}
Salt & Turmeric	14 days	B,O,S,D^{g}	R,O,S,D^{b}	R,B,S,D^{h}	R,B,O,D^{i}	R,B,O,S^{f}
Salt & Turmeric	15 days	B,O,S,D^{g}	R,O,S,D^{b}	R,B,S,D^{h}	R,B,O,D^{i}	R,B,O,S^{f}
KMS	24 hours	B,O,S,D^{g}	R,O,S^{k}	R,B,D^{l}	R,B,D^{l}	R,O,S^{k}
KMS	48 hours	B,O,S,D^{g}	R,O,D^{m}	R,B,S,D^{h}	R,O,D^{m}	R,B,O,S^{f}
KMS	14 days	B,O,S,D^{g}	R,O,S,D^{b}	R,B,S,D^{h}	R,B,Oj	R,B,O^{j}
KMS	15 days	B,O,S,D^{g}	R,O,S,D^{b}	R,B,S,D^{h}	R,B,O,D^{i}	R,B,O,S^{f}

R= Raw state, B= Boiling, O= Open pan dry roasting, S= Shallow frying, D= Deep frying. The same uppercase alphabets represent that there is no significant difference present among the variables.

This table shows the significant difference among the different variables such as cooking methods and preservation conditions. The raw state significantly differs from boiling, open pan dry roasting, shallow frying and deep frying in most of the preservation methods with preservatives and control conditions except in fresh condition, 24 hours, 48 hours control preservation without preservative. In fresh condition, the raw state and shallow frying significantly differ from boiling, open pan dry roasting and deep frying, whereas boiling significantly differs from the raw state, open pan dry roasting, shallow frying and deep frying in fresh condition, 14 days, 15 days control preservation without preservative, 24 hours, 48 hours, 14 days, 15 days salt and turmeric preservation and 14 days, 15 days KMS preservation. Moreover, open pan dry roasting and deep frying significantly differ from the raw state, boiling and shallow frying in fresh condition and 24 hours control preservation without preservative. The raw state, boiling and shallow frying significantly differ from open pan dry roasting and deep frying in 24 hours, 48 hours control preservation without preservative. Open pan dry roasting in 48 hours control preservation without preservative, significantly differs from the raw state, shallow frying and deep frying. Deep frying significantly differs from the raw state, boiling, open pan dry roasting and shallow frying in 48 hours, 14 days control preservation without preservative, 24 hours, 48 hours, 14 days, 15 days preservation with salt and turmeric as well as in 48 hours and 15 days KMS preservation.

Open pan dry roasting significantly differs from the raw state, boiling, shallow frying and deep frying in 14 days, 15 days control preservation without preservative, 24 hours, 48 hours, 14 days, 15 days salt and turmeric preservation as well as in 48 hours, 14 days, 15 days KMS preservation. Shallow frying significantly differs from the raw state, boiling and open pan dry roasting in 14 days control preservation without preservative, 24 hours, 48 hours, 14 days, 15 days salt and turmeric preservation and 15 days KMS preservation. Both shallow and deep frying significantly differ from the raw state, boiling and open pan dry roasting in 15 days control preservation without preservative and 14 days KMS preservation.

Boiling and deep frying in 24 hours KMS preservation significantly differ from the raw state, open pan dry roasting and shallow frying. Again open pan dry roasting and shallow frying significantly differ from the raw state, boiling and deep frying in 24 hours KMS preservation, whereas boiling and shallow frying significantly differ from the raw state, open pan dry roasting and deep frying in 48 hours KMS preservation.

Table no 5.1.4.5 Gradation of cooking methods from higher to lower restoration with respect to preservation days

Preservation	Duration	Method 1	Method 2	Method 3	Method 4	Method 5
Control	Fresh	R	SF	B	OPDR	DF
Control	24 hours	R	SF	B	DF	OPDR
Control	48 hours	SF	R	B	OPDR	DF
Control	14 days	R	DF	SF	OPDR	B
Control	15 days	R	DF	SF	OPDR	B
Salt & Turmeric	24 hours	R	DF	SF	OPDR	B
Salt & Turmeric	48 hours	R	DF	OPDR	SF	B
Salt & Turmeric	14 days	R	DF	SF	OPDR	B
Salt &Turmeric	15 days	R	DF	SF	OPDR	B
KMS	24 hours	R	DF	B	OPDR	SF
KMS	48 hours	R	DF	OPDR	B	SF
KMS	14 days	R	SF	DF	OPDR	B
KMS	15 days	DF	R	SF	OPDR	B

R= Raw state, B= Boiling, OPDR= Open pan dry roasting, SF= Shallow frying, DF= Deep frying. Same colour represents the similar order.

In all the preservation procedures and fresh condition, carbohydrate retention occurs mainly in the raw state than the other cooking methods. In fresh condition, retention occurs firstly in the raw state followed by shallow frying, boiling, open pan dry roasting and deep frying. In 24 hours control preservation without preservative, the order changes from the raw state to shallow frying, boiling, deep frying and open pan dry roasting. In 48 hours control preservation without preservative, the order is shallow frying, raw state, boiling, open pan dry roasting and deep frying. In 14 days, 15 days control preservation without preservative and 24 hours, 14 days, 15 days salt and turmeric preservation, the order becomes the raw state, deep frying, shallow frying, open pan dry roasting and boiling. In 48 hours salt and turmeric preservation, the order changes from the raw state to deep frying, open pan dry roasting, shallow frying and boiling.

In 24 hours KMS preservation, the order changes from raw state to deep frying, boiling, open pan dry roasting and shallow frying. In 48 hours KMS preservation, the order is the raw state, deep frying, open pan dry roasting, boiling and shallow frying. In 14 days KMS preservation, it changes in the order of the raw state, shallow frying, deep frying, open pan dry roasting and boiling. In 15 days KMS preservation, the order is deep frying, raw state, shallow frying, open pan dry roasting and boiling.

The overall analysis of carbohydrate content of lobster is mostly restored by the gradation of methods as the raw state>deep frying> shallow frying>open pan dry roasting>boiling.

Frying mainly restores[66] the nutrient as the oil can possibly create a protective layer so that the carbohydrate cannot be leached out, but in boiling the soluble carbohydrates get dissolved and the content is reduced, and discarding the boiling water can also be the possible cause for the loss of carbohydrate. In open pan dry roasting the carbohydrates possibly get charred, resulting in losses. Thus **deep frying** is the best method for cooking lobster to restore carbohydrate.

5.1.5 Pomfret (*Pampus argenteus*)

It has been reported that pomfret contains 1.8 gm carbohydrate per 100 gm[84] in the raw condition. This value changes due to the application of different cooking methods and preservation conditions (vide Table no **5.1.5.1**).

Table no 5.1.5.1 Carbohydrate content of Pomfret (gm/100gm)

Preservation	Duration	Raw state	Boiling	Dry roasting	Shallow frying	Deep frying
Control	Fresh	2.17±0.17	1.42±0.07	1.74±0.11	1.90±0.10	2.14±0.09
Control	24 hours	1.58±0.18	0.95±0.12	1.17±0.06	1.41±0.03	1.85.±0.11
Control	48 hours	1.55±0.13	0.68±0.11	0.89±0.06	1.18±0.10	1.52±0.07
Control	14 days	1.77±0.17	2.33±0.10	3.74±0.22	3.12±0.12	5.05±0.07
Control	15 days	2.63±0.11	1.33±0.12	2.59±0.09	2.60±0.07	4.33±0.10
Salt & Turmeric	24 hours	6.01±0.07	2.90±0.05	1.58±0.07	2.73±0.07	3.07±0.07
Salt & Turmeric	48 hours	3.15±0.05	1.65±0.05	3.40±0.05	3.11±0.10	4.01±0.06
Salt & Turmeric	14 days	4.80±0.05	3.78±0.07	1.75±0.05	3.46±0.07	4.21±0.06
Salt & Turmeric	15 days	4.19±0.11	2.08±0.08	2.08±0.07	2.76±0.04	3.20±0.05
KMS	24 hours	3.78±0.07	1.75±0.05	1.65±0.05	1.05±0.05	2.06±0.05
KMS	48 hours	3.15±0.05	2.05±0.05	1.50±0.05	1.72±0.08	1.25±0.05
KMS	14 days	3.78±0.08	1.04±0.05	0.71±0.06	1.69±0.03	1.25±0.05
KMS	15 days	1.80±0.05	1.25±0.05	1.56±0.07	1.01±0.07	1.10±0.10

Values are expressed as mean±SD. ☐ Loss ▒ Restoration

In fresh condition, 24 hours, 48 hours, 15 days control preservation without preservative and 48 hours, 15 days preservation with salt and turmeric, carbohydrate losses mainly occur by boiling, whereas 24 hours, 14 days, 15 days preservation with salt and turmeric as well as 14 days preservation with KMS, losses occur by open pan dry roasting. In 24 hours and 15 days KMS preservation, losses occur by shallow frying along with deep frying in 48 hours KMS preservation.

Most of the retention occurs by deep frying, but in 48 hours preservation with KMS, carbohydrate retention occurs by boiling and in 14 days and 15 days KMS preservation, retention occurs by shallow frying and open pan dry roasting respectively.

24 hours preservation with salt and turmeric shows the highest carbohydrate content in the raw state and boiled pomfret, and 14 days control preservation without preservative helps to increase the carbohydrate content in open pan dry roasting and deep frying, whereas 14 days salt and turmeric preservation shows that the maximum retention occurs in shallow frying.

Here the effects of the natural preservatives are prominent. These mostly help to increase the nutrient content. These probably help to modify the conformational change of carbohydrate, resulting in retention and in some cases the content is more than the raw state. The carbohydrate content becomes concentrated due to the loss of moisture for the effect of prolonged preservation with natural preservatives as well as the application of heat during cooking. 48 hours preservation with salt and turmeric helps in retention of carbohydrate more than the raw state by both open pan dry roasting and deep frying.

In 14 days control preservation without preservative, the carbohydrate content is increased over that in the raw state in all the cooking methods. In 15 days control preservation without preservative, carbohydrate content is increased by deep frying only. This happens probably due to the moisture loss from prolonged preservation and some chemical rearrangement may have also occurred so that the carbohydrates that are present in bound form may be released, the content becoming high after cooking.

Fig. 5.1.5.2 Graphical representation of Carbohydrate content of Pomfret with respect to different conditions

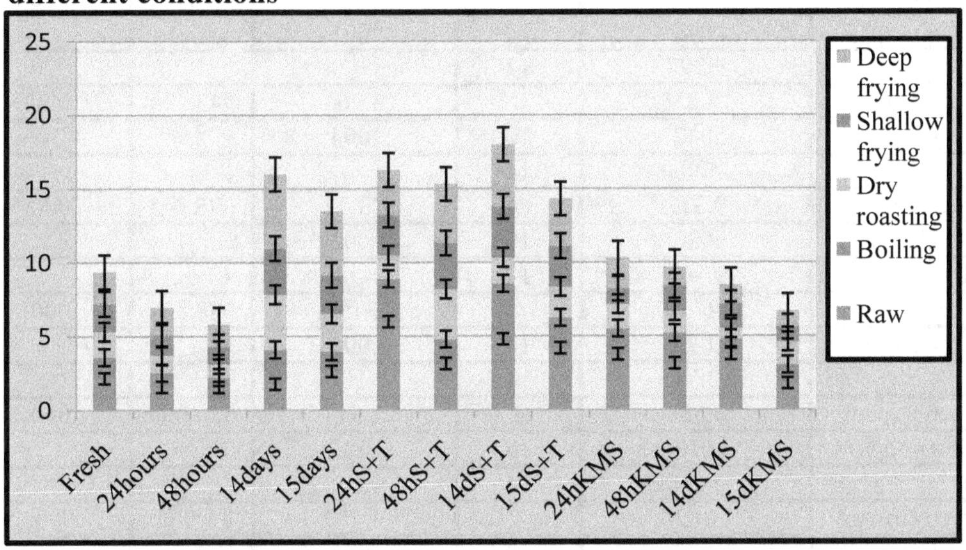

This graphical representation indicates that among all the preservation conditions, **14 days preservation with salt and turmeric**[55] helps to increase the carbohydrate content in all the cooking methods. The possible reason for this may be the moisture loss due to prolonged preservation that helps to concentrate the amount of carbohydrate and the efficiency of salt and turmeric to inhibit the microbial growth and in turn the restoration of carbohydrate[52]. The graph also shows that salt and turmeric preservation comparatively increases the carbohydrate content more than the control preservation without preservative and KMS preservation.

Table no 5.1.5.3 ANOVA with regard to cooking conditions and preservation methods

Condition	Differences	Sum of Squares	df	Mean Square	F	Sig.
Fresh (control)	Between Groups	1.159	4	.290	21.193	.000(S)
	Within Groups	.137	10	.014		
	Total	1.295	14			
24 hours (control)	Between Groups	1.461	4	.365	25.145	.000(S)
	Within Groups	.145	10	.015		
	Total	1.606	14			
48 hours (control)	Between Groups	1.768	4	.442	41.671	.000(S)
	Within Groups	.106	10	.011		
	Total	1.874	14			
14 days (control)	Between Groups	19.501	4	4.875	216.425	.000(S)
	Within Groups	.225	10	.023		
	Total	19.727	14			
15 days (control)	Between Groups	13.679	4	3.420	325.896	.000(S)
	Within Groups	.105	10	.010		
	Total	13.784	14			
24 hours (salt & turmeric)	Between Groups	32.553	4	8.138	1.587E3	.000(S)
	Within Groups	.051	10	.005		
	Total	32.604	14			
48 hours (salt & turmeric)	Between Groups	9.052	4	2.263	499.932	.000(S)
	Within Groups	.045	10	.005		
	Total	9.097	14			
14 days (salt & turmeric)	Between Groups	15.858	4	3.964	945.424	.000(S)
	Within Groups	.042	10	.004		
	Total	15.900	14			
15 days (salt & turmeric)	Between Groups	9.327	4	2.332	696.745	.000(S)
	Within Groups	.033	10	.003		
	Total	9.361	14			
24 hours (KMS)	Between Groups	12.763	4	3.191	988.831	.000(S)
	Within Groups	.032	10	.003		
	Total	12.795	14			
48 hours (KMS)	Between Groups	6.587	4	1.647	520.000	.000(S)
	Within Groups	.032	10	.003		
	Total	6.618	14			
14 days (KMS)	Between Groups	17.836	4	4.459	1.338E3	.000((S)
	Within Groups	.033	10	.003		
	Total	17.869	14			
15 days (KMS)	Between Groups	1.299	4	.325	60.891	.000(S)
	Within Groups	.053	10	.005		
	Total	1.352	14			

$p<0.05$ S= Significant, NS= Non-significant. All abbreviations are on page so and so.

This statistical ANOVA table shows that all the values are significant, which means there is significant difference present in the values of carbohydrate content of pomfret among different cooking methods and the raw state in respect to fresh condition along with different preservation methods.

Table no 5.1.5.4 Post hoc Duncan statistical analysis

Preservation	Duration	Raw state	Boiling	Dry roasting	Shallow frying	Deep frying
Control	Fresh	B,O,S^{a}	R,O,S,D^{b}	R,B,D^{c}	R,B,D^{c}	B,O,S^{a}
Control	24 hours	B,O,D^{d}	R,S,D^{e}	R,S,D^{e}	B,O,D^{d}	R,B,O,S^{i}
Control	48 hours	B,O,S^{a}	R,O,S,D^{b}	R,B,S,D^{f}	R,B,O,D^{g}	B,O,S^{a}
Control	14 days	B,O,S,D^{h}	R,O,S,D^{b}	R,B,S,D^{f}	R,B,O,D^{g}	R,B,O,S^{i}
Control	15 days	B,D^{j}	R,O,S,D^{b}	B,D^{j}	B,D^{j}	R,B,O,S^{i}
Salt & Turmeric	24 hours	B,O,S,D^{h}	R,O,S,D^{b}	R,B,S,D^{f}	R,B,O,D^{g}	R,B,O,S^{i}
Salt & Turmeric	48 hours	B,O,D^{d}	R,O,S,D^{b}	R,B,S,D^{f}	B,O,D^{d}	R,B,O,S^{i}
Salt & Turmeric	14 days	B,O,S,D^{h}	R,O,S,D^{b}	R,B,S,D^{f}	R,B,O,D^{g}	R,B,O,S^{i}
Salt & Turmeric	15 days	B,O,S,D^{h}	R,S,D^{e}	R,S,D^{e}	R,B,O,D^{g}	R,B,O,S^{i}
KMS	24 hours	B,O,S,D^{h}	R,S,D^{e}	R,S,D^{e}	R,B,O,D^{g}	R,B,O,S^{i}
KMS	48 hours	B,O,S,D^{h}	R,O,S,D^{b}	R,B,S,D^{f}	R,B,O,D^{g}	R,B,O,S^{i}
KMS	14 days	B,O,S,D^{h}	R,O,S,D^{b}	R,B,S,D^{f}	R,B,O,D^{g}	R,B,O,S^{i}
KMS	15 days	B,O,S,D^{h}	R,O,S,D^{b}	R,B,S,D^{f}	R,B,O^{k}	R,B,O^{k}

R= Raw state, B= Boiling, O= Open pan dry roasting, S= Shallow frying, D= Deep frying. The same uppercase alphabets represent that there is no significant difference present among the variables.

This table shows the significant difference among the different variables such as cooking methods and preservation conditions. The raw state significantly differs from boiling, open pan dry roasting, shallow frying and deep frying in most of the preservation methods with preservatives and control conditions except in fresh condition, 24 hours, 48 hours and 15 days control preservation without preservative, and in 48 hours salt and turmeric preservation. In fresh condition and 48 hours control preservation without preservative, the raw state along with deep frying significantly differ from boiling, open pan dry roasting and shallow frying, whereas boiling in all the preservation conditions except in 24 hours control preservation without preservative, 15 days salt and turmeric preservation as well as in 24 hours KMS preservation, significantly differs from the raw state, open pan dry roasting, shallow frying and deep frying.

Both shallow frying and open pan dry roasting significantly differ from the raw state, boiling and deep frying in fresh condition. In 24 hours control preservation without preservative and 48 hours salt and turmeric preservation, the raw state and shallow frying significantly differ from boiling, open pan dry roasting and deep frying. In 24 hours control preservation without preservative, 15 days salt and turmeric preservation, 24 hours KMS preservation, boiling and open pan dry roasting significantly differ from the raw state, shallow frying and deep frying. Open pan dry roasting in 48 hours, 14 days control preservation without preservative, 24 hours, 48 hours, 14 days salt and turmeric preservation and 48 hours, 14 days, 15 days KMS preservation, significantly differs from the raw state, boiling, shallow frying and deep frying. Shallow frying significantly differs from the raw state, boiling, open pan dry roasting and deep frying in 48 hours, 14 days control preservation without preservative, 24 hours, 14 days, 15 days salt and turmeric preservation as well as in 24 hours, 48 hours, 14 days KMS preservation. Deep frying significantly differs from the raw state, boiling, open pan dry roasting and shallow frying in all the preservation conditions except in fresh condition, 48 hours control preservation without preservative and 15 days KMS preservation. In 15 days control preservation without preservative, the raw state, open pan dry roasting and shallow frying significantly differ from boiling and deep frying. In 15 days KMS preservation, shallow frying and deep frying significantly differ from the raw state, boiling and open pan dry roasting.

Table no 5.1.5.5 Gradation of cooking methods from higher to lower restoration with respect to preservation days

Preservation	Duration	Method 1	Method 2	Method 3	Method 4	Method 5
Control	Fresh	R	DF	SF	OPDR	B
Control	24 hours	DF	R	SF	OPDR	B
Control	48 hours	R	DF	SF	OPDR	B
Control	14 days	DF	OPDR	SF	B	R
Control	15 days	DF	R	SF	OPDR	B
Salt & Turmeric	24 hours	R	DF	B	SF	OPDR
Salt & Turmeric	48 hours	DF	OPDR	R	SF	B
Salt & Turmeric	14 days	R	DF	B	SF	OPDR
Salt &Turmeric	15 days	R	DF	SF	B	OPDR
KMS	24 hours	R	DF	B	OPDR	SF
KMS	48 hours	R	B	SF	OPDR	DF
KMS	14 days	R	SF	DF	B	OPDR
KMS	15 days	R	OPDR	B	DF	SF

R= Raw state, B= Boiling, OPDR= Open pan dry roasting, SF= Shallow frying, DF= Deep frying. Same colours represent the similar order.

In all the preservation methods and fresh condition, carbohydrate retention occurs mainly in the raw state than the other cooking methods. In fresh condition and 48 hours control preservation without preservative, retention occurs firstly in the raw state then deep frying, shallow frying, open pan dry roasting and boiling. In 24 hours, 15 days control preservation without preservative, the order changes from shallow frying to the raw state, open pan dry roasting, boiling and then deep frying. In 14 days control preservation without preservative, the order becomes deep frying, open pan dry roasting, shallow frying, boiling and the raw state.

In 24 hours, 14 days salt and turmeric preservation, the order changes to the raw state, deep frying, boiling, shallow frying and open pan dry roasting. In 48 hours salt and turmeric preservation, the order becomes deep frying, open pan dry roasting, raw state, shallow frying and boiling. In 15 days salt and turmeric preservation, the order changes to the raw state, deep frying, shallow frying, boiling and open pan dry roasting.

In 24 hours KMS preservation, the order changes from the raw state to deep frying, boiling, open pan dry roasting and shallow frying. In 48 hours KMS preservation, the order is the raw state, boiling, shallow frying, open pan dry roasting and deep frying. In 14 days KMS preservation, the order changes to the raw state, shallow frying, deep frying, boiling and open pan dry roasting. In 15 days KMS preservation, the order becomes the raw state, open pan dry roasting, boiling, deep frying and shallow frying.

The overall analysis of carbohydrate content of pomfret is mostly restored by the gradation of methods as the raw state>deep frying> shallow frying>open pan dry roasting>boiling.

Frying mainly restores[66] the nutrients as the oil can possibly create a protective layer so that the carbohydrate cannot be leached out, but in boiling the soluble carbohydrates get dissolved and the content is reduced, and discarding this boiling water can also be the possible cause for the loss of carbohydrate. In open pan dry roasting the carbohydrates possibly get charred, resulting in losses. Thus among all the studied conventional cooking methods, **deep frying** is the best method for cooking pomfret to restore carbohydrate. Additionally pomfret is a sea fish and contains high amount of fatty tissues, being a possible reason for the reduction of carbohydrate loss in deep frying method.

5.1.6 *Hilsa* (*Tenualosa Ilisha*)

It has been reported that *hilsa* contains 2.9 gm of carbohydrate per 100 gm[84] in the raw condition. This value changes due to the application of different cooking methods and preservation conditions (vide Table no **5.1.6.1**).

Table no 5.1.6.1 Carbohydrate content of *Hilsa* (gm/100gm)

Preservation	Duration	Raw state	Boiling	Dry roasting	Shallow frying	Deep frying
Control	Fresh	3.59±0.14	2.37±0.15	1.72±0.09	2.30±0.10	3.25±0.10
Control	24 hours	1.52±0.13	1.03±0.10	0.99±0.17	1.22±0.14	1.17±0.07
Control	48 hours	1.04±0.08	0.98±0.05	0.76±0.08	0.72±0.08	2.05±0.05
Control	14 days	2.45±0.06	4.12±0.08	3.72±0.09	1.78±0.08	3.89±0.07
Control	15 days	1.72±0.08	2.40±0.10	1.27±0.08	2.05±0.05	2.50±0.08
Salt & Turmeric	24 hours	2.74±0.09	1.45±0.05	0.58±0.07	1.25±0.05	2.00±0.05
Salt & Turmeric	48 hours	2.66±0.17	0.50±0.05	1.00±0.05	1.58±0.08	3.27±0.05
Salt & Turmeric	14 days	2.82±0.08	0.35±0.05	1.32±0.10	3.30±0.05	3.38±0.08
Salt & Turmeric	15 days	3.25±0.05	0.65±0.05	1.65±0.05	1.75±0.05	2.62±0.13
KMS	24 hours	2.00±0.05	1.25±0.05	1.00±0.05	1.56±0.07	3.28±0.07
KMS	48 hours	1.65±0.05	1.93±0.07	1.25±0.05	1.93±0.07	1.98±0.07
KMS	14 days	3.55±0.05	1.25±0.05	2.05±0.05	1.90±0.05	0.70±0.05
KMS	15 days	2.30±0.05	0.40±0.05	1.95±0.05	1.00±0.05	2.05±0.05

Values are expressed as mean±SD. ☐ Loss ▨ Restoration

Red digits represent the significant highest values from the raw state in different conditions.

In 48 hours, 14 days, 15 days preservation with salt and turmeric and in 15 days KMS preservation, carbohydrate losses mainly occur by boiling, whereas in 24 hours, 15 days control preservation without preservative, 24 hours preservation with salt and turmeric as well as 24 hours, 48 hours preservation with KMS, losses occur by open pan dry roasting. In fresh condition, 48 hours 14 days control preservation without preservative, losses occur by shallow frying and in 14 days KMS preservation, deep frying causes most of the loss.

Most of the retention occurs by deep frying, but in 24 hours control preservation without preservative, carbohydrate retention occurs by shallow frying and in 14 days control preservation without preservative as well as in 14 days KMS preservation, retention occurs by boiling and open pan dry roasting respectively.

14 days control preservation without preservative shows the highest carbohydrate content in boiled, open pan dry roasted and deep fried *hilsa*, and 14 days salt and turmeric preservation helps to increase the carbohydrate content in shallow frying, whereas fresh condition shows the highest value in the raw state among the other preservation conditions.

In 48 hours, 14 days, 15 days control preservation without preservative, 48 hours, 14 days preservation with salt and turmeric, 24 hours, 48 hours KMS preservation helps in the retention of carbohydrate in deep frying, more than the raw state, whereas 15 days control preservation without preservative, 14 days salt and turmeric preservation, 48 hours KMS preservation help to increase the carbohydrate content in shallow frying, but 14 days control preservation without preservative increases the content by both boiling and open pan dry roasting. Again the carbohydrate content increases in 15 days control preservation without preservative and 48 hours KMS preservation by boiling only. As *hilsa* is a fatty fish, the carbohydrate loss is comparatively lower than the other fish in the conventional cooking methods.

In most of the preservation conditions, deep frying helps to increase the nutrient content mostly greater than the raw state. It can probably modify the structural rearrangement of carbohydrate and thus retention occurs and it can also create a layer of protection by the use of oil so that carbohydrates cannot be leached out. The carbohydrate content becomes concentrated possibly due to the loss of moisture for the effect of prolonged preservation with natural preservatives as well as the application of heat during cooking[48].

Fig. 5.1.6.2 Graphical representation of Carbohydrate content of *Hilsa* with respect to different conditions

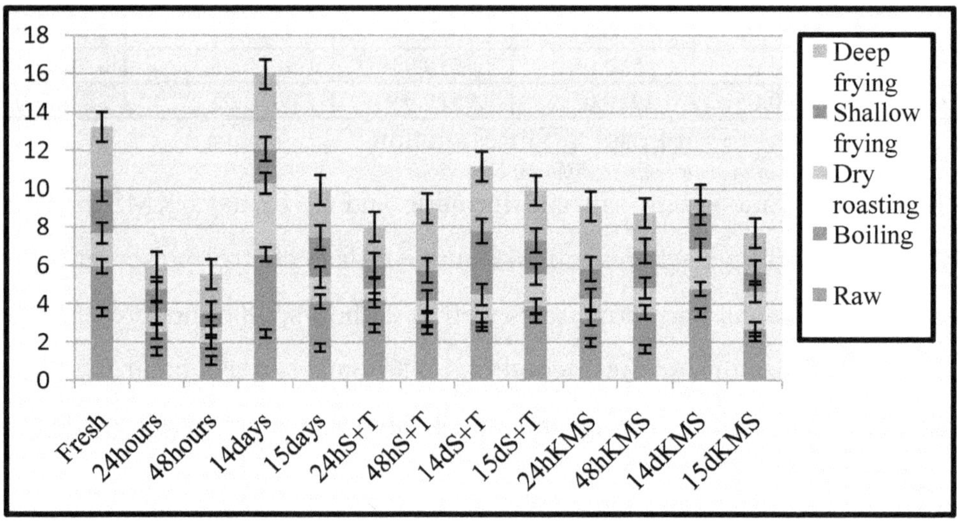

This graphical representation indicates that among all the preservation conditions, **14 days control preservation without preservative** helps to increase the carbohydrate content in all the cooking methods. The possible reason may be the moisture loss due to prolonged preservation that helps to concentrate the amount of carbohydrate. The graph also shows that without preservative control preservation comparatively increases the carbohydrate content more than the preservations with the combination of salt and turmeric and KMS.

Table no 5.1.6.3 ANOVA with regard to cooking conditions and preservation methods

Condition	Differences	Sum of Squares	df	Mean Square	F	Sig.
Fresh (control)	Between Groups	6.941	4	1.735	121.064	.000(S)
	Within Groups	.143	10	.014		
	Total	7.084	14			
24 hours (control)	Between Groups	.516	4	.129	9.298	.002(S)
	Within Groups	.139	10	.014		
	Total	.655	14			
48 hours (control)	Between Groups	3.546	4	.887	176.852	.000(S)
	Within Groups	.050	10	.005		
	Total	3.597	14			
14 days (control)	Between Groups	12.449	4	3.112	551.152	.000(S)
	Within Groups	.056	10	.006		
	Total	12.505	14			
15 days (control)	Between Groups	3.089	4	.772	126.322	.000(S)
	Within Groups	.061	10	.006		
	Total	3.150	14			
24 hours (salt & turmeric)	Between Groups	7.937	4	1.984	451.653	.000(S)
	Within Groups	.044	10	.004		
	Total	7.981	14			
48 hours (salt & turmeric)	Between Groups	15.692	4	3.923	444.104	.000(S)
	Within Groups	.088	10	.009		
	Total	15.780	14			
14 days (salt & turmeric)	Between Groups	21.563	4	5.391	980.152	.000(S)
	Within Groups	.055	10	.006		
	Total	21.618	14			
15 days (salt & turmeric)	Between Groups	11.847	4	2.962	573.226	.000(S)
	Within Groups	.052	10	.005		
	Total	11.898	14			
24 hours (KMS)	Between Groups	9.706	4	2.426	632.978	.000(S)
	Within Groups	.038	10	.004		
	Total	9.744	14			
48 hours (KMS)	Between Groups	1.145	4	.286	63.611	.000(S)
	Within Groups	.045	10	.004		
	Total	1.190	14			
14 days (KMS)	Between Groups	13.821	4	3.455	1.382E3	.000(S)
	Within Groups	.025	10	.002		
	Total	13.846	14			
15 days (KMS)	Between Groups	7.791	4	1.948	779.100	.000(S)
	Within Groups	.025	10	.003		
	Total	7.816	14			

$p<0.05$ S= Significant, NS= Non-significant. All abbreviations are on page so and so.

This statistical ANOVA table shows that all the values are significant, which means there is significant difference present in the values of carbohydrate content of *hilsa* among different cooking methods and the raw state in respect to fresh condition along with different preservation methods.

Table no 5.1.6.4 Post hoc Duncan statistical analysis

Preservation	Duration	Raw state	Boiling	Dry roasting	Shallow frying	Deep frying
Control	Fresh	B,O,S,D^{a}	R,O,D^{b}	R,B,S,D^{c}	R,O,D^{b}	R,B,O,S^{d}
Control	24 hours	B,O,S,D^{a}	R^{e}	R^{e}	R^{e}	R^{e}
Control	48 hours	O,S,D^{f}	O,S,D^{f}	R,B,D^{g}	R,B,D^{g}	R,B,O,S^{d}
Control	14 days	B,O,S,D^{a}	R,O,S,D^{h}	R,B,S,D^{c}	R,B,O,D^{i}	R,B,O,S^{d}
Control	15 days	B,O,S,D^{a}	R,O,S^{j}	R,B,S,D^{c}	R,B,O,D^{i}	R,O,S^{j}
Salt & Turmeric	24 hours	B,O,S,D^{a}	R,O,S,D^{h}	R,B,S,D^{c}	R,B,O,D^{i}	R,B,O,S^{d}
Salt & Turmeric	48 hours	B,O,S,D^{a}	R,O,S,D^{h}	R,B,S,D^{c}	R,B,O,D^{i}	R,B,O,S^{d}
Salt & Turmeric	14 days	B,O,S,D^{a}	R,O,S,D^{h}	R,B,S,D^{c}	R,B,O^{k}	R,B,O^{k}
Salt & Turmeric	15 days	B,O,S,D^{a}	R,O,S,D^{h}	R,B,D^{g}	R,B,D^{g}	R,B,O,S^{d}
KMS	24 hours	B,O,S,D^{a}	R,O,S,D^{h}	R,B,S,D^{c}	R,B,O,D^{i}	R,B,O,S^{d}
KMS	48 hours	B,O,S,D^{a}	R,O^{l}	R,B,S,D^{c}	R,O^{l}	R,O^{l}
KMS	14 days	B,O,S,D^{a}	R,O,S,D^{h}	R,B,S,D^{c}	R,B,O,D^{i}	R,B,O,S^{d}
KMS	15 days	B,O,S,D^{a}	R,O,S,D^{h}	R,B,S,D^{c}	R,B,O,D^{i}	R,B,O,S^{d}

R= Raw state, B= Boiling, O= Open pan dry roasting, S= Shallow frying, D= Deep frying. The same uppercase alphabets represent that there is no significant difference present among the variables.

This table shows the significant difference among the different variables such as cooking methods and preservation conditions. The raw state significantly differs from boiling, open pan dry roasting, shallow frying and deep frying in all of the preservation methods with preservatives and control conditions except in 48 hours control preservation without preservative. In fresh condition, boiling and shallow frying significantly differ from the raw state, open pan dry roasting, deep frying, whereas open pan dry roasting in all the preservation conditions except in 24 hours, 48 hours control preservation without preservative, 15 days salt and turmeric preservation significantly differs from the raw state, boiling, shallow frying and deep frying.

Deep frying significantly differs from the raw state, boiling, open pan dry roasting and shallow frying in all the preservation conditions except in 24 hours, 15 days control preservation without preservative and 14 days preservation by the combination of salt and turmeric and 48 hours KMS preservation. In 24 hours control preservation without preservative, boiling, open pan dry roasting and shallow frying, deep frying significantly differ from the raw state. In 48 hours control preservation without preservative, 15 days salt and turmeric preservation, open pan dry roasting and shallow frying significantly differ from the raw state, boiling and deep frying, whereas boiling significantly differs from the raw state, open pan dry roasting, shallow frying and deep frying in all conditions except in fresh condition, 24 hours, 48 hours, 15 days control preservation without preservative and also in 48 hours KMS preservation.

Shallow frying significantly differs from the raw state, boiling, open pan dry roasting and deep frying in all of the preservation conditions except in fresh, 24 hours, 48 hours control preservation without preservative, 14 and 15 days salt and turmeric preservation as well as 48 hours KMS preservation. In 15 days control preservation without preservative, boiling and deep frying significantly differ from the raw state, open pan dry roasting and shallow frying. In 14 days salt and turmeric preservation, shallow frying and deep frying significantly differ from the raw state, boiling and open pan dry roasting. Again boiling, shallow frying and deep frying significantly differ from the raw state and open pan dry roasting in 48 hours KMS preservation.

Table no 5.1.6.5 Gradation of cooking methods from higher to lower restoration with respect to preservation days

Preservation	Duration	Method 1	Method 2	Method 3	Method 4	Method 5
Control	Fresh	R	DF	B	SF	OPDR
Control	24 hours	R	SF	DF	B	OPDR
Control	48 hours	DF	R	B	OPDR	SF
Control	14 days	B	DF	OPDR	R	SF
Control	15 days	DF	B	SF	R	OPDR
Salt & Turmeric	24 hours	R	DF	B	SF	OPDR
Salt & Turmeric	48 hours	DF	R	SF	OPDR	B
Salt & Turmeric	14 days	DF	SF	R	OPDR	B
Salt &Turmeric	15 days	R	DF	SF	OPDR	B
KMS	24 hours	DF	R	SF	B	OPDR
KMS	48 hours	DF	SF	B	R	OPDR
KMS	14 days	R	OPDR	SF	DF	B
KMS	15 days	R	DF	OPDR	SF	B

R= Raw state, B= Boiling, OPDR= Open pan dry roasting, SF= Shallow frying, DF= Deep frying. Same colour represents the similar order.

In all the preservation techniques and fresh condition, carbohydrate retention mainly occurs in deep frying than the other cooking methods. In fresh condition and 24 hours salt and turmeric preservation, retention occurs firstly in the raw state then deep frying, boiling, shallow frying and open pan dry roasting. In 24 hours control preservation without preservative, the order changes from the raw state to shallow frying, deep frying, boiling and then open pan dry roasting. In 48 hours control preservation without preservative, it changes in the order of deep frying, raw state, boiling, open pan dry roasting and shallow frying. In 14 days control preservation without preservative, the order becomes boiling, deep frying, open pan dry roasting, raw state and shallow frying. In 15 days control preservation without preservative, the order is deep frying, boiling, shallow frying, raw state and open pan dry roasting.

In 48 hours salt and turmeric preservation, the order changes to deep frying, raw state, shallow frying, open pan dry roasting and boiling. In 14 days salt and turmeric preservation, the order changes from deep frying to shallow frying, raw state, open pan dry roasting and boiling. In 15 days salt and turmeric preservation, the order is the raw state, deep frying, shallow frying, open pan dry roasting and boiling.

In 24 hours KMS preservation, the order changes from deep frying to the raw state, shallow frying, boiling and open pan dry roasting. In 48 hours KMS preservation, the order becomes deep frying, shallow frying, boiling, raw state and open pan dry roasting. In 14 days KMS preservation, the order changes to the raw state, open pan dry roasting, shallow frying, deep frying and boiling. In 15 days KMS preservation, the order becomes the raw state, deep frying, open pan dry roasting, shallow frying and boiling.

The overall analysis of carbohydrate content of *hilsa* is mostly restored by the gradation of methods as deep frying> raw state>shallow frying> boiling >open pan dry roasting.

Frying mainly restores[66] the nutrients as the oil can possibly create a protective layer so that the carbohydrate cannot be leached out, but in boiling the soluble carbohydrates get dissolved and the content is reduced and discarding the boiling water can also be the possible cause for the loss of carbohydrate. *Hilsa* is a sea fish and it contains abundant adipose tissues. Here the loss in boiling is low due to the heavy fat content of the fish, which may restrict the carbohydrate to leach out in the cooking water. In open pan dry roasting the carbohydrates possibly get charred, resulting in losses. Here losses mostly occurs in open pan dry roasting as the fatty tissue melts due to the application of heat and the fat layer is eliminated to restore carbohydrate. Thus among all the studied conventional cooking methods, **deep frying** is the best method for cooking *hilsa* to restore carbohydrate.

5.2 Protein content

It has been reported that fish contains about 15- 16% of protein[1], this experiment is carried out to estimate the percentage of protein among the different fish and edible aquatic species. Changes in protein content due to the application of different cooking methods and preservation conditions are also estimated. Protein content estimation is carried out by Lowry method[69].

5.2.1 *Rohu (Labeo rohita)*

It has been reported that *rohu* contains 19.71 gm of protein per 100 gm[85] in the raw condition. This value changes due to the application of different cooking methods and preservation conditions (vide Table no **5.2.1.1**).

Table no 5.2.1.1 Protein content of *Rohu* (gm/100gm)

Preservation	Duration	Raw state	Boiling	Dry roasting	Shallow frying	Deep frying
Control	Fresh	17.52±0.53	2.96±0.06	5.73±0.12	5.03±0.15	7.36±0.4
Control	24 hours	16.72±0.29	4.44±0.04	5.64±0.19	4.48±0.05	7.41±0.14
Control	48 hours	13.09±0.53	3.34±0.04	5.62±0.23	4.09±0.10	5.05±0.50
Control	14 days	6.94±0.34	4.64±0.36	4.61±0.23	6.29±0.37	9.66±0.30
Control	15 days	5.25±0.25	3.57±0.36	4.64±0.28	4.81±0.37	5.91±0.34
Salt & Turmeric	24 hours	16.84±0.15	6.37±0.07	13.04±0.02	13.47±0.08	15.90±0.09
Salt & Turmeric	48 hours	15.53±0.04	7.06±0.04	9.94±0.13	5.83±0.04	8.75±0.08
Salt & Turmeric	14 days	14.03±0.04	5.06±0.04	8.07±0.06	5.81±0.04	8.72±0.02
Salt & Turmeric	15 days	12.03±0.04	4.11±0.90	6.05±0.04	5.79±0.03	8.70±0.08
KMS	24 hours	12.43±0.13	2.24±0.18	6.20±0.63	3.00±0.13	4.28±0.07
KMS	48 hours	8.76±0.04	2.14±0.04	4.59±0.20	1.85±0.03	2.65±0.03
KMS	14 days	14.03±0.04	5.05±0.04	8.06±0.06	5.81±0.03	8.72±0.02
KMS	15 days	12.03±0.04	4.10±0.09	6.05±0.04	5.79±0.03	8.71±0.08

Values are expressed as mean±SD. Loss Restoration

Red digits represent the significant highest values from the raw state in a single condition.

In all the preservation conditions except 48 hours preservation with salt and turmeric as well as KMS, protein losses mainly occur by boiling, whereas open pan dry roasting decreases the protein content in 48 hours preservation with salt and turmeric as well as with KMS.

Most of the retention occurs by deep frying, [32] but in 48 hours control preservation without preservative and 24 hours, 48 hours KMS preservation, protein retention occurs by open pan dry roasting.

24 hours preservation with salt and turmeric shows the highest protein content in all the cooking methods such as boiled, open pan dry roasted, shallow fried and deep fried *rohu*, but in fresh condition, the raw state shows the highest protein content.

Here the effects of the natural preservatives are prominent. They mostly help to increase the protein content. They probably help to modify the structure of protein leading to retention. In some cases the content is more than the raw state that is achieved by deep frying in 15 days control preservation without preservative. The protein becomes concentrated possibly due to the loss of moisture for the effect of prolonged preservation with natural preservatives as well as the application of heat during cooking[48]. There may be some chemical rearrangement so that the proteins that are present in bound form may get released, thus the content becomes high after cooking. Moreover, protein denaturation occurs due to the application of heat during cooking.

Fig. 5.2.1.2 Graphical representation of Protein content of *Rohu* with respect to different conditions

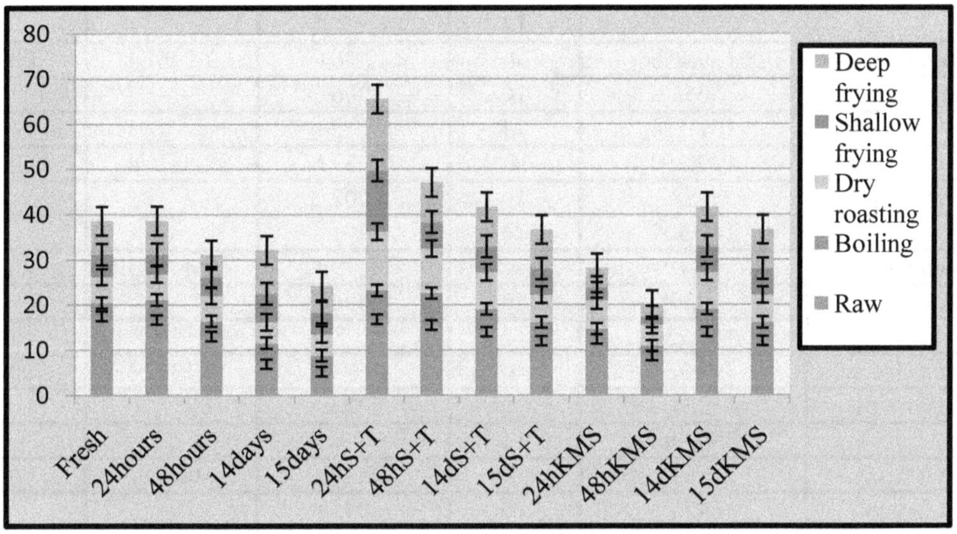

This graphical representation indicates that among all the preservation conditions, **24 hours preservation with salt and turmeric**[55] helps to increase the protein content in all the cooking methods. The possible reason may be the moisture loss due to prolonged preservation that helps to concentrate the amount of protein and the efficiency of salt and turmeric to inhibit the microbial growth and in turn the restoration of protein[34,52]. The graph also shows that salt and turmeric preservation comparatively increases the protein content more than the control preservation without preservative and KMS preservation.

Table no 5.2.1.3 ANOVA with regard to cooking conditions and preservation methods

Condition	Differences	Sum of Squares	df	Mean Square	F	Sig.
Fresh (control)	Between Groups	390.260	4	97.565	1.445E3	.000(S)
	Within Groups	.675	10	.068		
	Total	390.935	14			
24 hours (control)	Between Groups	320.089	4	80.022	2.807E3	.000(S)
	Within Groups	.285	10	.029		
	Total	320.374	14			
48 hours (control)	Between Groups	185.221	4	46.305	692.432	.000(S)
	Within Groups	.669	10	.067		
	Total	185.890	14			
14 days (control)	Between Groups	51.669	4	12.917	123.092	.000(S)
	Within Groups	1.049	10	.105		
	Total	52.719	14			
15 days (control)	Between Groups	8.947	4	2.237	21.223	.000(S)
	Within Groups	1.054	10	.105		
	Total	10.001	14			
24 hours (salt & turmeric)	Between Groups	201.840	4	50.460	6.021E3	.000(S)
	Within Groups	.084	10	.008		
	Total	201.924	14			
48 hours (salt & turmeric)	Between Groups	169.456	4	42.364	7.296E3	.000(S)
	Within Groups	.058	10	.006		
	Total	169.514	14			
14 days (salt & turmeric)	Between Groups	149.350	4	37.337	2.082E4	.000(S)
	Within Groups	.018	10	.002		
	Total	149.367	14			
15 days (salt & turmeric)	Between Groups	115.197	4	28.799	7.448E3	.000(S)
	Within Groups	.039	10	.004		
	Total	115.236	14			
24 hours (KMS)	Between Groups	199.761	4	49.940	2.137E3	.000(S)
	Within Groups	.234	10	.023		
	Total	199.994	14			
48 hours (KMS)	Between Groups	91.113	4	22.778	500.917	.000(S)
	Within Groups	.455	10	.045		
	Total	91.568	14			
14 days (KMS)	Between Groups	40.142	4	10.035	1.908E3	.000(S)
	Within Groups	.053	10	.005		
	Total	40.195	14			
15 days (KMS)	Between Groups	34.599	4	8.650	3.460E3	.000(S)
	Within Groups	.025	10	.003		
	Total	34.624	14			

$p<0.05$ S= Significant, NS= Non-significant. All abbreviations are on page so and so.

This statistical ANOVA table shows that all the values are significant, which means there is significant difference present in the values of protein content of *rohu* among different cooking methods and the raw state in respect to fresh condition along with different preservation methods.

Table no 5.2.1.4 Post hoc Duncan statistical analysis

Preservation	Duration	Raw state	Boiling	Dry roasting	Shallow frying	Deep frying
Control	Fresh	B,O,S,D^{a}	R,O,S,D^{b}	R,B,S,D^{c}	R,B,O,D^{d}	R,B,O,S^{e}
Control	24 hours	B,O,S,D^{a}	R,O,D^{f}	R,B,S,D^{c}	R,O,D^{f}	R,B,O,S^{e}
Control	48 hours	B,O,S,D^{a}	R,O,S,D^{b}	R,B,S,D^{c}	R,B,O,D^{d}	R,B,O,S^{e}
Control	14 days	B,O,S,D^{a}	R,S,D^{g}	R,S,D^{g}	R,B,O,D^{d}	R,B,O,S^{e}
Control	15 days	B,D^{h}	R,O,S,D^{b}	B,D^{h}	B,D^{h}	R,B,O,S^{e}
Salt & Turmeric	24 hours	B,O,S,D^{a}	R,O,S,D^{b}	R,B,S,D^{c}	R,B,O,D^{d}	R,B,O,S^{e}
Salt & Turmeric	48 hours	B,O,S,D^{a}	R,O,S,D^{b}	R,B,S,D^{c}	R,B,O,D^{d}	R,B,O,S^{e}
Salt & Turmeric	14 days	B,O,S,D^{a}	R,O,S,D^{b}	R,B,S,D^{c}	R,B,O,D^{d}	R,B,O,S^{e}
Salt & Turmeric	15 days	B,O,S,D^{a}	R,O,S,D^{b}	R,B,S,D^{c}	R,B,O,D^{d}	R,B,O,S^{e}
KMS	24 hours	B,O,S,D^{a}	R,O,S,D^{b}	R,B,S,D^{c}	R,B,O,D	R,B,O,S^{e}
KMS	48 hours	B,O,S,D^{a}	R,O,D^{f}	R,B,S,D^{c}	R,O,D^{f}	R,B,O,S^{e}
KMS	14 days	B,O,S,D^{a}	R,O,S,D^{b}	R,B,S,D^{c}	R,B,O,D^{d}	R,B,O,S^{e}
KMS	15 days	B,O,S,D^{a}	R,O,S^{i}	R,B,S,D^{c}	R,B,O,D^{d}	R,O,S^{i}

R= Raw state, B= Boiling, O= Open pan dry roasting, S= Shallow frying, D= Deep frying. The same uppercase alphabets represent that there is no significant difference present among the variables.

This table shows the significant difference among the different variables such as cooking methods and preservation conditions. The raw state significantly differs from boiling, open pan dry roasting, shallow frying and deep frying in all of the preservation methods with preservatives and control conditions except in 15 days control preservation without preservative. Boiling significantly differs from the raw state, open pan dry roasting, shallow frying and deep frying in all the preservation conditions except in 24 hours and 14 days control preservation without preservative and 48 hours, 15 days KMS preservation, whereas open pan dry roasting in all the preservation conditions except in 14 and 15 days control preservation without preservative, significantly differs from the raw state, boiling, shallow frying and deep frying. Shallow frying significantly differs from the raw state, boiling, open pan dry roasting and deep frying in most of the preservation conditions except in 24 hours, 15 days control preservation without preservative as well as in 48 hours KMS preservation. Deep frying significantly differs from the raw state, boiling, open pan dry roasting and shallow frying in all of the preservation conditions except in 15 days KMS preservation.

Shallow frying and boiling significantly differ from the raw state, open pan dry roasting and deep frying in 24 hours control preservation without preservative and 48 hours preservation by KMS. Boiling and open pan dry roasting significantly differ from the raw state, shallow frying and deep frying in 14 days control preservation without preservative. The raw state, open pan dry roasting and shallow frying significantly differ from boiling and deep frying in 15 days control preservation without preservative, whereas boiling and deep frying significantly differ from the raw state, open pan dry roasting and shallow frying in 15 days KMS preservation.

Table no 5.2.1.5 Gradation of cooking methods from higher to lower restoration with respect to preservation days

Preservation	Duration	Method 1	Method 2	Method 3	Method 4	Method 5
Control	Fresh	R	DF	OPDR	SF	B
Control	24 hours	R	DF	OPDR	SF	B
Control	48 hours	R	OPDR	DF	SF	B
Control	14 days	DF	R	SF	B	OPDR
Control	15 days	DF	R	SF	B	OPDR
Salt & Turmeric	24 hours	R	DF	SF	OPDR	B
Salt & Turmeric	48 hours	R	OPDR	DF	B	SF
Salt & Turmeric	14 days	R	DF	OPDR	SF	B
Salt &Turmeric	15 days	R	DF	OPDR	SF	B
KMS	24 hours	R	OPDR	DF	SF	B
KMS	48 hours	R	OPDR	DF	B	SF
KMS	14 days	R	DF	SF	B	OPDR
KMS	15 days	R	OPDR	SF	DF	B

R= Raw state, B= Boiling, OPDR= Open pan dry roasting, SF= Shallow frying, DF= Deep frying. Same colours represent the similar order.

In all the preservation methods and fresh condition, protein retention mainly occurs in the raw state than the other cooking methods. In fresh condition and 24 hours control preservation without preservative, retention occurs firstly in the raw state then deep frying, open pan dry roasting, shallow frying and boiling. In 48 hours control preservation without preservative and 24 hours KMS preservation, the order changes from the raw state to open pan dry roasting, deep frying, shallow frying and boiling. In 14 days, 15 days control preservation without preservative, the order is deep frying followed by the raw state, shallow frying, boiling and open pan dry roasting.

In 24 hours salt and turmeric the order changes to the raw state, deep frying, shallow frying, open pan dry roasting and boiling. In 48 hours salt and turmeric preservation, the order changes from the raw state to open pan dry roasting, deep frying, boiling and shallow frying. In 14 and 15 days salt and turmeric preservation, the order is the raw state, deep frying, open pan dry roasting, shallow frying and boiling.

In 48 hours KMS preservation, the order is the raw state, open pan dry roasting, deep frying, boiling and shallow frying. In 14 days KMS preservation, it changes in order of the raw state, deep frying, shallow frying, boiling and open pan dry roasting. In 15 days KMS preservation, the order changes from the raw state to open pan dry roasting, shallow frying, deep frying and boiling.

The overall analysis of protein content of *rohu* is mostly restored by the gradation of methods as the raw state>deep frying> open pan dry roasting> shallow frying>boiling.

Deep frying mainly restores[66] the nutrients as the oil can possibly create a protective layer so that the protein cannot be leached out, but in boiling the soluble protein parts get dissolved and the content is reduced, and discarding the boiling water can also be the possible cause for the loss of protein content. In open pan dry roasting the protein possibly gets charred, resulting in losses. Shallow frying can also reduce the protein content as small amount of oil is used to fry the fish which cannot cover the full surface area of the fish and so possibly less protection is created. Thus among all the studied conventional cooking methods, **deep frying** is the best method for cooking *rohu* to restore protein content.

5.2.2 *Katla* (*Catla catla*)

It has been reported that *katla* contains 17.94 gm of protein per 100 gm[85] in the raw condition. This value changes due to the application of different cooking methods and preservation conditions (vide Table no **5.2.2.1**).

Table no 5.2.2.1 Protein content of *Katla* (gm/100gm)

Preservation	Duration	Raw state	Boiling	Dry roasting	Shallow frying	Deep frying
Control	Fresh	21.20±0.28	2.75±0.03	6.25±0.05	10.92±0.02	5.03±0.04
Control	24 hours	16.37±0.58	5.46±0.07	7.10±0.13	7.24±0.05	4.28±0.10
Control	48 hours	14.34±0.29	2.72±0.03	6.17±0.08	5.570.22±	3.99±0.09
Control	14 days	12.33±1.23	5.71±0.20	5.30±0.27	4.00±0.20	7.19±0.80
Control	15 days	12.20±0.16	5.67±0.18	4.91±0.09	4.84±0.08	4.35±0.06
Salt & Turmeric	24 hours	17.09±0.10	6.23±0.13	5.96±0.04	8.03±0.04	10.84±0.04
Salt & Turmeric	48 hours	15.39±0.21	4.25±0.03	8.06±0.05	7.53±0.10	9.06±0.05
Salt & Turmeric	14 days	11.31±0.40	3.95±0.03	6.01±0.11	8.32±0.08	9.82±0.15
Salt & Turmeric	15 days	9.59±0.14	3.50±0.21	0.78±0.11	7.05±0.05	7.96±0.14
KMS	24 hours	12.09±0.10	4.28±0.07	6.78±0.15	7.46±0.25	10.34±0.43
KMS	48 hours	10.02±0.22	4.10±0.22	5.37±0.24	6.00±0.17	10.45±0.43
KMS	14 days	11.16±0.14	4.27±0.20	6.93±0.26	6.14±0.39	6.51±0.29
KMS	15 days	7.17±0.38	3.87±0.32	3.75±0.41	2.93±0.21	6.45±0.33

Values are expressed as mean±SD. Loss Restoration

Red digits represent the significant highest values from the raw state in a single condition.

In fresh condition, 48 hours control preservation without preservative and 48 hours, 14 days preservation with salt and turmeric as well as in 24 hours, 48 hours, 14 days KMS preservation, protein losses mainly occur by boiling, whereas in 24 hours and 15 days preservation with salt and turmeric, losses occur by open pan dry roasting. In 14 days control preservation without preservative and 15 days KMS preservation, losses occur by shallow frying along with deep frying in 24 hours and 15 days control preservation without preservative.

Most of the retention occurs by deep frying, [32] but in fresh condition and 24 hours control preservation without preservative, protein retention occurs by shallow frying, whereas in 48 hours control preservation without preservative and 14 days KMS preservation, retention occurs by open pan dry roasting and in 15 days control preservation without preservative, boiling helps to retain the protein content.

In fresh condition, the raw state and shallow fried *katla* shows the highest protein content, whereas 24 hours, 48 hours preservation with salt and turmeric shows the highest content in boiling and open pan dry roasting respectively. 48 hours KMS preservation helps to increase the protein content in deep frying.

Here the effects of the natural preservatives are prominent for boiling and open pan dry roasting. They mostly help to increase the protein content, whereas KMS preservation is effective for increasing protein content in deep frying. They probably help to modify the native structure and thus retention occurs and in some cases the content is more than the raw state. The content becomes concentrated possibly due to the loss of moisture for the effect of prolonged preservation with natural preservatives as well as the application of heat during cooking[48]. Some chemical rearrangement may also occur, thus the proteins that are present in bound form are released and the contents become high after cooking.

Fig. 5.2.2.2 Graphical representation of Protein content of *Katla* with respect to different conditions

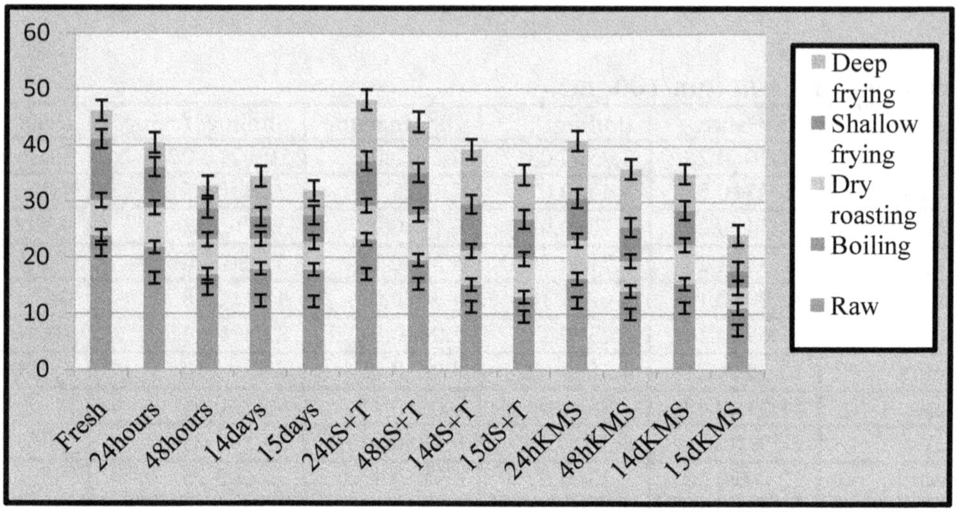

This graphical representation indicates that among all the preservation conditions, **24 hours preservation with salt and turmeric**[55] helps to increase the protein content in all the cooking methods. The possible reason for this may be the moisture loss due to prolonged preservation that helps to concentrate the amount of protein and the efficiency of salt and turmeric to inhibit the microbial growth and in turn the restoration of nutrient[52]. The graph also shows that salt and turmeric preservation comparatively increases the protein content more than that which is the control preservation without preservative and KMS preservation.

Table no 5.2.2.3 ANOVA with regard to cooking conditions and preservation methods

Condition	Differences	Sum of Squares	df	Mean Square	F	Sig.
Fresh (control)	Between Groups	644.037	4	161.009	9.599E3	.000(S)
	Within Groups	.168	10	.017		
	Total	644.205	14			
24 hours (control)	Between Groups	275.303	4	68.826	912.325	.000(S)
	Within Groups	.754	10	.075		
	Total	276.058	14			
48 hours (control)	Between Groups	248.870	4	62.217	2.056E3	.000(S)
	Within Groups	.303	10	.030		
	Total	249.173	14			
14 days (control)	Between Groups	125.819	4	31.455	67.813	.000(S)
	Within Groups	4.638	10	.464		
	Total	130.458	14			
15 days (control)	Between Groups	129.289	4	32.322	2.093E3	.000(S)
	Within Groups	.154	10	.015		
	Total	129.444	14			
24 hours (salt & turmeric)	Between Groups	253.891	4	63.473	9.876E3	.000(S)
	Within Groups	.064	10	.006		
	Total	253.956	14			
48 hours (salt & turmeric)	Between Groups	198.934	4	49.733	4.156E3	.000(S)
	Within Groups	.120	10	.012		
	Total	199.053	14			
14 days (salt & turmeric)	Between Groups	104.002	4	26.000	645.172	.000(S)
	Within Groups	.403	10	.040		
	Total	104.405	14			
15 days (salt & turmeric)	Between Groups	59.648	4	14.912	742.879	.000(S)
	Within Groups	.201	10	.020		
	Total	59.849	14			
24 hours (KMS)	Between Groups	112.939	4	28.235	476.564	.000(S)
	Within Groups	.592	10	.059		
	Total	113.532	14			
48 hours (KMS)	Between Groups	98.828	4	24.707	339.474	.000(S)
	Within Groups	.728	10	.073		
	Total	99.555	14			
14 days (KMS)	Between Groups	77.307	4	19.327	266.427	.000(S)
	Within Groups	.725	10	.073		
	Total	78.032	14			
15 days (KMS)	Between Groups	41.420	4	10.355	88.972	.000(S)
	Within Groups	1.164	10	.116		
	Total	42.584	14			

$p<0.05$ S= Significant, NS= Non-significant. All abbreviations are on page so and so.

This statistical ANOVA table shows that all the values are significant, which means there is significant difference present in the values of protein content of *katla* among different cooking methods and the raw state in respect to fresh condition along with different preservation methods.

Table no 5.2.2.4 Post hoc Duncan statistical analysis

Preservation	Duration	Raw state	Boiling	Dry roasting	Shallow frying	Deep frying
Control	Fresh	B,O,S,Da	R,O,S,Db	R,B,S,Dc	R,B,O,Dd	R,B,O,Se
Control	24 hours	B,O,S,Da	R,O,S,Db	R,B,Df	R,B,Df	R,B,O,Se
Control	48 hours	B,O,S,Da	R,O,S,Db	R,B,S,Dc	R,B,O,Dd	R,B,O,Se
Control	14 days	B,O,S,Da	R,S,Dg	R,S,Dg	R,B,O,Dd	R,B,O,Se
Control	15 days	B,O,S,Da	R,O,S,Db	R,B,Df	R,B,Df	R,B,O,Se
Salt & Turmeric	24 hours	B,O,S,Da	R,O,S,Db	R,B,S,Dc	R,B,O,Dd	R,B,O,Se
Salt & Turmeric	48 hours	B,O,S,Da	R,O,S,Db	R,B,S,Dc	R,B,O,Dd	R,B,O,Se
Salt & Turmeric	14 days	B,O,S,Da	R,O,S,Db	R,B,S,Dc	R,B,O,Dd	R,B,O,Se
Salt & Turmeric	15days	B,O,S,Da	R,O,S,Db	R,B,S,Dc	R,B,O,Dd	R,B,O,Se
KMS	24 hours	B,O,S,Da	R,O,S,Db	R,B,S,Dc	R,B,O,Dd	R,B,O,Se
KMS	48 hours	B,O,Sh	R,O,S,Db	R,B,S,Dc	R,B,O,Dd	B,O,Sh
KMS	14 days	B,O,S,Da	R,O,S,Db	R,B,Si	R,B,Oj	R,BK
KMS	15 days	B,O,S,Da	R,S,Dg	R,S,Dg	R,B,O,Dd	R,B,O,Se

R= Raw state, B= Boiling, O= Open pan dry roasting, S= Shallow frying, D= Deep frying. The same uppercase alphabets represent that there is no significant difference present among the variables.

This table shows the significant difference among the different variables such as cooking methods and preservation methods. The raw state significantly differs from boiling, open pan dry roasting, shallow frying and deep frying in all of the preservation methods with preservatives and control preservation without preservative except in 48 hours KMS preservation. Boiling significantly differs from the raw state, open pan dry roasting, shallow frying and deep frying in all the preservation conditions except in 14 days control preservation without preservative and 15 days KMS preservation. Open pan dry roasting significantly differs from the raw state, boiling, shallow frying and deep frying in all of the preservation conditions except in 24 hours, 14 days, and 15 days control preservation without preservative along with 14 days KMS preservation. Shallow frying significantly differs from the raw state, boiling, open pan dry roasting and deep frying in all the preservation conditions except in 24 hours and 15 days control preservation without preservative and 14 days KMS preservation. Deep frying significantly differs from the raw state, boiling, open pan dry roasting and shallow frying in all of the preservation conditions except in 48 hours and 14 days KMS preservation.

Shallow frying and open pan dry roasting significantly differ from the raw state, boiling and deep frying in 24 hours and 15 days control preservation without preservative. Boiling and open pan dry roasting significantly differ from the raw state, shallow frying and deep frying in 14 days control preservation without preservative and 15 days KMS preservation. The raw state and deep frying significantly differ from boiling, open pan dry roasting and shallow frying in 48 hours KMS preservation. Open pan dry roasting in 14 days KMS preservation significantly differs from the raw state, boiling and shallow frying. Shallow frying significantly differs from the raw state, boiling and open pan dry roasting in 14 days KMS preservation. Moreover, deep frying significantly differs from the raw state and boiling in 14 days KMS preservation.

Table no 5.2.2.5 Gradation of cooking methods from higher to lower restoration with respect to preservation days

Preservation	Duration	Method 1	Method 2	Method 3	Method 4	Method 5
Control	Fresh	R	SF	OPDR	DF	B
Control	24 hours	R	SF	OPDR	B	DF
Control	48 hours	R	OPDR	SF	DF	B
Control	14 days	R	DF	B	OPDR	SF
Control	15 days	R	B	OPDR	SF	DF
Salt & Turmeric	24 hours	R	DF	SF	B	OPDR
Salt & Turmeric	48 hours	R	DF	OPDR	SF	B
Salt & Turmeric	14 days	R	DF	SF	OPDR	B
Salt &Turmeric	15 days	R	DF	SF	OPDR	B
KMS	24 hours	R	DF	SF	OPDR	B
KMS	48 hours	DF	R	SF	OPDR	B
KMS	14 days	R	OPDR	DF	SF	B
KMS	15 days	R	DF	B	OPDR	SF

R= Raw state, B= Boiling, OPDR= Open pan dry roasting, SF= Shallow frying, DF= Deep frying. Same colour represents the similar order.

In all the preservation methods and fresh condition, protein retention mainly occurs in the raw state than the other cooking methods. In fresh condition, retention occurs firstly in the raw state then shallow frying, open pan dry roasting, deep frying and boiling. In 24 hours control preservation without preservative, the order changes from the raw state to shallow frying, open pan dry roasting, boiling and deep frying. In 48 hours control preservation without preservative, the order is the raw state, open pan dry roasting, shallow frying, deep frying and boiling. In 14 days control preservation without preservative, the order becomes the raw state, deep frying, boiling, open pan dry roasting and shallow frying. In 15 days control preservation without preservative, the order becomes the raw state, boiling, open pan dry roasting, shallow frying and deep frying.

In 24 hours salt and turmeric preservation, the order of retention changes from the raw state to deep frying, shallow frying, boiling and open pan dry roasting. In 48 hours salt and turmeric preservation, the order is the raw state, deep frying, open pan dry roasting, shallow frying and boiling. In 14 days, 15 days salt and turmeric preservation as well as 24 hours KMS preservation, the order changes from the raw state to deep frying, shallow frying, open pan dry roasting and boiling.

In 48 hours KMS preservation, it changes in the order of deep frying, raw state, shallow frying, open pan dry roasting and boiling. In 14 days KMS preservation, the order becomes the raw state, open pan dry roasting, deep frying, shallow frying and boiling. In 15 days KMS preservation, the order changes from the raw state to deep frying, boiling, open pan dry roasting and then shallow frying.

The overall analysis of protein content of *katla* is mostly restored by the gradation of methods as the raw state>deep frying> shallow frying>open pan dry roasting>boiling.

Frying mainly restores[66] the nutrients as the oil can possibly create a protective layer so that the protein cannot be leached out, but in boiling the soluble protein parts get dissolved, causing reduction in the content, and discarding the boiling water can also be the possible cause for the loss of protein content. In open pan dry roasting the protein possibly gets charred, resulting in losses. Moreover, *katla* contains more fat than *rohu,* so it is an additional protective layer for reduced elimination of protein in deep frying. Thus among the all the studied conventional cooking methods, **deep frying** is beneficial to restore protein in *katla.*

5.2.3 Prawn (*Fenneropenaeus indicus*)

It has been reported that prawn contains 19.1 gm of protein per 100 gm[85] in the raw condition. This value changes due to the application of different cooking methods and preservation conditions (vide Table no **5.2.3.1**).

Table no 5.2.3.1 Protein content of Prawn (gm/100gm)

Preservation	Duration	Raw state	Boiling	Dry roasting	Shallow frying	Deep frying
Control	Fresh	17.36±0.27	2.59±0.14	6.50±0.02	6.48±0.07	11.12±0.02
Control	24 hours	14.20±0.28	4.60±0.02	6.99±0.09	6.51±0.08	7.17±0.15
Control	48 hours	12.69±0.27	3.60±0.09	5.06±0.05	5.08±0.08	6.57±0.13
Control	14 days	17.00±0.25	6.40±0.08	12.35±0.22	10.20±0.20	14.95±0.31
Control	15 days	14.75±0.25	10.00±0.39	7.51±0.08	9.99±0.41	16.93±0.41
Salt & Turmeric	24 hours	16.75±0.25	7.30±0.39	11.30±0.44	8.88±0.25	9.41±0.59
Salt & Turmeric	48 hours	16.00±0.25	6.79±0.80	8.69±0.44	10.17±0.21	11.55±0.33
Salt & Turmeric	14 days	16.42±0.52	8.08±0.68	12.23±0.09	11.10±0.23	12.01±0.31
Salt & Turmeric	15 days	15.75±1.00	9.23±0.39	14.34±0.44	8.60±0.63	14.52±0.36
KMS	24 hours	18.25±0.25	15.76±0.39	14.63±0.66	8.75±0.41	14.34±0.32
KMS	48 hours	11.25±0.25	6.79±0.59	8.26±0.43	5.83±0.42	7.26±0.33
KMS	14 days	20.75±0.25	7.46±0.21	15.50±0.66	11.00±0.22	16.70±0.31
KMS	15 days	13.85±0.13	7.30±0.38	12.60±0.43	11.69±0.37	15.29±0.59

Values are expressed as mean±SD. ☐ Loss ☐ Restoration

Red digits represent the significant highest values from the raw state in two conditions.

In all the preservation conditions except in 15 days control preservation without preservative and 15 days salt and turmeric preservation and 24 hours, 48 hours KMS preservation, protein losses occur mainly by boiling, whereas open pan dry roasting decreases the protein content in 15 days control preservation without preservative. In 15 days salt and turmeric preservation and 24 hours, 48 hours KMS preservation, protein losses occurs by shallow frying.

Most of the retention occurs in deep frying,[32] but in 24 hours, 14 days salt and turmeric preservation and 24 hours, 48 hours KMS preservation, protein retention occurs by open pan dry roasting. 14 days preservation with KMS shows the highest protein content in all the cooking methods such as open pan dry roasted prawn as well as in the raw state, and 24 hours, 15 days KMS preservation shows the highest protein content in boiling and shallow frying respectively. Deep frying shows the highest protein content in 15 days control preservation without preservative. The highest values of protein present in the raw state in 14 days KMS preservation.

Here the effect of the synthetic preservative is prominent. It helps to increase mostly the protein content, probably because it helps to modify the structure of protein and thus retention occurs. In some cases the content is more than the raw state that is achieved by deep frying in 15 days KMS preservation and also in 15 days control preservation without preservative. The protein becomes concentrated possibly due to the loss of moisture for the effect of prolonged preservation with synthetic preservative as well as the application of heat during cooking[48]. There may be some chemical rearrangement occurring so that the proteins that are present in bound form may get released, the content becoming high after cooking. Moreover, protein denaturation occurs due to the application of heat during cooking.

Fig. 5.2.3.2 Graphical representation of Protein content of Prawn with respect to different conditions

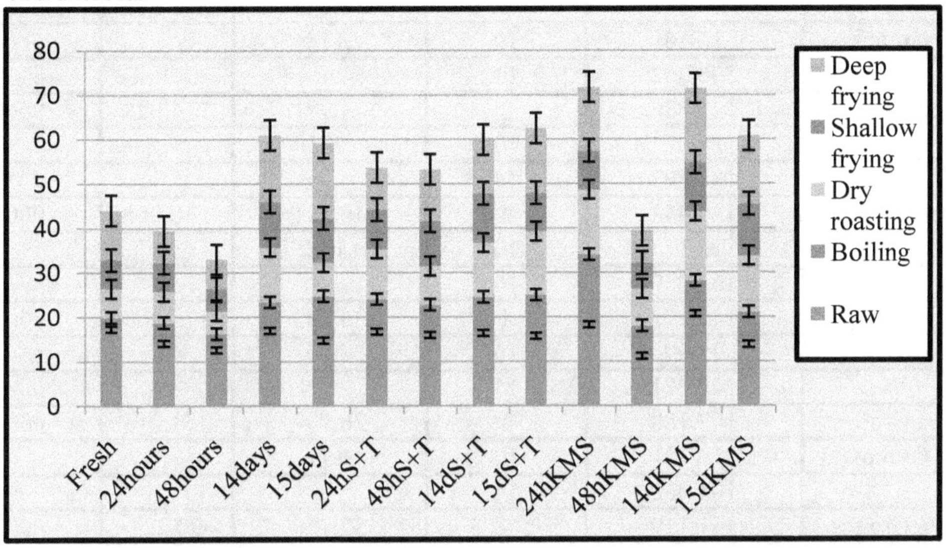

This graphical representation indicates that among all the preservation conditions, **24 hours and 14 days preservation with KMS**[59] help to increase the protein content in all the cooking methods. A possible reason for this may be the moisture loss due to prolonged preservation that helps to concentrate the amount of protein and the efficiency of KMS to inhibit the microbial growth in prawn and in turn the restoration of protein occurs[39]. The graph also shows that KMS preservation comparatively increases the protein contents more than that which is control preservation without preservative and salt and turmeric preservation.

Table no 5.2.3.3 ANOVA with regard to cooking conditions and preservation methods

Condition	Differences	Sum of Squares	df	Mean Square	F	Sig.
Fresh (control)	Between Groups	383.551	4	95.888	4.986E3	.000(S)
	Within Groups	.192	10	.019		
	Total	383.744	14			
24 hours (control)	Between Groups	161.643	4	40.411	1.730E3	.000(S)
	Within Groups	.234	10	.023		
	Total	161.877	14			
48 hours (control)	Between Groups	152.405	4	38.101	1.782E3	.000(S)
	Within Groups	.214	10	.021		
	Total	152.619	14			
14 days (control)	Between Groups	204.585	4	51.146	287.911	.000(S)
	Within Groups	1.776	10	.178		
	Total	206.362	14			
15 days (control)	Between Groups	179.886	4	44.971	224.028	.000(S)
	Within Groups	2.007	10	.201		
	Total	181.893	14			
24 hours (salt & turmeric)	Between Groups	160.442	4	40.111	248.055	.000(S)
	Within Groups	1.617	10	.162		
	Total	162.059	14			
48 hours (salt & turmeric)	Between Groups	145.172	4	36.293	172.868	.000(S)
	Within Groups	2.099	10	.210		
	Total	147.271	14			
14 days (salt & turmeric)	Between Groups	107.188	4	26.797	151.213	.000(S)
	Within Groups	1.772	10	.177		
	Total	108.960	14			
15 days (salt & turmeric)	Between Groups	131.119	4	32.780	90.223	.000(S)
	Within Groups	3.633	10	.363		
	Total	134.753	14			
24 hours (KMS)	Between Groups	146.056	4	36.514	197.879	.000(S)
	Within Groups	1.845	10	.185		
	Total	147.901	14			
48 hours (KMS)	Between Groups	51.809	4	12.952	73.721	.000(S)
	Within Groups	1.757	10	.176		
	Total	53.566	14			
14 days (KMS)	Between Groups	319.542	4	79.885	580.057	.000(S)
	Within Groups	1.377	10	.138		
	Total	320.919	14			
15 days (KMS)	Between Groups	109.971	4	27.493	162.800	.000(S)
	Within Groups	1.689	10	.169		
	Total	111.659	14			

$p<0.05$ S= Significant, NS= Non-significant. All abbreviations are on page so and so.

This statistical ANOVA table shows that all the values are significant, which means there is significant difference present in the values of protein content of prawn among different cooking methods and the raw state in respect to fresh condition along with different preservation methods.

Table no 5.2.3.4 Post hoc Duncan statistical analysis

Preservation	Duration	Raw state	Boiling	Dry roasting	Shallow frying	Deep frying
Control	Fresh	B,O,S,D^{a}	R,O,S,D^{b}	R,B,D^{c}	R,B,D^{c}	R,B,O,S^{d}
Control	24 hours	B,O,S,D^{a}	R,O,S,D^{b}	R,B,S^{e}	R,B,O,D^{f}	R,B,S^{e}
Control	48 hours	B,O,S,D^{a}	R,O,S,D^{b}	R,B,D^{c}	R,B,D^{c}	R,B,O,S^{d}
Control	14 days	B,O,S,D^{a}	R,O,S,D^{b}	R,B,S,D^{g}	R,B,O,D^{f}	R,B,O,S^{d}
Control	15 days	B,O,S,D^{a}	R,O,D^{h}	R,B,S,D^{g}	R,O,D^{h}	R,B,O,S^{d}
Salt & Turmeric	24 hours	B,O,S,D^{a}	R,O,S,D^{b}	R,B,S,D^{g}	R,B,O^{i}	R,B,O^{i}
Salt & Turmeric	48 hours	B,O,S,D^{a}	R,O,S,D^{b}	R,B,S,D^{g}	R,B,O,D^{f}	R,B,O,S^{d}
Salt & Turmeric	14 days	B,O,S,D^{a}	R,O,S,D^{b}	R,B,S^{j}	R,B,O,D^{f}	R,B,S^{j}
Salt & Turmeric	15 days	B,O,S,D^{a}	R,O,D^{h}	R,B,S^{j}	R,O,D^{h}	R,B,S^{j}
KMS	24 hours	B,O,S,D^{a}	R,O,S,D^{b}	R,B,S^{j}	R,B,O,D^{f}	R,B,S^{j}
KMS	48 hours	B,O,S,D^{a}	R,O,S^{k}	R,B,S,D^{g}	R,B,O,D^{f}	R,O,S^{k}
KMS	14 days	B,O,S,D^{a}	R,O,S,D^{b}	R,B,S,D^{g}	R,B,O,D^{f}	R,B,O,S^{d}
KMS	15 days	B,O,S,D^{a}	R,O,S,D^{b}	R,B,S,D^{g}	R,B,O,D^{f}	R,B,O,S^{d}

R= Raw state, B= Boiling, O= Open pan dry roasting, S= Shallow frying, D= Deep frying. The same uppercase alphabets represent that there is no significant difference present among the variables.

This table shows the significant difference among the different variables such as cooking methods and preservation conditions. The raw state significantly differs from boiling, open pan dry roasting, shallow frying and deep frying in all of the preservation methods with both the natural and synthetic preservatives and control preservation without preservative. Boiling significantly differs from the raw state, open pan dry roasting, shallow frying and deep frying in all the preservation conditions except in 15 days control preservation without preservative as well as salt and turmeric preservation and 48 hours KMS preservation.

Open pan dry roasting significantly differs from the raw state, boiling, shallow frying and deep frying in all the preservation conditions except in fresh condition, 24 hours, 48 hours control preservation without preservative along with 14 days, 15 days salt and turmeric preservation as well as in 24 hours KMS preservation. Shallow frying significantly differs from the raw state, boiling, open pan dry roasting, deep frying in all the preservation conditions except in fresh condition, 48 hours and 15 days control preservation without preservative and 24 hours, 15 days salt and turmeric preservation. Deep frying significantly differs from the raw state, boiling, open pan dry roasting and shallow frying in all of the preservation conditions except in 24 hours control preservation without preservative, 14 days, 15 days salt and turmeric preservation as well as in 24 hours, 48 hours KMS preservation.

Shallow frying and open pan dry roasting significantly differ from the raw state, boiling and deep frying in fresh condition and 48 hours control preservation without preservative. Both deep frying and open pan dry roasting significantly differ from the raw state, boiling and shallow frying in 24 hours control preservation without preservative. Boiling and shallow frying significantly differ from the raw state, open pan dry roasting and deep frying in 15 days control preservation without preservative as well as salt and turmeric preservation. Shallow frying and deep frying significantly differ from the raw state, boiling and open pan dry roasting in 24 hours salt and turmeric preservation. Moreover, open pan dry roasting and deep frying significantly differ from the raw state, boiling and shallow frying in 14 days and 15 days salt and turmeric preservation as well as in 24 hours KMS preservation. Boiling and deep frying significantly differ from the raw state, open pan dry roasting and shallow frying in 48 hours KMS preservation.

Table no 5.2.3.5 Gradation of cooking methods from higher to lower restoration with respect to preservation days

Preservation	Duration	Method 1	Method 2	Method 3	Method 4	Method 5
Control	Fresh	R	DF	OPDR	SF	B
Control	24 hours	R	DF	OPDR	SF	B
Control	48 hours	R	DF	SF	OPDR	B
Control	14 days	R	DF	OPDR	SF	B
Control	15 days	DF	R	B	SF	OPDR
Salt &Turmeric	24 hours	R	OPDR	DF	SF	B
Salt & Turmeric	48 hours	R	DF	SF	OPDR	B
Salt & Turmeric	14 days	R	OPDR	DF	SF	B
Salt &Turmeric	15 days	R	DF	OPDR	B	SF
KMS	24 hours	R	B	OPDR	DF	SF
KMS	48 hours	R	OPDR	DF	B	SF
KMS	14 days	R	DF	OPDR	SF	B
KMS	15 days	DF	R	OPDR	SF	B

R= Raw state, B= Boiling, OPDR= Open pan dry roasting, SF= Shallow frying, DF= Deep frying. Same colours represent the similar order.

In all the preservation methods and fresh condition, protein retention occurs mainly in the raw state than the other cooking methods. In fresh condition, 24 hours, 48 hours, 14 days control preservation without preservative as well as in 14 days KMS preservation, retention occurs firstly in the raw state followed by deep frying, open pan dry roasting, shallow frying and boiling. In 48 hours control preservation without preservative as well as salt and turmeric preservation, it changes in the following order: the raw state, deep frying, shallow frying, open pan dry roasting and boiling. In 15 days control preservation without preservative, the order changes to deep frying, raw state, boiling, shallow frying and open pan dry roasting. In 24 hours, 14 days salt and turmeric preservation, the order changes from the raw state, open pan dry roasting, deep frying, shallow frying and boiling. In 15 days salt and turmeric preservation, the order is the raw state, deep frying, open pan dry roasting, boiling and shallow frying.

In 24 hours KMS preservation, it changes in the order of the raw state, boiling, open pan dry roasting, deep frying and then shallow frying. In 48 hours KMS preservation, the order changes from the raw state to open pan dry roasting, deep frying, boiling and then shallow frying. In 15 days KMS preservation, it remains deep frying, raw state, open pan dry roasting, shallow frying and boiling.

The overall analysis of protein content of prawn is mostly restored by the gradation of methods as the raw state>deep frying> open pan dry roasting> shallow frying >boiling.

Deep frying mainly restores[66] the nutrients as the oil can possibly create a protective layer so that the protein cannot be leached out, but in boiling the soluble protein parts get dissolved and the content is reduced, and discarding the boiling water can also be the possible cause for the loss of protein content. In open pan dry roasting, loss occurs as the proteins possibly get charred. Shallow frying can also reduce the protein content as small amount of oil is used to fry prawn which cannot cover the full surface area and thus possibly the little protection is created. Thus among all the studied conventional cooking methods, **deep frying** is the best method for cooking prawn to restore protein content. Prawn is a rich source of protein.

5.2.4 Lobster (*Macrobrachium rosenbergii*)

It has been reported that lobster contains 20.5 gm of protein per 100 gm[85] in the raw condition. This value changes due to the application of different cooking methods and preservation conditions (vide Table no **5.2.4.1**).

Table no 5.2.4.1 Protein content of Lobster (gm/100gm)

Preservation	Duration	Raw state	Boiling	Dry roasting	Shallow frying	Deep frying
Control	Fresh	19.20±0.20	8.69±0.11	7.96±0.04	9.53±0.04	13.60±0.11
Control	24 hours	16.06±0.05	6.70±0.16	7.06±0.05	7.63±0.14	9.03±0.11
Control	48 hours	11.72±0.56	5.63±0.17	5.85±0.05	5.90±0.05	6.25±0.04
Control	14 days	15.36±0.31	6.11±0.51	10.27±0.61	8.33±0.59	10.00±0.48
Control	15 days	15.25±0.25	12.89±0.51	8.40±0.40	7.43±0.59	12.37±0.48
Salt & Turmeric	24 hours	15.33±1.23	7.00±0.34	10.30±0.27	6.42±0.24	8.57±0.48
Salt & Turmeric	48 hours	17.00±0.25	5.33±0.33	10.43±0.43	6.26±0.24	8.25±0.73
Salt & Turmeric	14 days	17.25±0.25	10.33±0.33	12.68±0.25	10.00±0.39	8.90±0.29
Salt & Turmeric	15 days	21.08±1.01	15.22±1.26	12.40±0.40	16.53±0.39	18.27±0.26
KMS	24 hours	12.83±0.28	6.66±0.34	10.80±0.40	9.53±0.27	8.55±0.50
KMS	48 hours	13.41±0.38	5.33±0.67	12.40±0.40	7.30±0.39	8.57±0.47
KMS	14 days	18.00±0.66	12.26±0.23	18.40±1.05	12.30±0.39	11.90±0.48
KMS	15 days	20.00±0.25	9.10±0.51	20.40±0.40	13.46±0.39	26.06±0.67

Values are expressed as mean±SD. ☐ Loss ▒ Restoration

Red digits represent the significant highest values from the raw state in a single condition.

In all the preservation conditions except fresh condtion, 15 days control preservation without preservative, 24 hours, 14 days, 15 days preservation with salt and turmeric, protein losses mainly occurs by boiling, whereas open pan dry roasting decreases the protein content in fresh condition and 15 days preservation with salt and turmeric. Shallow frying reduces the protein content in 15 days control preservation without preservative and 24 hours salt and turmeric preservation. Deep frying also decreases the protein content in 14 days salt and turmeric preservation.

Most of the retention occurs in open pan dry roasting, but in fresh condition, 24 hours, 48 hours control preservation without preservative and 15 days preservation with salt and turmeric as well as KMS preservation, protein retention occurs by deep frying, whereas in 15 days control preservation without preservative shows the highest protein content in boiling. 15 days preservation with salt and turmeric shows the highest protein content in the raw state as well as in boiled and shallow fried lobster, but 15 days KMS preservation shows the highest protein content in open pan dry roasting and deep frying.

Here the effects of both the natural and synthetic preservatives are prominent. They help to increase mostly the protein content, probably by modifying the structure of protein and thus helping retention. In some cases the content is more than the raw state that occurs by deep frying in 15 days KMS preservation. The protein becomes concentrated possibly due to the loss of moisture for the effect of prolonged preservation with natural and synthetic preservatives as well as the application of heat during cooking[48]. There may be some chemical rearrangement that also occurs so that the proteins that are present in bound form may get released, the content becoming higher after cooking. Moreover, protein denaturation occurs due to the application of heat during cooking.

Fig. 5.2.4.2 Graphical representation of Protein content of Lobster with respect to different conditions

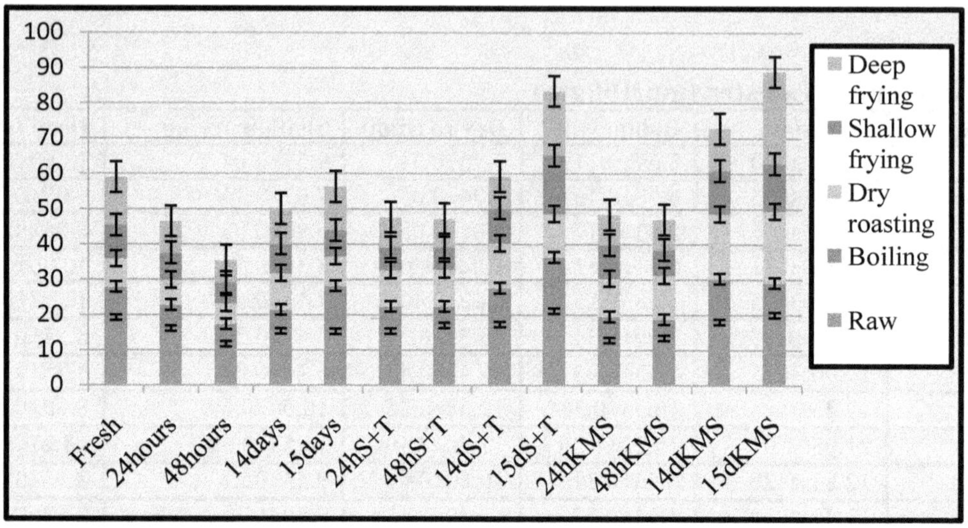

This graphical representation indicated that among all the preservation conditions, **15 days preservation with KMS**[59] helps to increase the protein content in all the cooking methods. The possible reason for this may be because of the moisture loss due to prolonged preservation that helps to concentrate the amount of protein and the efficiency of KMS to inhibit the microbial growth and in turn the restoration of nutrient. KMS is very much effective for both the crustaceans like prawn and lobster[39]. The graph also shows that KMS preservation comparatively increases the protein content more than that which is control preservation without preservative and salt and turmeric preservation.

Table no 5.2.4.3 ANOVA with regard to cooking conditions and preservation methods

Condition	Differences	Sum of Squares	df	Mean Square	F	Sig.
Fresh (control)	Between Groups	262.681	4	65.670	4.836E3	.000(S)
	Within Groups	.136	10	.014		
	Total	262.817	14			
24 hours (control)	Between Groups	181.024	4	45.256	3.575E3	.000(S)
	Within Groups	.127	10	.013		
	Total	181.151	14			
48 hours (control)	Between Groups	81.876	4	20.469	292.051	.000(S)
	Within Groups	.701	10	.070		
	Total	82.576	14			
14 days (control)	Between Groups	140.134	4	35.033	135.011	.000(S)
	Within Groups	2.595	10	.259		
	Total	142.729	14			
15 days (control)	Between Groups	127.984	4	31.996	152.207	.000(S)
	Within Groups	2.102	10	.210		
	Total	130.086	14			
24 hours (salt & turmeric)	Between Groups	153.899	4	38.475	96.858	.000(S)
	Within Groups	3.972	10	.397		
	Total	157.871	14			
48 hours (salt & turmeric)	Between Groups	259.704	4	64.926	346.395	.000(S)
	Within Groups	1.874	10	.187		
	Total	261.578	14			
14 days (salt & turmeric)	Between Groups	139.032	4	34.758	286.736	.000(S)
	Within Groups	1.212	10	.121		
	Total	140.245	14			
15 days (salt & turmeric)	Between Groups	127.190	4	31.797	53.225	.000(S)
	Within Groups	5.974	10	.597		
	Total	133.164	14			
24 hours (KMS)	Between Groups	64.792	4	16.198	119.408	.000(S)
	Within Groups	1.357	10	.136		
	Total	66.149	14			
48 hours (KMS)	Between Groups	140.367	4	35.092	155.466	.000(S)
	Within Groups	2.257	10	.226		
	Total	142.624	14			
14 days (KMS)	Between Groups	132.110	4	33.027	82.965	.000(S)
	Within Groups	3.981	10	.398		
	Total	136.090	14			
15 days (KMS)	Between Groups	522.798	4	130.700	602.765	.000(S)
	Within Groups	2.168	10	.217		
	Total	524.967	14			

$p<0.05$ S= Significant, NS= Non-significant. All abbreviations are on page so and so.

This statistical ANOVA table shows that all the values are significant, which means there is significant difference present in the values of protein content of lobster among different cooking methods and the raw state in respect to fresh condition along with different preservation methods.

Table no 5.2.4.4 Post hoc Duncan statistical analysis

Preservation	Duration	Raw state	Boiling	Dry roasting	Shallow frying	Deep frying
Control	Fresh	B,O,S,D^{a}	R,O,S,D^{b}	R,B,S,D^{c}	R,B,O,D^{d}	R,B,O,S^{e}
Control	24 hours	B,O,S,D^{a}	R,O,S,D^{b}	R,B,S,D^{c}	R,B,O,D^{d}	R,B,O,S^{e}
Control	48 hours	B,O,S,D^{a}	R,D^{f}	R^{g}	R^{g}	R,B^{h}
Control	14 days	B,O,S,D^{a}	R,O,S,D^{b}	R,B,S^{i}	R,B,O,D^{d}	R,B,S^{i}
Control	15 days	B,O,S,D^{a}	R,O,S^{j}	R,B,S,D^{c}	R,B,O,D^{d}	R,O,S^{j}
Salt & Turmeric	24 hours	B,O,S,D^{a}	R,O,D^{k}	R,B,S,D^{c}	R,O,D^{k}	R,B,O,S^{e}
Salt & Turmeric	48 hours	B,O,S,D^{a}	R,O,S,D^{b}	R,B,S,D^{c}	R,B,O,D^{d}	R,B,O,S^{e}
Salt & Turmeric	14 days	B,O,S,D^{a}	R,O,D^{k}	R,B,S,D^{c}	R,O,D^{k}	R,B,O,S^{e}
Salt & Turmeric	15 days	B,O,S,D^{a}	R,O,D^{k}	R,B,S,D^{c}	R,O,D^{k}	R,B,O,S^{e}
KMS	24 hours	B,O,S,D^{a}	R,O,S,D^{b}	R,B,S,D^{c}	R,B,O,D^{d}	R,B,O,S^{e}
KMS	48 hours	B,O,S,D^{a}	R,O,S,D^{b}	R,B,S,D^{c}	R,B,O,D^{d}	R,B,O,S^{e}
KMS	14 days	B,S,D^{l}	R,O^{m}	B,S,D^{l}	R,O^{m}	R,O^{m}
KMS	15 days	B,S,D^{l}	R,O,S,D^{b}	B,S,D^{l}	R,B,O,D^{d}	R,B,O,S^{e}

R= Raw state, B= Boiling, O= Open pan dry roasting, S= Shallow frying, D= Deep frying. The same uppercase alphabets signify that there is no significant difference present among the variables.

This table shows the significant difference among the different variables such as cooking methods and preservation conditions. The raw state significantly differs from boiling, open pan dry roasting, shallow frying and deep frying in all of the preservation methods with preservatives and control preservation without preservative except in 14 days and 15 days KMS preservation. Boiling significantly differs from the raw state, open pan dry roasting, shallow frying and deep frying in all of the preservation conditions except in 48 hours, 15 days control preservation without preservative and 24 hours, 14 days, 15 days salt and turmeric preservation as well as in 14 days KMS preservation. Open pan dry roasting significantly differs from the raw state, boiling, shallow frying and deep frying in all of the preservation conditions except in 48 hours control preservation without preservative and 14 days and 15 days KMS preservation. Shallow frying significantly differs from the raw state, boiling, open pan dry roasting, deep frying in all the preservation conditions except in 48 hours control preservation without preservative and 24 hours, 14 days, 15 days salt and turmeric preservation and 14 days KMS preservation. Deep frying significantly differs from the raw state, boiling, open pan dry roasting and shallow frying in all of the preservation conditions except in 48 hours, 14 days and 15 days control preservation without preservative and 14 days KMS preservation.

Boiling significantly differs from the raw state and deep frying in 48 hours control preservation without preservative. Shallow frying and open pan dry roasting significantly differ from the raw state in 48 hours control preservation without preservative. Deep frying significantly differs from the raw state, boiling in 48 hours control preservation without preservative. Open pan dry roasting and deep frying in 14 days control preservation without preservative significantly differ from the raw state, boiling and shallow frying, whereas boiling and deep frying significantly differ from the raw state, open pan dry roasting and shallow frying in 15 days control preservation without preservative. Again boiling and deep frying significantly differ from the raw state, open pan dry roasting and deep frying in 24 hours, 14 days and 15 days salt and turmeric preservation. Both the raw state and open pan dry roasting significantly differ from boiling, shallow frying and deep frying in 14 and 15 days KMS preservation. Moreover, boiling, shallow frying and deep frying significantly differ from the raw state and open pan dry roasting in 14 days KMS preservation.

Table no 5.2.4.5 Gradation of cooking methods from higher to lower restoration with respect to preservation days

Preservation	Duration	Method 1	Method 2	Method 3	Method 4	Method 5
Control	Fresh	R	DF	SF	B	OPDR
Control	24 hours	R	DF	SF	OPDR	B
Control	48 hours	R	DF	SF	OPDR	B
Control	14 days	R	OPDR	DF	SF	B
Control	15 days	R	B	DF	OPDR	SF
Salt & Turmeric	24 hours	R	OPDR	DF	B	SF
Salt & Turmeric	48 hours	R	OPDR	DF	SF	B
Salt & Turmeric	14 days	R	OPDR	B	SF	DF
Salt &Turmeric	15 days	R	DF	SF	B	OPDR
KMS	24 hours	R	OPDR	SF	DF	B
KMS	48 hours	R	OPDR	DF	SF	B
KMS	14 days	OPDR	R	SF	B	DF
KMS	15 days	DF	OPDR	R	SF	B

R= Raw state, B= Boiling, OPDR= Open pan dry roasting, SF= Shallow frying, DF= Deep frying. Same colours represent the similar order.

In all the preservation techniques and fresh condition, protein retention occurs mainly in the raw state rather than the other cooking methods. In fresh condition and 15 days salt and turmeric preservation, retention occurs firstly in the raw state then deep frying, shallow frying, boiling and open pan dry roasting. In 24 hours to 48 hours control preservation without preservative, the order changes to the raw state, deep frying, shallow frying, open pan dry roasting and boiling. In 14 days control preservation without preservative and 48 hours preservation with both salt and turmeric preservation as well as KMS preservation, the order is the raw state, open pan dry roasting, deep frying, shallow frying and boiling. In 15 days control preservation without preservative, the order becomes the raw state, boiling, deep frying, open pan dry roasting and shallow frying.

In 24 hours salt and turmeric preservation, the order changes from the raw state to open pan dry roasting, deep frying, boiling and then shallow frying. In 14 days salt and turmeric preservation, the order goes from the raw state to open pan dry roasting, boiling, shallow frying and deep frying.

In 24 hours KMS preservation, it changes in the order of the raw state, open pan dry roasting, shallow frying, deep frying and boiling. In 14 days KMS preservation, it remains in the order of open pan dry roasting, raw state, shallow frying, boiling and deep frying. In 15 days KMS preservation, the order changes to deep frying, open pan dry roasting, raw state, shallow frying and boiling.

The overall analysis of protein content of lobster is mostly restored by the gradation of methods as the raw state> open pan dry roasting > deep frying>shallow frying >boiling.

Open pan dry roasting helps to retain more nutrient as protein from lobster cannot be eliminated in this method. A possible reason may be the application of dry heat can help in molecular rearrangement, thus the complex protein structures are released, causing increased content of protein. Deep frying mainly restores[66] the nutrients as the oil can possibly create a protective layer so that the protein cannot be leached out, but in boiling the soluble protein parts get dissolved and the content is reduced, and discarding the boiling water can also be the possible cause for the loss of protein content. Shallow frying also reduces the protein content as small amount of oil is used for frying which cannot cover the full surface area of the lobster and thus possibly the little protection is created. Thus among the entire studied conventional cooking methods, **open pan dry roasting** is the best method for cooking lobster to restore protein content.

5.2.5 Pomfret (*Pampus argenteus*)

It has been reported that pomfret contains 19.02 gm of protein per 100 gm[85] in the raw condition. This value changes due to the application of different cooking methods and preservation conditions (vide Table no **5.2.5.1**).

Table no 5.2.5.1 Protein content of Pomfret (gm/100gm)

Preservation	Duration	Raw state	Boiling	Dry roasting	Shallow frying	Deep frying
Control	Fresh	16.36±0.31	4.22±0.20	6.24±0.04	6.82±0.02	7.93±0.12
Control	24 hours	15.06±0.05	3.36±0.05	5.74±0.10	5.97±0.02	7.42±0.19
Control	48 hours	10.49±0.09	2.74±0.04	5.11±0.10	5.23±0.20	6.53±0.13
Control	14 days	10.50±0.75	6.99±0.33	10.17±0.80	10.00±0.43	13.88±0.55
Control	15 days	7.50±0.25	6.66±0.33	11.04±0.52	10.43±0.43	10.00±0.55
Salt & Turmeric	24 hours	5.58±0.38	3.33±0.33	7.05±0.27	6.95±0.43	8.10±0.29
Salt &Turmeric	48 hours	6.13±0.12	2.83±0.17	5.55±0.26	6.52±0.43	7.23±0.55
Salt & Turmeric	14 days	5.50±0.25	4.00±0.33	10.52±0.52	6.52±0.43	8.51±0.85
Salt & Turmeric	15 days	7.50±0.25	3.33±0.33	8.40±0.55	6.95±0.43	7.75±0.25
KMS	24 hours	7.50±0.25	3.11±0.51	6.84±0.53	6.95±0.43	5.55±0.55
KMS	48 hours	6.12±0.13	2.44±0.51	5.26±0.53	6.95±0.44	7.45±0.29
KMS	14 days	5.50±0.25	3.33±0.33	6.31±0.53	4.34±0.44	6.11±0.55
KMS	15 days	6.25±0.25	3.77±0.30	6.84±0.53	9.13±0.44	13.86±0.56

Values are expressed as mean±SD. ☐ Loss ☐ Restoration

Red digits represent the significant highest values from the raw state in different conditions.

In all the preservation conditions both with and without preservatives including fresh condition, protein losses mainly occurs by boiling. Most of the retention occurs by deep frying, [32] but in 15 days control preservation and 14 days, 15 days salt and turmeric preservation as well as 14 days KMS preservation, protein retention occurs by open pan dry roasting, whereas in 24 hours KMS preservation, retention occurs by shallow frying.

15 days control preservation without preservative shows the highest protein content in open pan dry roasted and shallow fried pomfret, but in the raw state the highest protein content present in fresh condition, whereas 14 days control preservation without preservative shows the highest value of protein in boiling and deep frying methods.

The 15 days control preservation without preservative and 24 hours, 14 days, 15 days preservation with salt and turmeric, and 14 days, 15 days KMS preservation help to retain protein by open pan dry roasting more than the raw state, whereas 15 days control preservation without preservative, 24 hours, 48 hours, 14 days salt and turmeric preservation and 48 hours, 15 days KMS preservation, help to increase the protein content by shallow frying. The 14 days, 15 days control preservation without preservative, 24 hours, 48 hours, 14 days and 15 days salt and turmeric preservation, and 48 hours, 14 days, 15 days KMS preservation increase the protein content in deep fried pomfret more than the raw condition.

Here the effects of both the natural and synthetic preservatives are prominent, but the results show that the natural preservative is more effective than the synthetic preservative. They mostly help to increase the protein content compared to the raw state in open pan dry roasting, shallow frying and deep frying. They probably help to modify the conformation of protein, releasing the bound protein into free form, leading to retention. The protein becomes concentrated possibly due to the loss of moisture for the effect of prolonged preservation with natural and synthetic preservatives as well as the application of heat during cooking[48]. There may be some chemical rearrangement occurring due to cooking, so that the proteins that are present in bound form are liberated, the content becoming high after cooking. Moreover, protein denaturation occurs due to the application of heat during cooking.

Fig. 5.2.5.2 Graphical representation of Protein content of Pomfret with respect to different conditions

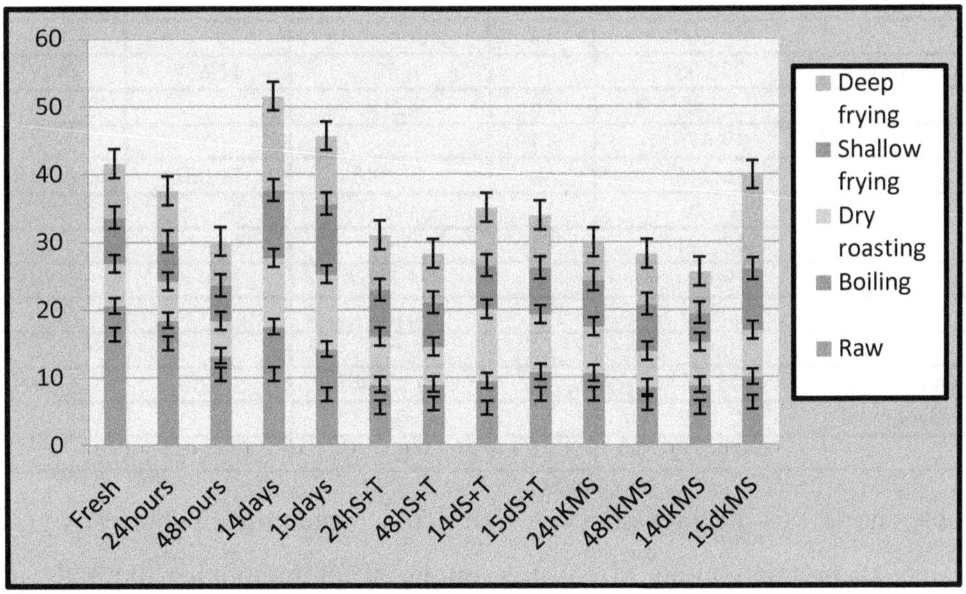

This graphical representation indicates that among all the preservation conditions, **14 days preservation without preservative** helps to increase the protein content in all the cooking methods. The possible reason for this may be because of the moisture loss due to prolonged preservation that helps to concentrate the amount of protein. The graph also shows that control preservation without preservative comparatively increases the protein content more than the salt and turmeric preservation and KMS preservation.

Table no 5.2.5.3 ANOVA with regard to cooking conditions and preservation methods

Condition	Differences	Sum of Squares	df	Mean Square	F	Sig.
Fresh (control)	Between Groups	264.543	4	66.136	2.096E3	.000(S)
	Within Groups	.315	10	.032		
	Total	264.858	14			
24 hours (control)	Between Groups	239.338	4	59.835	5.554E3	.000(S)
	Within Groups	.108	10	.011		
	Total	239.446	14			
48 hours (control)	Between Groups	97.358	4	24.340	1.506E3	.000(S)
	Within Groups	.162	10	.016		
	Total	97.520	14			
14 days (control)	Between Groups	71.700	4	17.925	49.281	.000(S)
	Within Groups	3.637	10	.364		
	Total	75.337	14			
15 days (control)	Between Groups	44.568	4	11.142	59.059	.000(S)
	Within Groups	1.887	10	.189		
	Total	46.455	14			
24 hours (salt & turmeric)	Between Groups	42.515	4	10.629	66.156	.000(S)
	Within Groups	1.607	10	.161		
	Total	44.121	14			
48 hours (salt & turmeric)	Between Groups	34.090	4	8.523	69.507	.000(S)
	Within Groups	1.226	10	.123		
	Total	35.316	14			
14 days (salt & turmeric)	Between Groups	78.622	4	19.655	72.155	.000(S)
	Within Groups	2.724	10	.272		
	Total	81.346	14			
15 days (salt & turmeric)	Between Groups	48.048	4	12.012	82.735	.000(S)
	Within Groups	1.452	10	.145		
	Total	49.500	14			
24 hours (KMS)	Between Groups	37.288	4	9.322	42.607	.000(S)
	Within Groups	2.188	10	.219		
	Total	39.476	14			
48 hours (KMS)	Between Groups	46.745	4	11.686	71.001	.000(S)
	Within Groups	1.646	10	.165		
	Total	48.391	14			
14 days (KMS)	Between Groups	19.024	4	4.756	25.043	.000(S)
	Within Groups	1.899	10	.190		
	Total	20.923	14			
15 days (KMS)	Between Groups	173.537	4	43.384	197.662	.000(S)
	Within Groups	2.195	10	.219		
	Total	175.732	14			

$p<0.05$ S= Significant, NS= Non-significant. All abbreviations are on page so and so.

This statistical ANOVA table shows that all the values are significant, which means there is significant difference present in the values of protein content of pomfret among different cooking methods and the raw state in respect to fresh condition along with different preservation methods.

Table no 5.2.5.4 Post hoc Duncan statistical analysis

Preservation	Duration	Raw state	Boiling	Dry roasting	Shallow frying	Deep frying
Control	Fresh	B,O,S,D^{a}	R,O,S,D^{b}	R,B,S,D^{c}	R,B,O,D^{d}	R,B,O,S^{e}
Control	24 hours	B,O,S,D^{a}	R,O,S,D^{b}	R,B,S,D^{c}	R,B,O,D^{d}	R,B,O,S^{e}
Control	48 hours	B,O,S,D^{a}	R,O,S,D^{b}	R,B,D^{f}	R,B,D^{f}	R,B,O,S^{e}
Control	14 days	B,D^{g}	R,O,S,D^{b}	B,D^{g}	B,D^{g}	R,B,O,S^{e}
Control	15 days	B,O,S,D^{a}	R,O,S,D^{b}	R,B,D^{f}	R,B^{h}	R,B,O^{i}
Salt & Turmeric	24 hours	B,O,S,D^{a}	R,O,S,D^{b}	R,B,D^{f}	R,B,D^{f}	R,B,O,S^{e}
Salt & Turmeric	48 hours	B,D^{g}	R,O,S,D^{b}	B,S,D^{j}	B,O,D^{k}	R,B,O,S^{e}
Salt & Turmeric	14 days	B,O,S,D^{a}	R,O,S,D^{b}	R,B,S,D^{c}	R,B,O,D^{d}	R,B,O,S^{e}
Salt & Turmeric	15 days	B,O^{l}	R,O,S,D^{b}	R,B,S^{m}	B,O,D^{k}	B,O^{l}
KMS	24 hours	B,D^{g}	R,O,S,D^{b}	B,D^{g}	B,D^{g}	R,B,O,S^{e}
KMS	48 hours	B,O,S,D^{a}	R,O,S,D^{b}	R,B,S,D^{c}	R,B,O^{i}	R,B,O^{i}
KMS	14 days	B,S^{n}	R,O,S,D^{b}	B,S^{n}	R,B,O,D^{d}	B,S^{n}
KMS	15 days	B,S,D^{j}	R,O,S,D^{b}	B,S,D^{j}	R,B,O,D^{d}	R,B,O,S^{e}

R= Raw state, B= Boiling, O= Open pan dry roasting, S= Shallow frying, D= Deep frying. The same uppercase alphabets represent that there is no significant difference present among the variables.

This table shows the significant difference among the different variables such as cooking methods and preservation conditions. The raw state significantly differs from boiling, open pan dry roasting, shallow frying and deep frying in all of the preservation methods with preservatives and control preservation without preservative except in 14 days control preservation without preservative, 48 hours, 15 days salt and turmeric preservation as well as 24 hours, 14 and 15 days KMS preservation. Boiling significantly differs from the raw state, open pan dry roasting, shallow frying and deep frying in all the preservation conditions. Open pan dry roasting significantly differs from the raw state, boiling, shallow and deep frying in fresh condition and 24 hours control preservation without preservative, 14 days salt and turmeric preservation along with 48 hours KMS preservation.

Shallow frying significantly differs from the raw state, boiling, open pan dry roasting and deep frying in fresh condition and 24 hours control preservation without preservative and 14 days salt and turmeric preservation as well as 14 days, 15 days KMS preservation. Deep frying significantly differs from the raw state, boiling, open pan dry roasting and shallow frying in all of the preservation conditions except in 15 days control preservation without preservative as well as salt and turmeric preservation and 48 hours, 14 days KMS preservation.

Shallow frying and open pan dry roasting significantly differ from the raw state, boiling and deep frying in 48 hours control preservation without preservative and 24 hours salt and turmeric preservation, whereas only open pan dry roasting significantly differs from the raw state, boiling and deep frying in 15 days control preservation without preservative. Again the raw state, shallow frying and open pan dry roasting significantly differ from boiling and deep frying in 14 days control preservation without preservative and 24 hours KMS preservation. The raw state significantly differs from boiling and deep frying in 48 hours salt and turmeric preservation. Shallow frying significantly differs from the raw state and boiling in 15 days control preservation without preservative, whereas deep frying significantly differs from the raw state, boiling and open pan dry roasting in 15 days control preservation without preservative. Both shallow frying and deep frying significantly differ from the raw state, boiling and open pan dry roasting in 48 hours KMS preservation. The raw state and open pan dry roasting significantly differ from boiling, shallow frying and deep frying in 15 days KMS preservation, and only open pan dry roasting significantly differs from boiling, shallow frying and deep frying in 48 hours salt and turmeric preservation.

Shallow frying in 48 hours and 15 days salt and turmeric preservation, significantly differs from boiling, open pan dry roasting and deep frying. The raw state and deep frying significantly differ from boiling and open pan dry roasting in 15 days salt and turmeric preservation. Open pan dry roasting significantly differs from the raw state, boiling, and shallow frying in 15 days salt and turmeric preservation. The raw state, open pan dry roasting and deep frying significantly differ from boiling and shallow frying in 14 days KMS preservation.

Table no 5.2.5.5 Gradation of cooking methods from higher to lower restoration with respect to preservation days

Preservation	Duration	Method 1	Method 2	Method 3	Method 4	Method 5
Control	Fresh	R	DF	SF	OPDR	B
Control	24 hours	R	DF	SF	OPDR	B
Control	48 hours	R	DF	SF	OPDR	B
Control	14 days	DF	R	OPDR	SF	B
Control	15 days	OPDR	SF	DF	R	B
Salt &Turmeric	24 hours	DF	OPDR	SF	R	B
Salt & Turmeric	48 hours	DF	SF	R	OPDR	B
Salt & Turmeric	14 days	OPDR	DF	SF	R	B
Salt &Turmeric	15 days	OPDR	DF	R	SF	B
KMS	24 hours	R	SF	OPDR	DF	B
KMS	48 hours	DF	SF	R	OPDR	B
KMS	14 days	R	OPDR	SF	DF	B
KMS	15 days	DF	SF	OPDR	R	B

R= Raw state, B= Boiling, OPDR= Open pan dry roasting, SF= Shallow frying, DF= Deep frying. Same colours represent the similar order.

In all the preservation methods and fresh condition, protein retention occurs mainly in the raw state than the other cooking methods. In fresh condition, 24 hours, 48 hours control preservation without preservative, retention occurs firstly in the raw state then deep frying, shallow frying, open pan dry roasting and boiling. In 14 days control preservation without preservative, the order changes from deep frying to the raw state, open pan dry roasting, shallow frying and boiling. In 15 days control preservation without preservative the order changes from open pan dry roasting to shallow frying, deep frying, raw state and boiling.

In 24 hours salt and turmeric preservation, the order is deep frying, open pan dry roasting shallow frying, raw state and boiling. In 48 hours salt and turmeric as well as 48 hours KMS preservation, the order changes from deep frying to shallow frying, raw state, open pan dry roasting and boiling. In 14 days salt and turmeric preservation, the order remains open pan dry roasting, deep frying, shallow frying, raw state and boiling. In 15 days salt and turmeric preservation, the order is open pan dry roasting, deep frying, raw state, shallow frying and boiling.

In 24 hours KMS preservation, the order becomes the raw state, shallow frying, open pan dry roasting, deep frying and boiling. In 14 days KMS preservation, the order remains the raw state, open pan dry roasting, shallow frying, deep frying and boiling. In 15 days KMS preservation, it remains in the order of deep frying, shallow frying, open pan dry roasting, raw state and boiling.

The overall analysis of protein content of pomfret is mostly restored by the gradation of methods as the raw state>deep frying > shallow frying > open pan dry roasting >boiling.

Frying mainly restores[66] the nutrients as the oil can possibly create a protective layer so that the protein cannot be leached out, but in boiling the soluble protein parts get dissolved, resulting in the reduction of content, and discarding the boiling water can also be the possible cause for the loss of protein content. In open pan dry roasting the protein possibly gets charred, resulting in losses and as pomfret is a sea fish, the application of dry heat can help to melt the protective layer of fat, causing the loss of protein. Thus among all the studied conventional cooking methods, **deep frying** is the best method for cooking pomfret to restore protein content.

5.2.6 *Hilsa* (*Tenualosa Ilisha*)

It has been reported that *hilsa* contains 21.80 gm of protein per 100 gm[84] in the raw condition. This value changes due to the application of different cooking methods and preservation conditions (vide Table no **5.2.6.1**).

Table no 5.2.6.1 Protein content of *Hilsa* (gm/100gm)

Preservation	Duration	Raw state	Boiling	Dry roasting	Shallow frying	Deep frying
Control	Fresh	24.07±0.11	6.58±0.20	9.64±0.18	10.73±0.17	11.92±0.11
Control	24 hours	20.53±0.04	3.92±0.09	6.10±0.02	6.56±0.12	7.90±0.12
Control	48 hours	17.42±0.20	3.53±0.04	5.56±0.04	5.89±0.04	7.85±0.05
Control	14 days	11.75±0.25	4.00±0.40	3.86±0.32	6.93±0.23	5.01±0.51
Control	15 days	11.42±0.87	4.84±0.41	4.09±0.19	2.96±0.37	3.85±0.30
Salt & Turmeric	24 hours	11.42±0.52	3.06±0.83	2.79±0.49	3.24±0.25	5.50±0.50
Salt & Turmeric	48 hours	14.66±0.38	4.53±0.61	3.02±0.17	5.92±0.37	10.50±0.50
Salt & Turmeric	14 days	14.16±0.63	2.93±0.61	3.37±0.16	3.33±0.37	5.50±0.50
Salt & Turmeric	15 days	5.25±0.25	2.80±0.40	2.98±0.44	3.36±0.40	3.50±0.50
KMS	24 hours	10.25±0.25	3.00±0.20	2.69±0.18	3.33±0.37	3.50±0.50
KMS	48 hours	11.75±0.25	4.81±0.40	3.22±0.32	4.74±0.28	14.28±0.26
KMS	14 days	8.25±0.25	4.80±0.40	4.45±0.24	2.71±0.57	8.95±0.51
KMS	15 days	3.12±0.13	1.20±0.40	2.06±0.17	2.85±0.23	3.50±0.50

Values are expressed as mean±SD. ☐ Loss ▨ Restoration

Red digits represent the significant highest values from the raw state in two conditions.

In most of the preservation conditions including fresh condition, protein losses mainly occurs by boiling, whereas in 14 days control preservation without preservative and 24 hours, 48 hours preservation with salt and turmeric as well as with KMS, losses occur by open pan dry roasting. In 15 days control preservation without preservative and 14 days KMS preservation, losses occur by shallow frying.

Most of the retention occurs by deep frying, [32] but in 14 days control preservation without preservative and 48 hours KMS preservation, protein retention occurs by shallow frying, whereas in 15 days control preservation without preservative, retention occurs by boiling.

Fresh condition shows the highest protein content in all the cooking methods such as boiling, open pan dry roasting, shallow frying and deep frying, including the raw state.

In 14 days and 15 days KMS preservation, deep frying shows the increased content of protein than the raw state. But the effect of natural technique is prominent as it helps to restore protein more than the other preservation conditions. It probably helps to modify the structure of protein leading to restoration. There may be some chemical rearrangement also occurs so that the proteins that are present in bound form may get released, the content becoming high after cooking. Moreover, protein denaturation occurs due to the application of heat during cooking.

Fig. 5.2.6.2 Graphical representation of Protein content of *Hilsa* with respect to different conditions

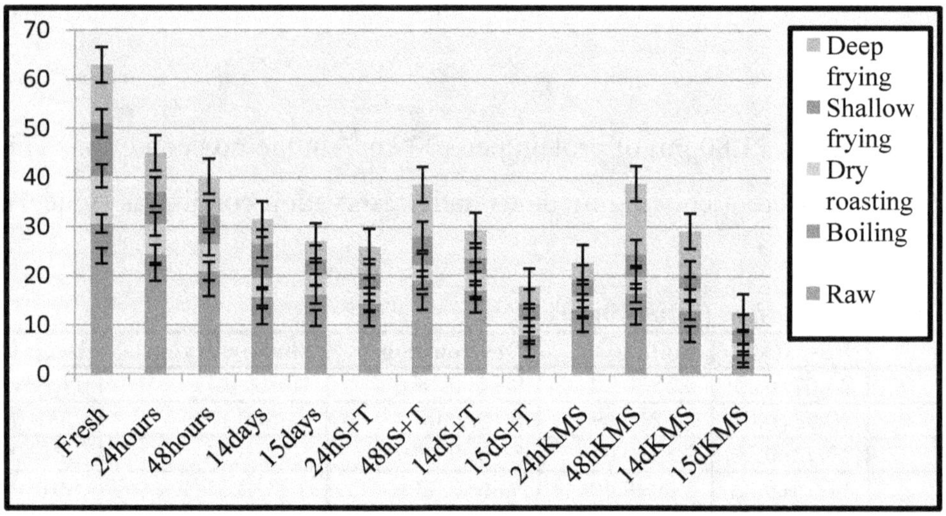

This graphical representation indicates that among all the preservation methods, the **fresh condition** helps to increase the protein content in all the cooking methods. The possible reason for this may be the moisture loss due to few days' preservation after catching the fish, as *hilsa* is a sea fish and it takes some time for transportation to Kolkata. So already it is preserved for a short time. Thus the protein content is highest in fresh condition in this study. The graph also shows that without preservative control preservation comparatively increases the protein content more than the salt and turmeric and KMS preservations.

Table no 5.2.6.3 ANOVA with regard to cooking conditions and preservation methods

Condition	Differences	Sum of Squares	df	Mean Square	F	Sig.
Fresh (control)	Between Groups	541.514	4	135.378	5.232E3	.000(S)
	Within Groups	.259	10	.026		
	Total	541.773	14			
24 hours (control)	Between Groups	522.999	4	130.750	1.555E4	.000(S)
	Within Groups	.084	10	.008		
	Total	523.083	14			
48 hours (control)	Between Groups	357.584	4	89.396	9.430E3	.000(S)
	Within Groups	.095	10	.009		
	Total	357.679	14			
14 days (control)	Between Groups	128.098	4	32.025	248.471	.000(S)
	Within Groups	1.289	10	.129		
	Total	129.387	14			
15 days (control)	Between Groups	139.705	4	34.926	144.145	.000(S)
	Within Groups	2.423	10	.242		
	Total	142.128	14			
24 hours (salt & turmeric)	Between Groups	158.735	4	39.684	130.221	.000(S)
	Within Groups	3.047	10	.305		
	Total	161.782	14			
48 hours (salt & turmeric)	Between Groups	274.313	4	68.578	366.454	.000(S)
	Within Groups	1.871	10	.187		
	Total	276.185	14			
14 days (salt & turmeric)	Between Groups	270.890	4	67.723	286.482	.000(S)
	Within Groups	2.364	10	.236		
	Total	273.254	14			
15 days (salt & turmeric)	Between Groups	11.453	4	2.863	17.412	.000(S)
	Within Groups	1.644	10	.164		
	Total	13.097	14			
24 hours (KMS)	Between Groups	122.928	4	30.732	293.432	.000(S)
	Within Groups	1.047	10	.105		
	Total	123.976	14			
48 hours (KMS)	Between Groups	290.724	4	72.681	778.003	.000(S)
	Within Groups	.934	10	.093		
	Total	291.658	14			
14 days (KMS)	Between Groups	84.809	4	21.202	123.985	.000(S)
	Within Groups	1.710	10	.171		
	Total	86.519	14			
15 days (KMS)	Between Groups	10.128	4	2.532	25.058	.000(S)
	Within Groups	1.010	10	.101		
	Total	11.139	14			

$p<0.05$ S= Significant, NS= Non-significant. All abbreviations are on page so and so.

This statistical ANOVA table shows that all the values are significant, which means there is significant difference present in the values of protein content of *hilsa* among different cooking methods and the raw state in respect to fresh condition along with different preservation methods.

Table no 5.2.6.4 Post hoc Duncan statistical analysis

Preservation	Duration	Raw state	Boiling	Dry roasting	Shallow frying	Deep frying
Control	Fresh	B,O,S,D^{a}	R,O,S,D^{b}	R,B,S,D^{c}	R,B,O,D^{d}	R,B,O,S^{e}
Control	24 hours	B,O,S,D^{a}	R,O,S,D^{b}	R,B,S,D^{c}	R,B,O,D^{d}	R,B,O,S^{e}
Control	48 hours	B,O,S,D^{a}	R,O,S,D^{b}	R,B,S,D^{c}	R,B,O,D^{d}	R,B,O,S^{e}
Control	14 days	B,O,S,D^{a}	R,S,D^{f}	R,S,D^{f}	R,B,O,D^{d}	R,B,O,S^{e}
Control	15 days	B,O,S,D^{a}	R,S,D^{f}	R,S^{g}	R,B,O^{h}	R,B,O,S^{e}
Salt &Turmeric	24 hours	B,O,S,D^{a}	R,D^{i}	R,D^{i}	R,D^{i}	R,B^{j}
Salt & Turmeric	48 hours	B,O,S,D^{a}	R,O,S,D^{b}	R,B,S,D^{c}	R,B,O,D^{d}	R,B,O,S^{e}
Salt & Turmeric	14 days	B,O,S,D^{a}	R,D^{i}	R,D^{i}	R,D^{i}	R,B,O,S^{e}
Salt & Turmeric	15 days	B,O,S,D^{a}	R^{k}	R^{k}	R^{k}	R^{k}
KMS	24 hours	B,O,S,D^{a}	R,D^{i}	R,S,D^{f}	R,O^{l}	R,O^{l}
KMS	48 hours	B,O,S,D^{a}	R,O,D^{m}	R,B,S,D^{c}	R,O,D^{m}	R,B,O,S^{e}
KMS	14 days	B,O,S^{n}	R,S,D^{f}	R,S,D^{f}	R,B,O,D^{d}	B,O,S^{n}
KMS	15 days	B,O^{o}	R,O,S,D^{b}	R,B,S,D^{c}	B,O,D^{p}	B,O,S^{n}

R= Raw state, B= Boiling, O= Open pan dry roasting, S= Shallow frying, D= Deep frying. The same uppercase alphabets represent that there is no significant difference present among the variables.

This table shows the significant difference among the different variables such as cooking methods and preservation conditions. The raw state significantly differs from boiling, open pan dry roasting, shallow frying and deep frying in all of the preservation methods with preservatives and control preservation without preservative except in 14 days, 15 days KMS preservation. Boiling significantly differs from the raw state, open pan dry roasting, shallow frying and deep frying in all of the preservation conditions except in 14 days, 15 days control preservation without preservative, 24 hours, 14 days, 15 days salt and turmeric preservation as well as 24 hours, 48 hours and 14 days KMS preservation. Open pan dry roasting significantly differs from the raw state, boiling, shallow frying and deep frying in all the preservation conditions except in 14 days, 15 days control preservation without preservative, 24 hours, 14 days, 15 days salt and turmeric preservation as well as 24 hours and 14 days KMS preservation. Shallow frying significantly differs from the raw state, boiling, open pan dry roasting and deep frying in all the preservation conditions except in 15 days control preservation without preservative, and 24 hours, 48 hours, 15 days salt and turmeric preservation as well as 24 hours, 48 hours and 15 days KMS preservation. Deep frying significantly differs from the raw state, boiling, open pan dry roasting and shallow frying in all the preservation conditions except in 24 hours, 15 days salt and turmeric preservation as well as 24 hours and 14 days, 15 days KMS preservation.

Boiling and open pan dry roasting significantly differ from the raw state, shallow frying and deep frying in 14 days control preservation without preservative as well as 24 hours and 14 days KMS preservation, whereas boiling and open pan dry roasting significantly differ from the raw state, shallow frying and deep frying in 15 days control preservation without preservative and 24 hours KMS preservation respectively. Again open pan dry roasting significantly differs from the raw state and shallow frying in 15 days control preservation without preservative. Shallow frying significantly differs from the raw state, boiling and open pan dry roasting in 15 days control preservation without preservative.

Boiling, open pan dry roasting, shallow frying significantly differ from the raw state and deep frying in 24 hours, 14 days salt and turmeric preservation, whereas only boiling significantly differs from the raw state and deep frying in 24 hours KMS preservation. Deep frying significantly differs from the raw state, boiling in 24 hours salt and turmeric preservation. Boiling, open pan dry roasting, shallow frying and deep frying significantly differ from the raw state in 15 days salt and turmeric preservation. Both shallow frying and deep frying significantly differ from the raw state and open pan dry roasting in 24 hours KMS preservation.

Boiling and shallow frying in 48 hours KMS preservation significantly differ from the raw state, open pan dry roasting and deep frying. The raw condition and deep frying significantly differ from boiling, open pan dry roasting and shallow frying in 14 days KMS preservation, whereas only deep frying significantly differs from boiling, open pan dry roasting, shallow frying in 15 days KMS preservation The raw state significantly differs from boiling and open pan dry roasting in 15 days KMS preservation, whereas shallow frying significantly differs from boiling, open pan dry roasting and shallow frying in 15 days KMS preservation.

Table no 5.2.6.5 Gradation of cooking methods from higher to lower restoration with respect to preservation days

Preservation	Duration	Method 1	Method 2	Method 3	Method 4	Method 5
Control	Fresh	R	DF	SF	OPDR	B
Control	24 hours	R	DF	SF	OPDR	B
Control	48 hours	R	DF	SF	OPDR	B
Control	14 days	R	DF	SF	OPDR	B
Control	15 days	R	B	OPDR	DF	SF
Salt &Turmeric	24 hours	R	DF	SF	B	OPDR
Salt & Turmeric	48 hours	R	DF	SF	B	OPDR
Salt & Turmeric	14 days	R	DF	OPDR	SF	B
Salt &Turmeric	15 days	R	DF	SF	OPDR	B
KMS	24 hours	R	DF	SF	B	OPDR
KMS	48 hours	DF	R	B	OPDR	SF
KMS	14 days	DF	R	B	OPDR	SF
KMS	15 days	DF	R	SF	OPDR	B

R= Raw state, B= Boiling, OPDR= Open pan dry roasting, SF= Shallow frying, DF= Deep frying. Same colours represent the similar order.

In all the preservation methods and fresh condition, protein retention occurs mainly in the raw state than the other cooking methods. In fresh condition, 24 hours, 48 hours, 14 days control preservation without preservative, retention occurs firstly in the raw state followed by deep frying, shallow frying, open pan dry roasting and boiling. In 15 days control preservation without preservative, the order changes to the raw state, boiling, open pan dry roasting, deep frying and shallow frying.

In 24 hours, 48 hours salt and turmeric preservation as well as 48 hours KMS preservation, the order is the raw state, deep frying, shallow frying, boiling and open pan dry roasting. In 14 days salt and turmeric preservation, it remains in the order of the raw state, deep frying, open pan dry roasting, shallow frying and boiling. In 15 days salt and turmeric preservation, the order remains the raw state, deep frying, shallow frying, open pan dry roasting and boiling.

In 48 hours and 14 days KMS preservation, it changes in the order of deep frying, raw state, boiling, open pan dry roasting and shallow frying. In 15 days KMS preservation, the order remains deep frying, raw state, shallow frying, open pan dry roasting and boiling.

The overall analysis of protein content of *hilsa* is mostly restored by the gradation of methods as the raw state>deep frying > shallow frying > open pan dry roasting >boiling.

Frying mainly restores[66] the nutrient as the oil can possibly create a protective layer so that the protein cannot be leached out, but in boiling the soluble protein parts get dissolved and the content is reduced, and discarding the boiling water can also be the possible cause for the loss of protein content. In open pan dry roasting the protein possibly gets charred, resulting in losses. Moreover, *hilsa* is a fatty fish, so the application of dry heat can help to melt the protective layer of fat leading to protein loss. Thus among the entire studied conventional cooking methods, **deep frying** is the best method for cooking *hilsa* to restore protein content.

5.3 Fat content

It has been reported that generally fish contains 2-13% of fat[1]. This experiment is carried out to estimate the percentage of fat content and also the changes of it in different cooking and preservation methods among different edible fish and aquatic species. Fat content is estimated by Soxhlet method[70].

5.3.1 *Rohu* (*Labeo rohita*)

It has been reported that *rohu* contains 2.39 gm of fat per 100 gm[85] in the raw condition. This value changes due to the application of different cooking methods and preservation conditions (vide Table no **5.3.1.1**).

Table no 5.3.1.1 Fat content of *Rohu* (gm/100gm)

Preservation	Duration	Raw state	Boiling	Dry roasting	Shallow frying	Deep frying
Control	Fresh	4.36±0.09	3.48±0.05	1.86±0.06	10.82±0.03	5.62±0.03
Control	24 hours	1.28±0.05	5.80±0.02	6.02±0.03	9.74±0.10	8.65±0.05
Control	48 hours	10.22±0.03	3.82±0.03	3.62±0.04	7.32±0.03	6.24±0.04
Control	14 days	2.42±0.08	2.10±0.15	2.60±0.02	7.56±0.07	2.44±0.05
Control	15 days	2.40±0.02	4.98±0.05	9.83±0.04	8.65±0.03	5.09±0.06
Salt & Turmeric	24 hours	5.82±0.03	4.03±0.04	5.40±0.02	10.57±0.07	9.25±0.05
Salt &Turmeric	48 hours	9.63±0.04	5.40±0.02	4.59±0.03	11.34±0.07	8.85±0.04
Salt & Turmeric	14 days	8.42±0.03	2.22±0.03	5.96±0.08	13.23±0.04	7.02±0.03
Salt & Turmeric	15 days	8.22±0.03	3.02±0.03	4.00±0.02	9.62±0.03	5.55±0.06
KMS	24 hours	6.22±0.03	5.46±0.07	5.82±0.03	7.82±0.03	7.57±0.05
KMS	48 hours	3.26±0.04	3.16±0.06	1.02±0.03	9.82±0.03	8.18±0.08
KMS	14 days	10.06±0.05	6.39±0.04	4.18±0.05	9.14±0.09	8.34±0.07
KMS	15 days	7.83±0.04	6.62±0.03	7.37±0.52	8.67±0.04	8.35±0.06

Values are expressed as mean±SD. Loss Restoration

Red digits represent the significant highest values from the raw state in different conditions.

In most of the preservation conditions, fat losses mainly occurs by boiling, whereas in fresh condition, 48 hours control preservation without preservative, 48 hours salt and turmeric preservation as well as KMS preservation and 14 days KMS preservation, fat content is reduced by open pan dry roasting. Retention of fat occurs by shallow frying[38].

The raw state shows the highest fat content in 48 hours control preservation without preservative, boiling in 15 days KMS preservation, open pan dry roasting in 15 days salt and turmeric preservation, whereas shallow frying in 14 days salt and turmeric preservation, and deep frying in 24 hours salt and turmeric preservation. Most of the retention of fat occurs in salt and turmeric preservation.

In 24 hours and 15 days control preservation without preservative, the fat content increases by boiling and open pan dry roasting as compared to the raw state. Open pan dry roasting also increases the fat content than the raw state in 24 hours salt and turmeric preservation. Shallow fried and deep fried *rohu* shows the increased content of fat as compared to the raw state in all the preservation conditions including fresh condition due to the addition of edible oil for frying[48]. Here the effect of natural preservative is prominent as it helps to restore the fat content more than the other preservation conditions. It probably helps to modify the structure of lipid, causing restoration.

Fig. 5.3.1.2 Graphical representation of Fat content of *Rohu* with respect to different conditions

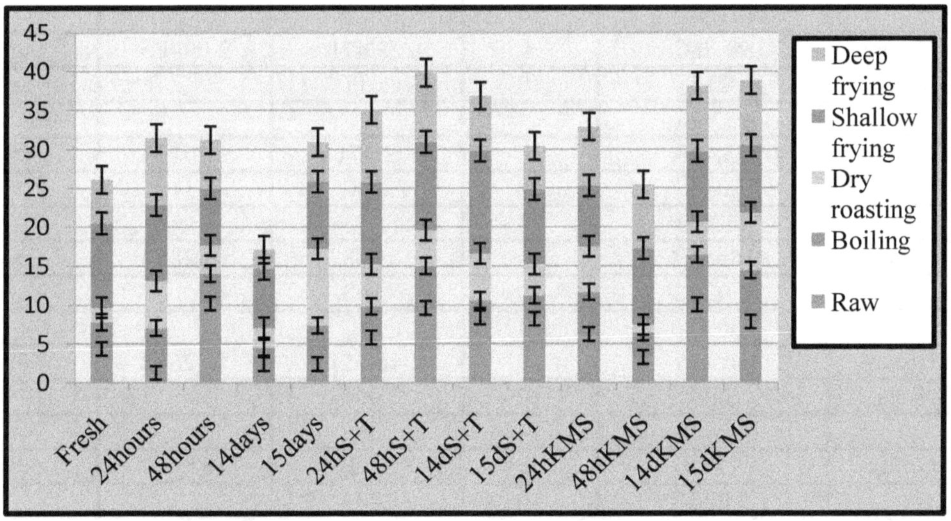

This graphical representation indicates that among all the preservation conditions, **48 hours salt and turmeric preservation**[55] helps to increase the fat content in all the cooking methods. The possible reason for this may be the moisture loss due to preservation and the efficiency of natural preservatives salt and turmeric, as they help to prevent the microbial growth and delays the lipid deterioration[34, 52]. The graph also shows that salt and turmeric preservation increases the fat content more than the control preservation without preservative and KMS preservation.

Table no 5.3.1.3 ANOVA with regard to cooking conditions and preservation methods

Condition	Differences	Sum of Squares	df	Mean Square	F	Sig.
Fresh (control)	Between Groups	140.025	4	35.006	1.024E4	.000(S)
	Within Groups	.034	10	.003		
	Total	140.059	14			
24 hours (control)	Between Groups	128.571	4	32.143	9.272E3	.000(S)
	Within Groups	.035	10	.003		
	Total	128.605	14			
48 hours (control)	Between Groups	89.208	4	22.302	2.215E4	.000(S)
	Within Groups	.010	10	.001		
	Total	89.218	14			
14 days (control)	Between Groups	64.600	4	16.150	5.660E3	.000(S)
	Within Groups	.029	10	.003		
	Total	64.629	14			
15 days (control)	Between Groups	108.966	4	27.242	1.362E4	.000(S)
	Within Groups	.020	10	.002		
	Total	108.986	14			
24 hours (salt & turmeric)	Between Groups	91.508	4	22.877	1.234E4	.000(S)
	Within Groups	.019	10	.002		
	Total	91.526	14			
48 hours (salt & turmeric)	Between Groups	98.714	4	24.679	1.381E4	.000(S)
	Within Groups	.018	10	.002		
	Total	98.732	14			
14 days (salt & turmeric)	Between Groups	192.282	4	48.071	2.341E4	.000(S)
	Within Groups	.021	10	.002		
	Total	192.303	14			
15 days (salt & turmeric)	Between Groups	93.886	4	23.471	2.094E3	.000(S)
	Within Groups	.112	10	.011		
	Total	93.998	14			
24 hours (KMS)	Between Groups	13.483	4	3.371	1.901E3	.000(S)
	Within Groups	.018	10	.002		
	Total	13.500	14			
48 hours (KMS)	Between Groups	166.754	4	41.689	1.628E4	.000(S)
	Within Groups	.026	10	.003		
	Total	166.780	14			
14 days (KMS)	Between Groups	66.446	4	16.611	4.326E3	.000(S)
	Within Groups	.038	10	.004		
	Total	66.484	14			
15 days (KMS)	Between Groups	8.889	4	2.222	863.569	.000(S)
	Within Groups	.026	10	.003		
	Total	8.915	14			

$p<0.05$ S= Significant, NS= Non-significant. All abbreviations are on page so and so.

This statistical ANOVA table shows that all the values are significant, which means there is significant difference present in the values of fat content of *rohu* among different cooking methods and the raw state in respect to fresh condition along with different preservation methods.

Table no 5.3.1.4 Post hoc Duncan statistical analysis

Preservation	Duration	Raw state	Boiling	Dry roasting	Shallow frying	Deep frying
Control	Fresh	B,O,S,D^{a}	R,O,S,D^{b}	R,B,S,D^{c}	R,B,O,D^{d}	R,B,O,S^{e}
Control	24 hours	B,O,S,D^{a}	R,O,S,D^{b}	R,B,S,D^{c}	R,B,O,D^{d}	R,B,O,S^{e}
Control	48 hours	B,O,S,D^{a}	R,O,S,D^{b}	R,B,S,D^{c}	R,B,O,D^{d}	R,B,O,S^{e}
Control	14 days	B,O,S^{f}	R,O,S,D^{b}	R,B,S,D^{c}	R,B,O,D^{d}	R,B,O,S^{e}
Control	15 days	B,O,S,D^{a}	R,O,S,D^{b}	R,B,S,D^{c}	R,B,O,D^{d}	R,B,O,S^{e}
Salt & Turmeric	24 hours	B,O,S,D^{a}	R,O,S,D^{b}	R,B,S,D^{c}	R,B,O,D^{d}	R,B,O,S^{e}
Salt & Turmeric	48 hours	B,O,S,D^{a}	R,O,S,D^{b}	R,B,S,D^{c}	R,B,O,D^{d}	R,B,O,S^{e}
Salt & Turmeric	14 days	B,O,S,D^{a}	R,O,S,D^{b}	R,B,S,D^{c}	R,B,O,D^{d}	R,B,O,S^{e}
Salt & Turmeric	15 days	B,O,S,D^{a}	R,O,S,D^{b}	R,B,S,D^{c}	R,B,O,D^{d}	R,B,O,S^{e}
KMS	24 hours	B,O,S,D^{a}	R,O,S,D^{b}	R,B,S,D^{c}	R,B,O,D^{d}	R,B,O,S^{e}
KMS	48 hours	B,O,S,D^{a}	R,O,S,D^{b}	R,B,S,D^{c}	R,B,O,D^{d}	R,B,O,S^{e}
KMS	14 days	B,O,S,D^{a}	R,O,S,D^{b}	R,B,S,D^{c}	R,B,O,D^{d}	R,B,O,S^{e}
KMS	15 days	B,O,S,D^{a}	R,O,S,D^{b}	R,B,S,D^{c}	R,B,O,D^{d}	R,B,O,S^{e}

R= Raw state, B= Boiling, O= Open pan dry roasting, S= Shallow frying, D= Deep frying. The same uppercase alphabets represent that there is no significant difference present among the variables.

This table shows the significant difference among the different variables such as cooking methods and preservation conditions. The raw state significantly differs from boiling, open pan dry roasting, shallow frying and deep frying in all of the preservation methods with preservatives and control preservation without preservative except in 14 days control preservation.

Boiling significantly differs from the raw state, open pan dry roasting, shallow frying and deep frying in all the preservation conditions. Open pan dry roasting significantly differs from the raw state, boiling, shallow frying and deep frying in all the preservation conditions. Shallow frying significantly differs from the raw state, boiling, open pan dry roasting and deep frying in all the preservation conditions. Deep frying significantly differs from the raw state, boiling, open pan dry roasting and shallow frying in all the preservation conditions. Again the raw state significantly differs from boiling, open pan dry roasting and shallow frying in 14 days control preservation without preservative.

Table no 5.3.1.5 Gradation of cooking methods from higher to lower restoration with respect to preservation days

Preservation	Duration	Method 1	Method 2	Method 3	Method 4	Method 5
Control	Fresh	SF	DF	R	B	OPDR
Control	24 hours	SF	DF	OPDR	B	R
Control	48 hours	R	SF	DF	B	OPDR
Control	14 days	SF	OPDR	DF	R	B
Control	15 days	OPDR	SF	DF	B	R
Salt & Turmeric	24 hours	SF	DF	R	OPDR	B
Salt & Turmeric	48 hours	SF	R	DF	B	OPDR
Salt & Turmeric	14 days	SF	R	DF	OPDR	B
Salt &Turmeric	15 days	SF	R	DF	OPDR	B
KMS	24 hours	SF	DF	R	OPDR	B
KMS	48 hours	SF	DF	R	B	OPDR
KMS	14 days	R	SF	DF	B	OPDR
KMS	15 days	SF	DF	R	OPDR	B

R= Raw state, B= Boiling, OPDR= Open pan dry roasting, SF= Shallow frying, DF= Deep frying. Same colours represent the similar order.

In all the preservation methods and fresh condition, fat retention occurs mainly in shallow frying than the other cooking methods. In fresh condition and 48 hours KMS preservation, retention occurs firstly in shallow frying followed by deep frying, raw state, boiling and open pan dry roasting. In 24 hours control preservation without preservative, it changes in the order of shallow frying, deep frying, open pan dry roasting, boiling and the raw state. In 48 hours control preservation without preservative and 14 days KMS preservation, the order changes to the raw state, shallow frying, deep frying, boiling and open pan dry roasting. In 14 days control preservation without preservative, the order is shallow frying, open pan dry roasting, deep frying, raw state and boiling. In 15 days control preservation without preservative, it changes in the order of open pan dry roasting, shallow frying, deep frying, boiling and the raw state.

In 24 hours salt and turmeric preservation as well as 24 hours KMS and 15 days KMS preservation, it remains in the order of shallow frying, deep frying, raw state, open pan dry roasting and boiling. In 48 hours salt and turmeric preservation, the order remains shallow frying, raw state, deep frying, boiling and open pan dry roasting. In 14 days and 15 days salt and turmeric preservation, the order becomes shallow frying, raw state, deep frying, open pan dry roasting and boiling.

The overall analysis of fat content of *rohu* is mostly restored by the gradation of methods as shallow frying>deep frying > raw state >boiling> open pan dry roasting.

Frying mainly restores[66] the fat content as the oil can possibly create a protective layer so that the lipid molecules cannot be leached out, but in open pan dry roasting, the fat content is reduced due to the application of direct dry heat so that the lipid molecules present in the fish get melted leading to reduction. Boiling also reduces the fat content, but the percentage is lower as lipid molecules cannot be dissolved in the water. Thus among all the studied conventional cooking methods, **shallow frying** is the best method for cooking *rohu* to restore fat content.

5.3.2 *Katla* (*Catla catla*)

It has been reported that *katla* contains 2.15 gm of fat per 100 gm[85] in the raw condition. This value changes due to the application of different cooking methods and preservation conditions (vide Table no **5.3.2.1**).

Table no 5.3.2.1 Fat content of *Katla* (gm/100gm)

Preservation	Duration	Raw state	Boiling	Dry roasting	Shallow frying	Deep frying
Control	Fresh	9.17±0.07	8.02±0.03	3.43±0.07	9.04±0.04	8.76±0.14
Control	24 hours	7.45±0.04	8.23±0.04	9.04±0.05	11.63±0.04	7.82±0.03
Control	48 hours	10.62±0.04	9.45±0.03	5.59±0.04	10.43±0.04	9.62±0.05
Control	14 days	12.04±0.04	9.87±0.04	2.96±0.04	6.64±0.04	8.28±0.04
Control	15 days	10.04±0.04	6.28±0.05	8.30±0.11	8.63±0.01	5.43±0.04
Salt & Turmeric	24 hours	10.25±0.04	9.38±0.08	6.42±0.03	9.31±0.09	6.24±0.03
Salt &Turmeric	48 hours	19.56±0.09	8.75±0.12	7.31±0.10	13.77±0.03	9.68±0.07
Salt & Turmeric	14 days	10.55±0.05	10.80±0.05	4.71±0.07	5.66±0.06	8.18±0.08
Salt & Turmeric	15 days	9.65±0.03	5.42±0.03	9.64±0.03	11.17±0.10	10.82±0.08
KMS	24 hours	9.33±0.07	6.44±0.06	4.31±0.10	12.43±0.04	10.24±0.09
KMS	48 hours	19.31±0.10	7.07±0.07	6.24±0.04	11.33±0.12	8.68±0.05
KMS	14 days	9.88±0.05	12.82±0.03	4.28±0.08	6.22±0.03	10.33±0.09
KMS	15 days	7.09±0.04	8.47±0.06	5.17±0.06	8.24±0.05	7.97±0.05

Values are expressed as mean±SD. ☐ Loss ☐ Restoration

Red digits represent the significant highest values from the raw state in different conditions.

In most of the preservation methods including fresh condition, fat losses mainly occurs by open pan dry roasting except in 24 hours, 15 days control preservation without preservative and 24 hours, 15 days salt and turmeric preservation, whereas boiling reduces fat content in 24 hours control preservation without preservative and 15 days salt and turmeric preservation. Deep frying reduces fat content in 24 hours salt and turmeric preservation and 15 days control preservation without preservative. Most of the retention occurs by shallow frying,[38] but in 14 days control preservation without preservative, 24 hours, 14 days salt and turmeric preservation as well as in 14 days, 15 days KMS preservation, retention occurs by boiling.

48 hours salt and turmeric preservation shows the highest fat content in the raw state and shallow frying, while 14 days KMS preservation shows the highest fat content in boiling. 15 days salt and turmeric shows the highest fat content in both open pan dry roasting and deep frying.

In 24 hours control preservation without preservative, 14 days salt and turmeric preservation and 14 days, 15 days KMS preservation, boiled *katla* shows the increased content of fat than the raw state. As *katla* is a fatty fish than *rohu*, fat is not leached out in boiling water. Here the effect of natural preservative is prominent as it helps to restore fat content more than the other preservation conditions. It probably helps to modify the structure of lipid molecule and thus restoration occurs.

Fig. 5.3.2.2 Graphical representation of Fat content of *Katla* with respect to different conditions

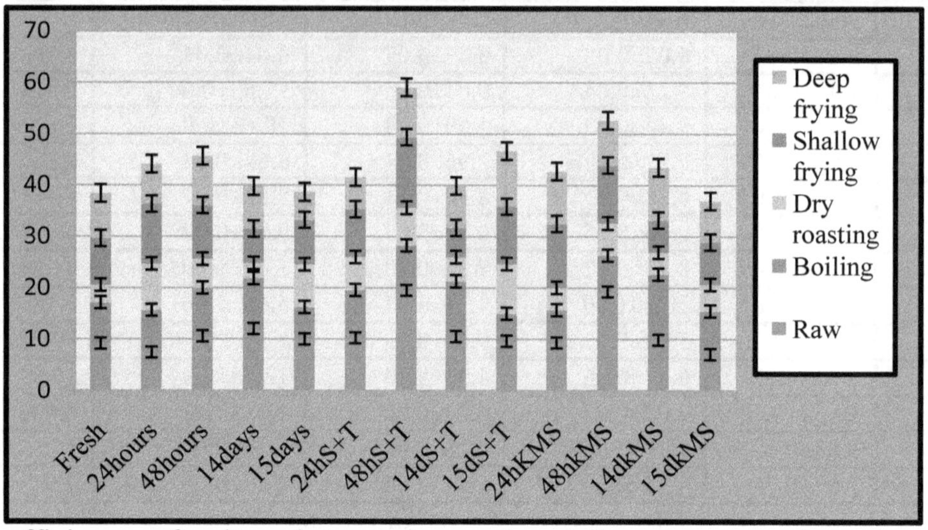

This graphical representation indicates that among all the preservation conditions, **48 hours salt and turmeric preservation**[55] helps to increase the fat content in all the cooking methods. The possible reason for this may be the moisture loss due to preservation and the efficiency of salt and turmeric, as they help to prevent the microbial growth and delays the lipid deterioration[34, 52]. The graph also shows that combination of salt and turmeric preservation increases the fat content more than that which is control preservation without preservative and KMS preservation.

Table no 5.3.2.3 ANOVA with regard to cooking conditions and preservation methods

Condition	Differences	Sum of Squares	df	Mean Square	F	Sig.
Fresh (control)	Between Groups	72.515	4	18.129	2.927E3	.000(S)
	Within Groups	.062	10	.006		
	Total	72.577	14			
24 hours (control)	Between Groups	33.426	4	8.357	5.698E3	.000(S)
	Within Groups	.015	10	.001		
	Total	33.441	14			
48 hours (control)	Between Groups	50.427	4	12.607	8.837E3	.000(S)
	Within Groups	.014	10	.001		
	Total	50.442	14			
14 days (control)	Between Groups	141.573	4	35.393	2.082E4	.000(S)
	Within Groups	.017	10	.002		
	Total	141.590	14			
15 days (control)	Between Groups	41.561	4	10.390	2.870E3	.000(S)
	Within Groups	.036	10	.004		
	Total	41.597	14			
24 hours (salt & turmeric)	Between Groups	41.254	4	10.314	2.644E3	.000(S)
	Within Groups	.039	10	.004		
	Total	41.293	14			
48 hours (salt & turmeric)	Between Groups	294.595	4	73.649	9.691E3	.000(S)
	Within Groups	.076	10	.008		
	Total	294.671	14			
14 days (salt & turmeric)	Between Groups	92.012	4	23.003	6.118E3	.000(S)
	Within Groups	.038	10	.004		
	Total	92.049	14			
15 days (salt & turmeric)	Between Groups	63.262	4	15.816	4.097E3	.000(S)
	Within Groups	.039	10	.004		
	Total	63.301	14			
24 hours (KMS)	Between Groups	123.033	4	30.758	5.592E3	.000(S)
	Within Groups	.055	10	.005		
	Total	123.088	14			
48 hours (KMS)	Between Groups	334.441	4	83.610	1.302E4	.000(S)
	Within Groups	.064	10	.006		
	Total	334.505	14			
14 days (KMS)	Between Groups	140.075	4	35.019	1.018E4	.000(S)
	Within Groups	.034	10	.003		
	Total	140.109	14			
15 days (KMS)	Between Groups	21.708	4	5.427	1.971E3	.000(S)
	Within Groups	.028	10	.003		
	Total	21.736	14			

$p<0.05$ S= Significant, NS= Non-significant. All abbreviations are on page so and so.

This statistical ANOVA table shows that all the values are significant, which means there is significant difference present in the values of fat content of *katla* among different cooking methods and the raw state in respect to fresh condition along with different preservation methods.

Table no 5.3.2.4 Post hoc Duncan statistical analysis

Preservation	Duration	Raw state	Boiling	Dry roasting	Shallow frying	Deep frying
Control	Fresh	B,O,D^{a}	R,O,S,D^{b}	R,B,S,D^{c}	B,O,D^{a}	R,B,O,S^{d}
Control	24 hours	B,O,S,D^{e}	R,O,S,D^{b}	R,B,S,D^{c}	R,B,O,D^{f}	R,B,O,S^{d}
Control	48 hours	B,O,S,D^{e}	R,O,S,D^{b}	R,B,S,D^{c}	R,B,O,D^{f}	R,B,O,S^{d}
Control	14 days	B,O,S,D^{e}	R,O,S,D^{b}	R,B,S,D^{c}	R,B,O,D^{f}	R,B,O,S^{d}
Control	15 days	B,O,S,D^{e}	R,O,S,D^{b}	R,B,S,D^{c}	R,B,O,D^{f}	R,B,O,S^{d}
Salt &Turmeric	24 hours	B,O,S,D^{e}	R,O,D^{g}	R,B,S,D^{c}	R,O,D^{g}	R,B,O,S^{d}
Salt & Turmeric	48 hours	B,O,S,D^{e}	R,O,S,D^{b}	R,B,S,D^{c}	R,B,O,D^{f}	R,B,O,S^{d}
Salt & Turmeric	14 days	B,O,S,D^{e}	R,O,S,D^{b}	R,B,S,D^{c}	R,B,O,D^{f}	R,B,O,S^{d}
Salt & Turmeric	15 days	B,S,D^{h}	R,O,S,D^{b}	B,S,D^{h}	R,B,O,D^{f}	R,B,O,S^{d}
KMS	24 hours	B,O,S,D^{e}	R,O,S,D^{b}	R,B,S,D^{c}	R,B,O,D^{f}	R,B,O,S^{d}
KMS	48 hours	B,O,S,D^{e}	R,O,S,D^{b}	R,B,S,D^{c}	R,B,O,D^{f}	R,B,O,S^{d}
KMS	14 days	B,O,S,D^{e}	R,O,S,D^{b}	R,B,S,D^{c}	R,B,O,D^{f}	R,B,O,S^{d}
KMS	15 days	B,O,S,D^{e}	R,O,S,D^{b}	R,B,S,D^{c}	R,B,O,D^{f}	R,B,O,S^{d}

R= Raw state, B= Boiling, O= Open pan dry roasting, S= Shallow frying, D= Deep frying. The same uppercase alphabets represent that there is no significant difference present among the variables.

This table shows the significant difference among the different variables such as cooking methods and preservation conditions. The raw state significantly differs from boiling, open pan dry roasting, shallow frying and deep frying in all of the preservation methods with preservatives and control preservation without preservative except in fresh condition and 15 days salt and turmeric preservation. Boiling significantly differs from the raw state, open pan dry roasting, shallow frying and deep frying in all the preservation conditions except in 24 hours salt and turmeric preservation. Open pan dry roasting significantly differs from the raw state, boiling, shallow frying and deep frying in all of the preservation conditions except in 15 days salt and turmeric preservation. Shallow frying significantly differs from the raw state, boiling, open pan dry roasting and deep frying in all the preservation conditions except in fresh condition and 15 days salt and turmeric preservation. Deep frying significantly differs from the raw state, boiling, open pan dry roasting and shallow frying in all of the preservation conditions.

Again both the raw state and shallow frying significantly differ from boiling, open pan dry roasting and shallow frying in fresh condition. Both boiling and shallow frying significantly differ from the raw state, open pan dry roasting and deep frying in 24 hours salt and turmeric preservation. Both the raw state and open pan dry roasting significantly differ from boiling, shallow frying and deep frying in 15 days salt and turmeric preservation.

Table no 5.3.2.5 Gradation of cooking methods from higher to lower restoration with respect to preservation days

Preservation	Duration	Method 1	Method 2	Method 3	Method 4	Method 5
Control	Fresh	R	SF	DF	B	OPDR
Control	24 hours	SF	DF	OPDR	B	R
Control	48 hours	R	SF	DF	B	OPDR
Control	14 days	SF	OPDR	DF	R	B
Control	15 days	OPDR	SF	DF	B	R
Salt & Turmeric	24 hours	R	B	SF	OPDR	DF
Salt & Turmeric	48 hours	R	SF	DF	B	OPDR
Salt & Turmeric	14 days	B	R	DF	SF	OPDR
Salt &Turmeric	15 days	SF	DF	R	OPDR	B
KMS	24 hours	SF	DF	R	B	OPDR
KMS	48 hours	R	SF	DF	B	OPDR
KMS	14 days	B	DF	R	SF	OPDR
KMS	15 days	B	SF	DF	R	OPDR

R= Raw state, B= Boiling, OPDR= Open pan dry roasting, SF= Shallow frying, DF= Deep frying. Same colour represents similar order.

In all the preservation methods and fresh condition, fat retention occurs mainly in the raw state than the other cooking methods. In fresh condition, 48 hours control preservation without preservative, 48 hours salt and turmeric preservation as well as KMS preservation, retention occurs firstly in the raw state followed by shallow frying, deep frying, boiling and open pan dry roasting. In 24 hours control preservation without preservative, it changes in the order of shallow frying, deep frying, open pan dry roasting, boiling and the raw state. In 14 days control preservation without preservative, the order is shallow frying, open pan dry roasting, deep frying, raw state and boiling. In 15 days control preservation without preservative, the order becomes open pan dry roasting, shallow frying, deep frying, boiling and the raw state.

In 24 hours salt and turmeric preservation, the order of retention is the raw state, boiling, shallow frying, open pan dry roasting and deep frying. In 14 days salt and turmeric preservation, it remains in the order of boiling, raw state, deep frying, shallow frying and open pan dry roasting. In 15 days salt and turmeric preservation, the order becomes shallow frying, deep frying, raw state, open pan dry roasting and boiling.

In 24 hours KMS preservation, the order of retention changes from shallow frying to deep frying, raw state, boiling and then open pan dry roasting. In 14 days KMS preservation, it remains in the order of boiling, deep frying, raw state, shallow frying and open pan dry roasting. In 15 days KMS preservation, the order is boiling, shallow frying, deep frying, raw state and open pan dry roasting.

The overall analysis of fat content of *katla* is mostly restored by the gradation of methods as the raw state>shallow frying > deep frying>boiling> open pan dry roasting.

Frying mainly restores[66] the fat content as the oil can possibly create a protective layer so that the lipid molecules cannot be leached out, but in open pan dry roasting the fat content reduces due to the application of direct dry heat so the lipid molecules present in the fish get melted and thus reduction occurs. Boiling also reduces the fat content, but the percentage is lower as the lipid molecules cannot be dissolved in water. Moreover, *katla* contains more fatty tissues than *rohu*. Thus among all the studied conventional cooking methods, **shallow frying** is best for cooking *katla* to restore fat content.

5.3.3 Prawn (*Fenneropenaeus indicus*)

It has been reported that prawn contains 1.0 gm of fat per 100 gm[85] in the raw condition. This value changes due to the application of different cooking methods and preservation conditions (vide Table no **5.3.3.1**).

Table no 5.3.3.1 Fat content of Prawn (gm/100gm)

Preservation	Duration	Raw state	Boiling	Dry roasting	Shallow frying	Deep frying
Control	Fresh	2.46±0.04	3.02±0.04	3.04±0.05	6.46±0.04	4.35±0.07
Control	24 hours	1.85±0.03	1.59±0.03	1.94±0.05	9.78±0.03	9.29±0.01
Control	48 hours	0.86±0.04	0.76±0.04	1.56±0.06	2.57±0.04	3.62±0.03
Control	14 days	0.90±0.05	0.80±0.02	1.04±0.04	4.42±0.03	2.04±0.04
Control	15 days	0.78±0.06	0.63±0.02	0.97±0.06	6.40±0.02	2.04±0.04
Salt & Turmeric	24 hours	0.60±0.03	0.52±0.03	0.37±0.02	2.53±0.03	3.40±0.02
Salt & Turmeric	48 hours	0.51±0.03	0.44±0.02	0.62±0.02	5.03±0.04	4.06±0.04
Salt & Turmeric	14 days	0.65±0.03	2.36±0.04	0.40±0.02	5.08±0.05	3.65±0.03
Salt & Turmeric	15 days	1.13±0.04	1.00±0.02	0.62±0.02	5.82±0.03	5.45±0.03
KMS	24 hours	1.34±0.03	2.84±0.02	2.45±0.04	4.35±0.07	3.04±0.04
KMS	48 hours	0.67±0.03	3.69±0.04	0.52±0.06	5.15±0.05	5.37±0.04
KMS	14 days	1.08±0.03	2.80±0.07	2.85±0.05	6.49±0.06	3.57±0.06
KMS	15 days	3.04±0.05	0.36±0.06	2.35±0.03	4.55±0.06	3.04±0.04

Values are expressed as mean±SD. Loss Restoration

Red digits represent the significant highest values from the raw state for each different condition.

In most of the preservation conditions, fat losses mainly occur by boiling, whereas in 24 hours, 14 days, 15 days salt and turmeric preservation as well as 24 hours, 48 hours KMS preservation, fat content is reduced by open pan dry roasting.

Retention of fat occurs by shallow frying[38] mostly, but in 48 hours control preservation without preservative, 24 hours salt and turmeric preservation and 48 hours KMS preservation, fat retention occurs by deep frying.

Both shallow frying and deep frying show the highest fat content in 24 hours control preservation without preservative, boiling in 48 hours KMS preservation, open pan dry roasting in fresh condition, and the raw state in 15 days KMS preservation.

In fresh condition, 14 days salt and turmeric preservation as well as 24 hours, 48 hours and 14 days KMS preservation, the fat content increases by boiling and in fresh condition, 24 hours, 48 hours, 14 and 15 days control preservation without preservative, 48 hours salt and turmeric preservation as well as 24 hours, 14 days and 15 days KMS preservation, the fat content increases in open pan dry roasting than the raw state.

Shallow fried and deep fried prawn show the increased content of fat than the raw state in all the preservation conditions including fresh condition due to the addition of edible oil for frying[48]. There is no prominent effect of both the natural and synthetic preservatives. Prawn preservation in the raw state, without preservative shows the effective result.

Fig. 5.3.3.2 Graphical representation of Fat content of Prawn with respect to different conditions

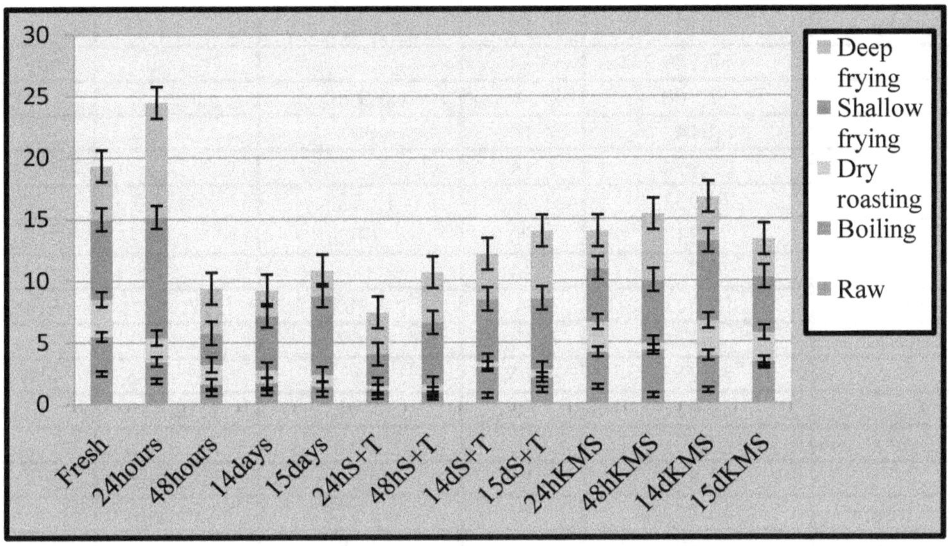

This graphical representation indicates that among all the preservation conditions, **24 hours control preservation without preservative** helps to increase the fat content in all the cooking methods. The possible reason may be the moisture loss due to preservation. Here the graph shows that salt and turmeric preservation reduces the fat content, whereas KMS preservation comparatively increases the fat content[39]. So prawn can be preserved by KMS rather than salt and turmeric. KMS can help to prevent the microbial growth and delays the lipid deterioration.

Table no 5.3.3.3 ANOVA with regard to cooking conditions and preservation methods

Condition	Differences	Sum of Squares	df	Mean Square	F	Sig.
Fresh (control)	Between Groups	31.039	4	7.760	3.538E3	.000(S)
	Within Groups	.022	10	.002		
	Total	31.060	14			
24 hours (control)	Between Groups	216.155	4	54.039	5.035E4	.000(S)
	Within Groups	.011	10	.001		
	Total	216.166	14			
48 hours (control)	Between Groups	17.772	4	4.443	2.563E3	.000(S)
	Within Groups	.017	10	.002		
	Total	17.789	14			
14 days (control)	Between Groups	27.960	4	6.990	5.165E3	.000(S)
	Within Groups	.014	10	.001		
	Total	27.974	14			
15 days (control)	Between Groups	70.931	4	17.733	8.417E3	.000(S)
	Within Groups	.021	10	.002		
	Total	70.952	14			
24 hours (salt & turmeric)	Between Groups	19.541	4	4.885	72.660	.000(S)
	Within Groups	.672	10	.067		
	Total	20.213	14			
48 hours (salt & turmeric)	Between Groups	59.672	4	14.918	1.522E4	.000(S)
	Within Groups	.010	10	.001		
	Total	59.682	14			
14 days (salt & turmeric)	Between Groups	45.272	4	11.318	166.540	.000(S)
	Within Groups	.680	10	.068		
	Total	45.952	14			
15 days (salt & turmeric)	Between Groups	80.683	4	20.171	2.909E4	.000(S)
	Within Groups	.007	10	.001		
	Total	80.690	14			
24 hours (KMS)	Between Groups	14.116	4	3.529	1.911E3	.000(S)
	Within Groups	.018	10	.002		
	Total	14.135	14			
48 hours (KMS)	Between Groups	66.794	4	16.698	8.820E3	.000(S)
	Within Groups	.019	10	.002		
	Total	66.813	14			
14 days (KMS)	Between Groups	46.963	4	11.741	3.594E3	.000(S)
	Within Groups	.033	10	.003		
	Total	46.996	14			
15 days (KMS)	Between Groups	27.765	4	6.941	2.740E3	.000(S)
	Within Groups	.025	10	.003		
	Total	27.790	14			

$p<0.05$ S= Significant, NS= Non-significant. All abbreviations are on page so and so.

This statistical ANOVA table shows that all the values are significant, which means there is significant difference present in the values of fat content of prawn among different cooking methods and the raw state in respect to fresh condition along with different preservation methods.

Table no 5.3.3.4 Post hoc Duncan statistical analysis

Preservation	Duration	Raw state	Boiling	Dry roasting	Shallow frying	Deep frying
Control	Fresh	B,O,S,D^{a}	R,S,D^{b}	R,S,D^{b}	R,B,O,D^{c}	R,B,O,S^{d}
Control	24 hours	B,O,S,D^{a}	R,O,S,D^{e}	R,B,S,D^{f}	R,B,O,D^{c}	R,B,O,S^{d}
Control	48 hours	B,O,S,D^{a}	R,O,S,D^{e}	R,B,S,D^{f}	R,B,O,D^{c}	R,B,O,S^{d}
Control	14 days	B,O,S,D^{a}	R,O,S,D^{e}	R,B,S,D^{f}	R,B,O,D^{c}	R,B,O,S^{d}
Control	15 days	B,O,S,D^{a}	R,O,S,D^{e}	R,B,S,D^{f}	R,B,O,D^{c}	R,B,O,S^{d}
Salt &Turmeric	24 hours	S,D^{g}	S,D^{g}	S,D^{g}	R,B,O,D^{c}	R,B,O,S^{d}
Salt & Turmeric	48 hours	B,O,S,D^{a}	R,O,S,D^{e}	R,B,S,D^{f}	R,B,O,D^{c}	R,B,O,S^{d}
Salt & Turmeric	14 days	B,S,D^{h}	R,O,S,D^{e}	B,S,D^{h}	R,B,O,D^{c}	R,B,O,S^{d}
Salt & Turmeric	15 days	B,O,S,D^{a}	R,O,S,D^{e}	R,B,S,D^{f}	R,B,O,D^{c}	R,B,O,S^{d}
KMS	24 hours	B,O,S,D^{a}	R,O,S,D^{e}	R,B,S,D^{f}	R,B,O,D^{c}	R,B,O,S^{d}
KMS	48 hours	B,O,S,D^{a}	R,O,S,D^{e}	R,B,S,D^{f}	R,B,O,D^{c}	R,B,O,S^{d}
KMS	14 days	B,O,S,D^{a}	R,S,D^{b}	R,S,D^{b}	R,B,O,D^{c}	R,B,O,S^{d}
KMS	15 days	B,O,S^{i}	R,O,S,D^{e}	R,B,S,D^{f}	R,B,O,D^{c}	B,O,S^{i}

R= Raw state, B= Boiling, O= Open pan dry roasting, S= Shallow frying, D= Deep frying. The same uppercase alphabets represent that there is no significant difference present among the variables.

This table shows the significant difference among the different variables such as cooking methods and preservation conditions. The raw state significantly differs from boiling, open pan dry roasting, shallow frying and deep frying in all of the preservation methods with preservatives and control preservation without preservative except in 24 hours, 14 days salt and turmeric preservation and 15 days KMS preservation. Boiling significantly differs from the raw state, open pan dry roasting, shallow frying and deep frying in all of the preservation conditions except in fresh condition, 24 hours salt and turmeric preservation and 14 days KMS preservation. Open pan dry roasting significantly differs from the raw state, boiling, shallow frying and deep frying in all the preservation conditions except in fresh condition, 24 hours salt and turmeric preservation and 14 days KMS preservation. Shallow frying significantly differs from the raw state, boiling, open pan dry roasting and deep frying in all the preservation conditions. Deep frying significantly differs from the raw state, boiling, open pan dry roasting and shallow frying in all of the preservation conditions except in 15 days KMS preservation.

Boiling and open pan dry roasting significantly differ from the raw state, shallow frying and deep frying in fresh condition and 14 days KMS preservation, whereas the raw state, boiling, open pan dry roasting significantly differ from both shallow frying and deep frying in 24 hours salt and turmeric preservation. Again the raw state and open pan dry roasting significantly differ from boiling, shallow frying and deep frying in 14 days salt and turmeric preservation. The raw state and deep frying significantly differs from boiling, open pan dry roasting and shallow frying in 15 days KMS preservation.

Table no 5.3.3.5 Gradation of cooking methods from higher to lower restoration with respect to preservation days

Preservation	Duration	Method 1	Method 2	Method 3	Method 4	Method 5
Control	Fresh	SF	DF	OPDR	B	R
Control	24 hours	SF	DF	OPDR	R	B
Control	48 hours	DF	SF	OPDR	R	B
Control	14 days	SF	DF	OPDR	R	B
Control	15 days	SF	DF	OPDR	R	B
Salt & Turmeric	24 hours	DF	SF	R	B	OPDR
Salt & Turmeric	48 hours	SF	DF	OPDR	R	B
Salt & Turmeric	14 days	SF	DF	B	R	OPDR
Salt &Turmeric	15 days	SF	DF	R	B	OPDR
KMS	24 hours	SF	DF	B	OPDR	R
KMS	48 hours	DF	SF	B	R	OPDR
KMS	14 days	SF	DF	OPDR	B	R
KMS	15 days	SF	R	DF	OPDR	B

R= Raw state, B= Boiling, OPDR= Open pan dry roasting, SF= Shallow frying, DF= Deep frying. Same colours represent similar order.

In all the preservation methods and fresh condition, fat retention occurs mainly in shallow frying as compared to the other cooking methods. In fresh condition and 14 days KMS preservation, retention occurs firstly in shallow frying then the raw state, deep frying, open pan dry roasting and boiling. In 24 hours, 14 days, 15 days control preservation without preservative, it changes in the order of shallow frying, deep frying, open pan dry roasting, raw state and boiling. In 48 hours control preservation without preservative, the order changes to deep frying, shallow frying, open pan dry roasting, raw state and boiling.

In 24 hours salt and turmeric preservation, the order of retention remains deep frying, shallow frying, raw state, boiling and open pan dry roasting. In 48 hours salt and turmeric preservation, the order changes to shallow frying, deep frying, open pan dry roasting, raw state and boiling. In 14 days salt and turmeric preservation, the order remains shallow frying, deep frying, boiling, raw state and open pan dry roasting. In 15 days salt and turmeric preservation, the order becomes shallow frying, deep frying, raw state, boiling and open pan dry roasting.

In 24 hours KMS preservation, it remains in the order of shallow frying, deep frying, boiling, open pan dry roasting and the raw state. In 48 hours KMS preservation, the order is deep frying, shallow frying, boiling, raw state and open pan dry roasting. In 15 days KMS preservation, it changes in the order of shallow frying, raw state, deep frying, open pan dry roasting and boiling.

The overall analysis of fat content of prawn is mostly restored by the gradation of methods as shallow frying > deep frying> open pan dry roasting> raw state> boiling.

Frying mainly restores[66] the fat content as the oil can possibly create a protective layer so that the lipid molecules cannot be leached out, but in boiling the fat content is reduced if the cooking water is discarded. Open pan dry roasting reduces the fat content due to the application of direct dry heat so the lipid molecules present in prawn get melted, leading to reduction. Thus among all the studied conventional cooking methods, **shallow frying** is the best method for cooking prawn to restore fat content.

5.3.4 Lobster (*Macrobrachium rosenbergii*)

It has been reported that lobster contains 0.9 gm of fat per 100 gm[84] in the raw condition. This value changes due to the application of different cooking methods and preservation conditions (vide Table no **5.3.4.1**).

Table no 5.3.4.1 Fat content of Lobster (gm/100gm)

Preservation	Duration	Raw state	Boiling	Dry roasting	Shallow frying	Deep frying
Control	Fresh	2.09±0.07	2.58±0.05	2.02±0.02	6.75±0.06	6.14±0.06
Control	24 hours	0.88±0.02	0.58±0.03	0.63±0.01	4.20±0.05	4.07±0.04
Control	48 hours	1.09±0.07	1.39±0.04	0.56±0.04	5.78±0.05	7.76±0.03
Control	14 days	1.20±0.05	1.59±0.04	0.59±0.01	4.90±0.03	4.69±0.07
Control	15 days	1.01±0.04	1.14±0.04	0.98±0.09	7.72±0.07	4.68±0.03
Salt & Turmeric	24 hours	2.49±0.02	5.90±0.05	0.70±0.10	5.78±0.02	6.15±0.05
Salt & Turmeric	48 hours	2.98±0.03	1.07±0.06	4.73±0.09	5.47±0.07	6.62±0.03
Salt & Turmeric	14 days	1.42±0.03	2.40±0.02	0.95±0.05	4.82±0.03	1.48±0.03
Salt & Turmeric	15 days	1.05±0.04	0.75±0.05	0.67±0.03	3.87±0.11	3.29±0.03
KMS	24 hours	0.85±0.05	0.72±0.02	0.44±0.05	1.45±0.06	3.05±0.22
KMS	48 hours	1.72±0.02	3.64±0.05	2.54±0.06	9.81±0.08	4.06±0.05
KMS	14 days	0.95±0.04	2.55±0.05	1.79±0.03	7.55±0.04	3.92±0.03
KMS	15 days	0.78±0.03	0.87±0.02	0.98±0.01	2.11±0.10	1.95±0.04

Values are expressed as mean±SD. Loss Restoration
Red digits represent the significant highest values from the raw state for each different condition.

In most of the preservation conditions, fat losses mainly occur by open pan dry roasting, whereas in 24 hours control preservation without preservative, 48 hours salt and turmeric preservation as well as 15 days KMS preservation, fat content is reduced by boiling.

Retention of fat occurs in shallow frying[38] mostly, but in 48 hours control preservation without preservative, 48 hours salt and turmeric preservation and 24 hours KMS preservation, fat retention occurs by deep frying.

Both the raw state and open pan dry roasting show the highest fat content in 48 hours salt and turmeric preservation, boiling shows the highest fat content in 24 hours salt and turmeric preservation, whereas shallow frying in 48 hours KMS preservation and deep frying in 48 hours control preservation without preservative.

In fresh condition, 48 hours, 14 days, 15 days control preservation without preservative, 24 hours, 14 days salt and turmeric preservation as well as 48 hours and 14 days, 15 days KMS preservation, the fat content increases in boiling and in 48 hours salt and turmeric preservation as well as 48 hours, 14 days KMS preservation, the fat content increases in open pan dry roasting than the raw state.

Shallow fried and deep fried lobster show the increased content of fat than the raw state in all the preservation conditions including fresh condition due to the addition of edible oil for frying[48]. There is prominent effect of both the natural and synthetic preservative. They may help to modify the structure of fat so that deterioration reduces to some extent.

Fig. 5.3.4.2 Graphical representation of Fat content of Lobster with respect to different conditions

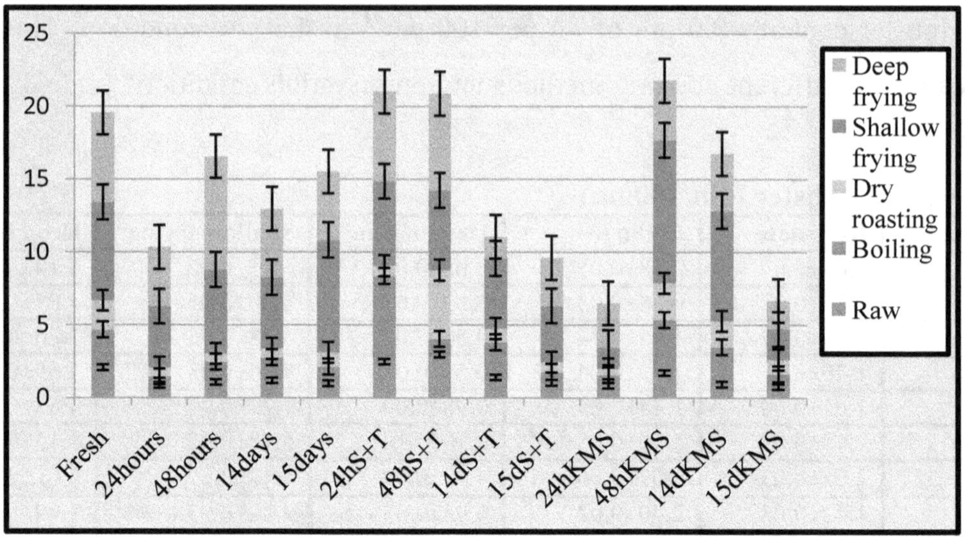

This graphical representation indicates that among all the preservation conditions, **48 hours KMS preservation**[59] helps to increase the fat content in all the cooking methods. The possible reason may be the moisture loss due to preservation. Here the graph shows that salt and turmeric preservation also increases the fat content, whereas KMS preservation comparatively increases the fat content more than salt and turmeric preservation[39]. Thus lobster can be better preserved by KMS than salt and turmeric. KMS can help to prevent the microbial growth and delays the lipid deterioration.

Table no 5.3.4.3 ANOVA with regard to cooking conditions and preservation methods

Condition	Differences	Sum of Squares	df	Mean Square	F	Sig.
Fresh (control)	Between Groups	65.195	4	16.299	5.433E3	.000(S)
	Within Groups	.030	10	.003		
	Total	65.225	14			
24 hours (control)	Between Groups	42.690	4	10.673	9.473E3	.000(S)
	Within Groups	.011	10	.001		
	Total	42.701	14			
48 hours (control)	Between Groups	126.170	4	31.542	1.300E4	.000(S)
	Within Groups	.024	10	.002		
	Total	126.194	14			
14 days (control)	Between Groups	49.988	4	12.497	7.074E3	.000(S)
	Within Groups	.018	10	.002		
	Total	50.006	14			
15 days (control)	Between Groups	109.560	4	27.390	9.274E3	.000(S)
	Within Groups	.030	10	.003		
	Total	109.590	14			
24 hours (salt & turmeric)	Between Groups	73.126	4	18.281	1.576E4	.000(S)
	Within Groups	.012	10	.001		
	Total	73.137	14			
48 hours (salt & turmeric)	Between Groups	57.024	4	14.256	3.738E3	.000(S)
	Within Groups	.038	10	.004		
	Total	57.062	14			
14 days (salt & turmeric)	Between Groups	28.822	4	7.205	8.378E3	.000(S)
	Within Groups	.009	10	.001		
	Total	28.831	14			
15 days (salt & turmeric)	Between Groups	28.071	4	7.018	1.876E3	.000(S)
	Within Groups	.037	10	.004		
	Total	28.109	14			
24 hours (KMS)	Between Groups	12.085	4	3.021	1.382E3	.000(S)
	Within Groups	.022	10	.002		
	Total	12.107	14			
48 hours (KMS)	Between Groups	121.857	4	30.464	1.022E4	.000(S)
	Within Groups	.030	10	.003		
	Total	121.887	14			
14 days (KMS)	Between Groups	80.744	4	20.186	1.251E4	.000(S)
	Within Groups	.016	10	.002		
	Total	80.760	14			
15 days (KMS)	Between Groups	4.871	4	1.218	2.348E3	.000(S)
	Within Groups	.005	9	.001		
	Total	4.876	13			

$p<0.05$ S= Significant, NS= Non-significant. All abbreviations are on page so and so.

This statistical ANOVA table shows that all the values are significant, which means there is significant difference present in the values of fat content of lobster among different cooking methods and the raw state in respect to fresh condition along with different preservation methods.

Table no 5.3.4.4 Post hoc Duncan statistical analysis

Preservation	Duration	Raw state	Boiling	Dry roasting	Shallow frying	Deep frying
Control	Fresh	B,S,D^{a}	R,O,S,D^{b}	B,S,D^{a}	R,B,O,D^{c}	R,B,O,S^{d}
Control	24 hours	B,O,S,D^{e}	R,S,D^{f}	R,S,D^{f}	R,B,O,D^{c}	R,B,O,S^{d}
Control	48 hours	B,O,S,D^{e}	R,O,S,D^{b}	R,B,S,D^{g}	R,B,O,D^{c}	R,B,O,S^{d}
Control	14 days	B,O,S,D^{e}	R,O,S,D^{b}	R,B,S,D^{g}	R,B,O,D^{c}	R,B,O,S^{d}
Control	15 days	B,S,D^{a}	R,O,S,D^{b}	R,B,S,D^{g}	R,B,O,D^{c}	R,B,O,S^{d}
Salt & Turmeric	24 hours	B,O,S,D^{e}	R,O,S,D^{b}	B,S,D^{a}	R,B,O,D^{c}	R,B,O,S^{d}
Salt & Turmeric	48 hours	B,O,S,D^{e}	R,O,S,D^{b}	R,B,S,D^{g}	R,B,O,D^{c}	R,B,O,S^{d}
Salt & Turmeric	14 days	B,O,S,D^{e}	R,O,S,D^{b}	R,S,D^{f}	R,B,O,D^{c}	R,B,O,S^{d}
Salt & Turmeric	15days	B,O,S,D^{e}	R,S,D^{f}	R,B,S,D^{g}	R,B,O,D^{c}	R,B,O,S^{d}
KMS	24 hours	B,O,S,D^{e}	R,O,S,D^{b}	R,B,S,D^{g}	R,B,O,D^{c}	R,B,O,S^{d}
KMS	48 hours	B,O,S,D^{e}	R,O,S,D^{b}	R,B,S,D^{g}	R,B,O,D^{c}	R,B,O,S^{d}
KMS	14 days	B,O,S,D^{e}	R,O,S,D^{b}	R,B,S,D^{g}	R,B,O,D^{c}	R,B,O,S^{d}
KMS	15 days	B,O,S,D^{e}	R,O,S,D^{b}	R,B,S,D^{g}	R,B,O,D^{c}	B,O,S^{g}

R= Raw state, B= Boiling, O= Open pan dry roasting, S= Shallow frying, D= Deep frying. The same uppercase alphabets represent that there is no significant difference present among the variables.

This table shows the significant difference among the different variables such as cooking methods and preservation conditions. The raw state significantly differs from boiling, open pan dry roasting, shallow frying and deep frying in all of the preservation methods with preservatives and control preservation without preservative except in fresh condition and 15 days control preservation without preservative. Boiling significantly differs from the raw state, open pan dry roasting, shallow frying and deep frying in all the preservation conditions except in fresh condition, 24 hours control preservation without preservative and 15 days salt and turmeric preservation. Open pan dry roasting significantly differs from the raw state, boiling, shallow frying and deep frying in all of the preservation conditions except in 24 hours control preservation without preservative, 24 hours, 14 days salt and turmeric preservation. Shallow frying significantly differs from the raw state, boiling, open pan dry roasting and deep frying in all of the preservation conditions. Deep frying significantly differs from the raw state, boiling, open pan dry roasting and shallow frying in all the preservation conditions except in 15 days KMS preservation.

The raw state and open pan dry roasting significantly differ from boiling, shallow frying and deep frying in fresh condition, whereas the raw state and open pan dry roasting significantly differ from boiling, shallow frying and deep frying in 15 days control preservation without preservative and 24 hours salt and turmeric preservation respectively. Boiling and open pan dry roasting significantly differ from the raw state, shallow frying and deep frying in 24 hours control preservation without preservative, whereas boiling and open pan dry roasting significantly differ from the raw state, shallow frying and deep frying in 15 days salt and turmeric preservation and 14 days salt and turmeric preservation respectively. Again deep frying significantly differs from boiling, open pan dry roasting and shallow frying in 15 days KMS preservation.

Table no 5.3.4.5 Gradation of cooking methods from higher to lower restoration with respect to preservation days

Preservation	Duration	Method 1	Method 2	Method 3	Method 4	Method 5
Control	Fresh	SF	DF	B	R	OPDR
Control	24 hours	SF	DF	R	OPDR	B
Control	48 hours	DF	SF	B	R	OPDR
Control	14 days	SF	DF	B	R	OPDR
Control	15 days	SF	DF	B	R	OPDR
Salt &Turmeric	24 hours	DF	B	SF	R	OPDR
Salt & Turmeric	48 hours	DF	SF	OPDR	R	B
Salt & Turmeric	14 days	SF	B	DF	R	OPDR
Salt &Turmeric	15 days	SF	DF	R	B	OPDR
KMS	24 hours	DF	SF	R	B	OPDR
KMS	48 hours	SF	DF	B	OPDR	R
KMS	14 days	SF	DF	B	OPDR	R
KMS	15 days	SF	DF	OPDR	R	B

R= Raw state, B= Boiling, OPDR= Open pan dry roasting, SF= Shallow frying, DF= Deep frying. Same colours represent the similar order.

In all the preservation methods and fresh condition, fat retention occurs mainly in shallow frying as compared to the other cooking methods. In fresh condition, 14 days and 15 days control preservation without preservative, fat retention occurs firstly in shallow frying followed by deep frying, boiling, raw state and open pan dry roasting. In 24 hours control preservation without preservative, it changes in the order of shallow frying, deep frying, raw state, open pan dry roasting and boiling. In 48 hours control preservation without preservative, the order changes to deep frying, shallow frying, boiling, raw state and open pan dry roasting.

In 24 hours salt and turmeric preservation, the order remains deep frying, boiling, shallow frying, raw state and open pan dry roasting. In 48 hours salt and turmeric preservation, the order remains deep frying, shallow frying, open pan dry roasting, raw state and boiling. In 14 days salt and turmeric preservation, it remains in the order of shallow frying, boiling, deep frying, raw state and open pan dry roasting. In 15 days salt and turmeric preservation, the order is shallow frying, deep frying, raw state, boiling and open pan dry roasting.

In 24 hours KMS preservation, the order is deep frying, shallow frying, raw state, boiling and open pan dry roasting. In 48 hours and 14 days KMS preservation, the order remains shallow frying, deep frying, boiling, open pan dry roasting and the raw state. In 15 days KMS preservation, the order becomes shallow frying, deep frying, open pan dry roasting, raw state and boiling.

The overall analysis of fat content of lobster is mostly restored by the gradation of methods as shallow frying > deep frying> boiling> raw state> open pan dry roasting.

Frying mainly restores[66] the fat content as the oil can possibly create a protective layer so that the lipid molecules cannot be leached out, but in boiling the fat content is reduced if the cooking water is discarded. Open pan dry roasting reduces the fat content due to the application of direct dry heat so the lipid molecules present in lobster get melted, leading to reduction. Thus among all the studied conventional cooking methods, **shallow frying** is the best method for cooking lobster to restore fat content.

5.3.5 Pomfret (*Pampus argenteus*)

It has been reported that pomfret contains 5.12 gm of fat per 100 gm[85] in the raw condition. This value changes due to the application of different cooking methods and preservation conditions (vide Table no **5.3.5.1**).

Table no 5.3.5.1 Fat content of Pomfret (gm/100gm)

Preservation	Duration	Raw state	Boiling	Dry roasting	Shallow frying	Deep frying
Control	Fresh	6.71±0.09	2.78±0.07	5.78±0.08	5.43±0.04	4.47±0.04
Control	24 hours	5.59±0.08	6.25±0.05	2.42±0.03	8.43±0.04	5.15±0.05
Control	48 hours	16.62±0.03	18.02±0.03	10.80±0.10	18.06±0.02	9.65±0.03
Control	14 days	14.34±0.06	11.92±0.03	4.76±0.06	2.33±0.03	3.24±0.04
Control	15 days	13.07±0.03	8.83±0.04	11.76±0.07	12.59±0.03	7.38±0.04
Salt & Turmeric	24 hours	19.40±0.08	21.26±0.05	14.40±0.08	16.92±0.03	18.82±0.03
Salt & Turmeric	48 hours	19.84±0.05	14.17±0.06	15.50±0.02	16.82±0.03	13.25±0.13
Salt & Turmeric	14 days	14.32±0.03	18.72±0.03	12.06±0.03	7.92±0.03	9.45±0.05
Salt & Turmeric	15 days	21.95±0.04	9.69±0.07	13.88±0.08	15.65±0.05	9.06±0.05
KMS	24 hours	25.93±0.07	14.54±0.05	18.84±0.05	39.42±0.03	17.18±0.08
KMS	48 hours	23.25±0.05	12.15±0.05	13.94±0.04	23.46±0.06	16.79±0.07
KMS	14 days	20.52±0.02	18.35±0.06	12.38±0.05	11.95±0.05	14.04±0.06
KMS	15 days	22.89±0.04	11.90±0.10	16.82±0.06	16.90±0.04	10.12±0.10

Values are expressed as mean±SD. ☐ Loss ☐ Restoration
Red digits represent the significant highest values from the raw state in different conditions.

In most of the preservation conditions, fat losses mainly occur by deep frying, whereas in fresh condition, 24 hours, 48 hours KMS preservation, fat content is reduced by boiling. In 24 hours control preservation without preservative as well as 24 hours salt and turmeric preservation, fat loss occurs by open pan dry roasting. In 14 days control preservation without preservative, salt and turmeric preservation as well as KMS preservation, fat loss occurs by shallow frying.

Retention of fat occurs mostly by shallow frying, [38] but in 14 days control preservation without preservative, 24 hours, 14 days salt and turmeric preservation and 14 days KMS preservation, fat retention occurs by boiling. In fresh condition and 15 days KMS preservation, fat retention occurs by open pan dry roasting.

The raw state, open pan dry roasting, shallow frying and deep frying show the highest fat content in 24 hours KMS preservation, whereas boiling shows the highest fat content in 24 hours salt and turmeric preservation.

In 24 hours, 48 hours control preservation without preservative, 24 hours, 14 days salt and turmeric preservation, the fat content increases by boiling than the raw state. This may occur due to the molecular rearrangement during cooking or as fat is not get dissolved in the water so there is no elimination of lipid, but some other water soluble nutrients may get eliminated, increasing the concentration of lipid.

Shallow fried pomfret shows the increased content of fat than the raw state in all the preservation conditions including fresh condition due to the addition of edible oil for frying[48]. There is prominent effect of synthetic preservative. It may probably help to modify the structure of lipid so that deterioration is reduced. Pomfret is a fatty fish so the deep frying reduces the fat content more than the other cooking methods.

Fig. 5.3.5.2 Graphical representation of Fat content of Pomfret with respect to different conditions

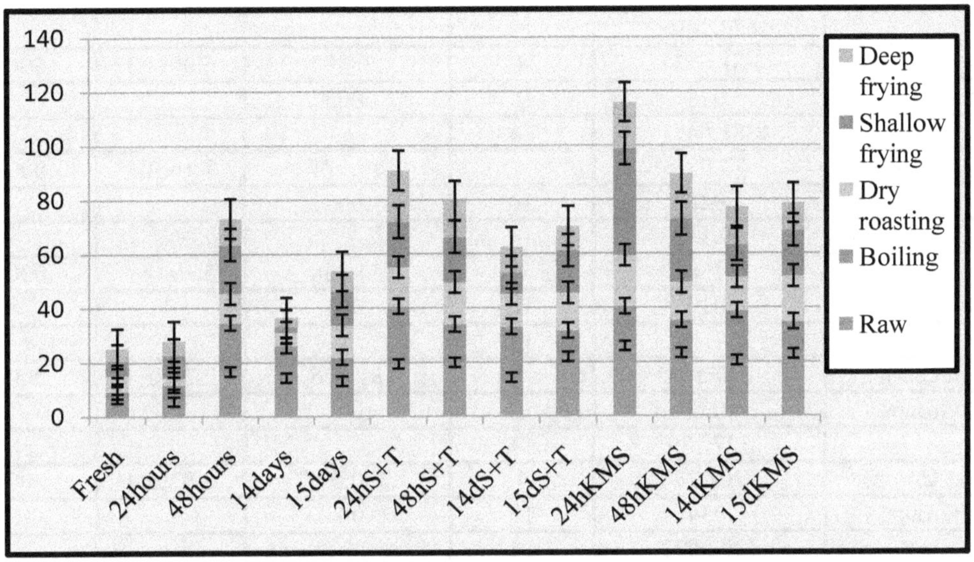

This graphical representation indicates that among all the preservation conditions, **24 hours KMS preservation** helps to increase the fat content in all the cooking methods. The possible reason for this may be the moisture loss due to preservation. Here the graph shows that salt and turmeric preservation also increases the fat content, whereas KMS preservation comparatively increases the fat content more than that which is control preservation without preservative and salt and turmeric preservation. KMS can probably help to prevent the microbial growth and delays the lipid deterioration.

Table no 5.3.5.3 ANOVA with regard to cooking conditions and preservation methods

Condition	Differences	Sum of Squares	df	Mean Square	F	Sig.
Fresh (control)	Between Groups	36.558	4	9.140	2.109E3	.000(S)
	Within Groups	.043	10	.004		
	Total	36.602	14			
24 hours (control)	Between Groups	56.281	4	14.070	5.049E3	.000(S)
	Within Groups	.028	10	.003		
	Total	56.309	14			
48 hours (control)	Between Groups	200.335	4	50.084	2.064E4	.000(S)
	Within Groups	.024	10	.002		
	Total	200.359	14			
14 days (control)	Between Groups	355.872	4	88.968	4.618E4	.000(S)
	Within Groups	.019	10	.002		
	Total	355.891	14			
15 days (control)	Between Groups	74.248	4	18.562	8.728E3	.000(S)
	Within Groups	.021	10	.002		
	Total	74.269	14			
24 hours (salt & turmeric)	Between Groups	81.613	4	20.403	6.001E3	.000(S)
	Within Groups	.034	10	.003		
	Total	81.647	14			
48 hours (salt & turmeric)	Between Groups	79.085	4	19.771	7.163E3	.000(S)
	Within Groups	.028	10	.003		
	Total	79.112	14			
14 days (salt & turmeric)	Between Groups	217.472	4	54.368	5.194E4	.000(S)
	Within Groups	.010	10	.001		
	Total	217.482	14			
15 days (salt & turmeric)	Between Groups	327.103	4	81.776	2.247E4	.000(S)
	Within Groups	.036	10	.004		
	Total	327.139	14			
24 hours (KMS)	Between Groups	1202.788	4	300.697	8.879E4	.000(S)
	Within Groups	.034	10	.003		
	Total	1202.822	14			
48 hours (KMS)	Between Groups	328.342	4	82.085	2.818E4	.000(S)
	Within Groups	.029	10	.003		
	Total	328.371	14			
14 days (KMS)	Between Groups	173.545	4	43.386	1.517E4	.000(S)
	Within Groups	.029	10	.003		
	Total	173.573	14			
15 days (KMS)	Between Groups	298.821	4	74.705	1.896E4	.000(S)
	Within Groups	.039	10	.004		
	Total	298.860	14			

$p<0.05$ S= Significant, NS= Non-significant. All abbreviations are on page so and so.

This statistical ANOVA table shows that all the values are significant, which means there is significant difference present in the values of fat content of pomfret among different cooking methods and the raw state in respect to fresh condition along with different preservation methods.

Table no 5.3.5.4 Post hoc Duncan statistical analysis

Preservation	Duration	Raw state	Boiling	Dry roasting	Shallow frying	Deep frying
Control	Fresh	B,O,S,D[a]	R,O,S,D[b]	R,B,S,D[c]	R,B,O,D[d]	R,B,O,S[e]
Control	24 hours	B,O,S,D[a]	R,O,S,D[b]	R,B,S,D[c]	R,B,O,D[d]	R,B,O,S[e]
Control	48 hours	B,O,S,D[a]	R,O,D[f]	R,B,S,D[c]	R,O,D[f]	R,B,O,S[e]
Control	14 days	B,O,S,D[a]	R,O,S,D[b]	R,B,S,D[c]	R,B,O,D[d]	R,B,O,S[e]
Control	15 days	B,O,S,D[a]	R,O,S,D[b]	R,B,S,D[c]	R,B,O,D[d]	R,B,O,S[e]
Salt & Turmeric	24 hours	B,O,S,D[a]	R,O,S,D[b]	R,B,S,D[c]	R,B,O,D[d]	R,B,O,S[e]
Salt & Turmeric	48 hours	B,O,S,D[a]	R,O,S,D[b]	R,B,S,D[c]	R,B,O,D[d]	R,B,O,S[e]
Salt & Turmeric	14 days	B,O,S,D[a]	R,O,S,D[b]	R,B,S,D[c]	R,B,O,D[d]	R,B,O,S[e]
Salt & Turmeric	15 days	B,O,S,D[a]	R,O,S,D[b]	R,B,S,D[c]	R,B,O,D[d]	R,B,O,S[e]
KMS	24 hours	B,O,S,D[a]	R,O,S,D[b]	R,B,S,D[c]	R,B,O,D[d]	R,B,O,S[e]
KMS	48 hours	B,O,S,D[a]	R,O,S,D[b]	R,B,S,D[c]	R,B,O,D[d]	R,B,O,S[e]
KMS	14 days	B,O,S,D[a]	R,O,S,D[b]	R,B,S,D[c]	R,B,O,D[d]	R,B,O,S[e]
KMS	15 days	B,O,S,D[a]	R,O,S,D[b]	R,B,D[g]	R,B,D[g]	R,B,O,S[e]

R= Raw state, B= Boiling, O= Open pan dry roasting, S= Shallow frying, D= Deep frying. The same uppercase alphabets signify that there is no significant difference present among the variables.

This table shows the significant difference among the different variables such as cooking methods and preservation conditions. The raw state significantly differs from boiling, open pan dry roasting, shallow frying and deep frying in all of the preservation conditions i.e. with preservatives and control preservation without preservative. Boiling significantly differs from the raw state, open pan dry roasting, shallow frying and deep frying in all the preservation conditions except in 48 hours control preservation without preservative. Open pan dry roasting significantly differs from the raw state, boiling, shallow frying and deep frying in all the preservation conditions except in 15 days KMS preservation. Shallow frying significantly differs from the raw state, boiling, open pan dry roasting and deep frying in all of the preservation conditions except in 48 hours control preservation without preservative and 15 days KMS preservation. Deep frying significantly differs from the raw state, boiling, open pan dry roasting and shallow frying in all the preservation conditions.

Boiling and shallow frying significantly differ from the raw state, open pan dry roasting and deep frying in 48 hours control preservation without preservative, whereas shallow frying and open pan dry roasting significantly differ from the raw state, boiling and deep frying in 15 days KMS preservation.

Table no 5.3.5.5 Gradation of cooking methods from higher to lower restoration with respect to preservation days

Preservation	Duration	Method 1	Method 2	Method 3	Method 4	Method 5
Control	Fresh	OPDR	SF	DF	B	R
Control	24 hours	SF	B	R	DF	OPDR
Control	48 hours	SF	B	R	OPDR	DF
Control	14 days	R	B	OPDR	DF	SF
Control	15 days	R	SF	OPDR	B	DF
Salt & Turmeric	24 hours	B	R	DF	SF	OPDR
Salt & Turmeric	48 hours	R	SF	OPDR	B	DF
Salt & Turmeric	14 days	B	R	OPDR	DF	SF
Salt &Turmeric	15 days	R	SF	OPDR	B	DF
KMS	24 hours	SF	R	OPDR	DF	B
KMS	48 hours	SF	R	DF	OPDR	B
KMS	14 days	R	B	DF	OPDR	SF
KMS	15 days	R	SF	OPDR	B	DF

R= Raw state, B= Boiling, OPDR= Open pan dry roasting, SF= Shallow frying, DF= Deep frying. Same colour represents the similar order.

In all the preservation techniques and fresh condition, fat retention occurs mainly in the raw state than the other cooking methods. In fresh condition, retention occurs firstly in open pan dry roasting followed by shallow frying, deep frying, boiling and the raw state. In 24 hours control preservation without preservative, it changes in the order of shallow frying, boiling, raw state, deep frying and open pan dry roasting. In 48 hours control preservation without preservative, the order changes to shallow frying, boiling, raw state, open pan dry roasting and deep frying. In 14 days control preservation without preservative, the order is the raw state, boiling, open pan dry roasting, deep frying and shallow frying. In 15 days control preservation without preservative, 48 hours, 15 days salt and turmeric preservation as well as 15 days KMS preservation, the order changes to the raw state, shallow frying, open pan dry roasting, boiling and deep frying.

In 24 hours salt and turmeric preservation, the order remains boiling, raw state, deep frying, shallow frying and open pan dry roasting. In 14 days salt and turmeric preservation, it changes in the order of boiling, raw state, open pan dry roasting, deep frying and shallow frying.

In 24 hours KMS preservation, the order is shallow frying, raw state, open pan dry roasting deep frying and boiling. In 48 hours KMS preservation, the order becomes shallow frying, raw state, deep frying, open pan dry roasting and boiling. In 14 days KMS preservation, the order is the raw state, boiling, deep frying, open pan dry roasting and shallow frying.

The overall analysis of fat content of pomfret is mostly is restored by the gradation of methods as the raw state> shallow frying> open pan dry roasting> boiling> deep frying.

Shallow frying mainly restores[66] the fat content as the oil can possibly create a protective layer so that the lipid molecules cannot be leached out, but in boiling the fat content is reduced if the water, in which the fish is cooked, is discarded. Open pan dry roasting reduces the fat content due to the application of direct dry heat, so the lipid molecules present in pomfret are melted, resulting in the reduction. Deep frying mostly reduces the fat content as lipid of the fish gets eliminated from the flesh due to higher concentration of cooking oil and also due to the application of heat that melts the tissue fat during deep frying. Thus among all the studied conventional cooking methods, **shallow frying** is the best method for cooking pomfret in order to restore fat content.

5.3.6 *Hilsa* (*Tenualosa Ilisha*)

It has been reported that *hilsa* contains 18.49 gm of fat per 100 gm[85] in the raw condition. This value changes due to the application of different cooking methods and preservation conditions (vide Table no **5.3.6.1**).

Table no 5.3.6.1 Fat content of *Hilsa* (gm/100gm)

Preservation	Duration	Raw state	Boiling	Dry roasting	Shallow frying	Deep frying
Control	Fresh	13.21±0.17	13.12±0.10	6.28±0.03	6.14±0.04	3.62±0.04
Control	24 hours	26.71±0.30	13.20±0.16	6.43±0.04	8.16±0.13	5.37±0.03
Control	48 hours	29.49±0.03	13.10±0.03	12.07±0.04	9.64±0.07	10.20±0.05
Control	14 days	28.90±0.09	18.10±0.10	11.98±0.08	16.04±0.04	11.57±0.06
Control	15 days	29.10±0.10	20.52±0.03	14.89±0.09	13.18±0.03	9.64±0.06
Salt & Turmeric	24 hours	23.45±0.05	22.72±0.08	9.24±0.01	18.60±0.10	11.20±0.12
Salt & Turmeric	48 hours	25.48±0.08	27.18±0.08	13.60±0.10	12.10±0.10	9.96±0.05
Salt & Turmeric	14 days	23.33±0.07	27.30±0.10	12.90±0.10	13.51±0.10	6.82±0.03
Salt & Turmeric	15 days	21.98±0.04	20.37±0.06	14.62±0.10	16.10±0.10	10.81±0.10
KMS	24 hours	26.41±0.09	26.10±0.10	12.61±0.09	9.85±0.06	10.20±0.11
KMS	48 hours	29.71±0.09	28.00±0.10	10.52±0.09	14.50±0.11	13.82±0.07
KMS	14 days	29.10±0.10	25.19±0.08	13.50±0.10	17.31±0.11	11.61±0.11
KMS	15 days	30.53±0.09	33.72±0.09	24.21±0.10	15.61±0.11	17.14±0.09

Values are expressed as mean±SD. Loss Restoration

Red digits represent the significant highest values from the raw state in different conditions.

In most of the preservation conditions, fat losses mainly occurs by deep frying, whereas in 48 hours control preservation without preservative, 24 hours, 15 days KMS preservation, fat content is reduced by shallow frying. Again in 24 hours salt and turmeric preservation and 48 hours KMS preservation, fat content is reduced by open pan dry roasting. Retention of fat content occurs by boiling in all the preservation methods.

The raw state, boiling, open pan dry roasting and deep frying show the highest fat content in 15 days KMS preservation, whereas shallow frying in 24 hours salt and turmeric preservation. In 48 hours, 14 days salt and turmeric preservation and 15 days KMS preservation, the fat content increases by boiling than the raw state.

Boiled *hilsa* shows the increased content of fat as fat molecules cannot be dissolved in cooking water, but the other nutrients get dissolved and eliminated, increasing the concentration of fat. There is a prominent effect of synthetic preservative on the restoration of fat content of *hilsa*. It may help to modify the structure of fat in such a way so that deterioration is reduced.

Fig. 5.3.6.2 Graphical representation of Fat content of *Hilsa* with respect to different conditions

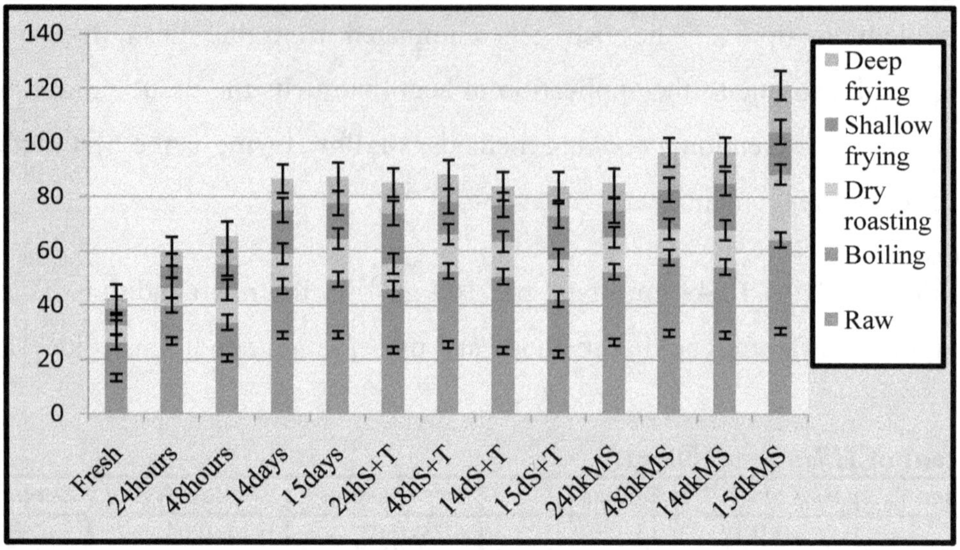

This graphical representation indicates that among all the preservation conditions, **15 days KMS preservation** helps to increase the fat content in all the cooking methods. The possible reason may be the moisture loss due to prolonged preservation. Here the graph shows that salt and turmeric preservation also increases the fat content, whereas KMS preservation comparatively increases the fat content more than that which is control preservation without preservative and salt and turmeric preservation. KMS can probably help to prevent the microbial growth and delays the lipid deterioration.

Table no 5.3.6.3 ANOVA with regard to cooking conditions and preservation methods

Condition	Differences	Sum of Squares	df	Mean Square	F	Sig.
Fresh (control)	Between Groups	234.558	4	58.639	1.705E4	.000(S)
	Within Groups	.034	10	.003		
	Total	234.592	14			
24 hours (control)	Between Groups	921.349	4	230.337	1.223E4	.000(S)
	Within Groups	.188	10	.019		
	Total	921.538	14			
48 hours (control)	Between Groups	821.878	4	205.470	8.682E4	.000(S)
	Within Groups	.024	10	.002		
	Total	821.902	14			
14 days (control)	Between Groups	594.061	4	148.515	2.462E4	.000(S)
	Within Groups	.060	10	.006		
	Total	594.121	14			
15 days (control)	Between Groups	694.548	4	173.637	2.747E4	.000(S)
	Within Groups	.063	10	.006		
	Total	694.611	14			
24 hours (salt & turmeric)	Between Groups	512.607	4	128.152	1.907E4	.000(S)
	Within Groups	.067	10	.007		
	Total	512.674	14			
48 hours (salt & turmeric)	Between Groups	775.913	4	193.978	2.758E4	.000(S)
	Within Groups	.070	10	.007		
	Total	775.983	14			
14 days (salt & turmeric)	Between Groups	835.630	4	208.908	2.833E4	.000(S)
	Within Groups	.074	10	.007		
	Total	835.704	14			
15 days (salt & turmeric)	Between Groups	242.043	4	60.511	8.320E3	.000(S)
	Within Groups	.073	10	.007		
	Total	242.116	14			
24 hours (KMS)	Between Groups	863.916	4	215.979	2.673E4	.000(S)
	Within Groups	.081	10	.008		
	Total	863.997	14			
48 hours (KMS)	Between Groups	942.203	4	235.551	2.645E4	.000(S)
	Within Groups	.089	10	.009		
	Total	942.293	14			
14 days (KMS)	Between Groups	681.950	4	170.487	1.681E4	.000(S)
	Within Groups	.101	10	.010		
	Total	682.051	14			
15 days (KMS)	Between Groups	762.652	4	190.663	1.978E4	.000(S)
	Within Groups	.096	10	.010		
	Total	762.748	14			

$p<0.05$ S= Significant, NS= Non-significant. All abbreviations are on page so and so.

This statistical ANOVA table shows that all the values are significant, which means there is significant difference present in the values of fat content of *hilsa* among different cooking methods and the raw state in respect to fresh condition along with different preservation methods.

Table no 5.3.6.4 Post hoc Duncan statistical analysis

Preservation	Duration	Raw state	Boiling	Dry roasting	Shallow frying	Deep frying
Control	Fresh	B,O,S,D[a]	R,O,S,D[b]	R,B,S,D[c]	R,B,O,D[d]	R,B,O,S[e]
Control	24 hours	B,O,S,D[a]	R,O,S,D[b]	R,B,S,D[c]	R,B,O,D[d]	R,B,O,S[e]
Control	48 hours	B,O,S,D[a]	R,O,S,D[b]	R,B,S,D[c]	R,B,O,D[d]	R,B,O,S[e]
Control	14 days	B,O,S,D[a]	R,O,S,D[b]	R,B,S,D[c]	R,B,O,D[d]	R,B,O,S[e]
Control	15 days	B,O,S,D[a]	R,O,S,D[b]	R,B,S,D[c]	R,B,O,D[d]	R,B,O,S[e]
Salt & Turmeric	24 hours	B,O,S,D[a]	R,O,S,D[b]	R,B,S,D[c]	R,B,O,D[d]	R,B,O,S[e]
Salt & Turmeric	48 hours	B,O,S,D[a]	R,O,S,D[b]	R,B,S,D[c]	R,B,O,D[d]	R,B,O,S[e]
Salt & Turmeric	14 days	B,O,S,D[a]	R,O,S,D[b]	R,B,S,D[c]	R,B,O,D[d]	R,B,O,S[e]
Salt & Turmeric	15days	B,O,S,D[a]	R,O,S,D[b]	R,B,S,D[c]	R,B,O,D[d]	R,B,O,S[e]
KMS	24 hours	B,O,S,D[a]	R,O,S,D[b]	R,B,S,D[c]	R,B,O,D[d]	R,B,O,S[e]
KMS	48 hours	B,O,S,D[a]	R,O,S,D[b]	R,B,S,D[c]	R,B,O,D[d]	R,B,O,S[e]
KMS	14 days	B,O,S,D[a]	R,O,S,D[b]	R,B,S,D[c]	R,B,O,D[d]	R,B,O,S[e]
KMS	15 days	B,O,S,D[a]	R,O,S,D[b]	R,B,S,D[c]	R,B,O,D[d]	R,B,O,S[e]

R= Raw state, B= Boiling, O= Open pan dry roasting, S= Shallow frying, D= Deep frying. The same uppercase alphabets represent that there is no significant difference present among the variables.

This table shows the significant difference among the different variables such as cooking methods and preservation conditions. The raw state significantly differs from boiling, open pan dry roasting, shallow frying and deep frying in all of the preservation methods with preservatives and control preservation without preservative. Boiling significantly differs from the raw state, open pan dry roasting, shallow frying and deep frying in all the preservation conditions. Open pan dry roasting significantly differs from the raw state, boiling, shallow frying and deep frying in all the preservation conditions. Shallow frying significantly differs from the raw state, boiling, open pan dry roasting and deep frying in all the preservation conditions. Deep frying significantly differs from the raw state, boiling, open pan dry roasting and shallow frying in all the preservation conditions.

Table no 5.3.6.5 Gradation of cooking methods from higher to lower restoration with respect to preservation days

Preservation	Duration	Method 1	Method 2	Method 3	Method 4	Method 5
Control	Fresh	R	B	OPDR	SF	DF
Control	24 hours	R	B	SF	OPDR	DF
Control	48 hours	R	B	OPDR	DF	SF
Control	14 days	R	B	SF	OPDR	DF
Control	15 days	R	B	OPDR	SF	DF
Salt & Turmeric	24 hours	R	B	SF	DF	OPDR
Salt & Turmeric	48 hours	B	R	OPDR	SF	DF
Salt & Turmeric	14 days	B	R	SF	OPDR	DF
Salt &Turmeric	15 days	R	B	SF	OPDR	DF
KMS	24 hours	R	B	OPDR	DF	SF
KMS	48 hours	R	B	SF	DF	OPDR
KMS	14 days	R	B	SF	OPDR	DF
KMS	15 days	B	R	OPDR	DF	SF

R= Raw state, B= Boiling, OPDR= Open pan dry roasting, SF= Shallow frying, DF= Deep frying. Same colours represent similar order.

In all the preservation methods and fresh condition, fat retention occurs mainly in the raw state than the other cooking methods. In fresh condition, 15 days control preservation without preservative, retention occurs firstly in the raw state followed by boiling, open pan dry roasting, shallow frying and deep frying.

In 24 hours, 14 days control preservation without preservative, it changes in the order of the raw state, boiling, shallow frying, open pan dry roasting and deep frying. In 48 hours control preservation without preservative and 24 hours KMS preservation, the order changes to the raw state, boiling, open pan dry roasting, deep frying and shallow frying.

In 24 hours salt and turmeric preservation and 48 hours KMS preservation, the order remains the raw state, boiling, shallow frying, deep frying and open pan dry roasting. In 48 hours salt and turmeric preservation, it remains in the order of boiling, raw state, open pan dry roasting, shallow frying and deep frying. In 14 days salt and turmeric preservation, the order is boiling, raw state, shallow frying, open pan dry roasting and deep frying. In 15 days salt and turmeric and 14 days KMS preservation, it remains in the order of the raw state, boiling, shallow frying, open pan dry roasting and deep frying. In 15 days KMS preservation, the order is boiling, raw state, open pan dry roasting, deep frying and shallow frying.

The overall analysis of fat content of *hilsa* is mostly restored by the gradation of methods as the raw state> boiling> shallow frying> open pan dry roasting> deep frying.

Hilsa is a fatty fish so that the lipid molecule can be restored best in boiling[56]. Fat cannot be dissolved in water so boiling can restore fat content, whereas shallow frying also restores the fat content as the oil can possibly create a protective layer so that the lipid molecules cannot be leached out. Open pan dry roasting reduces the fat content due to the application of direct dry heat so the lipid molecules present in *hilsa* get melted, resulting in reduction. Deep frying mostly reduces the fat content as lipid of the fish gets eliminated from the flesh possibly due to the higher concentration of cooking oil and the application of heat also melts the fatty tissue during deep frying. Thus among all the studied conventional cooking methods, **boiling** is the best method for cooking *hilsa* in order to restore fat content.

5.4 Moisture content

It has been reported that generally fish contains 60 - 80% of moisture[1]. This experiment is carried out to estimate the percentage of moisture content and also its changes in different cooking and preservation methods among different fish and edible aquatic species. Moisture content is estimated by wet difference method[72].

5.4.1 *Rohu* (*Labeo rohita*)

It has been reported that *rohu* contains 76.34 gm of moisture per 100 gm[85] in the raw condition. This value changes due to the application of different cooking methods and preservation conditions (vide Table no **5.4.1.1**).

Table no 5.4.1.1 Moisture content of *Rohu* (gm/100gm)

Preservation	Duration	Raw state	Boiling	Dry roasting	Shallow frying	Deep frying
Control	Fresh	77.27±1.41	55.63±1.62	36.40±1.31	41.53±1.20	21.51±0.31
Control	24 hours	75.40±2.44	69.97±2.94	41.30±3.21	40.24±0.58	24.20±1.92
Control	48 hours	76.00±2.10	61.53±6.65	35.90±5.10	30.62±4.22	21.20±1.59
Control	14 days	79.14±2.36	57.62±3.03	36.53±5.75	30.00±9.80	30.10±0.36
Control	15 days	79.90±2.19	52.00±7.00	41.83±3.95	40.81±0.90	23.48±0.05
Salt & Turmeric	24 hours	78.60±0.85	69.44±0.89	49.26±1.16	55.97±0.14	45.84±1.00
Salt &Turmeric	48 hours	80.98±0.40	69.17±0.56	44.57±0.64	59.66±0.66	42.84±0.31
Salt & Turmeric	14 days	77.38±0.75	67.58±0.77	45.01±1.00	47.40±2.53	35.21±0.71
Salt & Turmeric	15 days	76.38±1.69	69.49±0.95	49.38±0.79	50.97±0.50	41.34±1.03
KMS	24 hours	76.94±1.75	68.41±0.79	43.44±0.86	45.47±0.91	35.00±0.81
KMS	48 hours	79.60±0.61	64.34±0.76	45.52±1.00	49.37±0.52	37.28±0.68
KMS	14 days	79.74±0.77	65.60±0.88	38.98±0.55	50.85±0.51	38.57±0.61
KMS	15 days	76.87±1.10	62.48±1.34	40.41±0.87	40.10±1.56	35.50±0.88

Values are expressed as mean±SD. ☐ Loss ☐ Restoration

In most of the preservation conditions, moisture losses mainly occurs by deep frying, whereas in 14 days control preservation without preservative moisture content is reduced by shallow frying. Retention of moisture content occurs by boiling in all of the preservation methods.

The raw state and shallow frying show the highest moisture content in 48 hours salt and turmeric preservation, whereas boiling shows it in 24 hours control preservation without preservative. Open pan dry roasting and deep frying show the highest moisture content in 24 hours salt and turmeric preservation. There is a prominent effect of the natural preservative on the restoration of moisture content of *rohu*. It may occur due to the water absorption capacity of salt. Thus moisture content increases during salt and turmeric preservation.

Fig. 5.4.1.2 Graphical representation of Moisture content of *Rohu* with respect to different conditions

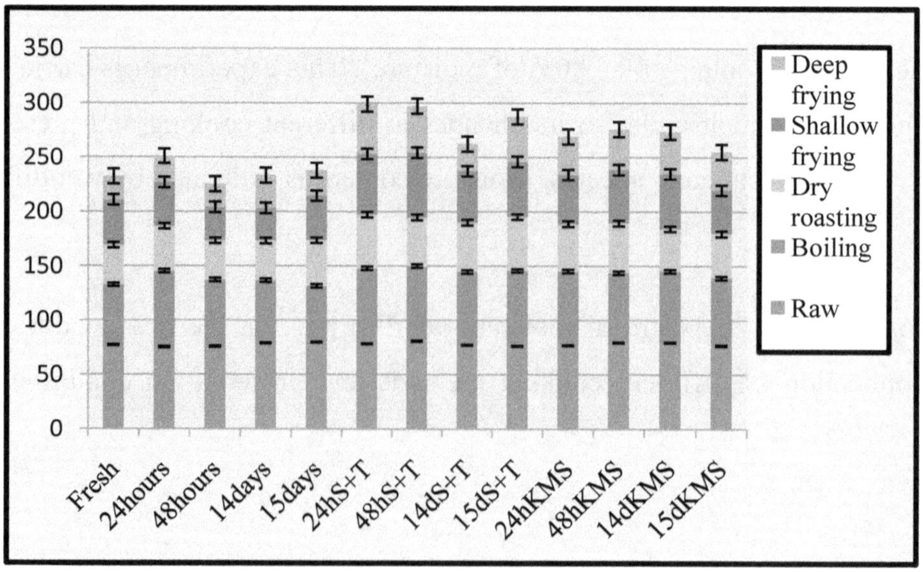

This graphical representation indicates that among all the preservation conditions, **24 hours, 48 hours salt and turmeric preservation**[55] help to increase the moisture content in all the cooking methods[34, 52]. The possible reason may be the water absorption capacity of salt and turmeric for prolonged preservation. Here the graph shows that KMS preservation also increases the moisture content, whereas salt and turmeric preservation comparatively increases the moisture content more than the control preservation without preservative and KMS preservation.

Table no 5.4.1.3 ANOVA with regard to cooking conditions and preservation methods

Condition	Differences	Sum of Squares	df	Mean Square	F	Sig.
Fresh (control)	Between Groups	5342.257	4	1335.564	861.402	.000(S)
	Within Groups	15.505	10	1.550		
	Total	5357.761	14			
24 hours (control)	Between Groups	4705.294	4	1176.324	228.546	.000(S)
	Within Groups	51.470	10	5.147		
	Total	4756.764	14			
48 hours (control)	Between Groups	5966.589	4	1491.647	120.887	.000(S)
	Within Groups	123.392	10	12.339		
	Total	6089.981	14			
14 days (control)	Between Groups	5488.227	4	1372.057	47.646	.000(S)
	Within Groups	287.971	10	28.797		
	Total	5776.197	14			
15 days (control)	Between Groups	5172.505	4	1293.126	93.151	.000(S)
	Within Groups	138.821	10	13.882		
	Total	5311.325	14			
24 hours (salt & turmeric)	Between Groups	2300.528	4	575.132	734.887	.000(S)
	Within Groups	7.826	10	.783		
	Total	2308.355	14			
48 hours (salt & turmeric)	Between Groups	3165.915	4	791.479	2.762E3	.000(S)
	Within Groups	2.865	10	.287		
	Total	3168.780	14			
14 days (salt & turmeric)	Between Groups	3620.885	4	905.221	497.491	.000(S)
	Within Groups	18.196	10	1.820		
	Total	3639.081	14			
15 days (salt & turmeric)	Between Groups	2782.041	4	695.510	69.542	.000(S)
	Within Groups	100.013	10	10.001		
	Total	2882.054	14			
24 hours (KMS)	Between Groups	3837.463	4	959.366	811.738	.000(S)
	Within Groups	11.819	10	1.182		
	Total	3849.282	14			
48 hours (KMS)	Between Groups	3384.368	4	846.092	1.580E3	.000(S)
	Within Groups	5.354	10	.535		
	Total	3389.722	14			
14 days (KMS)	Between Groups	3803.786	4	950.947	2.048E3	.000(S)
	Within Groups	4.642	10	.464		
	Total	3808.429	14			
15 days (KMS)	Between Groups	3815.929	4	953.982	680.315	.000(S)
	Within Groups	14.023	10	1.402		
	Total	3829.952	14			

$p<0.05$ S= Significant, NS= Non-significant. All abbreviations are on page so and so.

This statistical ANOVA table shows that all the values are significant, which means there is significant difference present in the values of moisture content of *rohu* among different cooking methods and the raw state in respect to fresh condition along with different preservation methods.

Table no 5.4.1.4 Post hoc Duncan statistical analysis

Preservation	Duration	Raw state	Boiling	Dry roasting	Shallow frying	Deep frying
Control	Fresh	B,O,S,D^{a}	R,O,S,D^{b}	R,B,S,D^{c}	R,B,O,D^{d}	R,B,O,S^{e}
Control	24 hours	B,O,S,D^{a}	R,O,S,D^{b}	R,B,D^{f}	R,B,D^{f}	R,B,O,S^{e}
Control	48 hours	B,O,S,D^{a}	R,O,S,D^{b}	R,B,D^{f}	R,B,D^{f}	R,B,O,S^{e}
Control	14 days	B,O,S,D^{a}	R,O,S,D^{b}	R,B^{g}	R,B^{g}	R,B^{g}
Control	15 days	B,O,S,D^{a}	R,O,S,D^{b}	R,B,D^{f}	R,B,D^{f}	R,B,O,S^{e}
Salt & Turmeric	24 hours	B,O,S,D^{a}	R,O,S,D^{b}	R,B,S,D^{c}	R,B,O,D^{d}	R,B,O,S^{e}
Salt & Turmeric	48 hours	B,O,S,D^{a}	R,O,S,D^{b}	R,B,S,D^{c}	R,B,O,D^{d}	R,B,O,S^{e}
Salt & Turmeric	14 days	B,O,S,D^{a}	R,O,S,D^{b}	R,B,D^{f}	R,B,D^{f}	R,B,O,S^{e}
Salt & Turmeric	15 days	O,S,D^{h}	O,S,D^{h}	R,B,D^{f}	R,B,D^{f}	R,B,O,S^{e}
KMS	24 hours	B,O,S,D^{a}	R,O,S,D^{b}	R,B,S,D^{c}	R,B,O,D^{d}	R,B,O,S^{e}
KMS	48 hours	B,O,S,D^{a}	R,O,S,D^{b}	R,B,S,D^{c}	R,B,O,D^{d}	R,B,O,S^{e}
KMS	14 days	B,O,S,D^{a}	R,O,S,D^{b}	R,B,S^{i}	R,B,O,D^{d}	R,B,S^{i}
KMS	15 days	B,O,S,D^{a}	R,O,S,D^{b}	R,B,D^{f}	R,B,D^{f}	R,B,O,S^{e}

R= Raw state, B= Boiling, O= Open pan dry roasting, S= Shallow frying, D= Deep frying. The same uppercase alphabets represent that there is no significant difference present among the variables.

This table shows the significant difference among the different variables such as cooking methods and preservation conditions. The raw state significantly differs from boiling, open pan dry roasting, shallow frying and deep frying in all of the preservation with preservatives and control preservations without preservative except in 15 days salt and turmeric preservation. Boiling significantly differs from the raw state, open pan dry roasting, shallow and deep frying in all the preservation conditions except in 15 days salt and turmeric preservation. Open pan dry roasting significantly differs from the raw state, boiling, shallow and deep frying in all of the preservation conditions except in 24 hours, 48 hours, 14 days and 15 days control preservation without preservative and 14 and 15 days salt and turmeric preservation as well as KMS preservation. Shallow frying significantly differs from the raw state, boiling, open pan dry roasting and deep frying in all the preservation conditions except in 24 hours, 48 hours, 14 days and 15 days control preservation without preservative and 14 days and 15 days salt and turmeric preservation as well as 15 days KMS preservation. Deep frying significantly differs from the raw state, boiling, open pan dry roasting and shallow frying in all the preservation conditions except in 14 days control preservation without preservative as well as 14 days KMS preservation.

The raw state and boiling significantly differ from open pan dry roasting, shallow frying and deep frying in 15 days salt and turmeric preservation, whereas shallow frying and open pan dry roasting significantly differ from the raw state, boiling and deep frying in 24 hours, 48 hours, 15 days control preservation without preservative and 14 days, 15 days salt and turmeric preservation as well as 15 days KMS preservation. Again shallow frying, deep frying and open pan dry roasting significantly differ from the raw state and boiling in 14 days control preservation without preservative. Deep frying and open pan dry roasting significantly differ from the raw state, boiling and shallow frying in 14 days KMS preservation.

Table no 5.4.1.5 Gradation of cooking methods from higher to lower restoration with respect to preservation days

Preservation	Duration	Method 1	Method 2	Method 3	Method 4	Method 5
Control	Fresh	R	B	SF	OPDR	DF
Control	24 hours	R	B	OPDR	SF	DF
Control	48 hours	R	B	OPDR	SF	DF
Control	14 days	R	B	OPDR	DF	SF
Control	15 days	R	B	OPDR	SF	DF
Salt &Turmeric	24 hours	R	B	SF	OPDR	DF
Salt & Turmeric	48 hours	R	B	SF	OPDR	DF
Salt & Turmeric	14 days	R	B	SF	OPDR	DF
Salt &Turmeric	15 days	R	B	SF	OPDR	DF
KMS	24 hours	R	B	SF	OPDR	DF
KMS	48 hours	R	B	SF	OPDR	DF
KMS	14 days	R	B	SF	OPDR	DF
KMS	15 days	R	B	OPDR	SF	DF

R= Raw state, B= Boiling, OPDR= Open pan dry roasting, SF= Shallow frying, DF= Deep frying. Same colours represent similar order.

In all the preservation methods and fresh condition, moisture retention occurs mainly in the raw state as compared to the other cooking methods. In fresh condition, 24 hours, 48 hours, 14 days, 15 days salt and turmeric preservation as well as 24 hours, 48 hours, 14 days KMS preservation, retention occurs firstly in the raw state followed by boiling, shallow frying, open pan dry roasting and deep frying.

In 24 hours, 48 hours control preservation without preservative, the order changes to the raw state, boiling, open pan dry roasting, shallow frying and deep frying. In 14 days control preservation without preservative, it changes in the order of the raw state, boiling, open pan dry roasting, deep frying and shallow frying. In 15 days control preservation without preservative as well as 15 days KMS preservation, the order remains the raw state, boiling, open pan dry roasting, shallow frying and deep frying.

The overall analysis of moisture content of *rohu* is mostly restored by the gradation of methods as the raw state> boiling> shallow frying> open pan dry roasting> deep frying.

Boiling can restore more moisture content due to the absorption of water during cooking, whereas shallow frying also restores moisture content as the oil can possibly create a protective layer so that the water molecules cannot be leached out. Open pan dry roasting reduces the moisture content possibly due to the application of direct dry heat so the water molecules present in *rohu* get eliminated, resulting in reduction. Deep frying mostly reduces the moisture content as total dryness occurs during deep frying possibly due to the elimination of water molecules. Thus among all the studied conventional cooking methods, **boiling** is the best method for cooking *rohu* to restore moisture content.

5.4.2 *Katla* (*Catla catla*)

It has been reported that *katla* contains 78.43 gm of moisture per 100 gm[85] in the raw condition. This value changes due to the application of different cooking methods and preservation conditions (vide Table no **5.4.2.1**).

Table no 5.4.2.1 Moisture content of *Katla* (gm/100gm)

Preservation	Duration	Raw state	Boiling	Dry roasting	Shallow frying	Deep frying
Control	Fresh	77.86±0.66	63.90±1.70	35.77±1.72	42.40±0.53	25.91±3.25
Control	24 hours	79.68±1.80	62.78±1.28	44.60±4.22	49.40±3.53	29.15±4.90
Control	48 hours	79.07±0.20	58.76±0.93	45.74±3.56	40.74±3.66	25.64±2.71
Control	14 days	71.77±0.78	60.02±0.62	38.76±0.48	38.76±0.40	30.98±0.88
Control	15 days	78.48±2.84	60.23±1.69	40.85±3.36	38.20±5.02	27.25±1.18
Salt & Turmeric	24 hours	76.74±0.34	70.33±0.85	70.33±0.85	44.60±1.16	46.54±0.76
Salt & Turmeric	48 hours	34.65±0.61	69.40±0.59	51.43±0.91	57.36±1.11	49.25±0.85
Salt & Turmeric	14 days	76.21±0.90	66.54±1.09	45.74±0.51	42.47±1.45	39.27±0.88
Salt & Turmeric	15 days	74.19±0.75	68.06±0.49	42.37±0.69	55.12±0.84	40.74±1.05
KMS	24 hours	75.59±0.29	68.61±0.75	48.44±1.21	54.43±0.51	32.40±1.84
KMS	48 hours	79.17±1.04	70.90±0.35	44.33±1.19	53.58±0.64	41.60±1.05
KMS	14 days	78.48±0.50	58.50±0.36	43.00±1.82	46.71±0.19	36.37±0.45
KMS	15 days	79.01±0.64	61.31±1.25	50.94±0.67	52.00±1.00	50.54±0.41

Values are expressed as mean±SD. Loss Restoration

In most of the preservation conditions, moisture losses mainly occurs by deep frying, whereas in 24 hours salt and turmeric preservation, moisture content is reduced by shallow frying. Retention of moisture content mainly occurs by boiling in all of the preservation methods, but in 24 hours salt and turmeric preservation, moisture retention also occurs by open pan dry roasting.

The raw state shows the highest moisture content in 24 hours control preservation without preservative, whereas boiling in 48 hours KMS preservation. Open pan dry roasting and shallow frying show the highest moisture content in 24 hours and 48 hours salt and turmeric preservation respectively. Deep frying shows the highest moisture content in 15 days KMS preservation.

There is a prominent effect of both the natural and synthetic preservatives on the restoration of moisture content of *katla*. It may occur due to the water absorption capacity of the preservatives.

Fig. 5.4.2.2 Graphical representation of Moisture content of *Katla* with respect to different conditions

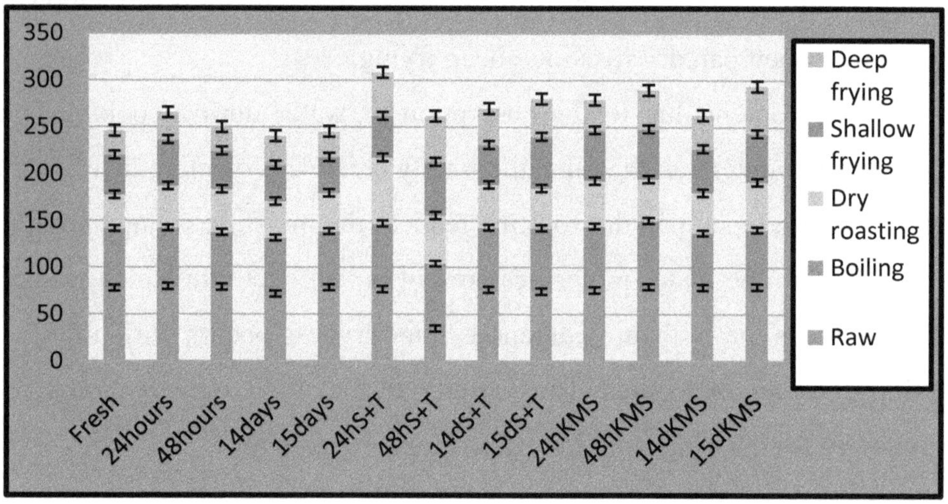

This graphical representation indicates that among all the preservation conditions, **24 hours salt and turmeric preservation**[55] helps to increase the moisture content in all the cooking methods[52]. The possible reason may be the water absorption capacity of salt and turmeric for prolonged preservation. Here the graph shows that KMS preservation also increases the moisture content, whereas salt and turmeric preservation comparatively increases the moisture content more than the control preservation without preservative and KMS preservation.

Table no 5.4.2.3 ANOVA with regard to cooking conditions and preservation methods

Condition	Differences	Sum of Squares	df	Mean Square	F	Sig.
Fresh (control)	Between Groups	5406.028	4	1351.507	408.917	.000(S)
	Within Groups	33.051	10	3.305		
	Total	5439.079	14			
24 hours (control)	Between Groups	4378.396	4	1094.599	92.273	.000(S)
	Within Groups	118.626	10	11.863		
	Total	4497.023	14			
48 hours (control)	Between Groups	4857.713	4	1214.428	176.298	.000(S)
	Within Groups	68.885	10	6.889		
	Total	4926.598	14			
14 days (control)	Between Groups	3509.976	4	877.494	2.002E3	.000(S)
	Within Groups	4.383	10	.438		
	Total	3514.358	14			
15 days (control)	Between Groups	4952.729	4	1238.182	125.979	.000(S)
	Within Groups	98.285	10	9.828		
	Total	5051.013	14			
24 hours (salt & turmeric)	Between Groups	3901.319	4	975.330	1.545E3	.000(S)
	Within Groups	6.313	10	.631		
	Total	3907.632	14			
48 hours (salt & turmeric)	Between Groups	2036.802	4	509.201	342.682	.000(S)
	Within Groups	14.859	10	1.486		
	Total	2051.661	14			
14 days (salt & turmeric)	Between Groups	3206.083	4	801.521	779.892	.000(S)
	Within Groups	10.277	10	1.028		
	Total	3216.361	14			
15 days (salt & turmeric)	Between Groups	2682.349	4	670.587	1.075E3	.000(S)
	Within Groups	6.241	10	.624		
	Total	2688.589	14			
24 hours (KMS)	Between Groups	3597.447	4	899.362	780.420	.000(S)
	Within Groups	11.524	10	1.152		
	Total	3608.971	14			
48 hours (KMS)	Between Groups	3271.435	4	817.859	976.882	.000(S)
	Within Groups	8.372	10	.837		
	Total	3279.807	14			
14 days (KMS)	Between Groups	3283.954	4	820.989	1.045E3	.000(S)
	Within Groups	7.855	10	.785		
	Total	3291.809	14			
15 days (KMS)	Between Groups	1773.457	4	443.364	614.492	.000(S)
	Within Groups	7.215	10	.722		
	Total	1780.672	14			

$p<0.05$ S= Significant, NS= Non-significant. All abbreviations are on page so and so.

This statistical ANOVA table shows that all the values are significant, which means there is significant difference present in the values of moisture content of *katla* among different cooking methods and the raw state in respect to fresh condition along with different preservation methods.

Table no 5.4.2.4 Post hoc Duncan statistical analysis

Preservation	Duration	Raw state	Boiling	Dry roasting	Shallow frying	Deep frying
Control	Fresh	B,O,S,D^{a}	R,O,S,D^{b}	R,B,S,D^{c}	R,B,O,D^{d}	R,B,O,S^{e}
Control	24 hours	B,O,S,D^{a}	R,O,S,D^{b}	R,B,D^{f}	R,B,D^{f}	R,B,O,S^{e}
Control	48 hours	B,O,S,D^{a}	R,O,S,D^{b}	R,B,S,D^{c}	R,B,O,D^{d}	R,B,O,S^{e}
Control	14 days	B,O,S,D^{a}	R,O,S,D^{b}	R,B,D^{f}	R,B,D^{f}	R,B,O,S^{e}
Control	15 days	B,O,S,D^{a}	R,O,S,D^{b}	R,B,D^{f}	R,B,D^{f}	R,B,O,S^{e}
Salt & Turmeric	24 hours	B,O,S,D^{a}	R,O,S,D^{b}	R,B,S,D^{c}	R,B,O,D^{d}	R,B,O,S^{e}
Salt & Turmeric	48 hours	B,O,S,D^{a}	R,O,S,D^{b}	R,B,S^{g}	R,B,O,D^{d}	R,B,S^{g}
Salt & Turmeric	14 days	B,O,S,D^{a}	R,O,S,D^{b}	R,B,S,D^{c}	R,B,O,D^{d}	R,B,O,S^{e}
Salt & Turmeric	15 days	B,O,S,D^{a}	R,O,S,D^{b}	R,B,S,D^{c}	R,B,O,D^{d}	R,B,O,S^{e}
KMS	24 hours	B,O,S,D^{a}	R,O,S,D^{b}	R,B,S,D^{c}	R,B,O,D^{d}	R,B,O,S^{e}
KMS	48 hours	B,O,S,D^{a}	R,O,S,D^{b}	R,B,S,D^{c}	R,B,O,D^{d}	R,B,O,S^{e}
KMS	14 days	B,O,S,D^{a}	R,O,S,D^{b}	R,B,S,D^{c}	R,B,O,D^{d}	R,B,O,S^{e}
KMS	15 days	B,O,S,D^{a}	R,O,S,D^{b}	R,B^{h}	R,B^{h}	R,B^{h}

R= Raw state, B= Boiling, O= Open pan dry roasting, S= Shallow frying, D= Deep frying. The same uppercase alphabets represent that there is no significant difference present among the variables.

This table shows the significant difference among the different variables such as cooking methods and preservation conditions. The raw state significantly differs from boiling, open pan dry roasting, shallow frying and deep frying in all of the preservation methods with preservatives and control preservation without preservative except in 15 days salt and turmeric preservation. Boiling significantly differs from the raw state, open pan dry roasting, shallow frying and deep frying in all the preservation conditions. Open pan dry roasting significantly differs from the raw state, boiling, shallow frying and deep frying in all of the preservation conditions except in 24 hours, 14 days and 15 days control preservation without preservative and 48 hours salt and turmeric preservation as well as 15 days KMS preservation. Shallow frying significantly differs from the raw state, boiling, open pan dry roasting and deep frying in all the preservation conditions except in 24 hours, 14 days and 15 days control preservation without preservative and 15 days KMS preservation. Deep frying significantly differs from the raw state, boiling, open pan dry roasting and shallow frying in all of the preservation conditions except in 48 hours salt and turmeric preservation as well as 15 days KMS preservation.

Shallow frying and open pan dry roasting significantly differ from the raw state, boiling and deep frying in 24 hours, 14 days, 15 days control preservation without preservative. Again open pan dry roasting and deep frying significantly differ from the raw state, boiling and shallow frying in 48 hours salt and turmeric preservation. Deep frying, shallow frying and open pan dry roasting significantly differ from the raw state and boiling in 15 days KMS preservation.

Table no 5.4.2.5 Gradation of cooking methods from higher to lower restoration with respect to preservation days

Preservation	Duration	Method 1	Method 2	Method 3	Method 4	Method 5
Control	Fresh	R	B	SF	OPDR	DF
Control	24 hours	R	B	SF	OPDR	DF
Control	48 hours	R	B	OPDR	SF	DF
Control	14 days	R	B	SF	OPDR	DF
Control	15 days	R	B	OPDR	SF	DF
Salt & Turmeric	24 hours	R	B	SF	OPDR	DF
Salt & Turmeric	48 hours	R	B	SF	OPDR	DF
Salt & Turmeric	14 days	R	B	OPDR	SF	DF
Salt &Turmeric	15 days	R	B	SF	OPDR	DF
KMS	24 hours	R	B	SF	OPDR	DF
KMS	48 hours	R	B	SF	OPDR	DF
KMS	14 days	R	B	SF	OPDR	DF
KMS	15 days	R	B	SF	OPDR	DF

R= Raw state, B= Boiling, OPDR= Open pan dry roasting, SF= Shallow frying, DF= Deep frying. Same colours represent similar order.

In all the preservation techniques and fresh condition, moisture retention occurs mainly in the raw state than the other cooking methods. In almost all the preservation conditions including fresh condition, retention occurs firstly in the raw state then boiling, shallow frying, open pan dry roasting and deep frying, whereas in 48 hours, 15 days control preservation without preservative as well as 14 days salt and turmeric preservation, retention occurs in the raw state followed by boiling, open pan dry roasting, shallow frying and deep frying.

The overall analysis of moisture content of *katla* is mostly restored by the gradation of methods as the raw state> boiling> shallow frying> open pan dry roasting> deep frying.

Boiling can restore more moisture content due to the absorption of water during cooking, whereas shallow frying also restores moisture content as the oil can possibly create a protective layer so that the water molecules cannot be leached out. Open pan dry roasting reduces the moisture content due to the application of direct dry heat so the water molecules present in *katla* get eliminated, leading to reduction. Deep frying mostly reduces the moisture content as total dryness occurs during deep frying possibly due to the elimination of water molecules. Thus among all the studied conventional cooking methods, **boiling** is the best method for cooking *katla* to restore moisture content.

5.4.3 Prawn (*Fenneropenaeus indicus*)

It has been reported that prawn contains 77.4 gm of moisture per 100 gm[84] in the raw condition. This value changes due to the application of different cooking methods and preservation conditions (vide Table no **5.4.3.1**).

Table no 5.4.3.1 Moisture content of Prawn (gm/100gm)

Preservation	Duration	Raw state	Boiling	Dry roasting	Shallow frying	Deep frying
Control	Fresh	79.84±1.25	52.93±0.30	35.67±0.91	39.50±0.87	23.90±0.51
Control	24 hours	79.81±0.5	48.97±0.44	42.96±0.15	31.21±0.52	25.17±0.39
Control	48 hours	82.62±0.55	43.00±0.50	30.87±0.81	34.44±0.50	20.45±0.52
Control	14 days	82.00±0.50	5.40±0.53	49.02±0.50	43.48±0.57	37.76±1.15
Control	15 days	82.86±0.15	60.50±0.88	53.00±0.91	49.02±1.04	51.40±1.08
Salt & Turmeric	24 hours	82.40±0.36	73.51±0.10	51.24±1.12	49.54±0.56	52.64±0.41
Salt & Turmeric	48 hours	78.90±0.65	70.51±0.69	56.68±0.70	56.56±1.30	43.64±0.62
Salt & Turmeric	14 days	78.36±0.73	70.91±0.78	58.77±0.81	54.56±0.49	44.83±0.35
Salt & Turmeric	15 days	80.28±0.67	66.93±0.23	56.34±0.57	50.53±0.35	52.21±0.25
KMS	24 hours	84.40±0.45	52.96±0.36	38.97±0.24	40.61±0.27	21.65±1.07
KMS	48 hours	80.94±0.58	52.94±0.24	49.11±0.36	51.05±0.56	47.64±0.31
KMS	14 days	79.89±1.70	59.18±1.27	51.37±1.18	46.14±1.00	26.00±1.32
KMS	15 days	80.30±1.48	53.24±1.38	45.78±0.36	46.32±0.02	39.28±1.34

Values are expressed as mean±SD. ☐ Loss ☐ Restoration

In most of the preservation conditions including fresh condition, moisture losses mainly occur by deep frying, whereas in 14 days control preservation without preservative, loss occurs by boiling, and in 15 days control preservation without preservative, 24 hours, 15 days salt and turmeric preservation moisture content is reduced by shallow frying. Retention of moisture content occurs by boiling in all of the preservation methods, but in 14 days control preservation without preservative, moisture retention occurs by open pan dry roasting.

The raw state shows the highest moisture content in 24 hours KMS preservation, whereas boiling and deep frying show the highest moisture content in 24 hours salt and turmeric preservation. Open pan dry roasting and shallow frying show the highest moisture content in 14 days, 48 hours salt and turmeric preservation respectively.

There is a prominent effect of the natural preservative on the restoration of moisture content of Prawn. It may occur due to the water absorption capacity of the salt.

Fig. 5.4.3.2 Graphical representation of Moisture content of Prawn with respect to different conditions

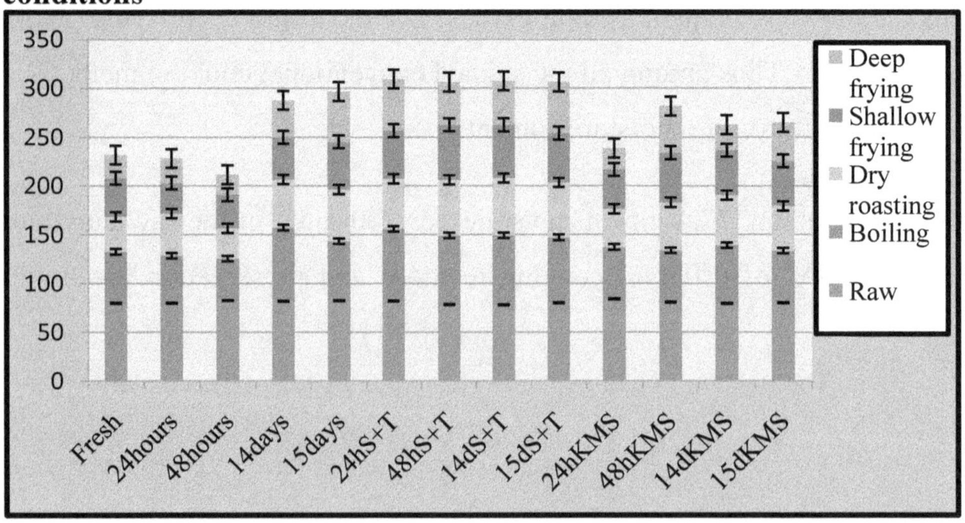

This graphical representation indicates that among all the preservation conditions, **24 hours salt and turmeric preservation**[55] helps to increase the moisture content in all the cooking methods[52]. The possible reason may be the water absorption capacity of salt and turmeric for prolonged preservation. Here the graph shows that KMS preservation also increases the moisture content, whereas salt and turmeric preservation comparatively increases the moisture content more than the control preservation without preservative and KMS preservation.

Table no 5.4.3.3 ANOVA with regard to cooking conditions and preservation methods

Condition	Differences	Sum of Squares	df	Mean Square	F	Sig.
Fresh (control)	Between Groups	5555.984	4	1388.996	2.731E3	.000(S)
	Within Groups	5.086	10	.509		
	Total	5561.070	14			
24 hours (control)	Between Groups	5440.521	4	1360.130	7.371E3	.000(S)
	Within Groups	1.845	10	.185		
	Total	5442.366	14			
48 hours (control)	Between Groups	6887.075	4	1721.769	4.930E3	.000(S)
	Within Groups	3.493	10	.349		
	Total	6890.567	14			
14 days (control)	Between Groups	4735.589	4	1183.897	2.428E3	.000(S)
	Within Groups	4.876	10	.488		
	Total	4740.465	14			
15 days (control)	Between Groups	2293.769	4	573.442	732.678	.000(S)
	Within Groups	7.827	10	.783		
	Total	2301.596	14			
24 hours (salt & turmeric)	Between Groups	2725.498	4	681.375	1.774E3	.000(S)
	Within Groups	3.840	10	.384		
	Total	2729.339	14			
48 hours (salt & turmeric)	Between Groups	2250.786	4	562.696	806.834	.000(S)
	Within Groups	6.974	10	.697		
	Total	2257.760	14			
14 days (salt & turmeric)	Between Groups	2119.135	4	529.784	1.211E3	.000(S)
	Within Groups	4.377	10	.438		
	Total	2123.512	14			
15 days (salt & turmeric)	Between Groups	1969.067	4	492.267	80.911	.000(S)
	Within Groups	60.840	10	6.084		
	Total	2029.907	14			
24 hours (KMS)	Between Groups	6538.290	4	1634.572	5.055E3	.000(S)
	Within Groups	3.234	10	.323		
	Total	6541.524	14			
48 hours (KMS)	Between Groups	2317.962	4	579.491	3.074E3	.000(S)
	Within Groups	1.885	10	.189		
	Total	2319.847	14			
14 days (KMS)	Between Groups	4616.452	4	1154.113	663.769	.000(S)
	Within Groups	17.387	10	1.739		
	Total	4633.839	14			
15 days (KMS)	Between Groups	3091.966	4	772.992	639.463	.000(S)
	Within Groups	12.088	10	1.209		
	Total	3104.054	14			

$p<0.05$ S= Significant, NS= Non-significant. All abbreviations are on page so and so.

This statistical ANOVA table shows that all the values are significant, which means there is significant difference present in the values of moisture content of prawn among different cooking methods and the raw state in respect to fresh condition along with different preservation methods.

Table no 5.4.3.4 Post hoc Duncan statistical analysis

Preservation	Duration	Raw state	Boiling	Dry roasting	Shallow frying	Deep frying
Control	Fresh	B,O,S,D^{a}	R,O,S,D^{b}	R,B,S,D^{c}	R,B,O,D^{d}	R,B,O,S^{e}
Control	24 hours	B,O,S,D^{a}	R,O,S,D^{b}	R,B,S,D^{c}	R,B,O,D^{d}	R,B,O,S^{e}
Control	48 hours	B,O,S,D^{a}	R,O,S,D^{b}	R,B,S,D^{c}	R,B,O,D^{d}	R,B,O,S^{e}
Control	14 days	B,O,S,D^{a}	R,O,S,D^{b}	R,B,S,D^{c}	R,B,O,D^{d}	R,B,O,S^{e}
Control	15 days	B,O,S,D^{a}	R,O,S,D^{b}	R,B,S^{f}	R,B,O,D^{d}	R,B,S^{f}
Salt & Turmeric	24 hours	B,O,S,D^{a}	R,O,S,D^{b}	R,B,S,D^{c}	R,B,O,D^{d}	R,B,O,S^{e}
Salt & Turmeric	48 hours	B,O,S,D^{a}	R,O,S,D^{b}	R,B,D^{g}	R,B,D^{g}	R,B,O,S^{e}
Salt & Turmeric	14 days	B,O,S,D^{a}	R,O,S,D^{b}	R,B,S,D^{c}	R,B,O,D^{d}	R,B,O,S^{e}
Salt & Turmeric	15 days	B,O,S,D^{a}	R,O,S,D^{b}	R,B,S^{f}	R,B,O^{h}	R,B^{i}
KMS	24 hours	B,O,S,D^{a}	R,O,S,D^{b}	R,B,S,D^{c}	R,B,O,D^{d}	R,B,O,S^{e}
KMS	48 hours	B,O,S,D^{a}	R,O,S,D^{b}	R,B,S,D^{c}	R,B,O,D^{d}	R,B,O,S^{e}
KMS	14 days	B,O,S,D^{a}	R,O,S,D^{b}	R,B,S,D^{c}	R,B,O,D^{d}	R,B,O,S^{e}
KMS	15 days	B,O,S,D^{a}	R,O,S,D^{b}	R,B,D^{g}	R,B,D^{g}	R,B,O,S^{e}

R= Raw state, B= Boiling, O= Open pan dry roasting, S= Shallow frying, D= Deep frying. The same uppercase alphabets represent that there is no significant difference present among the variables.

This table shows the significant difference among the different variables such as cooking methods and preservation conditions. The raw state significantly differs from boiling, open pan dry roasting, shallow frying and deep frying in all of the preservation conditions with preservatives and control preservation without preservative. Boiling significantly differs from the raw state, open pan dry roasting, shallow frying and deep frying in all the preservation conditions. Open pan dry roasting significantly differs from the raw state, boiling, shallow frying and deep frying in all the preservation conditions except in 15 days control preservation without preservative, 48 hours and 15 days salt and turmeric preservation as well as 15 days KMS preservation. Shallow frying significantly differs from the raw state, boiling, open pan dry roasting and deep frying in all the preservation conditions except in 48 hours, 15 days salt and turmeric preservation and 15 days KMS preservation. Deep frying significantly differs from the raw state, boiling, open pan dry roasting and shallow frying in all the preservation conditions except in 15 days control preservation without preservative as well as 15 days salt and turmeric preservation.

Deep frying and open pan dry roasting significantly differ from the raw state, boiling and shallow frying in 15 days control preservation without preservative, but only open pan dry roasting significantly differs from the raw state, boiling and shallow frying in 15 days salt and turmeric preservation. Again open pan dry roasting and shallow frying significantly differ from the raw state, boiling and deep frying in 48 hours salt and turmeric and 15 days KMS preservation. Deep frying significantly differs from the raw state and boiling in 15 days salt and turmeric preservation, whereas shallow frying significantly differs from the raw state, boiling and open pan dry roasting in 15 days salt and turmeric preservation.

Table no 5.4.3.5 Gradation of cooking methods from higher to lower restoration with respect to preservation days

Preservation	Duration	Method 1	Method 2	Method 3	Method 4	Method 5
Control	Fresh	R	B	SF	OPDR	DF
Control	24 hours	R	B	OPDR	SF	DF
Control	48 hours	R	B	SF	OPDR	DF
Control	14 days	R	B	OPDR	SF	DF
Control	15 days	R	B	OPDR	DF	SF
Salt & Turmeric	24 hours	R	B	DF	OPDR	SF
Salt & Turmeric	48 hours	R	B	OPDR	SF	DF
Salt & Turmeric	14 days	R	B	OPDR	SF	DF
Salt &Turmeric	15 days	R	B	OPDR	DF	SF
KMS	24 hours	R	B	SF	OPDR	DF
KMS	48 hours	R	B	SF	OPDR	DF
KMS	14 days	R	B	OPDR	SF	DF
KMS	15 days	R	B	SF	OPDR	DF

R= Raw state, B= Boiling, OPDR= Open pan dry roasting, SF= Shallow frying, DF= Deep frying. Same colours represent similar order.

In all the preservation methods and fresh condition, moisture retention occurs mainly in the raw state than the other cooking methods. In almost all preservation conditions including fresh condition, 48 hours control preservation without preservative and 24 hours, 48 hours, 15 days KMS preservation, retention occurs firstly in the raw state followed by boiling, shallow frying, open pan dry roasting and deep frying, whereas in 24 hours, 14 days control preservation without preservative and 48 hours, 14 days salt and turmeric preservation as well as 14 days KMS preservation, retention occurs firstly in the raw state then boiling, open pan dry roasting, shallow frying and deep frying.

In 15 days control preservation without preservative as well as salt and turmeric preservation, retention occurs in the order of the raw state followed by boiling, open pan dry roasting, deep frying and shallow frying. In 24 hours salt and turmeric preservation, the order is the raw state followed by boiling, deep frying, open pan dry roasting and shallow frying.

The overall analysis of moisture content of prawn is mostly restored by the gradation of methods as the raw state> boiling> open pan dry roasting>shallow frying> deep frying.

Boiling can restore more moisture content due to the absorption of water during cooking, whereas open pan dry roasting reduces the moisture content due to the application of direct dry heat so that the water molecules present in prawn gets eliminated, causing reduction. Shallow frying restores moisture content as the oil can possibly create a protective layer so that the water molecules cannot be leached out. Deep frying mostly reduces the moisture content as the total dryness possibly occurs during deep frying due to the elimination of water molecules. Thus among all the studied conventional cooking methods, **boiling** is the best method for cooking prawn to restore moisture content.

5.4.4 Lobster (*Macrobrachium rosenbergii*)

It has been reported that lobster contains 76.34 gm of moisture per 100 gm[85] in the raw condition. This value changes due to the application of different cooking methods and preservation conditions (vide Table no **5.4.4.1**).

Table no 5.4.4.1 Moisture content of Lobster (gm/100gm)

Preservation	Duration	Raw state	Boiling	Dry roasting	Shallow frying	Deep frying
Control	Fresh	74.97±0.56	67.43±0.49	40.50±0.50	30.37±0.63	41.11±0.94
Control	24 hours	81.44±0.84	63.14±0.71	45.46±0.45	48.38±0.58	39.47±0.42
Control	48 hours	85.06±0.21	67.10±0.10	47.14±0.31	42.20±0.26	40.26±0.25
Control	14 days	79.98±1.87	62.60±0.53	54.04±0.96	48.00±0.87	33.56±0.40
Control	15 days	83.13±0.32	64.11±0.92	41.46±1.00	58.76±0.93	49.13±2.89
Salt & Turmeric	24 hours	80.86±0.78	74.61±0.20	46.82±0.13	60.64±0.14	63.81±0.10
Salt & Turmeric	48 hours	84.14±0.32	67.78±0.24	61.82±0.10	62.81±0.23	61.97±0.96
Salt & Turmeric	14 days	83.37±0.15	71.31±0.55	55.81±0.19	54.57±0.20	52.84±0.20
Salt & Turmeric	15 days	80.14±1.31	75.16±1.05	61.24±0.25	60.48±0.34	56.71±0.29
KMS	24 hours	84.26±0.26	72.48±0.46	47.69±0.19	51.42±0.09	55.20±0.10
KMS	48 hours	82.77±0.72	65.05±0.83	53.15±0.57	57.11±0.86	47.30±0.54
KMS	14 days	82.53±0.47	66.78±0.19	48.57±0.57	52.70±0.44	49.77±0.86
KMS	15 days	80.19±0.88	68.48±0.46	47.01±0.57	29.00±1.00	32.36±0.69

Values are expressed as mean±SD. Loss Restoration

In most of the preservation conditions, moisture losses mainly occurs by deep frying, whereas in fresh condition, 24 hours, 15 days KMS preservation, loss occurs by shallow frying and in 15 days control preservation without preservative, 24 hours, 48 hours salt and turmeric preservation, moisture content is reduced by open pan dry roasting. Retention of moisture content occurs by boiling in all the preservation conditions.

Open pan dry roasting and shallow frying show the highest moisture content in 48 hours salt and turmeric preservation, whereas boiling shows the highest moisture content in 15 days salt and turmeric preservation. Deep frying shows the highest moisture content in 24 hours salt and turmeric preservation and raw lobster shows the highest moisture content in 48 hours control preservation without preservative.

There is a prominent effect of the natural preservative on the restoration of moisture content of lobster. It may occur due to the water absorption capacity of salt.

Fig. 5.4.4.2 Graphical representation of Moisture content of Lobster with respect to different conditions

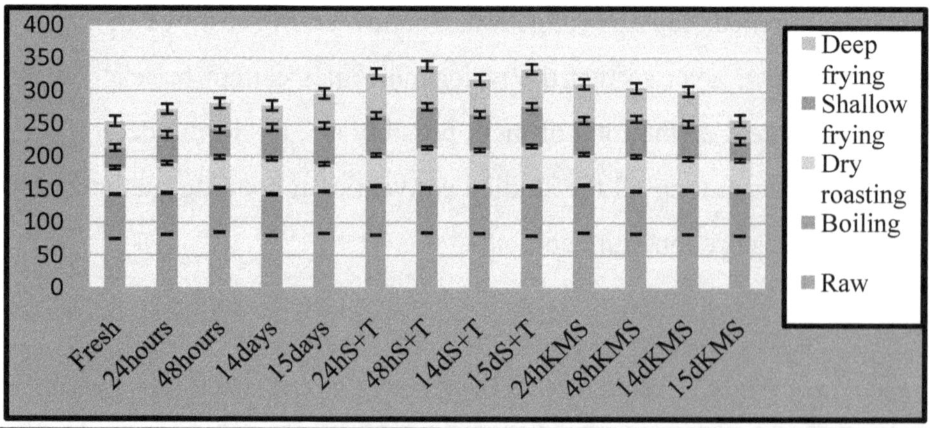

This graphical representation indicates that among all the preservation conditions, **48 hours salt and turmeric preservation**[55] helps to increase the moisture content in all the cooking methods[52]. The possible reason may be the water absorption capacity of salt and turmeric for prolonged preservation. Here the graph shows that KMS preservation also increases the moisture content, whereas salt and turmeric preservation comparatively increases the moisture content more than the control preservation without preservative and KMS preservation.

Table no 5.4.4.3 ANOVA with regard to cooking conditions and preservation methods

Condition	Differences	Sum of Squares	df	Mean Square	F	Sig.
Fresh (control)	Between Groups	4434.667	4	1108.667	2.652E3	.000(S)
	Within Groups	4.180	10	.418		
	Total	4438.846	14			
24 hours (control)	Between Groups	3418.471	4	854.618	2.225E3	.000(S)
	Within Groups	3.840	10	.384		
	Total	3422.311	14			
48 hours (control)	Between Groups	4451.789	4	1112.947	1.949E4	.000(S)
	Within Groups	.571	10	.057		
	Total	4452.360	14			
14 days (control)	Between Groups	3567.571	4	891.893	789.174	.000(S)
	Within Groups	11.302	10	1.130		
	Total	3578.873	14			
15 days (control)	Between Groups	3039.054	4	759.764	346.950	.000(S)
	Within Groups	21.898	10	2.190		
	Total	3060.952	14			
24 hours (salt & turmeric)	Between Groups	2080.408	4	520.102	3.808E3	.000(S)
	Within Groups	1.366	10	.137		
	Total	2081.774	14			
48 hours (salt & turmeric)	Between Groups	1084.585	4	271.146	1.171E3	.000(S)
	Within Groups	2.316	10	.232		
	Total	1086.901	14			
14 days (salt & turmeric)	Between Groups	2124.678	4	531.170	5.867E3	.000(S)
	Within Groups	.905	10	.091		
	Total	2125.583	14			
15 days (salt & turmeric)	Between Groups	1241.595	4	310.399	448.657	.000(S)
	Within Groups	6.918	10	.692		
	Total	1248.513	14			
24 hours (KMS)	Between Groups	2903.553	4	725.888	1.079E4	.000(S)
	Within Groups	.673	10	.067		
	Total	2904.226	14			
48 hours (KMS)	Between Groups	2264.925	4	566.231	1.104E3	.000(S)
	Within Groups	5.127	10	.513		
	Total	2270.052	14			
14 days (KMS)	Between Groups	2526.411	4	631.603	2.069E3	.000(S)
	Within Groups	3.053	10	.305		
	Total	2529.464	14			
15 days (KMS)	Between Groups	6008.705	4	1502.176	2.744E3	.000(S)
	Within Groups	5.474	10	.547		
	Total	6014.178	14			

$p<0.05$ S= Significant, NS= Non-significant. All abbreviations are on page so and so.

This statistical ANOVA table shows that all the values are significant, which means there is significant difference present in the values of moisture content of lobster among different cooking methods and the raw state in respect to fresh condition along with different preservation methods.

Table no 5.4.4.4 Post hoc Duncan statistical analysis

Preservation	Duration	Raw state	Boiling	Dry roasting	Shallow frying	Deep frying
Control	Fresh	B,O,S,D[a]	R,O,S,D[b]	R,B,S[c]	R,B,O,D[d]	R,B,S[c]
Control	24 hours	B,O,S,D[a]	R,O,S,D[b]	R,B,S,D[e]	R,B,O,D[d]	R,B,O,S[f]
Control	48 hours	B,O,S,D[a]	R,O,S,D[b]	R,B,S,D[e]	R,B,O,D[d]	R,B,O,S[f]
Control	14 days	B,O,S,D[a]	R,O,S,D[b]	R,B,S,D[e]	R,B,O,D[d]	R,B,O,S[f]
Control	15 days	B,O,S,D[a]	R,O,S,D[b]	R,B,S,D[e]	R,B,O,D[d]	R,B,O,S[f]
Salt & Turmeric	24 hours	B,O,S,D[a]	R,O,S,D[b]	R,B,S,D[e]	R,B,O,D[d]	R,B,O,S[f]
Salt & Turmeric	48 hours	B,O,S,D[a]	R,O,S,D[b]	R,B,S[g]	R,B,O,D[d]	R,B[h]
Salt & Turmeric	14 days	B,O,S,D[a]	R,O,S,D[b]	R,B,S,D[e]	R,B,O,D[d]	R,B,O,S[f]
Salt & Turmeric	15 days	B,O,S,D[a]	R,O,S,D[b]	R,B,D[i]	R,B,D[i]	R,B,O,S[f]
KMS	24 hours	B,O,S,D[a]	R,O,S,D[b]	R,B,S,D[e]	R,B,O,D[d]	R,B,O,S[f]
KMS	48 hours	B,O,S,D[a]	R,O,S,D[b]	R,B,S,D[e]	R,B,O,D[d]	R,B,O,S[f]
KMS	14 days	B,O,S,D[a]	R,O,S,D[b]	R,B,S,D[e]	R,B,O,D[d]	R,B,O,S[f]
KMS	15 days	B,O,S,D[a]	R,O,S,D[b]	R,B,S,D[e]	R,B,O,D[d]	R,B,O,S[f]

R= Raw state, B= Boiling, O= Open pan dry roasting, S= Shallow frying, D= Deep frying. The same uppercase alphabets signify that there is no significant difference present among the variables.

This table shows the significant difference among the different variables such as cooking methods and preservation conditions. The raw state significantly differs from boiling, open pan dry roasting, shallow frying and deep frying in all of the preservation conditions with preservatives and control preservation without preservative. Boiling significantly differs from the raw state, open pan dry roasting, shallow frying and deep frying in all of the preservation conditions. Open pan dry roasting significantly differs from the raw state, boiling, shallow frying and deep frying in all the preservation conditions except in fresh condition, 48 hours, 15 days salt and turmeric preservation. Shallow frying significantly differs from the raw state, boiling, open pan dry roasting and deep frying in all the preservation conditions except in 15 days salt and turmeric preservation. Deep frying significantly differs from the raw state, boiling, open pan dry roasting and shallow frying in all the preservation conditions except in fresh condition, 48 hours salt and turmeric preservation.

Deep frying and open pan dry roasting significantly differ from the raw state, boiling and shallow frying in fresh condition, but only open pan dry roasting significantly differs from the raw state, boiling and shallow frying in 48 hours salt and turmeric preservation . Again open pan dry roasting and shallow frying significantly differ from the raw state, boiling and deep frying in 15 days salt and turmeric preservation. Deep frying significantly differs from the raw state and boiling in 48 hours salt and turmeric preservation.

Table no 5.4.4.5 Gradation of cooking methods from higher to lower restoration with respect to preservation days

Preservation	Duration	Method 1	Method 2	Method 3	Method 4	Method 5
Control	Fresh	R	B	DF	OPDR	SF
Control	24 hours	R	B	SF	OPDR	DF
Control	48 hours	R	B	OPDR	SF	DF
Control	14 days	R	B	OPDR	SF	DF
Control	15 days	R	B	SF	DF	OPDR
Salt & Turmeric	24 hours	R	B	DF	SF	OPDR
Salt & Turmeric	48 hours	R	B	SF	DF	OPDR
Salt & Turmeric	14 days	R	B	OPDR	SF	DF
Salt &Turmeric	15 days	R	B	OPDR	SF	DF
KMS	24 hours	R	B	DF	SF	OPDR
KMS	48 hours	R	B	SF	OPDR	DF
KMS	14 days	R	B	SF	DF	OPDR
KMS	15 days	R	B	OPDR	DF	SF

R=Raw state, B=Boiling, OPDR=Open pan dry roasting, SF=Shallow frying, DF=Deep frying. Same colours represent similar order.

In all the preservation techniques and fresh condition, moisture retention occurs mainly in the raw state than the other cooking methods. In fresh condition, retention occurs firstly in the raw state followed by boiling, deep frying, open pan dry roasting and shallow frying, whereas in 24 hours control preservation without preservative and 48 hours KMS preservation, the order of retention is the raw state, boiling, shallow frying, deep frying and open pan dry roasting. In 48 hours, 14 days control preservation without preservative and 14 days, 15 days salt and turmeric preservation, retention occurs in the order of the raw state then boiling, open pan dry roasting, shallow frying and deep frying. In 15 days control preservation without preservative and 48 hours salt and turmeric as well as 14 days KMS preservation, the order changes to the raw state followed by boiling, shallow frying, deep frying and open pan dry roasting.

In 24 hours salt and turmeric preservation as well as KMS preservation, retention occurs in the following manner: the raw state, boiling, deep frying, shallow frying and open pan dry roasting. In 15 days preservation, the order is the raw state followed by boiling, open pan dry roasting, deep frying and shallow frying.

The overall analysis of moisture content of lobster is mostly restored by the gradation of methods as the raw state> boiling> open pan dry roasting>shallow frying> deep frying.

Boiling can restore more moisture content due to the absorption of water during cooking, whereas open pan dry roasting reduces the moisture content due to the application of direct dry heat so that the water molecules present in lobster get eliminated, leading to reduction. Shallow frying restores moisture content as the oil can possibly create a protective layer so that the water molecules cannot be leached out. Deep frying mostly reduces the moisture content as the total dryness occurs possibly during deep frying due to the elimination of water molecules. Thus among all the studied conventional cooking methods, **boiling** is the best method for cooking lobster to restore moisture content.

5.4.5 Pomfret (*Pampus argenteus*)

It has been reported that pomfret contains 75.91 gm of moisture per 100 gm[85] in the raw condition. This value changes due to the application of different cooking methods and preservation conditions (vide Table no **5.4.5.1**).

Table no 5.4.5.1 Moisture content of Pomfret (gm/100gm)

Preservation	Duration	Raw state	Boiling	Dry roasting	Shallow frying	Deep frying
Control	Fresh	80.74±1.97	55.78±0.05	25.31±0.10	31.64±0.14	8.41±0.07
Control	24 hours	77.65±0.53	52.27±1.49	36.25±4.63	38.51±2.46	21.86±1.20
Control	48 hours	75.71±0.10	52.41±0.03	56.57±0.06	52.98±0.07	33.96±0.05
Control	14 days	77.10±0.09	55.94±0.09	43.90±0.10	48.61±0.09	15.78±0.05
Control	15 days	76.03±0.0	51.02±0.62	42.93±0.52	45.21±0.50	30.77±0.24
Salt & Turmeric	24 hours	75.13±0.83	63.37±0.45	49.04±0.45	41.07±0.50	53.86±0.15
Salt & Turmeric	48 hours	73.90±0.71	56.90±0.40	48.74±1.16	60.70±0.43	40.82±0.20
Salt & Turmeric	14 days	76.84±0.20	60.54±0.35	38.94±0.61	46.50±0.50	31.92±0.07
Salt & Turmeric	15 days	75.36±0.47	39.90±0.26	46.98±0.58	43.53±0.31	29.60±0.36
KMS	24 hours	78.91±0.49	63.03±0.15	45.03±0.80	39.07±0.42	39.33±0.42
KMS	48 hours	75.80±0.10	57.66±0.32	50.30±0.10	57.14±2.56	29.60±0.37
KMS	14 days	76.31±0.56	57.60±0.43	38.11±0.46	37.67±1.08	39.37±0.15
KMS	15 days	73.37±0.52	38.61±0.37	49.46±0.46	44.21±0.90	31.03±0.54

Values are expressed as mean±SD. ☐ Loss ☐ Restoration

In most of the preservation conditions, moisture losses mainly occur by deep frying, whereas in 14 days control preservation without preservative, loss occurs by boiling. In 15 days control preservation without preservative, 24 hours, 15 days salt and turmeric preservation, moisture content is reduced by shallow frying. Retention of moisture content occurs by boiling in all of the preservation methods, but in 14 days control preservation, moisture retention occurs by open pan dry roasting.

The raw state shows the highest moisture content in fresh condition, whereas boiling shows that in 24 hours KMS preservation. Open pan dry roasting shows the highest moisture content in 48 hours control preservation without preservative. Shallow frying and deep frying show the highest moisture content in 48 hours and 24 hours salt and turmeric preservation respectively.

There is a prominent effect of the natural preservative on the restoration of moisture content of pomfret. It may occur due to the water absorption capacity of the salt.

Fig. 5.4.5.2 Graphical representation of Moisture content of Pomfret with respect to different conditions

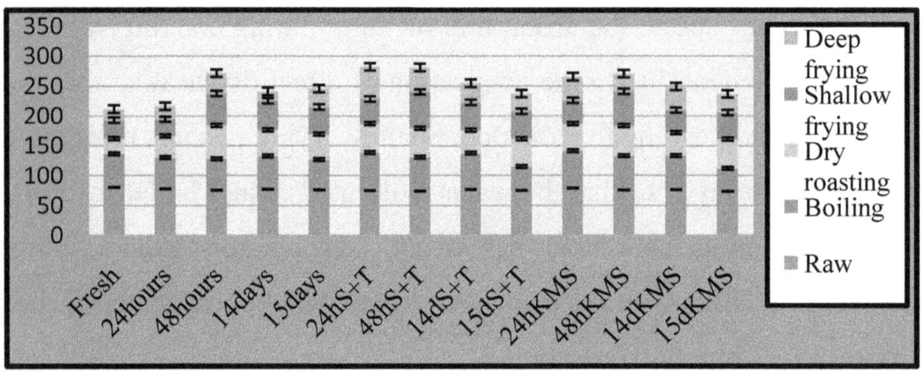

This graphical representation indicates that among all the preservation conditions, **24 hours, 48 hours salt and turmeric preservation**[55] help to increase the moisture content in all the cooking methods[52]. The possible reason may be the water absorption capacity of salt and turmeric for prolonged preservation. Here the graph shows that KMS preservation also increases the moisture content, whereas salt and turmeric preservation comparatively increases the moisture content more than the control preservation without preservative and KMS preservation.

Table no 5.4.5.3 ANOVA with regard to cooking conditions and preservation methods

Condition	Differences	Sum of Squares	df	Mean Square	F	Sig.
Fresh (control)	Between Groups	7895.299	4	1973.825	2.522E3	.000(S)
	Within Groups	7.827	10	.783		
	Total	7903.127	14			
24 hours (control)	Between Groups	5226.277	4	1306.569	90.650	.000(S)
	Within Groups	144.133	10	14.413		
	Total	5370.410	14			
48 hours (control)	Between Groups	2647.550	4	661.888	1.398E5	.000(S)
	Within Groups	.047	10	.005		
	Total	2647.598	14			
14 days (control)	Between Groups	5896.900	4	1474.225	1.967E5	.000(S)
	Within Groups	.075	10	.007		
	Total	5896.975	14			
15 days (control)	Between Groups	3354.140	4	838.535	4.364E3	.000(S)
	Within Groups	1.922	10	.192		
	Total	3356.062	14			
24 hours (salt & turmeric)	Between Groups	2084.737	4	521.184	1.892E3	.000(S)
	Within Groups	2.754	10	.275		
	Total	2087.492	14			
48 hours (salt & turmeric)	Between Groups	1879.264	4	469.816	1.040E3	.000(S)
	Within Groups	4.517	10	.452		
	Total	1883.781	14			
14 days (salt & turmeric)	Between Groups	3856.845	4	964.211	5.392E3	.000(S)
	Within Groups	1.788	10	.179		
	Total	3858.633	14			
15 days (salt & turmeric)	Between Groups	3476.256	4	869.064	5.078E3	.000(S)
	Within Groups	1.711	10	.171		
	Total	3477.968	14			
24 hours (KMS)	Between Groups	3649.009	4	912.252	3.642E3	.000(S)
	Within Groups	2.505	10	.250		
	Total	3651.513	14			
48 hours (KMS)	Between Groups	3322.689	4	830.672	609.411	.000(S)
	Within Groups	13.631	10	1.363		
	Total	3336.320	14			
14 days (KMS)	Between Groups	3467.376	4	866.844	2.293E3	.000(S)
	Within Groups	3.781	10	.378		
	Total	3471.157	14			
15 days (KMS)	Between Groups	3101.960	4	775.490	2.247E3	.000(S)
	Within Groups	3.451	10	.345		
	Total	3105.411	14			

$p<0.05$ S= Significant, NS= Non-significant. All abbreviations are on page so and so.

This statistical ANOVA table shows that all the values are significant, which means there is significant difference present in the values of moisture content of pomfret among different cooking methods and the raw state in respect to fresh condition along with different preservation methods.

Table no 5.4.5.4 Post hoc Duncan statistical analysis

Preservation	Duration	Raw state	Boiling	Dry roasting	Shallow frying	Deep frying
Control	Fresh	B,O,S,D^{a}	R,O,S,D^{b}	R,B,S,D^{c}	R,B,O,D^{d}	R,B,O,S^{e}
Control	24 hours	B,O,S,D^{a}	R,O,S,D^{b}	R,B,D^{f}	R,B,D^{f}	R,B,O,S^{e}
Control	48 hours	B,O,S,D^{a}	R,O,S,D^{b}	R,B,S,D^{c}	R,B,O,D^{d}	R,B,O,S^{e}
Control	14 days	B,O,S,D^{a}	R,O,S,D^{b}	R,B,S,D^{c}	R,B^{g}	R,B,O,S^{e}
Control	15 days	B,O,S,D^{a}	R,O,S,D^{b}	R,B,S,D^{c}	R,B,D^{f}	R,B,O,S^{e}
Salt & Turmeric	24 hours	B,O,S,D^{a}	R,O,S,D^{b}	R,B,S,D^{c}	R,B,O,D^{d}	R,B,O,S^{e}
Salt & Turmeric	48 hours	B,O,S,D^{a}	R,O,S,D^{b}	R,B,S,D^{c}	R,B,O,D^{d}	R,B,O,S^{e}
Salt & Turmeric	14 days	B,O,S,D^{a}	R,O,S,D^{b}	R,B,S,D^{c}	R,B,O,D^{d}	R,B,O,S^{e}
Salt & Turmeric	15 days	B,O,S,D^{a}	R,O,S,D^{b}	R,B,S,D^{c}	R,B,O,D^{d}	R,B,O,S^{e}
KMS	24 hours	B,O,S,D^{a}	R,O,S,D^{b}	R,B,S,D^{c}	R,B,O^{i}	R,B,O^{i}
KMS	48 hours	B,O,S,D^{a}	R,O,D^{h}	R,B,S,D^{c}	R,O,D^{h}	R,B,O,S^{e}
KMS	14 days	B,O,S,D^{a}	R,O,S,D^{b}	R,B,D^{f}	R,B,D^{f}	R,B,O,S^{e}
KMS	15 days	B,O,S,D^{a}	R,O,S,D^{b}	R,B,S,D^{c}	R,B,O,D^{d}	R,B,O,S^{e}

R= Raw state, B= Boiling, O= Open pan dry roasting, S= Shallow frying, D= Deep frying. The same uppercase alphabets represent that there is no significant difference present among the variables.

This table shows the significant difference among the different variables such as cooking methods and preservation conditions. The raw state significantly differs from boiling, open pan dry roasting, shallow frying and deep frying in all of the preservation conditions with preservatives and control preservation without preservative. Boiling significantly differs from the raw state, open pan dry roasting, shallow frying and deep frying in all the preservation conditions excluding 48 hours KMS preservation. Open pan dry roasting significantly differs from the raw state, boiling, shallow frying and deep frying in all the preservation conditions except in 24 hours control preservation without preservative and 14 days KMS preservation. Shallow frying significantly differs from the raw state, boiling, open pan dry roasting and deep frying in all the preservation conditions except in 24 hours, 14 days, 15 days control preservation without preservative and 24 hours, 48 hours, 14 days KMS preservation. Deep frying significantly differs from the raw state, boiling, open pan dry roasting and shallow frying in all the preservation conditions except in 24 hours KMS preservation.

Shallow frying and open pan dry roasting significantly differ from the raw state, boiling and deep frying in 24 hours control preservation without preservative and 14 days KMS preservation, but only shallow frying significantly differs from the raw state, boiling and deep frying in 15 days control preservation without preservative. Again boiling and shallow frying significantly differ from the raw state, open pan dry roasting and deep frying in 48 hours KMS preservation. Shallow frying significantly differs from the raw state and boiling in 14 days control preservation without preservative. Shallow frying and deep frying significantly differ from the raw state, boiling and open pan dry roasting in 24 hours KMS preservation.

Table no 5.4.5.5 Gradation of cooking methods from higher to lower restoration with respect to preservation days

Preservation	Duration	Method 1	Method 2	Method 3	Method 4	Method 5
Control	Fresh	R	B	SF	OPDR	DF
Control	24 hours	R	B	SF	OPDR	DF
Control	48 hours	R	OPDR	SF	B	DF
Control	14 days	R	B	SF	OPDR	DF
Control	15 days	R	B	SF	OPDR	DF
Salt & Turmeric	24 hours	R	B	DF	OPDR	SF
Salt & Turmeric	48 hours	R	SF	B	OPDR	DF
Salt & Turmeric	14 days	R	B	SF	OPDR	DF
Salt &Turmeric	15 days	R	OPDR	SF	B	DF
KMS	24 hours	R	B	OPDR	DF	SF
KMS	48 hours	R	B	SF	OPDR	DF
KMS	14 days	R	B	DF	OPDR	SF
KMS	15 days	R	OPDR	SF	B	DF

R= Raw state, B= Boiling, OPDR= Open pan dry roasting, SF= Shallow frying, DF= Deep frying. Same colours represent similar order.

In all the preservation methods and fresh condition, moisture retention occurs mainly in the raw state than the other cooking methods. In fresh condition, 24 hours, 14 days, 15 days control preservation without preservative, 14 days salt and turmeric and 48 hours KMS preservation, retention occurs firstly in the raw state then boiling, shallow frying, open pan dry roasting and deep frying. In 48 hours control preservation without preservative and 15 days salt and turmeric preservation as well as KMS preservation, the order is the raw state, open pan dry roasting, shallow frying, boiling and deep frying.

In 24 hours salt and turmeric and 14 days KMS preservation, retention occurs in the order of the raw state followed by boiling, deep frying, open pan dry roasting and shallow frying. In 48 hours salt and turmeric preservation, the order remains the raw state, shallow frying, boiling, open pan dry roasting and deep frying. In 24 hours KMS preservation, the order is the raw state then boiling, open pan dry roasting, deep frying and shallow frying.

The overall analysis of moisture content of pomfret is mostly restored by the gradation of methods as the raw state> boiling>shallow frying>open pan dry roasting> deep frying.

Boiling can restore more moisture content due to the absorption of water during cooking, whereas shallow frying restores moisture content as the oil can possibly create a protective covering so that the water molecules cannot be leached out. Open pan dry roasting reduces the moisture content possibly due to the application of direct dry heat so that the water molecules along with fatty tissues present in pomfret get eliminated, causing reduction. Deep frying mostly reduces the moisture content as the total dryness possibly occurs during deep frying due to the elimination of water molecules. Thus among all the studied conventional cooking methods, **boiling** is the best method for cooking pomfret in order to restore moisture content.

5.4.6 *Hilsa* (*Tenualosa Ilisha*)

It has been reported that *hilsa* contains 60.09 gm of moisture per 100 gm[85] in the raw condition. This value changes due to the application of different cooking methods and preservation conditions (vide Table no **5.4.6.1**).

Table no 5.4.6.1 Moisture content of *Hilsa* (gm/100gm)

Preservation	Duration	Raw state	Boiling	Dry roasting	Shallow frying	Deep frying
Control	Fresh	69.76±0.25	50.06±0.05	36.81±0.10	24.54±0.06	11.53±0.05
Control	24 hour	68.27±0.25	50.06±0.05	26.81±0.09	31.41±0.11	14.12±0.03
Control	48 hours	56.91±0.11	48.51±0.11	29.71±0.10	32.53±0.15	26.58±0.15
Control	14 day	54.74±0.06	46.75±0.22	33.80±0.10	36.05±0.05	29.77±0.06
Control	15 days	66.60±3.32	59.47±0.50	27.30±0.77	32.94±0.48	23.81±1.80
Salt & Turmeric	24 hours	53.53±0.45	53.03±0.15	29.20±0.29	46.72±0.29	24.90±0.35
Salt & Turmeric	48 hours	58.10±0.75	50.94±0.52	31.75±0.21	38.11±0.76	27.92±0.09
Salt & Turmeric	14 days	65.46±0.47	55.77±0.33	35.51±1.23	39.00±0.20	23.20±0.26
Salt & Turmeric	15 days	57.36±0.47	54.67±0.22	35.57±0.49	41.24±0.66	24.57±0.50
KMS	24 hours	52.81±0.80	48.59±0.38	26..78±0.24	23.44±0.04	28.00±0.51
KMS	48 hours	51.26±0.21	49.94±0.08	26.90±0.10	33.85±0.34	25.17±0.16
KMS	14 days	59.80±0.19	50.85±0.57	36.95±0.27	38.90±0.36	25.14±0.83
KMS	15 days	60.93±0.73	48.97±0.24	41.02±0.64	28.60±0.45	33.90±0.36

Values are expressed as mean±SD. Loss Restoration

In most of the preservation conditions, moisture loss mainly occurs by deep frying, whereas in 15 days KMS preservation, loss occurs by shallow frying. Retention of moisture content occurs by boiling in all the preservation conditions including fresh condition.

The raw state shows the highest moisture content in fresh condition, whereas boiling shows that in 15 days control preservation without preservative. Open pan dry roasting and deep frying show the highest moisture content in 15 days KMS preservation. Shallow frying shows the highest moisture content in 24 hours salt and turmeric preservation.

There is a prominent effect of both the natural and synthetic preservatives on the restoration of moisture content of *hilsa*. It may occur due to the water absorption capacity of the preservatives.

Fig. 5.4.6.2 Graphical representation of Moisture content of *Hilsa* with respect to different conditions

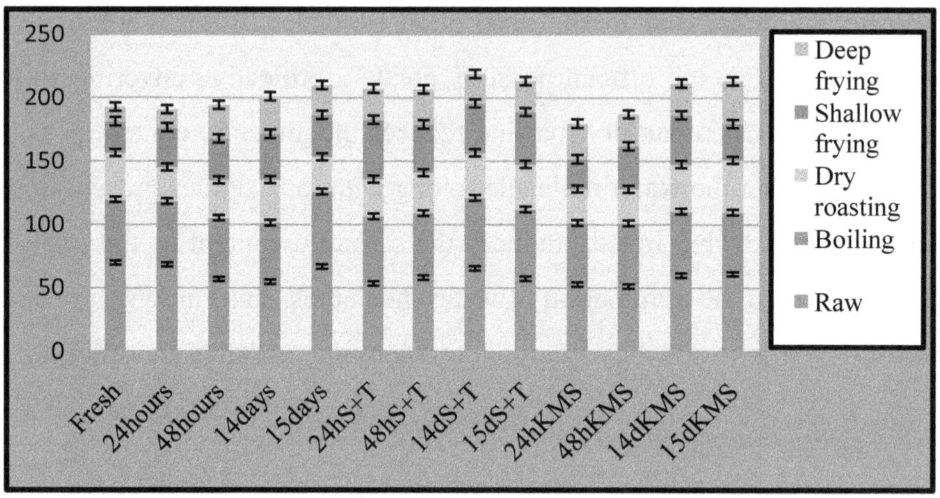

This graphical representation indicates that among all the preservation conditions, **14 days salt and turmeric preservation**[55] helps to increase the moisture content in all the cooking methods[52]. The possible reason for this may be the water absorption capacity of salt and turmeric for prolonged preservation. Here the graph shows that KMS preservation also increases the moisture content, whereas the combination of salt and turmeric preservation comparatively increases the moisture content more than the control preservation without preservative and KMS preservation.

Table no 5.4.6.3 ANOVA with regard to cooking conditions and preservation methods

Condition	Differences	Sum of Squares	df	Mean Square	F	Sig.
Fresh (control)	Between Groups	6107.369	4	1526.842	9.239E4	.000(S)
	Within Groups	.165	10	.017		
	Total	6107.535	14			
24 hours (control)	Between Groups	5401.337	4	1350.334	7.687E4	.000(S)
	Within Groups	.176	10	.018		
	Total	5401.513	14			
48 hours (control)	Between Groups	2080.426	4	520.107	3.271E4	.000(S)
	Within Groups	.159	10	.016		
	Total	2080.585	14			
14 days (control)	Between Groups	1174.886	4	293.721	6.067	.010(S)
	Within Groups	484.159	10	48.416		
	Total	1659.044	14			
15 days (control)	Between Groups	4228.084	4	1057.021	60.852	.000(S)
	Within Groups	173.704	10	17.370		
	Total	4401.788	14			
24 hours (salt & turmeric)	Between Groups	2188.836	4	547.209	4.790E3	.000(S)
	Within Groups	1.142	10	.114		
	Total	2189.978	14			
48 hours (salt & turmeric)	Between Groups	1966.130	4	491.533	1.673E3	.000(S)
	Within Groups	2.938	10	.294		
	Total	1969.068	14			
14 days (salt & turmeric)	Between Groups	3378.826	4	844.706	2.159E3	.000(S)
	Within Groups	3.913	10	.391		
	Total	3382.739	14			
15 days (salt & turmeric)	Between Groups	2219.903	4	554.976	2.300E3	.000(S)
	Within Groups	2.413	10	.241		
	Total	2222.316	14			
24 hours (KMS)	Between Groups	2243.311	4	560.828	2.434E3	.000(S)
	Within Groups	2.304	10	.230		
	Total	2245.616	14			
48 hours (KMS)	Between Groups	1865.316	4	466.329	1.155E4	.000(S)
	Within Groups	.404	10	.040		
	Total	1865.720	14			
14 days (KMS)	Between Groups	2143.030	4	535.757	2.109E3	.000(S)
	Within Groups	2.540	10	.254		
	Total	2145.570	14			
15 days (KMS)	Between Groups	1952.045	4	488.011	1.815E3	.000(S)
	Within Groups	2.688	10	.269		
	Total	1954.733	14			

$p<0.05$ S= Significant, NS= Non-significant. All abbreviations are on page so and so.

This statistical ANOVA table shows that all the values are significant, which means there is significant difference present in the values of moisture content of *hilsa* among different cooking methods and the raw state in respect to fresh condition along with different preservation methods.

Table no 5.4.6.4 Post hoc Duncan statistical analysis

Preservation	Duration	Raw state	Boiling	Dry roasting	Shallow frying	Deep frying
Control	Fresh	B,O,S,D^{a}	R,O,S,D^{b}	R,B,S,D^{c}	R,B,O,D^{d}	R,B,O,S^{e}
Control	24 hours	B,O,S,D^{a}	R,O,S,D^{b}	R,B,S,D^{c}	R,B,O,D^{d}	R,B,O,S^{e}
Control	48 hours	B,O,S,D^{a}	R,O,S,D^{b}	R,B,S,D^{c}	R,B,O,D^{d}	R,B,O,S^{e}
Control	14 days	S,D^{f}	S,D^{f}	---	R,B^{g}	R,B^{g}
Control	15 days	O,S,D^{h}	O,S,D^{h}	R,B^{g}	R,B,D^{i}	R,B,S^{j}
Salt & Turmeric	24 hours	O,S,D^{h}	O,S,D^{h}	R,B,S,D^{c}	R,B,O,D^{d}	R,B,O,S^{e}
Salt & Turmeric	48 hours	B,O,S,D^{a}	R,O,S,D^{b}	R,B,S,D^{c}	R,B,O,D^{d}	R,B,O,S^{e}
Salt & Turmeric	14 days	B,O,S,D^{a}	R,O,S,D^{b}	R,B,S,D^{c}	R,B,O,D^{d}	R,B,O,S^{e}
Salt & Turmeric	15 days	B,O,S,D^{a}	R,O,S,D^{b}	R,B,S,D^{c}	R,B,O,D^{d}	R,B,O,S^{e}
KMS	24 hours	B,O,S,D^{a}	R,O,S,D^{b}	R,B,S,D^{c}	R,B,O,D^{d}	R,B,O,S^{e}
KMS	48 hours	B,O,S,D^{a}	R,O,S,D^{b}	R,B,S,D^{c}	R,B,O,D^{d}	R,B,O,S^{e}
KMS	14 days	B,O,S,D^{a}	R,O,S,D^{b}	R,B,S,D^{c}	R,B,O,D^{d}	R,B,O,S^{e}
KMS	15 days	B,O,S,D^{a}	R,O,S,D^{b}	R,B,S,D^{c}	R,B,O,D^{d}	R,B,O,S^{e}

R= Raw state, B= Boiling, O= Open pan dry roasting, S= Shallow frying, D= Deep frying. The same uppercase alphabets represent that there is no significant difference present among the variables.

This table shows the significant difference among the different variables such as cooking methods and preservation conditions. The raw state significantly differs from boiling, open pan dry roasting, shallow frying and deep frying in all of the preservation conditions with preservatives and control preservation without preservative except in 14 days, 15 days control preservation and 24 hours salt and turmeric preservation. Boiling significantly differs from the raw state, open pan dry roasting, shallow and deep frying in all the preservation conditions except in 14 days, 15 days control preservation and 24 hours salt and turmeric preservation. Open pan dry roasting significantly differs from the raw state, boiling, shallow and deep frying in all the preservation conditions except in 14 days and 15 days control preservation. Shallow frying significantly differs from the raw state, boiling, open pan dry roasting and deep frying in all the preservation conditions except in 14 days, 15 days control preservation. Deep frying significantly differs from the raw state, boiling, open pan dry roasting and shallow frying in all the preservation conditions except in 14 days, 15 days control preservation without preservative.

The raw state and boiling significantly differ from shallow frying and deep frying in 14 days control preservation. Again deep frying and shallow frying significantly differ from the raw state and boiling in 14 days control preservation, but open pan dry roasting significantly differs from the raw state and boiling in 15 days control preservation. The raw state and boiling significantly differ from open pan dry roasting, shallow frying and deep frying in 15 days control and 24 hours salt and turmeric preservation. Shallow frying significantly differs from the raw state, boiling and deep frying in 15 days control preservation, whereas deep frying significantly differs from the raw state, boiling and shallow frying in 15 days control preservation.

Table no 5.4.6.5 Gradation of cooking methods from higher to lower restoration with respect to preservation days

Preservation	Duration	Method 1	Method 2	Method 3	Method 4	Method 5
Control	Fresh	R	B	OPDR	SF	DF
Control	24 hours	R	B	SF	OPDR	DF
Control	48 hours	R	B	SF	OPDR	DF
Control	14 days	R	B	OPDR	SF	DF
Control	15 days	R	B	SF	OPDR	DF
Salt & Turmeric	24 hours	R	B	SF	OPDR	DF
Salt & Turmeric	48 hours	R	B	SF	OPDR	DF
Salt & Turmeric	14 days	R	B	SF	OPDR	DF
Salt &Turmeric	15 days	R	B	SF	OPDR	DF
KMS	24 hours	R	B	DF	OPDR	SF
KMS	48 hours	R	B	SF	OPDR	DF
KMS	14 days	R	B	SF	OPDR	DF
KMS	15 days	R	B	OPDR	DF	SF

R= Raw state, B= Boiling, OPDR= Open pan dry roasting, SF= Shallow frying, DF= Deep frying. Same colours represent similar order.

In all the preservation methods and fresh condition, moisture retention occurs mainly in the raw state than the other cooking methods. In fresh condition, 14 days control preservation without preservative and 15 days KMS preservation, retention occurs firstly in the raw state then boiling, open pan dry roasting, deep frying and shallow frying. In 24 hours, 48 hours, 15 days control preservation without preservative and 24 hours, 48 hours, 14 days, 15 days salt and turmeric preservation as well as 48 hours, 14 days KMS preservation, retention occurs in the order of the raw state followed by boiling, shallow frying, open pan dry roasting and deep frying. In 24 hours KMS preservation, retention occurs in the order of the raw state then boiling, deep frying, open pan dry roasting and shallow frying.

The overall analysis of moisture content of *hilsa* is mostly restored by the gradation of methods as the raw state> boiling>shallow frying>open pan dry roasting> deep frying.

Boiling can restore more moisture content due to the absorption of water during cooking, whereas shallow frying restore moisture content as the oil can possibly create a protective layer so that the water molecules cannot be leached out. Open pan dry roasting reduces the moisture content due to the application of direct dry heat so that the water molecules present in *hilsa* get eliminated, leading to reduction. Deep frying mostly reduces the moisture content as the total dryness possibly occurs during deep frying due to the elimination of water molecules. Thus among all the studied conventional cooking methods, **boiling** is the best method for *hilsa* to restore moisture content.

5.5 Ash content

It has been reported that generally fish contains 0.1-1gm% of ash[86] in the raw state. This experiment is carried out to estimate the percentage of ash content and also the changes of it in different cooking and preservation methods among different fish and edible aquatic species. Ash content is estimated by weight difference method[72].

5.5.1 *Rohu* (*Labeo rohita*)

It has been reported that *rohu* contains 1.28 gm of fat per 100 gm[85] in the raw condition. This value changes due to the application of different cooking methods and preservation conditions (vide Table no **5.5.1.1**).

Table no 5.5.1.1 Ash content of *Rohu* (gm/100gm)

Preservation	Duration	Raw state	Boiling	Dry roasting	Shallow frying	Deep frying
Control	Fresh	2.29±0.04	1.06±0.05	3.63±0.10	4.15±0.13	1.25±0.03
Control	24 hours	2.31±0.04	1.94±0.08	1.29±0.04	1.12±0.10	0.78±0.03
Control	48 hours	2.29±0.07	1.71±0.09	2.19±0.08	2.77±0.05	6.24±0.04
Control	14 days	2.28±0.08	1.40±0.02	1.42±0.03	1.32±0.03	1.73±0.04
Control	15 days	3.25±0.04	2.08±0.07	1.28±0.08	1.66±0.04	0.72±0.07
Salt & Turmeric	24 hours	8.05±0.05	6.38±0.04	3.69±0.08	2.55±0.05	4.04±0.05
Salt & Turmeric	48 hours	6.40±0.02	3.59±0.08	3.74±0.11	4.64±0.04	4.52±0.03
Salt & Turmeric	14 days	5.45±0.05	1.17±0.06	4.06±0.05	3.35±0.03	2.20±0.05
Salt & Turmeric	15 days	3.74±0.06	3.28±0.07	3.24±0.05	3.31±0.10	3.12±0.03
KMS	24 hours	5.79±0.04	3.69±0.04	2.92±0.11	4.69±0.04	1.59±0.08
KMS	48 hours	0.92±0.08	3.92±0.03	4.02±0.05	1.22±0.03	1.47±0.03
KMS	14 days	1.59±0.07	1.36±0.05	0.92±0.04	0.86±0.08	2.52±0.03
KMS	15 days	0.82±0.12	0.62±0.03	1.35±0.08	0.45±0.04	1.02±0.12

Values are expressed as mean±SD. ☐ Loss ☐ Restoration

Red digits represent the significant highest values from the raw state in different conditions.

In most of the preservation methods and fresh condition, ash losses mainly occur by boiling, [38] whereas in 24 hours, 15 days control preservation without preservative and 15 days salt and turmeric preservation and 24 hours KMS preservation, ash content is reduced by deep frying. In 24 hours salt and turmeric preservation and 48 hours, 14 days, 15 days KMS preservation, ash loss occurs by shallow frying.

Retention of ash content occurs by shallow frying mostly, but in 24 hours, 15 days control preservation without preservative and 24 hours salt and turmeric preservation, ash retention occurs by boiling. In 48 hours and 15 days KMS preservation, ash retention occurs by open pan dry roasting, whereas in 48 hours, 14 days control preservation without preservative and 14 days KMS preservation, retention of ash content occurs by deep frying.

The raw state and boiling show the highest ash content in 24 hours salt and turmeric preservation, whereas open pan dry roasting shows that in 14 days salt and turmeric preservation. Shallow frying and deep frying show the highest ash content in 48 hours salt and turmeric and 48 hours control preservation without preservative respectively.

Boiling shows the increased ash content than the raw value in 48 hours KMS preservation, whereas open pan dry roasting shows the increased ash content than the raw value in fresh condition and 48 hours, 15 days KMS preservation and shallow frying in fresh condition and 48 hours KMS preservation. Deep frying shows the ash content more than the raw state in 48 hours control preservation without preservative and 48 hours, 14 days, 15 days KMS preservation.

This may occur due to the molecular rearrangement during cooking and the addition of cooking oil during frying or may be due to the addition of the natural and synthetic preservatives. Another reason may be the elimination of water during cooking[48] concentrates the minerals, thus increasing the ash content.

Fig. 5.5.1.2 Graphical representation of Ash content of *Rohu* with respect to different conditions

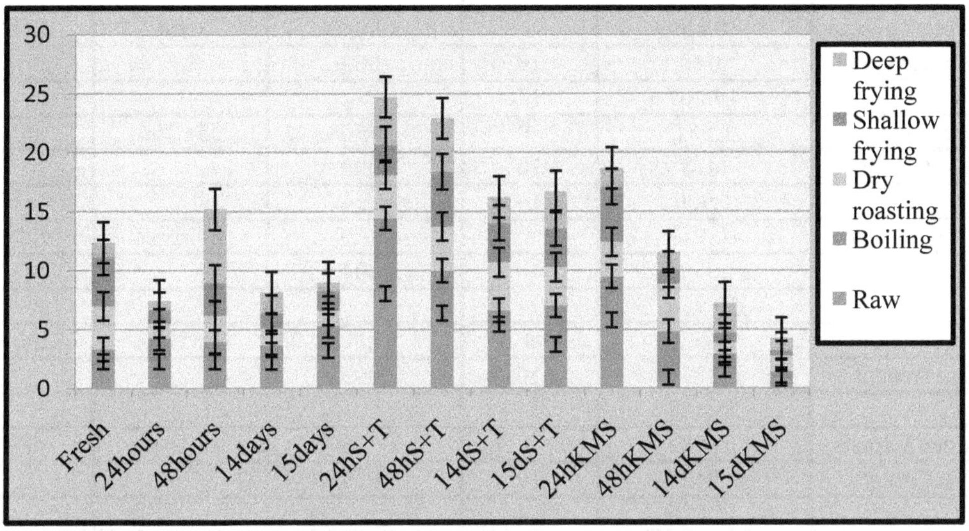

This graphical representation indicates that among all the preservation conditions, **24 hours salt and turmeric preservation**[55] helps to increase the ash content in all the cooking methods. The possible reason may be the moisture loss for prolonged preservation and the efficiency of salt and turmeric as preservatives[34, 52]. Here the graph shows that KMS preservation also increases the moisture content, whereas salt and turmeric preservation comparatively increases the ash content more than the control preservation without preservative and KMS preservation. Another possible reason may be that the natural preservative helps to modify the structure of minerals, thus the content is restored.

Table no 5.5.1.3 ANOVA with regard to cooking conditions and preservation methods

Condition	Differences	Sum of Squares	df	Mean Square	F	Sig.
Fresh (control)	Between Groups	23.030	4	5.758	877.674	.000(S)
	Within Groups	.066	10	.007		
	Total	23.096	14			
24 hours (control)	Between Groups	4.698	4	1.175	283.713	.000(S)
	Within Groups	.041	10	.004		
	Total	4.740	14			
48 hours (control)	Between Groups	40.159	4	10.040	2.086E3	.000(S)
	Within Groups	.048	10	.005		
	Total	40.207	14			
14 days (control)	Between Groups	1.881	4	.470	254.706	.000(S)
	Within Groups	.018	10	.002		
	Total	1.900	14			
15 days (control)	Between Groups	10.917	4	2.729	693.852	.000(S)
	Within Groups	.039	10	.004		
	Total	10.956	14			
24 hours (salt & turmeric)	Between Groups	59.520	4	14.880	4.852E3	.000(S)
	Within Groups	.031	10	.003		
	Total	59.550	14			
48 hours (salt & turmeric)	Between Groups	14.982	4	3.746	887.588	.000(S)
	Within Groups	.042	10	.004		
	Total	15.025	14			
14 days (salt & turmeric)	Between Groups	32.719	4	8.180	3.281E3	.000(S
	Within Groups	.025	10	.002		
	Total	32.744	14			
15 days (salt & turmeric)	Between Groups	.679	4	.170	36.050	.000(S)
	Within Groups	.047	10	.005		
	Total	.726	14			
24 hours (KMS)	Between Groups	31.213	4	7.803	1.721E3	.000(S)
	Within Groups	.045	10	.005		
	Total	31.258	14			
48 hours (KMS)	Between Groups	28.031	4	7.008	3.326E3	.000(S)
	Within Groups	.021	10	.002		
	Total	28.052	14			
14 days (KMS)	Between Groups	5.452	4	1.363	422.446	.000(S)
	Within Groups	.032	10	.003		
	Total	5.485	14			
15 days (KMS)	Between Groups	1.481	4	.370	48.774	.000(S)
	Within Groups	.076	10	.008		
	Total	1.557	14			

$p<0.05$ S= Significant, NS= Non-significant. All abbreviations are on page so and so

This statistical ANOVA table shows that all the values are significant, which means there is significant difference present in the values of ash content of *rohu* among different cooking methods and the raw state in respect to fresh condition along with different preservation methods.

Table no 5.5.1.4 Post hoc Duncan statistical analysis

Preservation	Duration	Raw state	Boiling	Dry roasting	Shallow frying	Deep frying
Control	Fresh	B,O,S,D^{a}	R,O,S,D^{b}	R,B,S,D^{c}	R,B,O,D^{d}	R,B,O,S^{e}
Control	24 hours	B,O,S,D^{a}	R,O,S,D^{b}	R,B,S,D^{c}	R,B,O,D^{d}	R,B,O,S^{e}
Control	48 hours	B,S,D^{f}	R,O,S,D^{b}	B,S,D^{f}	R,B,O,D^{d}	R,B,O,S^{e}
Control	14 days	B,O,S,D^{a}	R,D^{g}	R,S,D^{h}	R,O,D^{i}	R,B,O,S^{e}
Control	15 days	B,O,S,D^{a}	R,O,S,D^{b}	R,B,S,D^{c}	R,B,O,D^{d}	R,B,O,S^{e}
Salt & Turmeric	24 hours	B,O,S,D^{a}	R,O,S,D^{b}	R,B,S,D^{c}	R,B,O,D^{d}	R,B,O,S^{e}
Salt & Turmeric	48 hours	B,O,S,D^{a}	R,O,S,D^{b}	R,B,S,D^{c}	R,B,O,D^{d}	R,B,O,S^{e}
Salt & Turmeric	14 days	B,O,S,D^{a}	R,O,S,D^{b}	R,B,S,D^{c}	R,B,O,D^{d}	R,B,O,S^{e}
Salt & Turmeric	15 days	B,O,S,D^{a}	R,D^{g}	R^{j}	R,D^{k}	R,B,S^{l}
KMS	24 hours	B,O,S,D^{a}	R,O,S,D^{b}	R,B,S,D^{c}	R,B,O,D^{d}	R,B,O,S^{e}
KMS	48 hours	B,O,S,D^{a}	R,O,S,D^{b}	R,B,S,D^{c}	R,B,O,D^{d}	R,B,O,S^{e}
KMS	14 days	B,O,S,D^{a}	R,O,S,D^{b}	R,B,D^{m}	R,B,D^{m}	R,B,O,S^{e}
KMS	15 days	B,O,S,D^{a}	R,O,S,D^{b}	R,B,S,D^{c}	R,B,O,D^{d}	R,B,O,S^{e}

R= Raw state, B= Boiling, O= Open pan dry roasting, S= Shallow frying, D= Deep frying. The same uppercase alphabets represent that there is no significant difference present among the variables.

This table shows the significant difference among the different variables such as cooking methods and preservation conditions. The raw state significantly differs from boiling, open pan dry roasting, shallow frying and deep frying in all of the preservation conditions with preservatives and control preservation without preservative except in 48 hours control preservation. Boiling significantly differs from the raw state, open pan dry roasting, shallow frying and deep frying in all the preservation conditions except in 14 days control preservation without preservative and 15 days salt and turmeric preservation. Open pan dry roasting significantly differs from the raw state, boiling, shallow frying and deep frying in all the preservation conditions except in 48 hours, 14 days control preservation without preservative and 15 days salt and turmeric preservation. Shallow frying significantly differs from the raw state, boiling, open pan dry roasting and deep frying in all the preservation conditions except in 14 days control preservation without preservative, 15 days salt and turmeric preservation and 14 days KMS preservation. Deep frying significantly differs from the raw state, boiling, open pan dry roasting and shallow frying in all the preservation conditions except in 15 days salt and turmeric preservation.

The raw state and open pan dry roasting significantly differ from boiling, shallow frying and deep frying in 48 hours control preservation without preservative, whereas boiling and shallow frying significantly differ from the raw state and deep frying in 15 days salt and turmeric preservation, and only boiling significantly differs from the raw state and deep frying in 14 days control preservation without preservative. Again open pan dry roasting and shallow frying significantly differ from the raw state, boiling and deep frying in 14 days KMS preservation. Open pan dry roasting significantly differs from the raw state, shallow frying and deep frying in 14 days control preservation without preservative. Shallow frying significantly differs from the raw state, open pan dry roasting and deep frying in 14 days control preservation without preservative. Open pan dry roasting significantly differs from the raw state in 15 days salt and turmeric preservation. Deep frying significantly differs from the raw state, boiling and shallow frying in 15 days salt and turmeric preservation.

Table no 5.5.1.5 Gradation of cooking methods from higher to lower restoration with respect to preservation days

Preservation	Duration	Method 1	Method 2	Method 3	Method 4	Method 5
Control	Fresh	SF	OPDR	R	DF	B
Control	24 hours	R	B	OPDR	SF	DF
Control	48 hours	DF	SF	R	OPDR	B
Control	14 days	R	DF	OPDR	B	SF
Control	15 days	R	B	SF	OPDR	DF
Salt & Turmeric	24 hours	R	B	DF	OPDR	SF
Salt & Turmeric	48 hours	R	SF	DF	OPDR	B
Salt & Turmeric	14 days	R	OPDR	SF	DF	B
Salt &Turmeric	15 days	R	SF	B	OPDR	DF
KMS	24 hours	R	SF	B	OPDR	DF
KMS	48 hours	OPDR	B	DF	SF	R
KMS	14 days	DF	R	B	OPDR	SF
KMS	15 days	OPDR	DF	R	B	SF

R= Raw state, B= Boiling, OPDR= open pan dry roasting, SF= Shallow frying, DF= Deep frying. Same colour represents the similar order.

In all the preservation methods and fresh condition, ash retention occurs mainly in the raw state than the other cooking methods. In fresh condition, retention occurs firstly in shallow frying then open pan dry roasting, raw state, deep frying and boiling. In 24 hours control preservation without preservative, the order of retention is the raw state, boiling, open pan dry roasting, shallow frying and deep frying. In 48 hours control preservation without preservative, retention occurs in the order of deep frying then shallow frying, raw state, open pan dry roasting and boiling. In 14 days control preservation without preservative, the order is the raw state, deep frying, open pan dry roasting, boiling and shallow frying. In 15 days control preservation without preservative, the order of retention changes from the raw state to boiling, shallow frying, open pan dry roasting and deep frying.

In 24 hours salt and turmeric preservation, the order is the raw state, boiling, deep frying, open pan dry roasting and shallow frying. In 48 hours salt and turmeric preservation, the order remains the raw state, shallow frying, deep frying, open pan dry roasting and boiling. In 14 days salt and turmeric preservation, the order becomes the raw state, open pan dry roasting, shallow frying, deep frying and boiling. In 15 days salt and turmeric preservation and 24 hours KMS preservation, the order changes from the raw state to shallow frying, boiling, open pan dry roasting and deep frying.

In 48 hours KMS preservation, retention occurs firstly in open pan dry roasting followed by boiling, deep frying, shallow frying and the raw state. In 14 days KMS preservation, the order changes from deep frying to the raw state, boiling, open pan dry roasting and shallow frying. In 15 days KMS preservation, the order becomes open pan dry roasting, deep frying, raw state, boiling and shallow frying.

The overall analysis of ash content of *rohu* is mostly restored by the gradation of methods as the raw state> shallow frying> deep frying >open pan dry roasting> boiling.

Shallow frying and deep frying[66] can restore ash content as the oil can possibly create a protective layer so that the inorganic constituents cannot be leached out. Open pan dry roasting reduces the ash content due to the application of direct dry heat so the inorganic constituents present in *rohu* get charred and thus the reduction occurs, whereas boiling can reduce ash content as the inorganic constituents are dissolved in water during cooking and discarding this cooking water causes the reduction. Thus among all the studied conventional cooking methods, **shallow frying** is the best method for *rohu* to restore ash content.

5.5.2 *Katla* (*Catla catla*)

It has been reported that *katla* contains 0.94 gm of ash per 100 gm[84] in the raw condition. This value changes due to the application of different cooking methods and preservation conditions (vide Table no **5.5.2.1**).

Table no 5.5.2.1 Ash content of *Katla* (gm/100gm)

Preservation	Duration	Raw state	Boiling	Dry roasting	Shallow frying	Deep frying
Control	Fresh	3.35±0.06	2.32±0.03	2.06±0.05	1.65±0.44	1.19±0.04
Control	24 hours	3.89±0.03	3.72±0.03	4.16±0.07	5.13±0.08	4.69±0.10
Control	48 hours	4.79±0.07	2.38±0.02	7.65±0.06	6.24±0.04	10.09±0.01
Control	14 days	12.08±0.07	7.22±0.03	6.75±0.04	11.39±0.04	13.62±0.03
Control	15 days	15.11±0.10	7.35±0.08	8.10±0.10	13.12±0.03	10.55±0.06
Salt & Turmeric	24 hours	3.74±0.06	3.53±0.04	1.97±0.04	0.88±0.10	2.95±0.04
Salt & Turmeric	48 hours	2.38±0.07	3.60±0.10	3.82±0.02	4.35±0.52	6.75±0.08
Salt & Turmeric	14 days	4.59±0.07	3.43±0.09	3.15±0.00	5.12±0.10	5.35±0.06
Salt & Turmeric	15 days	1.18±0.07	1.87±0.06	4.69±0.07	5.08±0.08	3.18±0.08
KMS	24 hours	0.81±0.07	0.69±0.08	0.49±0.80	0.88±0.08	0.74±0.04
KMS	48 hours	3.28±0.08	2.14±0.04	2.61±0.04	2.81±0.04	3.52±0.09
KMS	14 days	3.86±0.08	2.34±0.04	1.80±0.08	1.87±0.03	3.63±0.04
KMS	15 days	2.35±0.04	2.96±0.05	3.05±0.05	3.27±0.03	5.55±0.08

Values are expressed as mean±SD. Loss Restoration

Red digits represent the significant highest values from the raw state in different conditions.

In most of the preservation conditions, ash losses mainly occur by boiling,[38] whereas in 14 days salt and turmeric preservation and 24 hours, 14 days KMS preservation, ash content is reduced by open pan dry roasting. In fresh condition, 24 hours salt and turmeric preservation, ash content is reduced by deep frying and shallow frying respectively.

Retention of ash content occurs by deep frying mostly, but in 24 hours, 15 days control preservation without preservative and 15 days salt and turmeric preservation, 24 hours KMS preservation, ash retention occurs by shallow frying, whereas in fresh condition, ash retention occurs by boiling. All the cooking conditions and the raw state show the highest ash content in 15 days control preservation without preservative.

Boiling shows the increased ash content than the raw state in 48 hours, 15 days salt and turmeric preservation and 15 days KMS preservation, whereas open pan dry roasting shows the increased ash content than the raw value in 24 hours, 48 hours control preservation without preservative, 48 hours, 15 days salt and turmeric preservation, 15 days KMS preservation. Again shallow frying shows the ash content more than the raw state in 24 hours, 48 hours control preservation without preservative, 48 hours, 14 days, 15 days salt and turmeric preservation as well as 24 hours, 15 days KMS preservation. Deep frying shows the ash content more than the raw value in 24 hours, 48 hours, 14 days control preservation without preservative, 48 hours, 14 days, 15 days salt and turmeric preservation as well as 48 hours, 15 days KMS preservation.

This is possible due to the molecular rearrangement during cooking and the addition of cooking oil during frying or may be due to the addition of the natural and synthetic preservatives. Another possible reason may be the elimination of water during cooking[48] that concentrates the ash, leading to its increased content.

Fig. 5.5.2.2 Graphical representation of Ash content of *Katla* with respect to different conditions

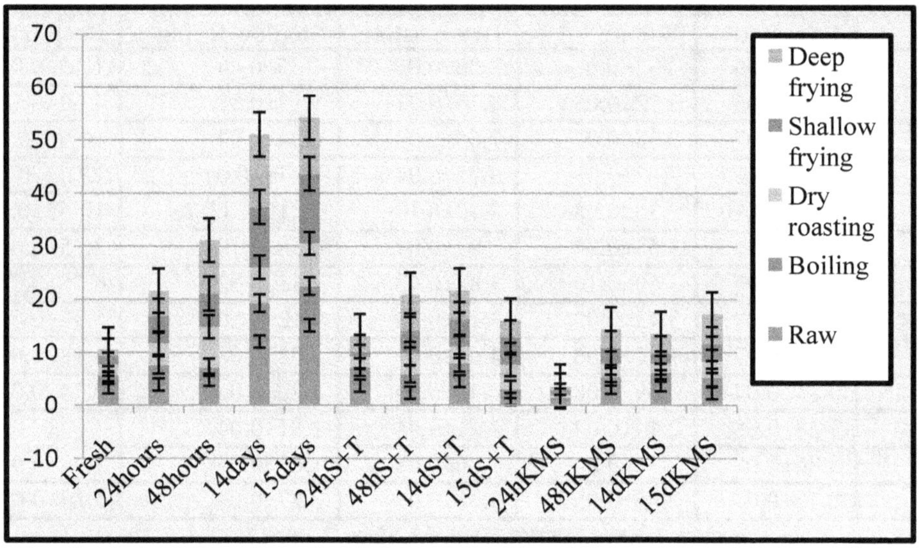

This graphical representation indicates that among all the preservation conditions, **15 days control preservation without preservative** helps to increase the ash content in all the cooking methods. The possible reason may be the moisture loss for prolonged preservation. Here the graph shows that there is no such prominent effect of preservatives found on *katla*.

Table no 5.5.2.3 ANOVA with regard to cooking conditions and preservation methods

Condition	Differences	Sum of Squares	df	Mean Square	F	Sig.
Fresh (control)	Between Groups	7.420	4	1.855	622.525	.000(S)
	Within Groups	.030	10	.003		
	Total	7.450	14			
24 hours (control)	Between Groups	4.107	4	1.027	209.231	.000(S)
	Within Groups	.049	10	.005		
	Total	4.156	14			
48 hours (control)	Between Groups	101.417	4	25.354	1.255E4	.000(S)
	Within Groups	.020	10	.002		
	Total	101.437	14			
14 days (control)	Between Groups	112.195	4	28.049	1.398E4	.000(S)
	Within Groups	.020	10	.002		
	Total	112.215	14			
15 days (control)	Between Groups	2236.753	4	559.188	1.037	.435(S)
	Within Groups	5389.863	10	538.986		
	Total	7626.617	14			
24 hours (salt & turmeric)	Between Groups	16.966	4	4.242	1.048E3	.000(S)
	Within Groups	.040	10	.004		
	Total	17.007	14			
48hours (salt & turmeric)	Between Groups	30.856	4	7.714	1.272E3	.000(S)
	Within Groups	.061	10	.006		
	Total	30.917	14			
14 days (salt & turmeric)	Between Groups	10.430	4	2.608	627.809	.000(S)
	Within Groups	.042	10	.004		
	Total	10.472	14			
15 days (salt & turmeric)	Between Groups	34.783	4	8.696	1.677E3	.000(S)
	Within Groups	.052	10	.005		
	Total	34.835	14			
24 hours (KMS)	Between Groups	.267	4	.067	13.707	.000(S)
	Within Groups	.049	10	.005		
	Total	.316	14			
48 hours (KMS)	Between Groups	3.578	4	.894	254.573	.000(S)
	Within Groups	.035	10	.004		
	Total	3.613	14			
14 days (KMS)	Between Groups	11.558	4	2.890	890.010	.000(S)
	Within Groups	.032	10	.003		
	Total	11.591	14			
15 days (KMS)	Between Groups	18.211	4	4.553	1.650E3	.000(S)
	Within Groups	.028	10	.003		
	Total	18.238	14			

$p<0.05$ S= Significant, NS= Non-significant. All abbreviations are on page so and so.

This statistical ANOVA table shows that all the values are significant, which means there is significant difference present in the values of ash content of *katla* among different cooking methods and the raw state in respect to fresh condition along with different preservation methods.

Table no 5.5.2.4 Post hoc Duncan statistical analysis

Preservation	Duration	Raw state	Boiling	Dry roasting	Shallow frying	Deep frying
Control	Fresh	B,O,S,D^{a}	R,O,S,D^{b}	R,B,S,D^{c}	R,B,O,D^{d}	R,B,O,S^{e}
Control	24 hours	B,O,S,D^{a}	R,O,S,D^{b}	R,B,S,D^{c}	R,B,O,D^{d}	R,B,O,S^{e}
Control	48 hours	B,O,S,D^{a}	R,O,S,D^{b}	R,B,S,D^{c}	R,B,O,D^{d}	R,B,O,S^{e}
Control	14 days	B,O,S,D^{a}	R,O,S,D^{b}	R,B,S,D^{c}	R,B,O,D^{d}	R,B,O,S^{e}
Control	15 days	--	--	--	--	--
Salt & Turmeric	24 hours	B,O,S,D^{a}	R,O,S,D^{b}	R,B,S,D^{d}	R,B,O,D^{d}	R,B,O,S^{e}
Salt & Turmeric	48 hours	B,O,S,D^{a}	R,O,S,D^{b}	R,B,S,D^{d}	R,B,O,D^{d}	R,B,O,S^{e}
Salt & Turmeric	14 days	B,O,S,D^{a}	R,S,D^{f}	R,S,D^{f}	R,B,O,D^{d}	R,B,O,S^{e}
Salt & Turmeric	15 days	B,O,S,D^{a}	R,O,S,D^{b}	R,B,O,D^{d}	R,B,O,D^{d}	R,B,O,S^{e}
KMS	24 hours	O^{g}	O,S^{h}	R,B,O,D^{d}	B,O,D^{i}	O,S^{h}
KMS	48 hours	B,O,S,D^{a}	R,O,S,D^{b}	R,B,O,D^{d}	R,B,O,D^{d}	R,B,O,S^{e}
KMS	14 days	B,O,S,D^{a}	R,O,S,D^{b}	R,B,D^{j}	R,B,D^{j}	R,B,O,S^{e}
KMS	15 days	B,O,S,D^{a}	R,S,D^{k}	R,S,D^{k}	R,B,O,D^{d}	R,B,O,S^{e}

R= Raw state, B= Boiling, O= Open pan dry roasting, S= Shallow frying, D= Deep frying. The same uppercase alphabets signify that there is no significant difference present among the variables.

This table shows the significant difference among the different variables such as cooking methods and preservation conditions. The raw state significantly differs from boiling, open pan dry roasting, shallow frying and deep frying in all of the preservation conditions with preservatives and control preservation without preservative except in 15 days control preservation and 24 hours KMS preservation. Boiling significantly differs from the raw state, open pan dry roasting, shallow frying and deep frying in all the preservation conditions except in 15 days control preservation without preservative and 24 hours KMS preservation. Open pan dry roasting significantly differs from the raw state, boiling, shallow frying and deep frying in all the preservation conditions except in 15 days control preservation without preservative and 14 days salt and turmeric preservation as well as 14 days, 15 days KMS preservation. Shallow frying significantly differs from the raw state, boiling, open pan dry roasting and deep frying in all the preservation conditions except in 15 days control preservation without preservative, 24 hours salt and turmeric preservation and 24 hours, 14 days KMS preservation. Deep frying significantly differs from the raw state, boiling, open pan dry roasting and shallow frying in all the preservation conditions except in 15 days control preservation without preservative and 24 hours KMS preservation.

Boiling and open pan dry roasting significantly differ from the raw state, shallow frying and deep frying in 14 days salt and turmeric preservation, whereas boiling and deep frying significantly differ from open pan dry roasting and shallow frying in 24 hours KMS preservation and only the raw state significantly differs from open pan dry roasting in 24 hours KMS preservation. Again open pan dry roasting and shallow frying significantly differ from the raw state, boiling and deep frying in 14 days KMS preservation. Both boiling and open pan dry roasting significantly differ from the raw state, shallow frying and deep frying in 15 days KMS preservation. Shallow frying significantly differs from boiling, open pan dry roasting and deep frying in 15 days KMS preservation.

Table no 5.5.2.5 Gradation of cooking methods from higher to lower restoration with respect to preservation days

Preservation	Duration	Method 1	Method 2	Method 3	Method 4	Method 5
Control	Fresh	R	B	OPDR	SF	DF
Control	24 hours	SF	DF	OPDR	R	B
Control	48 hours	DF	OPDR	SF	R	B
Control	14 days	DF	R	SF	B	OPDR
Control	15 days	DF	R	SF	OPDR	B
Salt & Turmeric	24 hours	R	B	DF	OPDR	SF
Salt & Turmeric	48 hours	DF	SF	R	OPDR	B
Salt & Turmeric	14 days	DF	SF	R	OPDR	B
Salt &Turmeric	15 days	SF	OPDR	DF	B	R
KMS	24 hours	SF	R	DF	B	OPDR
KMS	48 hours	DF	R	SF	OPDR	B
KMS	14 days	R	DF	B	SF	OPDR
KMS	15 days	DF	SF	OPDR	B	R

R= Raw state, B= Boiling, OPDR= Open pan dry roasting, SF= Shallow frying, DF= Deep frying. Same colour represents the similar order.

In all the preservation techniques and fresh condition, ash retention occurs mainly in deep frying than the raw state and the other cooking methods. In fresh condition, retention occurs firstly in the raw state followed by boiling, open pan dry roasting, shallow frying and deep frying. In 24 hours control preservation without preservative, retention occurs in the order of shallow frying, deep frying, open pan dry roasting, raw state and boiling. In 48 hours control preservation without preservative, the order of retention is deep frying, open pan dry roasting, shallow frying, raw state and boiling. In 14 days control preservation without preservative, the order becomes deep frying, raw state, shallow frying, boiling and open pan dry roasting. In 15 days control preservation without preservative, the order remains deep frying followed by the raw state, shallow frying, open pan dry roasting and boiling.

In 24 hours salt and turmeric preservation, retention occurs firstly in the raw state then boiling, deep frying, open pan dry roasting and shallow frying. In 48 hours, 14 days salt and turmeric preservation, the order is deep frying, shallow frying, raw state, open pan dry roasting and boiling. In 15 days salt and turmeric preservation, the order is shallow frying, open pan dry roasting, deep frying, boiling and the raw state.

In 24 hours KMS preservation, retention occurs in the following order: shallow frying, raw state, deep frying, boiling and open pan dry roasting. In 48 hours KMS preservation, the order is deep frying, raw state, shallow frying, open pan dry roasting and boiling. In 14 days KMS preservation, the order becomes the raw state, deep frying, boiling, shallow frying and open pan dry roasting. In 15 days KMS preservation, the order changes from deep frying to shallow frying, open pan dry roasting, boiling and the raw state.

The overall analysis of ash content of *katla* is mostly restored by the gradation of methods as deep frying> >raw state> shallow frying >open pan dry roasting> boiling.

Shallow frying and deep frying[66] can restore ash content as the oil can possibly create a protective layer, so that the inorganic constituents cannot be leached out. Open pan dry roasting reduces the ash content due to the application of direct dry heat, so the inorganic constituents present in *katla* possibly get charred, causing reduction, whereas boiling can reduce ash content as the inorganic constituents may dissolve in water during cooking and discarding the water reduces the ash content. Thus among all the studied conventional cooking methods, **deep frying** is the best method for *katla* to restore ash content.

5.5.3 Prawn (*Fenneropenaeus indicus*)

It has been reported that prawn contains 0.86 gm of ash per 100 gm[84] in the raw condition. This value changes due to the application of different cooking methods and preservation conditions (vide Table no **5.5.3.1**).

Table no 5.5.3.1 Ash content of Prawn (gm/100gm)

Preservation	Duration	Raw state	Boiling	Dry roasting	Shallow frying	Deep frying
Control	Fresh	4.82±0.03	2.07±0.04	2.53±0.04	3.81±0.08	3.56±0.06
Control	24 hours	4.70±0.19	2.96±0.05	3.87±0.06	5.41±0.03	2.85±0.04
Control	48 hours	2.56±0.04	1.24±0.04	1.34±0.11	0.45±0.05	1.01±0.07
Control	14 days	2.50±0.08	2.29±0.07	2.46±0.04	2.21±0.10	1.11±0.10
Control	15 day	4.17±0.04	3.55±0.05	3.17±0.03	2.41±0.08	8.83±0.06
Salt & Turmeric	24 hours	5.49±0.07	1.50±0.08	2.06±0.05	3.53±0.04	2.93±0.04
Salt & Turmeric	48 hours	5.49±0.04	4.25±0.05	4.60±0.09	5.70±0.02	3.32±0.03
Salt & Turmeric	14 days	5.44±0.04	4.34±0.04	3.62±0.10	9.92±0.03	3.44±0.04
Salt & Turmeric	15 days	1.60±0.09	0.70±0.09	1.76±0.04	4.60±0.05	1.60±0.80
KMS	24 hours	5.15±0.06	2.14±0.04	1.96±0.04	1.24±0.04	2.42±0.03
KMS	48 hours	3.25±0.08	2.17±0.08	2.95±0.04	3.67±0.04	2.71±0.60
KMS	14 days	4.11±0.04	3.82±0.03	3.16±0.04	5.21±0.03	6.61±0.04
KMS	15 days	8.18±0.03	3.79±0.07	4.16±0.06	3.27±0.03	4.52±0.06

Values are expressed as mean±SD. ☐ Loss ☐ Restoration
Red digits represent the significant highest values from the raw state in different conditions.

In fresh condition, 24 hours, 15 days salt and turmeric and 48 hours KMS preservation, ash content is reduced by boiling, whereas in 14 days KMS preservation, ash content is reduced by open pan dry roasting. In 48 hours, 15 days control preservation without preservative, 24 hours, 15 days KMS preservation, ash content is reduced by shallow frying and in 24 hours, 14 days control preservation without preservative, 48 hours, 14 days salt and turmeric preservation, losses occur by deep frying.

Retention of ash content occurs by shallow frying mostly, but in 48 hours, 14 days control preservation without preservative, ash retention occurs by open pan dry roasting, whereas in 15 days control preservation without preservative, 24 hours, 14 days, 15 days KMS preservation, ash retention occurs by deep frying.

The raw state and open pan dry roasting show the highest ash content in 15 days KMS preservation, whereas boiling and shallow frying show the highest ash content in 14 days salt and turmeric preservation. Deep fried Prawn shows the highest ash content in 15 days control preservation without preservative.

Open pan dry roasting shows the increased ash content than the raw state in 15 days salt and turmeric preservation, whereas shallow frying shows the increased ash content than the raw value in 24 hours control preservation without preservative, 48 hours, 14 days, 15 days salt and turmeric preservation as well as 48 hours, 14 days KMS preservation. Again deep frying increases the ash content than the raw value in 15 days control preservation without preservative and 14 days KMS preservation.

This may occur due to the molecular rearrangement during cooking and the addition of cooking oil during frying, or may be due to the addition of the natural and synthetic preservatives during prolonged preservation. Another possible reason may be the elimination of water during cooking[48] concentrates the minerals, resulting in the increased content of ash.

Fig. 5.5.3.2 Graphical representation of Ash content of Prawn with respect to different conditions

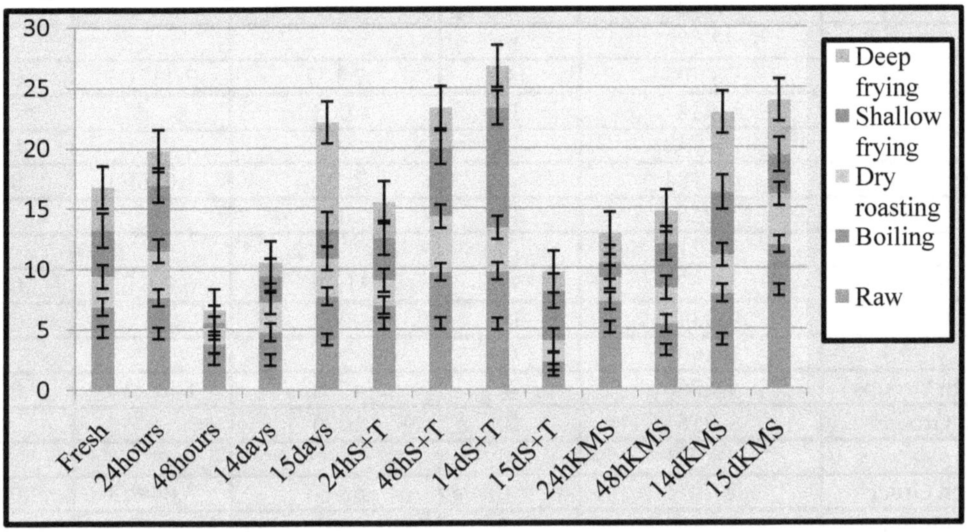

This graphical representation indicates that among all the preservation conditions, **14 days salt and turmeric preservation[55]** helps to increase the ash content in all the cooking methods[52]. The possible reason may be the moisture loss for prolonged preservation. Here the graph shows that there is prominent effect of both the natural and synthetic preservatives, but salt and turmeric preservation is more effective than KMS. The possible reason may be that the natural preservative helps to modify the structure of minerals, thus restoring the content.

Table no 5.5.3.3 ANOVA with regard to cooking conditions and preservation

Condition	Differences	Sum of Squares	df	Mean Square	F	Sig.
Fresh (control)	Between Groups	14.134	4	3.534	1.325E3	.000(S)
	Within Groups	.027	10	.003		
	Total	14.161	14			
24 hours (control)	Between Groups	14.763	4	3.691	403.814	.000(S)
	Within Groups	.091	10	.009		
	Total	14.855	14			
48 hours (control)	Between Groups	7.258	4	1.814	394.444	.000(S)
	Within Groups	.046	10	.005		
	Total	7.304	14			
14 days (control)	Between Groups	3.925	4	.981	150.637	.000(S)
	Within Groups	.065	10	.007		
	Total	3.990	14			
15 days (control)	Between Groups	77.638	4	19.409	6.104E3	.000(S)
	Within Groups	.032	10	.003		
	Total	77.670	14			
24 hours (salt & turmeric)	Between Groups	28.708	4	7.177	2.115E3	.000(S)
	Within Groups	.034	10	.003		
	Total	28.742	14			
48 hours (salt & turmeric)	Between Groups	11.184	4	2.796	1.056E3	.000(S)
	Within Groups	.026	10	.003		
	Total	11.211	14			
14 days (salt & turmeric)	Between Groups	85.571	4	21.393	6.207E3	.000(S)
	Within Groups	.034	10	.003		
	Total	85.605	14			
15 days (salt & turmeric)	Between Groups	18.866	4	4.716	846.244	.000(S)
	Within Groups	.056	10	.006		
	Total	18.921	14			
24 hours (KMS)	Between Groups	27.051	4	6.763	3.649E3	.000(S)
	Within Groups	.019	10	.002		
	Total	27.070	14			
48 hours (KMS)	Between Groups	2.091	4	.523	7.015	.006(S)
	Within Groups	.745	10	.074		
	Total	2.836	14			
14 days (KMS)	Between Groups	22.077	4	5.519	4.813E3	.000(S)
	Within Groups	.011	10	.001		
	Total	22.089	14			
15 days (KMS)	Between Groups	45.695	4	11.424	5.028E3	.000(S)
	Within Groups	.020	9	.002		
	Total	45.715	13			

$p<0.05$ S= Significant, NS= Non-significant. All abbreviations are on page so and so.

This statistical ANOVA table shows that all the values are significant, which means there is significant difference present in the values of ash content of prawn among different cooking methods and the raw state in respect to fresh condition along with different preservation methods.

Table no 5.5.3.4 Post hoc Duncan statistical analysis

Preservation	Duration	Raw state	Boiling	Dry roasting	Shallow frying	Deep frying
Control	Fresh	B,O,S,D^{a}	R,O,S,D^{b}	R,B,S,D^{c}	R,B,O,D^{d}	R,B,O,S^{e}
Control	24 hours	B,O,S,D^{a}	R,O,S^{f}	R,B,S,D^{c}	R,B,O,D^{d}	R,O,S^{f}
Control	48 hours	B,O,S,D^{a}	R,S,D^{g}	R,S,D^{g}	R,B,O,D^{d}	R,B,O,S^{e}
Control	14 days	B,S,D^{h}	R,O,D^{i}	B,S,D^{h}	R,O,D^{i}	R,B,O,S^{e}
Control	15 days	B,S,D^{h}	R,O,S,D^{b}	R,B,S,D^{c}	R,B,O,D^{d}	R,B,O,S^{e}
Salt & Turmeric	24 hours	B,O,S,D^{a}	R,O,S,D^{b}	R,B,S,D^{c}	R,B,O,D^{d}	R,B,O,S^{e}
Salt & Turmeric	48 hours	B,O,S,D^{a}	R,O,S,D^{b}	R,B,S,D^{c}	R,B,O,D^{d}	R,B,O,S^{e}
Salt & Turmeric	14 days	B,O,S,D^{a}	R,O,S,D^{b}	R,B,S,D^{c}	R,B,O,D^{d}	R,B,O,S^{e}
Salt & Turmeric	15 days	B,O,S^{J}	R,O,S,D^{b}	R,B,S,D^{c}	R,B,O,D^{d}	B,O,S^{J}
KMS	24 hours	B,O,S,D^{a}	R,O,S,D^{b}	R,B,S,D^{c}	R,B,O,D^{d}	R,B,O,S^{e}
KMS	48 hours	B,D^{k}	R,O,S,D^{b}	B^{l}	B^{l}	R,B^{m}
KMS	14 days	B,O,S,D^{a}	R,O,S,D^{b}	RB,S,D^{c}	R,B,O,D^{d}	R,B,O,S^{e}
KMS	15 days	B,O,S,D^{a}	R,O,S,D^{b}	R,B,S,D^{c}	R,B,O,D^{d}	R,B,O,S^{e}

R= Raw state, B= Boiling, O= Open pan dry roasting, S= Shallow frying, D= Deep frying. The same uppercase alphabets represent that there is no significant difference present among the variables.

This table shows the significant difference among the different variables such as cooking methods and preservation conditions. The raw state significantly differs from boiling, open pan dry roasting, shallow frying and deep frying in all of the preservation conditions with preservatives and control preservation without preservative except in 14 days, 15 days control preservation without preservative, 15 days salt and turmeric preservation and 48 hours KMS preservation. Boiling significantly differs from the raw state, open pan dry roasting, shallow frying and deep frying in all the preservation conditions except in 24 hours, 48 hours and 14 days control preservation without preservative. Open pan dry roasting significantly differs from the raw state, boiling, shallow frying and deep frying in all preservation conditions except in 48 hours and 14 days control preservation without preservative, and 48 hours KMS preservation. Shallow frying significantly differs from the raw state, boiling, open pan dry roasting and deep frying in all the preservation conditions except in 14 days control preservation without preservative as well as in 48 hours KMS preservation. Deep frying significantly differs from the raw state, boiling, open pan dry roasting and shallow frying in all the preservation conditions except in 24 hours control preservation without preservative, 15 days salt and turmeric preservation and 48 hours KMS preservation. Boiling and deep frying significantly differ from the raw state, open pan dry roasting and shallow frying in 24 hours control preservation without preservative, whereas boiling and open pan dry roasting significantly differ from the raw state, shallow frying and deep frying in 48 hours control preservation without preservative. Again boiling and shallow frying significantly differ from the raw state, open pan dry roasting and deep frying in 14 days control preservation without preservative. The raw state and open pan dry roasting significantly differ from boiling, shallow frying and deep frying in 14 days control preservation without preservative, and only the raw state significantly differs from boiling, shallow frying and deep frying in 15 days control preservation without preservative. The raw state and deep frying significantly differ from boiling, open pan dry roasting and shallow frying in 15 days salt and turmeric preservation. Shallow frying and open pan dry roasting significantly differ from boiling in 48 hours KMS preservation. The raw state significantly differs from boiling, deep frying in 48 hours KMS preservation, whereas deep frying significantly differs from the raw state and boiling in 48 hours KMS preservation.

Table no 5.5.3.5 Gradation of cooking methods from higher to lower restoration with respect to preservation days

Preservation	Duration	Method 1	Method 2	Method 3	Method 4	Method 5
Control	Fresh	R	SF	DF	OPDR	B
Control	24 hours	SF	R	OPDR	B	DF
Control	48 hours	R	OPDR	B	DF	SF
Control	14 days	R	OPDR	B	SF	DF
Control	15 days	DF	R	B	OPDR	SF
Salt & Turmeric	24 hours	R	SF	DF	OPDR	B
Salt & Turmeric	48 hours	SF	R	OPDR	B	DF
Salt & Turmeric	14 days	SF	R	B	OPDR	DF
Salt &Turmeric	15 days	SF	OPDR	DF	R	B
KMS	24 hours	R	DF	B	OPDR	SF
KMS	48 hours	R	SF	OPDR	DF	B
KMS	14 days	DF	SF	R	B	OPDR
KMS	15 days	R	DF	OPDR	B	SF

R= Raw state, B= Boiling, OPDR= Open pan dry roasting, SF= Shallow frying, DF= Deep frying. Same colours represent similar order.

In all the preservation methods and fresh condition, ash retention occurs mainly in the raw state than the other cooking methods. In fresh condition and 24 hours salt and turmeric preservation, retention occurs firstly in the raw state followed by shallow frying, deep frying, open pan dry roasting and boiling. In 24 hours control preservation without preservative and 48 hours salt and turmeric preservation, retention occurs in the order of shallow frying followed by the raw state, open pan dry roasting, boiling and deep frying. In 48 hours control preservation without preservative, the order of retention is the raw state, open pan dry roasting, boiling, deep frying and shallow frying. In 14 days control preservation without preservative, the order remains the raw state, open pan dry roasting, boiling, shallow frying and deep frying. In 15 days control preservation without preservative, retention changes in the order of deep frying, raw state, boiling, open pan dry roasting and shallow frying.

In 14 days salt and turmeric preservation, retention occurs in the order of shallow frying then the raw state, boiling, open pan dry roasting and deep frying. In 15 days salt and turmeric preservation, retention occurs firstly in shallow frying followed by open pan dry roasting, deep frying, raw state and boiling.

In 24 hours KMS preservation, retention occurs in the following manner: the raw state, deep frying, boiling, open pan dry roasting and shallow frying. In 48 hours KMS preservation, the order changes from the raw state to shallow frying, open pan dry roasting, deep frying and boiling. In 14 days KMS preservation, the order is deep frying, shallow frying, raw state, boiling and open pan dry roasting. In 15 days KMS preservation, the order beomes the raw state, deep frying, open pan dry roasting, boiling and shallow frying.

The overall analysis of ash content of prawn is mostly restored by the gradation of methods as the raw state >shallow frying >boiling>open pan dry roasting> deep frying.

Shallow frying[66] can restore ash content as the oil can possibly create a protective layer so that the inorganic constituents cannot be leached out. Open pan dry roasting reduces the ash content due to the application of direct dry heat, so that the inorganic constituents present in prawn may get charred, resulting in reduction, whereas boiling can reduce ash content as the inorganic constituents may dissolve in water during cooking and discarding the cooking water leads to the reduction of ash content. Deep frying possibly causes the total dryness and inorganic constituents may also get charred, causing reduction. Thus among all the studied conventional cooking methods, **shallow frying** is the best method for prawn in order to restore ash content.

5.5.4 Lobster (*Macrobrachium rosenbergii*)

It has been reported that lobster contains 0.84 gm of ash per 100 gm[85] in the raw condition. This value changes due to the application of different cooking methods and preservation conditions (vide Table no **5.5.4.1**).

Table no 5.5.4.1 Ash content of Lobster (gm/100gm)

Preservation	Duration	Raw state	Boiling	Dry roasting	Shallow frying	Deep frying
Control	Fresh	2.09±0.07	2.58±0.05	2.06±0.05	6.78±0.05	6.15±0.05
Control	24 hours	0.89±0.03	0.58±0.02	0.63±0.02	4.20±0.05	4.06±0.04
Control	48 hours	1.05±0.05	1.38±0.02	0.56±0.03	5.78±0.05	7.75±0.03
Control	14 days	1.20±0.05	1.59±0.04	0.59±0.01	4.89±0.03	4.68±0.06
Control	15 days	1.01±0.04	1.14±0.04	0.98±0.09	7.72±0.07	4.67±0.03
Salt & Turmeric	24 hours	5.78±0.07	0.81±0.04	0.51±0.07	3.07±0.08	3.23±0.05
Salt & Turmeric	48 hours	9.24±0.04	1.35±0.06	4.32±0.03	1.31±0.09	6.28±0.07
Salt & Turmeric	14 days	3.42±0.08	0.73±0.04	2.32±0.07	1.67±0.03	4.79±0.07
Salt & Turmeric	15 days	5.51±0.04	3.50±0.02	4.85±0.05	4.85±0.05	7.89±0.04
KMS	24 hours	1.11±0.09	0.50±0.08	0.66±0.04	0.25±0.05	0.70±0.08
KMS	48 hours	5.08±0.08	2.43±0.08	3.12±0.06	2.28±0.06	2.35±0.03
KMS	14 days	4.92±0.03	2.61±0.04	2.84±0.05	3.61±0.04	3.85±0.06
KMS	15 days	0.85±0.04	0.70±0.02	0.49±0.02	0.30±0.02	3.50±0.02

Values are expressed as mean±SD. ☐ Loss ▩ Restoration
Red digits represent the significant highest values from the raw state in different conditions.

In most of the conditions, ash content is mainly reduced by boiling, [38] whereas in fresh condition, 14 days, 15 days control preservation without preservative and 24 hours salt and turmeric preservation, ash content is reduced by open pan dry roasting. In 24 hours, 48 hours, 15 days KMS preservation, ash content is reduced by shallow frying. Retention of ash content occurs by deep frying mostly, but in fresh condition, 24 hours, 14 days and 15 days control preservation without preservative, ash retention occurs by shallow frying, whereas in 48 hours KMS preservation, ash retention occurs by open pan dry roasting. The raw state and open pan dry roasting show the highest ash content in 48 hours salt and turmeric preservation, whereas boiling and deep frying show the highest ash content in 15 days salt and turmeric preservation. Shallow fried lobster shows the highest ash content in fresh condition.

Boiling shows the increased ash content than the raw state in fresh condition, 48 hours, 14 days and 15 days control preservation without preservative, whereas shallow frying and deep frying show the increased ash content than the raw value in fresh condition, 24 hours, 48 hours, 14 days, 15 days control preservation without preservative. Again deep frying also increases the ash content in 15 days salt and turmeric preservation as well as 15 days KMS preservation.

This may occur due to the molecular rearrangement during cooking and the addition of cooking oil during frying or possibly may be due to the addition of the natural and synthetic preservatives. Another possible reason may be the elimination of water during cooking[48] concentrates the minerals, thus causing the increased content of ash.

Fig. 5.5.4.2 Graphical representation of Ash content of Lobster with respect to different conditions

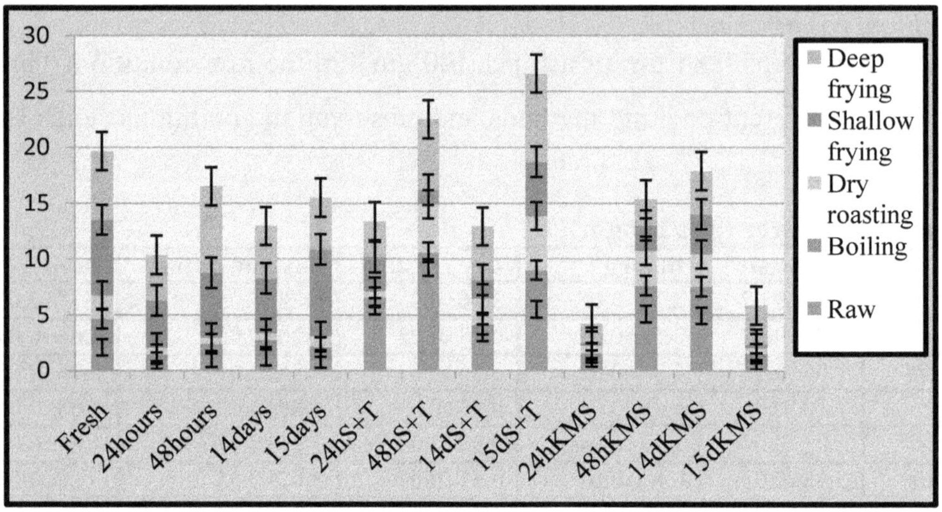

This graphical representation indicates that among all the preservation conditions, **15 days salt and turmeric preservation**[55] helps to increase the ash content in all the cooking methods[52]. The possible reason may be the moisture loss for prolonged preservation. Here the graph shows that control preservation without preservative also increases the ash content, but salt and turmeric preservation is more effective than the control preservation without preservative. The possible reason behind this condition is that the natural preservative may help to modify the structure of minerals, thus restoring the content.

Table no 5.5.4.3 ANOVA with regard to cooking conditions and preservation methods

Condition	Differences	Sum of Squares	df	Mean Square	F	Sig.
Fresh (control)	Between Groups	65.268	4	16.317	5.367E3	.000(S)
	Within Groups	.030	10	.003		
	Total	65.298	14			
24 hours (control)	Between Groups	42.643	4	10.661	8.738E3	.000(S)
	Within Groups	.012	10	.001		
	Total	42.655	14			
48 hours (control)	Between Groups	126.772	4	31.693	1.997E4	.000(S)
	Within Groups	.016	10	.002		
	Total	126.788	14			
14 days (control)	Between Groups	49.863	4	12.466	8.499E3	.000(S)
	Within Groups	.015	10	.001		
	Total	49.877	14			
15 days (control)	Between Groups	109.560	4	27.390	9.274E3	.000(S)
	Within Groups	.030	10	.003		
	Total	109.590	14			
24 hours (salt & turmeric)	Between Groups	54.836	4	13.709	3.801E3	.000(S)
	Within Groups	.036	10	.004		
	Total	54.872	14			
48 hours (salt & turmeric)	Between Groups	137.302	4	34.325	8.160E3	.000(S)
	Within Groups	.042	10	.004		
	Total	137.344	14			
14 days (salt & turmeric)	Between Groups	29.622	4	7.406	1.998E3	.000(S)
	Within Groups	.037	10	.004		
	Total	29.659	14			
15 days (salt & turmeric)	Between Groups	31.180	4	7.795	5.220E3	.000(S)
	Within Groups	.015	10	.001		
	Total	31.195	14			
24 hours (KMS)	Between Groups	3.964	4	.991	187.910	.000(S)
	Within Groups	.053	10	.005		
	Total	4.016	14			
48 hours (KMS)	Between Groups	16.441	4	4.110	942.693	.000(S)
	Within Groups	.044	10	.004		
	Total	16.484	14			
14 days (KMS)	Between Groups	9.832	4	2.458	1.341E3	.000(S)
	Within Groups	.018	10	.002		
	Total	9.850	14			
15 days (KMS)	Between Groups	14.945	4	3.736	3.603E3	.000(S)
	Within Groups	.009	9	.001		
	Total	14.954	13			

p<0.05 S= Significant, NS= Non-significant. All abbreviations are on page so and so.

This statistical ANOVA table shows that all the values are significant, which means there is significant difference present in the values of ash content of lobster among different cooking methods and the raw state in respect to fresh condition along with different preservation methods.

Table no 5.5.4.4 Post hoc Duncan statistical analysis

Preservation	Duration	Raw state	Boiling	Dry roasting	Shallow frying	Deep frying
Control	Fresh	B,S,D^{a}	R,O,S,D^{b}	B,S,D^{a}	R,B,O,D^{c}	R,B,O,S^{d}
Control	24 hours	B,O,S,D^{e}	R,S,D^{f}	R,S,D^{f}	R,B,O,D^{c}	R,B,O,S^{d}
Control	48 hours	B,O,S,D^{e}	R,O,S,D^{b}	R,B,S,D^{g}	R,B,O,D^{c}	R,B,O,S^{d}
Control	14 days	B,O,S,D^{e}	R,O,S,D^{b}	R,B,S,D^{g}	R,B,O,D^{c}	R,B,O,S^{d}
Control	15 days	B,S,D^{a}	R,O,S,D^{b}	B,S,D^{a}	R,B,O,D^{c}	R,B,O,S^{d}
Salt & Turmeric	24 hours	B,O,S,D^{e}	R,O,S,D^{b}	R,B,S,D^{g}	R,B,O,D^{c}	R,B,O,S^{d}
Salt & Turmeric	48 hours	B,O,S,D^{e}	R,O,D^{h}	R,B,S,D^{g}	R,O,D^{h}	R,B,O,S^{d}
Salt & Turmeric	14 days	B,O,S,D^{e}	R,O,S,D^{b}	R,B,S,D^{g}	R,B,O,D^{c}	R,B,O,S^{d}
Salt & Turmeric	15 days	B,O,S,D^{e}	R,O,S,D^{b}	R,B,D^{i}	R,B,D^{i}	R,B,O,S^{d}
KMS	24 hours	B,O,S,D^{e}	R,O,S,D^{b}	R,B,S,D^{g}	R,B,O,D^{c}	R,B,O,S^{d}
KMS	48 hours	B,O,S,D^{e}	R,O,S,D^{b}	R,B,S,D^{g}	R,B,O^{j}	R,B,O^{j}
KMS	14 days	B,O,S,D^{e}	R,O,S,D^{b}	R,B,S,D^{g}	R,B,O,D^{c}	R,B,O,S^{d}
KMS	15 days	B,O,S,D^{e}	R,O,S,D^{b}	R,B,S,D^{g}	R,B,O,D^{c}	R,B,O,S^{d}

R= Raw state, B= Boiling, O= Open pan dry roasting, S= Shallow frying, D= Deep frying. The same uppercase alphabets represent that there is no significant difference present among the variables.

This table shows the significant difference among the different variables such as cooking methods and preservation conditions. The raw state significantly differs from boiling, open pan dry roasting, shallow frying and deep frying in all of the preservation conditions with preservatives and control preservation without preservative except in fresh condition and 15 days control preservation without preservative. Boiling significantly differs from the raw state, open pan dry roasting, shallow frying and deep frying in all the preservation conditions except in 24 hours control preservation without preservative and 48 hours salt and turmeric preservation. Open pan dry roasting significantly differs from the raw state, boiling, shallow frying and deep frying in all the preservation conditions except in fresh condition, 24 hours, 15 days control preservation without preservative and 15 days salt and turmeric preservation. Shallow frying significantly differs from the raw state, boiling, open pan dry roasting and deep frying in all the preservation conditions except in 48 hours, 15 days salt and turmeric preservation as well as in 48 hours KMS preservation. Deep frying significantly differs from the raw state, boiling, open pan dry roasting and shallow frying in all the preservation conditions except in 48 hours KMS preservation.

The raw state and open pan dry roasting significantly differ from boiling, shallow frying and deep frying in fresh condition and 15 days control preservation without preservative, whereas boiling and open pan dry roasting significantly differ from the raw state, shallow frying and deep frying in 24 hours control preservation without preservative. Again boiling and shallow frying significantly differ from the raw state, open pan dry roasting and deep frying in 48 hours salt and turmeric preservation. Shallow frying and open pan dry roasting significantly differ from the raw state, boiling, shallow frying and deep frying in 15 days salt and turmeric preservation. Shallow frying and deep frying significantly differ from the raw state, boiling and open pan dry roasting in 48 hours KMS preservation.

Table no 5.5.4.5 Gradation of cooking methods from higher to lower restoration with respect to preservation days

Preservation	Duration	Method 1	Method 2	Method 3	Method 4	Method 5
Control	Fresh	SF	DF	B	R	OPDR
Control	24 hours	SF	DF	R	OPDR	B
Control	48 hours	DF	SF	B	R	OPDR
Control	14 days	SF	DF	B	R	OPDR
Control	15 days	SF	DF	B	R	OPDR
Salt & Turmeric	24 hours	R	DF	SF	B	OPDR
Salt & Turmeric	48 hours	R	DF	OPDR	B	SF
Salt & Turmeric	14 days	DF	R	OPDR	SF	B
Salt &Turmeric	15 days	DF	R	SF	OPDR	B
KMS	24 hours	DF	R	OPDR	B	SF
KMS	48 hours	R	OPDR	B	DF	SF
KMS	14 days	R	DF	SF	OPDR	B
KMS	15 days	DF	R	B	OPDR	SF

R= Raw state, B= Boiling, OPDR= Open pan dry roasting, SF= Shallow frying, DF= Deep frying. Same colour represents the similar order.

In all the preservation methods and fresh condition, ash retention occurs mainly in shallow frying than the raw state and the other cooking methods. In fresh condition and 14 days and 15 days control preservation without preservative, retention occurs firstly in shallow frying followed by deep frying, boiling, raw state and open pan dry roasting. In 24 hours control preservation without preservative, retention occurs in the order of shallow frying, deep frying, raw state, open pan dry roasting and boiling. In 48 hours control preservation without preservative, the order of retention is deep frying, shallow frying, boiling, raw state and open pan dry roasting.

In 24 hours salt and turmeric preservation, retention occurs in the order of the raw state, deep frying, shallow frying, boiling and open pan dry roasting. In 48 hours salt and turmeric preservation, the order of retention becomes the raw state, deep frying, open pan dry roasting, boiling and shallow frying. In 14 days salt and turmeric preservation, the order remains deep frying, raw state, open pan dry roasting, shallow frying and boiling. In 15 days salt and turmeric preservation, the order changes from deep frying to the raw state, shallow frying, open pan dry roasting and boiling.

In 24 hours KMS preservation, retention occurs in the order of deep frying, raw state, open pan dry roasting, boiling and shallow frying. In 48 hours KMS preservation, the order is the raw state, open pan dry roasting, boiling, deep frying and shallow frying. In 14 days KMS preservation, it changes in the order of the raw state, deep frying, shallow frying, open pan dry roasting and boiling. In 15 days KMS preservation, the order of retention remains deep frying, raw state, boiling, open pan dry roasting and shallow frying.

The overall analysis of ash content of lobster is mostly restored by the gradation of methods as shallow frying>deep frying >boiling> raw state>open pan dry roasting.

Shallow frying[66] can restore ash content as the oil can possibly create a protective layer, so that the inorganic constituents cannot be leached out. Deep frying possibly causes the total dryness and inorganic constituents may get charred, leading to reduction. Boiling can reduce ash content as the inorganic constituents may get dissolved in water during cooking and discarding this water causes reduction, whereas open pan dry roasting reduces the ash content possibly due to the application of direct dry heat, so the inorganic constituents present in lobster may get charred, leading to reduction. Thus among all the studied conventional cooking methods, **shallow frying** is the best method for lobster to restore ash content.

5.5.5 Pomfret (*Pampus argenteus*)

It has been reported that pomfret contains 1.01 gm of ash per 100 gm[85] in the raw condition. This value changes due to the application of different cooking methods and preservation conditions (vide Table no **5.5.5.1**).

Table no 5.5.5.1 Ash content of Pomfret (gm/100gm)

Preservation	Duration	Raw state	Boiling	Dry roasting	Shallow frying	Deep frying
Control	Fresh	4.11±0.10	1.68±0.05	1.08±0.07	0.97±0.03	1.06±0.05
Control	24 hours	2.74±0.04	2.14±0.04	1.70±0.08	1.08±0.08	2.80±0.03
Control	48 hours	1.50±0.02	0.56±0.10	0.58±0.07	0.52±0.05	1.68±0.05
Control	14 days	2.35±0.06	2.24±0.04	1.34±0.04	1.19±0.09	1.06±0.05
Control	15 days	3.05±0.05	1.03±0.04	1.27±0.04	2.65±0.05	3.35±0.03
Salt & Turmeric	24 hours	3.06±0.05	3.18±0.08	4.39±0.07	2.08±0.08	4.70±0.05
Salt & Turmeric	48 hours	3.77±0.03	1.69±0.07	2.52±0.03	2.39±0.08	5.08±0.08
Salt & Turmeric	14 days	8.36±0.13	1.82±0.03	1.18±0.08	1.90±0.02	1.30±0.05
Salt & Turmeric	15 days	2.30±0.05	1.59±0.08	1.40±0.05	1.82±0.03	3.24±0.04
KMS	24 hours	3.98±0.08	1.99±0.07	1.78±0.03	1.18±0.02	1.80±0.01
KMS	48 hours	1.52±0.03	0.61±0.07	1.02±0.05	1.18±0.08	0.57±0.08
KMS	14 days	1.17±0.06	1.06±0.05	1.09±0.08	0.79±0.07	0.54±0.04
KMS	15 days	2.92±0.03	0.81±0.09	1.48±0.05	1.28±0.08	0.93±0.04

Values are expressed as mean±SD. ☐ Loss ☐ Restoration
Red digits represent the significant highest values from the raw state in different conditions.

In most of the conditions, ash content is mainly reduced by shallow frying, whereas in 15 days control preservation without preservative, 48 hours salt and turmeric preservation and 15 days KMS preservation, ash content is reduced by boiling. In 14 days 15 days salt and turmeric preservation, ash content is reduced by open pan dry roasting and in 14 days control preservation without preservative, 48 hours, 14 days KMS preservation ash content is reduced by deep frying.

Retention of ash content occurs by deep frying mostly, but in fresh condition, 14 days control preservation without preservative, 24 hours KMS preservation, ash retention occurs by boiling, whereas in 14 days, 15 days KMS preservation, ash retention occurs by open pan dry roasting. In 14 days salt and turmeric preservation as well as 48 hours KMS preservation, ash content is retained by shallow frying.

Boiling and open pan dry roasting show the highest ash content in 24 hours salt and turmeric preservation, whereas shallow frying and deep frying show the highest ash content in 48 hours salt and turmeric preservation. Pomfret, in raw state shows the highest ash content in fresh condition.

Boiling and open pan dry roasting show the increased ash content than the raw value in 24 hours salt and turmeric preservation, whereas deep frying shows the increased ash content than the raw value in 24 hours, 48 hours, 15 days control preservation without preservative as well as in 24 hours, 48 hours and 15 days salt and turmeric preservation.

The possible mechanism for this condition may be due to the molecular rearrangement during cooking and the addition of cooking oil during frying or may be due to the addition of both the natural and synthetic preservatives. Another possible reason may be the elimination of water during[48] cooking concentrates the minerals, thus increasing the content of ash.

Fig. 5.5.5.2 Graphical representation of Ash content of Pomfret with respect to different conditions

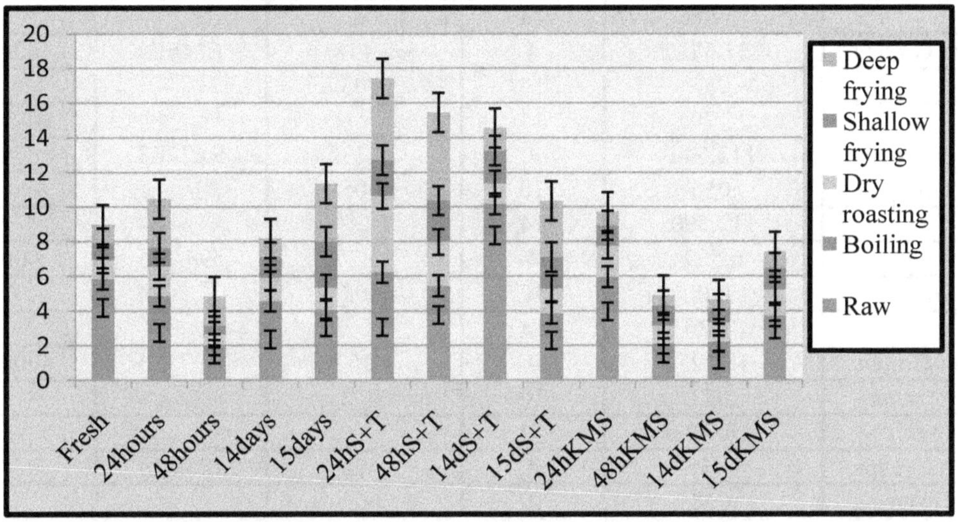

This graphical representation indicates that among all the preservation conditions, **24 hours salt and turmeric preservation** helps to increase the ash content in all the cooking methods[52]. The possible reason may be the moisture loss due to prolonged preservation. Here the graph shows that the control preservation without preservative also increases the ash content, but salt and turmeric preservation is more effective than the control preservation without preservative. KMS preservation does not have a prominent effect on the ash content of pomfret. The possible reason may be that the natural preservative helps to modify the structure of minerals, hence restoring the content.

Table no 5.5.5.3 ANOVA with regard to cooking conditions and preservation methods

Condition	Differences	Sum of Squares	df	Mean Square	F	Sig.
Fresh (control)	Between Groups	21.357	4	5.339	1.166E3	.000(S)
	Within Groups	.046	10	.005		
	Total	21.403	14			
24 hours (control)	Between Groups	5.658	4	1.415	79.262	.000(S)
	Within Groups	.178	10	.018		
	Total	5.837	14			
48 hours (control)	Between Groups	3.898	4	.974	259.627	.000(S)
	Within Groups	.038	10	.004		
	Total	3.935	14			
14 days (control)	Between Groups	4.505	4	1.126	315.745	.000(S)
	Within Groups	.036	10	.004		
	Total	4.540	14			
15 days (control)	Between Groups	13.329	4	3.332	1.991E3	.000(S)
	Within Groups	.017	10	.002		
	Total	13.345	14			
24 hours (salt & turmeric)	Between Groups	13.643	4	3.411	796.926	.000(S)
	Within Groups	.043	10	.004		
	Total	13.686	14			
48 hours (salt & turmeric)	Between Groups	21.671	4	5.418	1.566E3	.000(S)
	Within Groups	.035	10	.003		
	Total	21.705	14			
14 days (salt & turmeric)	Between Groups	112.540	4	28.135	5.627E3	.000(S)
	Within Groups	.050	10	.005		
	Total	112.590	14			
15 days (salt & turmeric)	Between Groups	6.509	4	1.627	599.746	.000(S)
	Within Groups	.027	10	.003		
	Total	6.536	14			
24 hours (KMS)	Between Groups	18.227	4	4.557	1.975E3	.000(S)
	Within Groups	.023	10	.002		
	Total	18.250	14			
48 hours (KMS)	Between Groups	1.913	4	.478	124.550	.000(S)
	Within Groups	.038	10	.004		
	Total	1.951	14			
14 days (KMS)	Between Groups	.807	4	.202	51.724	.000(S)
	Within Groups	.039	10	.004		
	Total	.846	14			
15 days (KMS)	Between Groups	8.337	4	2.084	502.471	.000(S)
	Within Groups	.037	9	.004		
	Total	8.375	13			

$p<0.05$ S= Significant, NS= Non-significant. All abbreviations are on page so and so.

This statistical ANOVA table shows that all the values are significant, which means there is significant difference present in the values of ash content of pomfret among different cooking methods and the raw state in respect to fresh condition along with different preservation methods.

Table no 5.5.5.4 Post hoc Duncan statistical analysis

Preservation	Duration	Raw state	Boiling	Dry roasting	Shallow frying	Deep frying
Control	Fresh	B,O,S,D^{a}	R,O,S,D^{b}	R,B^{c}	R,B^{c}	R,B^{c}
Control	24 hours	B,O,S^{d}	R,O,S,D^{b}	R,B,S,D^{e}	R,B,O,D^{f}	B,O,S^{d}
Control	48 hours	B,O,S,D^{a}	R,,D^{g}	R,D^{g}	R,D^{g}	R,B,O,S^{h}
Control	14 days	B,O,S,D^{a}	R,O,S,D^{b}	R,B,S,D^{e}	R,B,O,D^{f}	R,B,O,S^{h}
Control	15 days	B,O,S,D^{a}	R,O,S,D^{b}	R,B,S,D^{e}	R,B,O,D^{f}	R,B,O,S^{h}
Salt &Turmeric	24 hours	B,O,S,D^{a}	R,O,S,D^{b}	R,B,S,D^{e}	R,B,O,D^{f}	R,B,O,S^{h}
Salt & Turmeric	48 hours	B,O,S,D^{a}	R,O,S,D^{b}	R,B,S^{j}	R,B,O,D^{f}	R,B,O,S^{h}
Salt & Turmeric	14 days	B,O,S,D^{a}	R,O,D^{i}	R,B,S,D^{e}	R,O,D^{i}	R,B,S^{j}
Salt & Turmeric	15 days	B,O,S,D^{a}	R,O,S,D^{b}	R,B,S,D^{e}	R,B,O,D^{f}	R,B,O,S^{h}
KMS	24 hours	B,O,S,D^{a}	R,O,S,D^{b}	R,B,S,D^{e}	R,B,O,D^{f}	R,B,O,S^{h}
KMS	48 hours	B,O,S,D^{a}	R,O,S^{k}	R,B,S,D^{e}	R,B,O,D^{f}	R,O,S^{k}
KMS	14 days	S,D^{l}	S,D^{l}	S,D^{l}	R,B,O,D^{f}	R,B,O,S^{h}
KMS	15 days	B,O,S,D^{a}	R,O,S^{k}	R,B,S,D^{e}	R,B,O,D^{f}	R,O,S^{k}

R= Raw state, B= Boiling, O= Open pan dry roasting, S= Shallow frying, D= Deep frying. The same uppercase alphabets represent that there is no significant difference present among the variables.

This table shows the significant difference among the different variables such as cooking methods and preservation conditions. The raw state significantly differs from boiling, open pan dry roasting, shallow frying and deep frying in all of the preservation conditions with preservatives and control preservation without preservative except in 24 hours control preservation and 14 days KMS preservation. Boiling significantly differs from the raw state, open pan dry roasting, shallow frying and deep frying in all the preservation conditions except in 48 hours control preservation without preservative and 14 days salt and turmeric preservation and 48 hours, 14 days, 15 days KMS preservation. Open pan dry roasting significantly differs from the raw state, boiling, shallow frying and deep frying in all the preservation conditions except in fresh condition, 48 hours control preservation without preservative and 48 hours salt and turmeric preservation and 14 days KMS preservation. Shallow frying significantly differs from the raw state, boiling, open pan dry roasting and deep frying in all the preservation conditions except in fresh condition, 48 hours control preservation without preservative and 14 days salt and turmeric preservation. Deep frying significantly differs from the raw state, boiling, open pan dry roasting and shallow frying in all the preservation conditions except in fresh condition, 24 hours control preservation without preservative, 14 days salt and turmeric preservation as well as 48 hours, 15 days KMS preservation.

Open pan dry roasting, shallow frying and deep frying significantly differ from the raw state and boiling in fresh condition, whereas the raw state and deep frying significantly differ from boiling, open pan dry roasting and shallow frying in 24 hours control preservation without preservative. Again boiling, open pan dry roasting and shallow frying significantly differ from the raw state and deep frying in 48 hours control preservation without preservative. Boiling and shallow frying significantly differ from the raw state, open pan dry roasting and deep frying in 14 days salt and turmeric preservation. Boiling and deep frying significantly differ from the raw state, open pan dry roasting and shallow frying in 48 hours, 15 days KMS preservation. The raw state, boiling and open pan dry roasting significantly differ from shallow frying and deep frying in 14 days KMS preservation. Open pan dry roasting and deep frying significantly differ from the raw state, boiling and shallow frying in 48 hours and 14 days salt and turmeric preservation respectively.

Table no 5.5.5.5 Gradation of cooking methods from higher to lower restoration with respect to preservation days

Preservation	Duration	Method 1	Method 2	Method 3	Method 4	Method 5
Control	Fresh	R	B	OPDR	DF	SF
Control	24 hours	R	DF	B	OPDR	SF
Control	48 hours	DF	R	OPDR	B	SF
Control	14 days	R	B	OPDR	SF	DF
Control	15 days	DF	R	SF	OPDR	B
Salt & Turmeric	24 hours	DF	OPDR	B	R	SF
Salt & Turmeric	48 hours	DF	R	OPDR	SF	B
Salt & Turmeric	14 days	R	SF	B	DF	OPDR
Salt &Turmeric	15 days	DF	R	SF	B	OPDR
KMS	24 hours	R	B	OPDR	SF	DF
KMS	48 hours	R	SF	OPDR	B	DF
KMS	14 days	R	OPDR	B	SF	DF
KMS	15 days	R	OPDR	SF	DF	B

R= Raw state, B= Boiling, OPDR= Open pan dry roasting, SF= Shallow frying, DF= Deep frying. Same colour represents the similar order.

In all the preservation methods and fresh condition, ash retention occurs mainly in the raw state than the other cooking methods. In fresh condition, retention occurs firstly in the raw state followed by boiling, open pan dry roasting, deep frying and shallow frying. In 24 hours control preservation without preservative, the order of retention is the raw state, deep frying, boiling, open pan dry roasting and shallow frying. In 48 hours control preservation without preservative, the order is deep frying, raw state, open pan dry roasting, boiling and shallow frying. In 14 days control preservation without preservative and 24 hours KMS preservation, the order of retention becomes the raw state, boiling, open pan dry roasting, shallow frying and deep frying. In 15 days control preservation without preservative, the order remains deep frying, raw state, shallow frying, open pan dry roasting and boiling.

In 24 hours salt and turmeric preservation, the order of retention is deep frying, open pan dry roasting, boiling, raw state and shallow frying. In 48 hours salt and turmeric preservation, the order is deep frying, raw state, open pan dry roasting, shallow frying and boiling. In 14 days salt and turmeric preservation, the order remains the raw state followed by shallow frying, boiling, deep frying and open pan dry roasting. In 15 days salt and turmeric preservation, it changes in the order of deep frying, raw state, shallow frying, boiling and open pan dry roasting.

In 48 hours KMS preservation, retention occurs firstly in the raw state followed by shallow frying, open pan dry roasting, boiling and deep frying. In 14 days KMS preservation, the order becomes the raw state followed by open pan dry roasting, boiling, shallow frying and deep frying. In 15 days KMS preservation, the order of retention changes from the raw state to open pan dry roasting, shallow frying, deep frying and boiling.

The overall analysis of ash content of pomfret is mostly restored by the gradation of methods as the raw state>boiling>open pan dry roasting> shallow frying> deep frying.

Boiling can restore ash content as the inorganic constituents cannot be dissolved in water during cooking due to the high fat content of pomfret. Fatty tissues can possibly protect the inorganic constituents by creating a barrier that prevent the elimination of minerals in cooking water[50] and thus discarding the cooking water cannot reduce the ash content, whereas open pan dry roasting reduces the ash content due to the application of direct dry heat. As a result the inorganic constituents may get charred, leading to reduction. Shallow frying can reduce the inorganic constituents as the application of heat probably melts the protective covering of fatty layer. Deep frying probably causes the total dryness, reducing the inorganic constituents. Thus among all the studied conventional cooking methods, **boiling** is the best method for pomfret to restore ash content.

5.5.6 *Hilsa* (*Tenualosa Ilisha*)

It has been reported that *hilsa* contains 1.1 gm of ash per 100 gm[85] in the raw condition. This value changes due to the application of different cooking methods and preservation conditions (vide Table no **5.5.6.1**).

Table no 5.5.6.1 Ash content of *Hilsa* (gm/100gm)

Preservation	Duration	Raw state	Boiling	Dry roasting	Shallow frying	Deep frying
Control	Fresh	2.07±0.06	1.08±0.08	1.49±0.07	1.10±0.10	3.69±0.07
Control	24 hours	2.75±0.05	0.53±0.04	0.52±0.03	0.65±0.04	0.59±0.08
Control	48 hours	2.83±0.05	2.42±0.03	1.46±0.04	1.65±0.03	2.34±0.04
Control	14 days	0.59±0.08	0.48±0.05	1.35±0.04	0.72±0.03	6.32±0.03
Control	15 days	1.25±0.08	0.60±0.10	0.34±0.03	0.34±0.02	0.93±0.04
Salt & Turmeric	24 hours	2.67±0.05	1.09±0.08	1.47±0.06	2.81±0.08	1.47±0.06
Salt & Turmeric	48 hours	3.44±0.05	2.04±0.04	1.91±0.04	1.46±0.05	1.96±0.04
Salt & Turmeric	14 days	3.94±0.04	3.81±0.03	2.44±0.03	1.97±0.03	2.31±0.10
Salt & Turmeric	15 days	3.36±0.06	2.75±0.03	1.78±0.08	2.43±0.04	2.66±0.06
KMS	24 hours	2.69±0.07	1.44±0.07	1.85±0.03	1.55±0.03	1.78±0.04
KMS	48 hours	3.08±0.08	1.06±0.05	1.36±0.05	2.06±0.05	2.32±0.06
KMS	14days	0.58±0.08	0.57±0.04	0.39±0.08	0.47±0.03	0.30±0.07
KMS	15 days	1.25±0.03	1.00±0.10	1.26±0.04	1.12±0.03	1.35±0.03

Values are expressed as mean±SD. ☐ Loss ☐ Restoration

Red digits represent the significant highest values from the raw state in different conditions.

In most of the conditions, ash content is mainly reduced by boiling, [38] whereas in 24 hours, 48 hours control preservation without preservative, 15 days salt and turmeric preservation ash content is reduced by open pan dry roasting. In 15 days control preservation without preservative, 48 hours, 14 days salt and turmeric preservation and 24 hours KMS preservation, ash content is reduced by shallow frying and 14 days KMS preservation, ash content is reduced by deep frying.

Retention of ash content occurs by deep frying mostly, but in 48 hours, 14 days, 15 days salt and turmeric preservation as well as 14 days KMS preservation, ash retention occurs by boiling, whereas in 24 hours salt and turmeric preservation as well as KMS preservation, ash retention occurs by shallow frying.

The raw state, boiling and open pan dry roasting show the highest ash content in 14 days salt and turmeric preservation, whereas shallow frying and deep frying show the highest ash content in 24 hours salt and turmeric preservation and 14 days control preservation without preservative.

Open pan dry roasting shows the increased ash content than the raw value in 14 days control preservation without preservative and 15 days KMS preservation, whereas shallow frying shows the increased ash content than the raw state in 24 hours salt and turmeric preservation. Deep frying shows the increased ash content than the raw value in fresh condition, 14 days control preservation without preservative and 15 days KMS preservation.

This happens may be due to the molecular rearrangement during cooking and the addition of cooking oil during frying or may be due to the addition of the natural and synthetic preservatives. Another possible reason may be the elimination of water during cooking[48] concentrates the inorganic constituents, hence increasing the content of ash.

Fig. 5.5.6.2 Graphical representation of Ash content of *Hilsa* with respect to different conditions

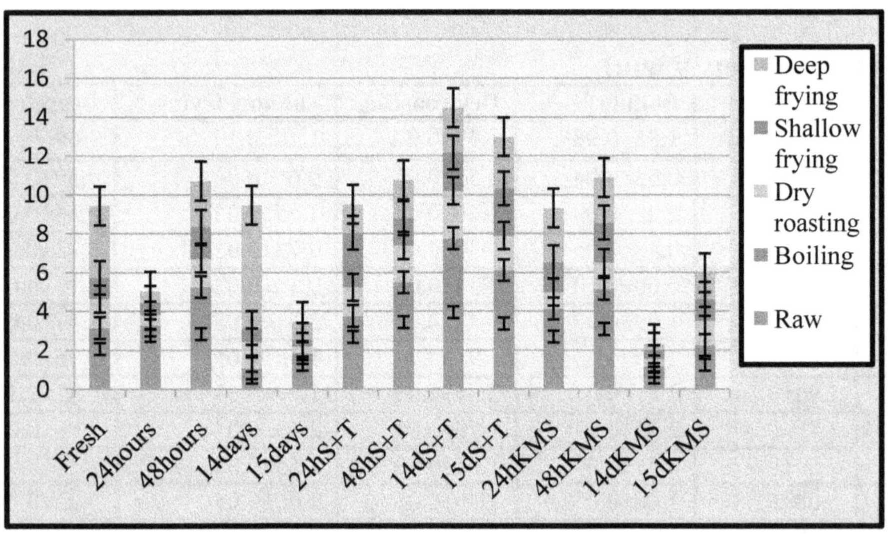

This graphical representation indicates that among all the preservation conditions, **14 days salt and turmeric preservation**[55] helps to increase the ash content in all the cooking methods[52]. The possible reason may be the moisture loss for prolonged preservation. Here the graph shows that the control preservation without preservative and KMS also increase the ash content, but salt and turmeric preservation is more effective than that which is control preservation without preservative and KMS preservation. The natural preservative possibly helps to modify the structure of minerals, causing restoration of the content.

Table no 5.5.6.3 ANOVA with regard to cooking conditions and preservation methods

Condition	Differences	Sum of Squares	df	Mean Square	F	Sig.
Fresh (control)	Between Groups	14.121	4	3.530	627.435	.000(S)
	Within Groups	.056	10	.006		
	Total	14.178	14			
24 hours (control)	Between Groups	11.379	4	2.845	1.111E3	.000(S)
	Within Groups	.026	10	.003		
	Total	11.404	14			
48 hours (control)	Between Groups	3.911	4	.978	643.206	.000(S)
	Within Groups	.015	10	.002		
	Total	3.926	14			
14 days (control)	Between Groups	74.908	4	18.727	7.412E3	.000(S)
	Within Groups	.025	10	.003		
	Total	74.933	14			
15 days (control)	Between Groups	1.889	4	.472	119.073	.000(S)
	Within Groups	.040	10	.004		
	Total	1.929	14			
24 hours (salt & turmeric)	Between Groups	7.453	4	1.863	356.924	.000(S)
	Within Groups	.052	10	.005		
	Total	7.505	14			
48 hours (salt & turmeric)	Between Groups	6.988	4	1.747	876.360	.000(S)
	Within Groups	.020	10	.002		
	Total	7.007	14			
14 days (salt & turmeric)	Between Groups	9.917	4	2.479	2.282E3	.000(S)
	Within Groups	.011	10	.001		
	Total	9.928	14			
15 days (salt & turmeric)	Between Groups	3.928	4	.982	308.185	.000(S)
	Within Groups	.032	10	.003		
	Total	3.960	14			
24 hours (KMS)	Between Groups	8.485	4	2.121	924.988	.000(S)
	Within Groups	.023	10	.002		
	Total	8.508	14			
48 hours (KMS)	Between Groups	4.591	4	1.148	329.823	.000(S)
	Within Groups	.035	10	.003		
	Total	4.626	14			
14 days (KMS)	Between Groups	.166	4	.041	10.750	.001(S)
	Within Groups	.039	10	.004		
	Total	.205	14			
15 days (KMS)	Between Groups	.188	4	.047	15.742	.000(S)
	Within Groups	.027	9	.003		
	Total	.215	13			

$p<0.05$ S= Significant, NS= Non-significant. All abbreviations are on page so and so.

This statistical ANOVA table shows that all the values are significant, which means there is significant difference present in the values of ash content of *hilsa* among different cooking methods and the raw state in respect to fresh condition along with different preservation methods.

Table no 5.5.6.4 Post hoc Duncan statistical analysis

Preservation	Duration	Raw state	Boiling	Dry roasting	Shallow frying	Deep frying
Control	Fresh	B,O,S,D^{a}	R,O,D^{b}	R,B,S,D^{c}	R,O,D^{b}	R,B,O,S^{d}
Control	24 hours	B,O,S,D^{a}	R,S^{e}	R,S^{e}	R,B,O^{f}	R^{g}
Control	48 hours	B,O,S,D^{a}	R,O,S,D^{h}	R,B,S,D^{c}	R,B,O,D^{i}	R,B,O,S^{d}
Control	14 days	B,O,S,D^{a}	R,O,S,D^{h}	R,B,S,D^{c}	R,B,O,D^{i}	R,B,O,S^{d}
Control	15 days	B,O,S,D^{a}	R,O,S,D^{h}	R,B,D^{j}	R,B,D^{j}	R,B,O,S^{d}
Salt & Turmeric	24 hours	B,O,S,D^{a}	R,O,S,D^{h}	R,B,S^{k}	B,O,D^{l}	R,B,S^{k}
Salt & Turmeric	48 hours	B,O,S,D^{a}	R,O,S^{m}	R,B,S^{k}	R,B,O,D^{i}	R,S^{e}
Salt & Turmeric	14 days	B,O,S,D^{a}	R,O,S,D^{h}	R,B,S,D^{c}	R,B,O,D^{i}	R,B,O,S^{d}
Salt & Turmeric	15 days	B,O,S,D^{a}	R,O,S^{m}	R,B,S,D^{c}	R,B,O,D^{i}	RO,S^{m}
KMS	24 hours	B,O,S,D^{a}	R,O,S,D^{h}	R,B,S,D^{c}	R,B,O,D^{i}	R,B,O,S^{d}
KMS	48 hours	B,O,S,D^{a}	R,O,D^{b}	R,B,S,D^{c}	R,O,D^{b}	R,B,O,S^{d}
KMS	14 days	O,D^{n}	O,D^{n}	R,B^{o}	R,B,D^{j}	R,B,S^{k}
KMS	15 days	B,S^{p}	R,O,S,D^{h}	B,S^{p}	R,B,O,D^{i}	B,S^{p}

R= Raw state, B= Boiling, O= Open pan dry roasting, S= Shallow frying, D= Deep frying. The same uppercase alphabets signify that there is no significant difference present among the variables.

This table shows the significant difference among the different variables such as cooking methods and preservation conditions. The raw state significantly differs from boiling, open pan dry roasting, shallow frying and deep frying in all of the preservation conditions with preservatives and control preservation without preservative except in 14 days and 15 days KMS preservation. Boiling significantly differs from the raw state, open pan dry roasting, shallow frying and deep frying in all the preservation conditions except in fresh condition, 24 hours control preservation without preservative and 48 hours, 15 days salt and turmeric preservation and 48 hours, 14 days KMS preservation. Open pan dry roasting significantly differs from the raw state, boiling, shallow frying and deep frying in all the preservation conditions except in 24 hours, 15 days control preservation without preservative and 24 hours, 48 hours salt and turmeric preservation and 14 days, 15 days KMS preservation. Shallow frying significantly differs from the raw state, boiling, open pan dry roasting and deep frying in all the preservation conditions except in 24 hours, 15 days control preservation without preservative and 24 hours, 48 hours salt and turmeric preservation and 48 hours, 14 days KMS preservation. Deep frying significantly differs from the raw state, boiling, open pan dry roasting and shallow frying in all the preservation conditions except in 24 hours control preservation without preservative, 24 hours, 48 hours, 15 days salt and turmeric preservation as well as 14 days, 15 days KMS preservation.

Boiling and shallow frying significantly differ from the raw state, open pan dry roasting and deep frying in fresh condition and 48 hours KMS preservation, whereas boiling and open pan dry roasting significantly differ from the raw state and shallow frying in 24 hours control preservation without preservative, and only deep frying significantly differs from the raw state and shallow frying in 48 hours salt and turmeric preservation. Again open pan dry roasting and shallow frying significantly differ from the raw state, boiling and deep frying in 15 days control preservation without preservative. Open pan dry roasting significantly differs from the raw state, boiling and shallow frying in 24 hours, 48 hours salt and turmeric preservation, and only deep frying significantly differs from the raw state, boiling and shallow frying in 24 hours salt and turmeric preservation and 14 days KMS preservation. Boiling significantly differs from the raw state, open pan dry roasting and shallow frying in 48 hours, 15 days salt and turmeric preservation, and only deep frying significantly differs from the raw state, open pan dry roasting and shallow frying in 15 days salt and turmeric preservation. The raw state and boiling significantly differ from open pan dry roasting and deep frying in 14 days KMS preservation. Open pan dry roasting, raw state and deep frying significantly differ from boiling and shallow frying in 15 days KMS preservation. Deep frying significantly differs from the raw state in 24 hours control preservation without preservative.

Table no 5.5.6.5 Gradation of cooking methods from higher to lower with respect to preservation days

Preservation	Duration	Method 1	Method 2	Method 3	Method 4	Method 5
Control	Fresh	DF	R	OPDR	SF	B
Control	24 hours	R	SF	DF	B	OPDR
Control	48 hours	R	B	DF	SF	OPDR
Control	14 days	DF	OPDR	SF	R	B
Control	15 days	R	DF	B	OPDR	SF
Salt & Turmeric	24 hours	SF	R	DF	OPDR	B
Salt & Turmeric	48 hours	R	B	DF	OPDR	SF
Salt & Turmeric	14 days	R	B	OPDR	DF	SF
Salt &Turmeric	15 days	R	B	DF	SF	OPDR
KMS	24 hours	DF	R	SF	B	OPDR
KMS	48 hours	R	DF	SF	B	OPDR
KMS	14 days	R	B	SF	OPDR	DF
KMS	15 days	DF	OPDR	R	SF	B

R= Raw state, B= Boiling, OPDR= open pan dry roasting, SF= Shallow frying, DF= Deep frying. Same colour represents the similar order.

In all the preservation methods and fresh condition, ash retention occurs mainly in the raw state than the other cooking methods. In fresh condition, retention occurs firstly in deep frying followed by the raw state, open pan dry roasting, shallow frying and boiling. In 24 hours control preservation without preservative, retention occurs in the order of the raw state then shallow frying, deep frying, boiling and open pan dry roasting. In 48 hours control preservation without preservative and 15 days salt and turmeric preservation, retention occurs in the following order: the raw state, boiling, deep frying, shallow frying and open pan dry roasting. In 14 days control preservation without preservative, it changes from deep frying to open pan dry roasting, shallow frying, raw state and boiling. In 15 days control preservation without preservative, the order is the raw state, deep frying, boiling, open pan dry roasting and shallow frying.

In 24 hours salt and turmeric preservation, retention occurs firstly in shallow frying followed by the raw state, deep frying, open pan dry roasting and boiling. In 48 hours salt and turmeric preservation, the order becomes the raw state followed by boiling, deep frying, open pan dry roasting and shallow frying. In 14 days salt and turmeric preservation, the order is the raw state, boiling, open pan dry roasting, deep frying and shallow frying.

In 24 hours KMS preservation, retention occurs firstly in deep frying followed by the raw state, shallow frying, boiling, open pan dry roasting and boiling. In 48 hours KMS preservation, the order becomes the raw state, deep frying, shallow frying, boiling and open pan dry roasting. In 14 days KMS preservation, the order changes from the raw state to boiling, shallow frying, open pan dry roasting and deep frying. In 15 days KMS preservation, the order becomes deep frying, open pan dry roasting, raw state, shallow frying and boiling.

The overall analysis of ash content of *hilsa* is mostly restored by the gradation of methods as the raw state>boiling>deep frying> shallow frying>open pan dry roasting.

Boiling can restore ash content as the inorganic constituents cannot be dissolved in water during cooking due to the high fat content of *hilsa*. Fatty tissues can possibly protect the inorganic constituents by creating a barrier that prevents the elimination of minerals in cooking water[50] and thus discarding the cooking water reduces the ash content to some extent, whereas deep frying probably causes the total dryness, reducing the inorganic constituents. Shallow frying can reduce the inorganic constituents as the application of heat probably melts the protective covering of fatty layer. Open pan dry roasting reduces the ash content due to the application of direct dry heat so that the inorganic constituents may get charred, resulting in the reduction. Thus among all the studied conventional cooking methods, **boiling** is the best method for *hilsa* to restore ash content.

5.6 Iron content

It has been reported that generally fish contains 0.2-2.3mg of iron[86] in the raw state. This experiment is carried out to estimate the iron content along with the changes of it in different cooking and preservation methods among different fish and edible aquatic species. Iron content is estimated by AOAC method[71].

5.6.1 *Rohu* (*Labeo rohita*)

It has been reported that *rohu* contains 1.04 mg of iron per 100 gm[85] in the raw condition. This value changes due to the application of different cooking methods and preservation conditions (vide Table no **5.6.1.1**)

Table no 5.6.1.1 Iron content of *Rohu* (mg/100gm)

Preservation	Duration	Raw state	Boiling	Dry roasting	Shallow frying	Deep frying
Control	Fresh	2.71±0.03	3.15±0.06	1.67±0.02	1.49±0.03	7.05±0.04
Control	24 hours	0.37±0.02	1.08±0.03	2.04±0.03	2.43±0.08	1.05±0.05
Control	48 hours	1.39±0.06	0.94±0.04	0.61±0.08	3.92±00.02	4.79±0.07
Control	14 days	1.41±0.06	1.97±0.02	1.86±0.01	4.94±0.06	1.49±0.03
Control	15 days	2.79±0.06	1.52±0.02	1.75±0.04	1.58±0.07	1.72±0.02
Salt & Turmeric	24 hours	1.12±0.02	0.37±0.02	0.72±0.02	0.77±0.02	1.27±0.02
Salt & Turmeric	48 hours	2.72±0.02	2.17±0.01	4.54±0.04	3.52±0.02	2.14±0.04
Salt & Turmeric	14 days	0.82±0.02	1.92±0.02	2.04±0.04	1.81±0.01	2.32±0.02
Salt & Turmeric	15 days	1.82±0.02	1.61±0.01	1.72±0.02	1.62±0.02	2.11±0.01
KMS	24 hours	1.75±0.04	2.54±0.04	2.57±0.01	2.43±0.04	2.02±0.02
KMS	48 hours	1.21±0.06	1.25±0.03	1.14±0.04	0.72±0.02	1.34±0.04
KMS	14 days	0.77±0.02	0.54±0.04	1.47±0.02	0.54±0.04	1.03±0.04
KMS	15 days	4.04±0.04	1.24±0.04	1.34±0.04	2.23±0.04	1.62±0.02

Values are expressed as mean±SD. Loss Restoration

Red digits represent the significant highest values from the raw state in different conditions.

In most of the conditions, iron content is mainly reduced by boiling, whereas in fresh condition, 14 days salt and turmeric preservation without preservative, 48 hours, 14 days KMS preservation, iron content is reduced by shallow frying. In 24 hours, 14 days control preservation without preservative, 48 hours salt and turmeric preservation and 24 hours KMS preservation, iron content is reduced by deep frying.

Retention of iron content occurs by deep frying[66] mostly, but in 24 hours, 14 days KMS preservation, iron retention occurs by open pan dry roasting, whereas in 24 hours, 14 days control preservation without preservative, 48 hours salt and turmeric preservation as well as 15 days KMS preservation, iron retention occurs by shallow frying.

Boiling and deep frying show the highest iron content in fresh condition, whereas shallow frying and open pan dry roasting show the highest iron content in 14 days control preservation without preservative and 48 hours salt and turmeric preservation respectively. The raw state shows the highest iron content in 15 days KMS preservation.

Boiling shows the increased iron content than the raw value in fresh condition, 24 hours, 14 days control preservation without preservative, 14 days salt and turmeric preservation and 24 hours, 48 hours KMS preservation. Open pan dry roasting shows the increased iron content than the raw state in fresh condition, 24 hours, 14 days control preservation without preservative, 48 hours, 14 days salt and turmeric preservation and 24 hours, 14 days KMS preservation, whereas shallow frying shows the increased iron content than the raw state in 24 hours, 48 hours, 14 days control preservation without preservative, 48 hours, 14 days salt and turmeric preservation and 24 hours KMS preservation. Deep frying shows the increased iron content than the raw value in fresh condition, 24 hours, 48 hours, 14 days control preservation without preservative, 14 days, 15 days salt and turmeric preservation and 24 hours, 48 hours, 14 days KMS preservation.

This happens may be due to the molecular rearrangement during cooking and the addition of cooking oil during frying or may be due to the addition of the natural and synthetic preservatives. Another possible reason may be the elimination of water during cooking[48] that concentrates the inorganic constituents, thus increasing the content of iron. Another possible reason for increasing the iron content is due to the use of iron pan for cooking, that leads to iron absorption by the fish, and thus the content is increased.

Fig. 5.6.1.2 Graphical representation of Iron content of *Rohu* with respect to different conditions

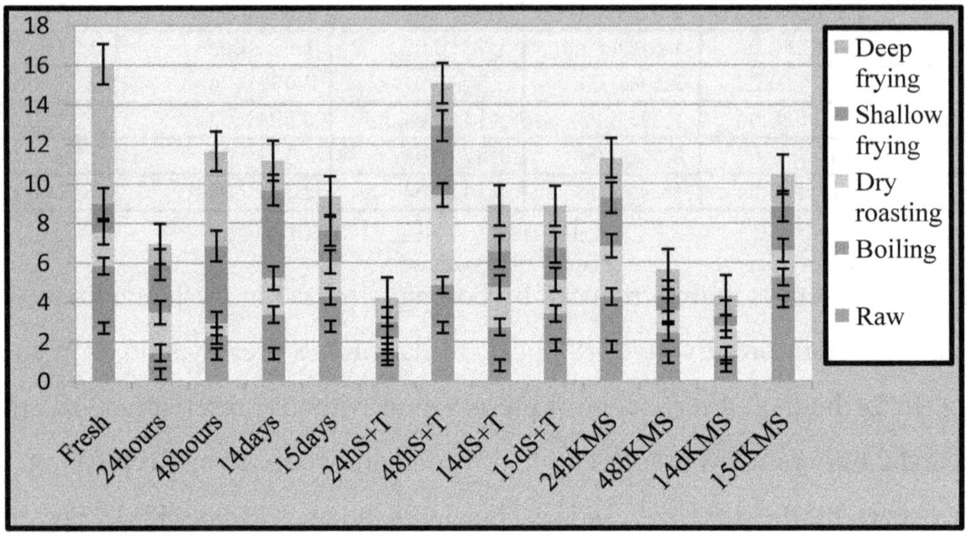

This graphical representation indicates that among all the preservation conditions, **fresh condition** helps to increase the iron content in all the cooking methods. The possible reason may be that the preservation can hamper the iron content as it is a very vulnerable mineral. Here the graph shows that the control preservation without preservative and both salt-turmeric and KMS preservation also increase the iron content but preservatives are not so effective here.

Table no 5.6.1.3 ANOVA with regard to cooking conditions and preservation methods

Condition	Differences	Sum of Squares	df	Mean Square	F	Sig.
Fresh (control)	Between Groups	61.087	4	15.272	9.274E3	.000(S)
	Within Groups	.016	10	.002		
	Total	61.104	14			
24 hours (control)	Between Groups	8.463	4	2.116	1.339E3	.000(S)
	Within Groups	.016	10	.002		
	Total	8.479	14			
48 hours (control)	Between Groups	42.997	4	10.749	2.674E3	.000(S)
	Within Groups	.040	10	.004		
	Total	43.037	14			
14 days (control)	Between Groups	18.691	4	4.673	2.239E3	.000(S)
	Within Groups	.021	10	.002		
	Total	18.712	14			
15 days (control)	Between Groups	3.249	4	.812	311.596	.000(S)
	Within Groups	.026	10	.003		
	Total	3.275	14			
24 hours (salt & turmeric)	Between Groups	1.506	4	.377	594.568	.000(S)
	Within Groups	.006	10	.001		
	Total	1.513	14			
48 hours (salt & turmeric)	Between Groups	12.459	4	3.115	3.222E3	.000(S)
	Within Groups	.010	10	.001		
	Total	12.468	14			
14 days (salt & turmeric)	Between Groups	3.904	4	.976	1.331E3	.000(S)
	Within Groups	.007	10	.001		
	Total	3.911	14			
15 days (salt & turmeric)	Between Groups	2.175	4	.544	1.359E3	.000(S)
	Within Groups	.004	10	.000		
	Total	2.179	14			
24 hours (KMS)	Between Groups	1.567	4	.392	304.560	.000(S)
	Within Groups	.013	10	.001		
	Total	1.580	14			
48 hours (KMS)	Between Groups	.698	4	.174	88.717	.000(S)
	Within Groups	.020	10	.002		
	Total	.718	14			
14 days (KMS)	Between Groups	1.850	4	.463	331.981	.000(S)
	Within Groups	.014	10	.001		
	Total	1.864	14			
15 days (KMS)	Between Groups	15.984	4	3.996	2.750E3	.000(S)
	Within Groups	.015	10	.001		
	Total	15.998	14			

$p<0.05$ S= Significant, NS= Non-significant. All abbreviations are on page so and so.

This statistical ANOVA table shows that all the values are significant, which means there is significant difference present in the values of iron content of *rohu* among different cooking methods and the raw state in respect to fresh condition along with different preservation methods.

Table no 5.6.1.4 Post hoc Duncan statistical analysis

Preservation	Duration	Raw state	Boiling	Dry roasting	Shallow frying	Deep frying
Control	Fresh	B,O,S,D^{a}	R,O,S,D^{b}	R,B,S,D^{c}	R,B,O,D^{d}	R,B,O,S^{e}
Control	24 hours	B,O,S,D^{a}	R,O,S^{f}	R,B,S,D^{c}	R,B,O,D^{d}	R,O,S^{f}
Control	48 hours	B,O,S,D^{a}	R,O,S,D^{b}	R,B,S,D^{c}	R,B,O,D^{d}	R,B,O,S^{e}
Control	14 days	B,O,S^{g}	R,O,S,D^{b}	R,B,S,D^{c}	R,B,O,D^{d}	B,O,S^{g}
Control	15 days	B,O,S,D^{a}	R,O,D^{h}	R,B,S^{i}	R,O,D^{h}	R,B,S^{i}
Salt &Turmeric	24 hours	B,O,S,D^{a}	R,O,S,D^{b}	R,B,S,D^{c}	R,B,O,D^{d}	R,B,O,S^{e}
Salt & Turmeric	48 hours	B,O,S,D^{a}	R,O,S^{f}	R,B,S,D^{c}	R,B,O,D^{d}	R,O,S^{f}
Salt & Turmeric	14 days	B,O,S,D^{a}	R,O,S,D^{b}	R,B,S,D^{c}	R,B,O,D^{d}	R,B,O,S^{e}
Salt & Turmeric	15 days	B,O,S,D^{a}	R,O,D^{h}	R,B,S,D^{c}	R,O,D^{h}	R,B,O,S^{e}
KMS	24 hours	B,O,S,D^{a}	R,S,D^{j}	R,S,D^{j}	R,B,O,D^{d}	R,B,O,S^{e}
KMS	48 hours	B,O,S,D^{a}	O,S,D^{l}	B,S,D^{m}	R,B,O,D^{d}	R,B,O,S^{e}
KMS	14 days	S,D^{K}	R,O,D^{h}	R,B,S,D^{c}	R,O,D^{h}	R,B,O,S^{e}
KMS	15 days	B,O,S,D^{a}	R,O,S,D^{b}	R,B,S,D^{c}	R,B,O,D^{d}	R,B,O,S^{e}

R= Raw state, B= Boiling, O= Open pan dry roasting, S= Shallow frying, D= Deep frying. The same uppercase alphabets represent that there is no significant difference present among the variables.

This table shows the significant difference among the different variables such as cooking methods and preservation conditions. The raw state significantly differs from boiling, open pan dry roasting, shallow frying and deep frying in all of the preservation conditions with preservatives and control preservation without preservative except in 14 days control preservation and 14 days KMS preservation. Boiling significantly differs from the raw state, open pan dry roasting, shallow frying and deep frying in all the preservation conditions except in 24 hours, 15 days control preservation without preservative and 48 hours, 15 days salt and turmeric preservation and 24 hours, 48 hours, 14 days KMS preservation. Open pan dry roasting significantly differs from the raw state, boiling, shallow frying and deep frying in all the preservation conditions except in 15 days control preservation without preservative and 24 hours, 48 hours KMS preservation. Shallow frying significantly differs from the raw state, boiling, open pan dry roasting and deep frying in all the preservation conditions except in 15 days control preservation without preservative and 15 days salt and turmeric preservation and 14 days KMS preservation. Deep frying significantly differs from the raw state, boiling, open pan dry roasting and shallow frying in all the preservation conditions except in 24 hours, 14 days, 15 days control preservation without preservative, 48 hours salt and turmeric preservation.

Boiling and deep frying significantly differ from the raw state, open pan dry roasting and shallow frying in 24 hours control preservation without preservative and 48 hours salt and turmeric preservation, whereas the raw state and deep frying significantly differ from boiling, open pan dry roasting and shallow frying in 14 days control preservation without preservative. Boiling and shallow frying significantly differ from the raw state, open pan dry roasting and deep frying in 15 days control preservation without preservative, 15 days salt and turmeric preservation and 14 days KMS preservation. Again both open pan dry roasting and deep frying significantly differ from the raw state, boiling and shallow frying in 15 days control preservation without preservative. Open pan dry roasting and boiling significantly differ from the raw state, shallow frying and deep frying in 24 hours KMS preservation. Boiling significantly differs from open pan dry roasting, shallow frying and deep frying in 48 hours KMS preservation. Open pan dry roasting significantly differs from boiling, shallow frying and deep frying in 48 hours KMS preservation. The raw state significantly differs from shallow frying and deep frying in 14 days KMS preservation.

Table no 5.6.1.5 Gradation of cooking methods from higher to lower restoration with respect to preservation days

Preservation	Duration	Method 1	Method 2	Method 3	Method 4	Method 5
Control	Fresh	DF	B	R	OPDR	SF
Control	24 hours	SF	OPDR	B	DF	R
Control	48 hours	DF	SF	R	B	OPDR
Control	14 days	SF	B	OPDR	DF	R
Control	15 days	R	OPDR	DF	SF	B
Salt &Turmeric	24 hours	DF	R	SF	OPDR	B
Salt & Turmeric	48 hours	OPDR	SF	R	B	DF
Salt & Turmeric	14 days	DF	OPDR	B	SF	R
Salt &Turmeric	15 days	SF	B	DF	R	OPDR
KMS	24 hours	OPDR	B	SF	DF	R
KMS	48 hours	DF	B	R	OPDR	SF
KMS	14 days	OPDR	DF	R	SF	B
KMS	15 days	R	SF	DF	OPDR	B

R= Raw state, B= Boiling, OPDR= Open pan dry roasting, SF= Shallow frying, DF= Deep frying. Same colour represents the similar order.

In all the preservation methods and fresh condition, iron retention occurs mainly by deep frying than the other cooking methods. In fresh condition and 48 hours KMS preservation, retention occurs firstly in deep frying then boiling, raw state, open pan dry roasting and shallow frying. In 24 hours control preservation without preservative, retention occurs in the order of shallow frying, open pan dry roasting, boiling, deep frying and the raw state. In 48 hours control preservation without preservative, the order is deep frying, shallow frying, raw state, boiling and open pan dry roasting. In 14 days control preservation without preservative, the order remains shallow frying, boiling, open pan dry roasting, deep frying and the raw state. In 15 days control preservation without preservative, the order is the raw state, open pan dry roasting, deep frying, shallow frying and boiling.

In 24 hours salt and turmeric preservation, retention occurs firstly in deep frying followed by the raw state, shallow frying, open pan dry roasting and boiling. In 48 hours salt and turmeric preservation, the order is open pan dry roasting, shallow frying, raw state, boiling and deep frying. In 14 days salt and turmeric preservation, it changes in the order of deep frying, open pan dry roasting, boiling, shallow frying and the raw state. In 15 days salt and turmeric preservation, the order becomes shallow frying, boiling, deep frying, raw state and open pan dry roasting.

In 24 hours KMS preservation, retention occurs firstly in open pan dry roasting followed by boiling, shallow frying, deep frying and the raw state. In 14 days KMS preservation, the order is open pan dry roasting, deep frying, raw state, shallow frying and boiling. In 15 days KMS preservation, the order is the raw state, shallow frying, deep frying, open pan dry roasting and boiling.

The overall analysis of iron content of *rohu* is mostly restored by the gradation of methods as deep frying>boiling>raw state>open pan dry roasting> shallow frying.

Deep frying can restore[66] iron rather than the other cooking methods probably due to the protective covering of cooking oil and the other possible reason is the use of iron pan for frying. Boiling can reduce some of the iron loss as iron pan is used and little amount of iron is eliminated possibly due to the solubility property of iron in the cooking water, hence discarding this water, iron content is reduced. Open pan dry roasting reduces the iron content due to the application of direct dry heat, so that the iron may get charred, resulting in reduction. Shallow frying can reduce the iron content as the amount of oil used for frying probably is not sufficient to cover the total surface of the fish, so iron is eliminated and charred due to the application of direct heat. Thus among all the studied conventional cooking methods, **deep frying** is the best method for *rohu* to restore iron content.

5.6.2 *Katla (Catla catla)*

It has been reported that *katla* contains 1.14 mg of iron per 100 gm[85] in the raw state. This value changes due to the application of different cooking methods and preservation conditions (vide Table no **5.6.2.1**).

Table no 5.6.2.1 Iron content of *Katla* (mg/100gm)

Preservation	Duration	Raw state	Boiling	Dry roasting	Shallow frying	Deep frying
Control	Fresh	2.85±0.03	1.35±0.06	5.64±0.06	2.42±0.11	4.19±0.06
Control	24 hours	0.84±0.08	1.06±0.05	1.14±0.04	2.44±0.12	2.55±0.03
Control	48 hours	0.81±0.08	2.09±0.09	3.19±0.06	3.06±0.05	2.13±0.05
Control	14 days	1.35±0.06	3.05±0.04	0.95±0.04	1.42±0.02	4.52±0.02
Control	15 days	1.15±0.05	1.45±0.03	1.82±0.08	4.95±0.05	1.65±0.03
Salt & Turmeric	24 hours	1.51±0.01	0.97±0.02	0.51±0.01	0.95±0.03	1.35±0.03
Salt &Turmeric	48 hours	0.37±0.02	0.67±0.02	0.75±0.03	0.95±0.03	2.01±0.01
Salt & Turmeric	14 days	0.84±0.04	0.87±0.02	0.72±0.02	0.61±0.01	1.02±0.02
Salt & Turmeric	15 days	1.94±0.04	1.72±0.02	1.34±0.04	1.07±0.02	3.01±0.02
KMS	24 hours	2.23±0.04	1.92±0.02	0.84±0.04	0.67±0.02	1.92±0.02
KMS	48 hours	1.63±0.04	0.84±0.04	0.82±0.02	0.53±0.04	0.92±0.02
KMS	14 days	1.04±0.04	0.84±0.04	0.82±0.02	0.74±0.04	0.34±0.04
KMS	15 days	0.94±0.04	0.92±0.02	0.65±0.03	0.42±0.02	1.12±0.02

Values are expressed as mean±SD. Loss Restoration

Red digits represent the significant highest values from the raw state in different conditions.

In most of the conditions, iron content is mainly reduced by shallow frying, whereas in 14 days control preservation without preservative, iron content is reduced by open pan dry roasting. In fresh condition, 24 hours, 48 hours, 15 days control preservation without preservative and 48 hours salt and turmeric preservation, iron content is reduced by boiling. In 48 hours KMS preservation, iron content is reduced by deep frying.

Retention of iron content occurs by deep frying[66] mostly, but in fresh condition and 48 hours control preservation without preservative, iron retention occurs by open pan dry roasting, whereas in 24 hours, 14 days, 15 days KMS preservation, iron retention occurs by boiling. In 15 days control preservation without preservative, iron retention occurs by shallow frying.

Boiling and deep frying show the highest iron content in 14 days control preservation without preservative, whereas shallow frying shows the highest iron content in 15 days control preservation without preservative. Both the raw state and open pan dry roasting show the highest iron content in the fresh conditions.

Boiling shows the increased iron content than the raw state in fresh condition, 24 hours, 48 hours, 14 days, 15 days control preservation without preservative and 48 hours,14 days salt and turmeric preservation. Open pan dry roasting shows the increased iron content than the raw value in fresh condition, 24 hours, 48 hours, 15 days control preservation without preservative and 48 hours salt and turmeric preservation, whereas shallow frying shows the increased iron content than the raw state in 24 hours, 48 hours, 14 days, 15 days control preservation without preservative and 48 hours salt and turmeric preservation. Deep frying shows the increased iron content than the raw state in fresh condition, 24 hours, 48 hours, 14 days, 15 days control preservation without preservative and 48 hours, 14 days, 15 days salt and turmeric preservation as well as 15 days KMS preservation.

This happens may be due to the molecular rearrangement during cooking and the addition of cooking oil during frying or may be due to the addition of natural preservative. Another possible reason may be the elimination of water during cooking[48] that concentrates the iron, thus increasing the content of iron. The use of iron pan for cooking can also be one of the mechanisms for increasing the iron content as iron is absorbed by the fish.

Fig. 5.6.2.2 Graphical representation of Iron content of *Katla* with respect to different conditions

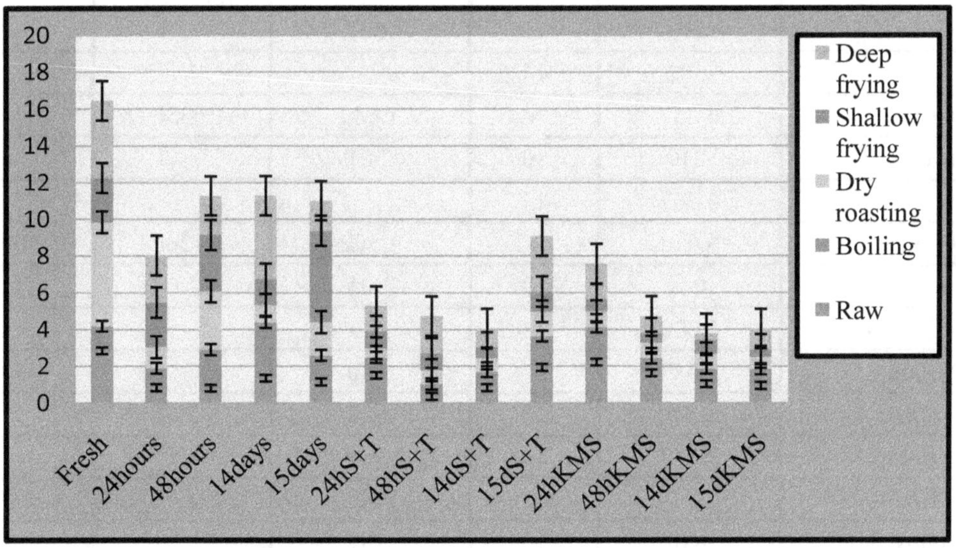

This graphical representation indicates that among all the preservation conditions, **fresh condition** helps to increase the iron content in all the cooking methods. The possible reason may be that the preservation can hamper the iron content as it is a very vulnerable mineral. Here the graph shows that the control preservation without preservative and both salt-turmeric and KMS preservation also increase the iron content, but preservatives are not so effective here.

Table no 5.6.2.3 ANOVA with regard to cooking conditions and preservation methods

Condition	Differences	Sum of Squares	df	Mean Square	F	Sig.
Fresh (control)	Between Groups	33.139	4	8.285	1.618E3	.000(S)
	Within Groups	.051	10	.005		
	Total	33.190	14			
24 hours (control)	Between Groups	8.228	4	2.057	499.270	.000(S)
	Within Groups	.041	10	.004		
	Total	8.269	14			
48 hours (control)	Between Groups	10.975	4	2.744	559.213	.000(S)
	Within Groups	.049	10	.005		
	Total	11.025	14			
14 days (control)	Between Groups	26.968	4	6.742	3.428E3	.000(S)
	Within Groups	.020	10	.002		
	Total	26.988	14			
15 days (control)	Between Groups	29.015	4	7.254	2.513E3	.000(S)
	Within Groups	.029	10	.003		
	Total	29.044	14			
24 hours (salt & turmeric)	Between Groups	1.860	4	.465	704.712	.000(S)
	Within Groups	.007	10	.001		
	Total	1.867	14			
48 hours (salt & turmeric)	Between Groups	4.701	4	1.175	1.856E3	.000(S)
	Within Groups	.006	10	.001		
	Total	4.707	14			
14 days (salt & turmeric)	Between Groups	.294	4	.074	95.904	.000(S)
	Within Groups	.008	10	.001		
	Total	.302	14			
15 days (salt & turmeric)	Between Groups	6.757	4	1.689	1.635E3	.000(S)
	Within Groups	.010	10	.001		
	Total	6.767	14			
24 hours (KMS)	Between Groups	6.010	4	1.502	1.426E3	.000(S)
	Within Groups	.011	10	.001		
	Total	6.020	14			
48 hours (KMS)	Between Groups	2.633	4	.658	407.981	.000(S)
	Within Groups	.016	10	.002		
	Total	2.649	14			
14 days (KMS)	Between Groups	.797	4	.199	125.015	.000(S)
	Within Groups	.016	10	.002		
	Total	.813	14			
15 days (KMS)	Between Groups	.912	4	.228	257.038	.000(S)
	Within Groups	.009	10	.001		
	Total	.920	14			

$p<0.05$ S= Significant, NS= Non-significant. All abbreviations are on page so and so.

This statistical ANOVA table shows that all the values are significant, which means there is significant difference present in the values of iron content of *katla* among different cooking methods and the raw state in respect to fresh condition along with different preservation methods.

Table no 5.6.2.4 Post hoc Duncan statistical analysis

Preservation	Duration	Raw state	Boiling	Dry roasting	Shallow frying	Deep frying
Control	Fresh	B,O,S,D^{a}	R,O,S,D^{b}	R,B,S,D^{c}	R,B,O,D^{d}	R,B,O,S^{e}
Control	24 hours	B,O,S,D^{a}	R,S,D^{f}	R,S,D^{f}	R,B,O^{g}	R,B,O^{g}
Control	48 hours	B,O,S,D^{a}	R,O,S^{h}	R,B,S,D^{c}	R,B,O,D^{d}	R,O,S^{h}
Control	14 days	B,O,D^{i}	R,O,S,D^{b}	R,B,S,D^{c}	B,O,D^{i}	R,B,O,S^{e}
Control	15 days	B,O,S,D^{a}	R,O,S,D^{b}	R,B,S,D^{c}	R,B,O,D^{d}	R,B,O,S^{e}
Salt & Turmeric	24 hours	B,O,S,D^{a}	R,O,D^{j}	R,B,S,D^{c}	R,O,D^{j}	R,B,O,S^{e}
Salt & Turmeric	48 hours	B,O,S,D^{a}	R,O,S,D^{b}	R,B,S,D^{c}	R,B,O,D^{d}	R,B,O,S^{e}
Salt & Turmeric	14 days	O,S,D^{k}	O,S,D^{k}	R,B,S,D^{c}	R,B,O,D^{d}	R,B,O,S^{e}
Salt & Turmeric	15 days	B,O,S,D^{a}	R,O,S,D^{b}	R,B,S,D^{c}	R,B,O,D^{d}	R,B,O,S^{e}
KMS	24 hours	B,O,S,D^{a}	R,O,S^{h}	R,B,S,D^{c}	R,B,O,D^{d}	R,O,S^{h}
KMS	48 hours	B,O,S,D^{a}	R,S,D^{f}	R,S,D^{f}	R,B,O,D^{d}	R,B,O,S^{e}
KMS	14 days	B,O,S,D^{a}	R,S,D^{f}	R,S,D^{f}	R,B,O,D^{d}	R,B,O,S^{e}
KMS	15 days	O,S,D^{k}	O,S,D^{k}	R,B,S,D^{c}	R,B,O,D^{d}	R,B,O,S^{e}

R= Raw state, B= Boiling, O= Open pan dry roasting, S= Shallow frying, D= Deep frying. The same uppercase alphabets signify that there is no significant difference present among the variables.

This table shows the significant difference among the different variables such as cooking methods and preservation conditions. The raw state significantly differs from boiling, open pan dry roasting, shallow frying and deep frying in all of the preservation conditions with preservatives and control preservation without preservative except in 14 days control preservation, 14 days salt and turmeric preservation and 15 days KMS preservation. Boiling significantly differs from the raw state, open pan dry roasting, shallow frying and deep frying in all the preservation conditions except in 24 hours, 48 hours control preservation without preservative and 24 hours, 14 days salt and turmeric preservation and 24 hours, 48 hours, 14 days, 15 days KMS preservation. Open pan dry roasting significantly differs from the raw state, boiling, shallow frying and deep frying in all the preservation conditions except in 24 hours control preservation without preservative and 48 hours, 14 days KMS preservation. Shallow frying significantly differs from the raw state, boiling, open pan dry roasting and deep frying in all of the preservation conditions except in 24 hours, 14 days control preservation without preservative and 24 hours salt and turmeric preservation.

Deep frying significantly differs from the raw state, boiling, open pan dry roasting and shallow frying in all the preservation conditions except in 24 hours, 48 hours control preservation without preservative and 24 hours KMS preservation. Boiling and open pan dry roasting significantly differ from the raw state, shallow frying and deep frying in 24 hours control preservation without preservative and 48 hours, 14 days KMS preservation, whereas shallow frying and deep frying significantly differ from the raw state, boiling and open pan dry roasting in 24 hours control preservation without preservative. Boiling and deep frying significantly differ from the raw state, open pan dry roasting and shallow frying in 48 hours control preservation without preservative and 24 hours KMS preservation. Again the raw state and shallow frying significantly differ from boiling, open pan dry roasting and deep frying in 14 days control preservation without preservative.

Shallow frying and boiling significantly differ from the raw state, open pan dry roasting and deep frying in 24 hours salt and turmeric preservation. Boiling and the raw state significantly differ from open pan dry roasting, shallow frying and deep frying in 14 days salt and turmeric and 15 days KMS preservation.

Table no 5.6.2.5 Gradation of cooking methods from higher to lower restoration with respect to preservation days

Preservation	Duration	Method 1	Method 2	Method 3	Method 4	Method 5
Control	Fresh	OPDR	DF	R	SF	B
Control	24 hours	DF	SF	OPDR	B	R
Control	48 hours	OPDR	SF	B	DF	R
Control	14 days	DF	B	SF	R	OPDR
Control	15 days	SF	OPDR	DF	B	R
Salt &Turmeric	24 hours	R	DF	B	SF	OPDR
Salt & Turmeric	48 hours	DF	SF	OPDR	B	R
Salt & Turmeric	14 days	DF	B	R	OPDR	SF
Salt &Turmeric	15 days	DF	R	B	OPDR	SF
KMS	24 hours	R	DF	B	OPDR	SF
KMS	48 hours	R	B	OPDR	SF	DF
KMS	14 days	R	B	OPDR	SF	DF
KMS	15 days	DF	R	B	OPDR	SF

R= Raw state, B= Boiling, OPDR= Open pan dry roasting, SF= Shallow frying, DF= Deep frying. Same colours represent the similar order.

In all the preservation methods and fresh condition, iron retention occurs mainly in deep frying than the other cooking methods. In fresh condition, retention occurs firstly in open pan dry roasting followed by deep frying followed by the raw state, shallow frying, boiling. In 24 hours control preservation without preservative and 48 hours salt and turmeric preservation, the order is deep frying, shallow frying, open pan dry roasting, boiling and the raw state. In 48 hours control preservation without preservative, the order becomes open pan dry roasting, shallow frying, boiling, deep frying and the raw state. In 14 days control preservation without preservative, it changes in the order of deep frying, boiling, shallow frying, raw state and open pan dry roasting. In 15 days control preservation without preservative, the order is shallow frying, open pan dry roasting, deep frying, boiling and the raw state.

In 24 hours salt and turmeric preservation, retention occurs firstly in the raw state followed by deep frying, boiling, shallow frying and open pan dry roasting. In 14 days salt and turmeric preservation, the order changes from deep frying to boiling, raw state, open pan dry roasting and shallow frying. In 15 days salt and turmeric preservation and 15 days KMS preservation, the order becomes deep frying, raw state, boiling, open pan dry roasting and shallow frying.

In 24 hours KMS preservation, retention occurs firstly in the raw state then deep frying, boiling, open pan dry roasting and shallow frying. In 48 hours and 14 days KMS preservation, the order is the raw state, boiling, open pan dry roasting, shallow frying and deep frying.

The overall analysis of iron content of *katla* is mostly restored by the gradation of methods as deep frying>shallow frying>boiling>open pan dry roasting> raw state.

Deep frying and shallow frying can restore[66] iron rather than the other cooking methods possibly due to the protective covering of cooking oil and the other possible reason is the use of iron pan for frying. Boiling can reduce some of the iron loss as iron pan is used and possibly little amount iron is eliminated due to the lower solubility of iron in the cooking water as *katla* contains lots of fatty tissues, thus discarding the cooking water reduces the iron content. Open pan dry roasting reduces the iron content due to the application of direct dry heat so that the iron may get charred, leading to the reduction. Thus among all the studied conventional cooking methods, **deep frying** is the best method for *katla* to restore iron content.

5.6.3 Prawn (*Fenneropenaeus indicus*)

It has been reported that prawn contains 5.3 mg of iron per 100 gm[85] in the raw state. This value changes due to the application of different cooking methods and preservation conditions (vide Table no **5.6.2.1**).

Table no 5.6.3.1 Iron content of Prawn (mg/100gm)

Preservation	Duration	Raw state	Boiling	Dry roasting	Shallow frying	Deep frying
Control	Fresh	1.40±0.01	1.45±0.02	1.51±0.01	0.93±0.01	0.67±0.05
Control	24 hours	2.52±0.02	1.80±0.08	1.74±0.05	3.45±0.03	2.50±0.02
Control	48 hours	1.58±0.05	1.32±0.02	2.03±0.04	2.32±0.02	2.23±0.04
Control	14 days	4.03±0.04	3.44±0.06	4.52±0.02	1.53±0.04	1.52±0.02
Control	15 days	3.12±0.02	2.16±0.05	1.41±0.01	2.65±0.03	2.84±0.04
Salt & Turmeric	24 hours	2.02±0.02	2.52±0.02	2.22±0.02	1.24±0.04	1.84±0.04
Salt & Turmeric	48 hours	1.82±0.02	1.41±0.01	1.65±0.03	0.94±0.04	1.51±0.01
Salt & Turmeric	14 days	0.82±0.02	0.26±0.01	0.95±0.03	1.02±0.02	0.63±0.02
Salt & Turmeric	15 days	0.52±0.02	1.45±0.03	0.94±0.02	0.53±0.01	0.62±0.02
KMS	24 hours	0.46±0.05	2.72±0.02	3.22±0.02	2.14±0.04	1.54±0.04
KMS	48 hours	0.92±0.02	0.62±0.02	0.93±0.04	0.93±0.02	0.84±0.03
KMS	14 days	0.47±0.02	0.87±0.02	0.86±0.04	1.13±0.04	0.74±0.04
KMS	15 days	2.82±0.02	2.65±0.03	2.97±0.02	3.08±0.07	3.82±0.02

Values are expressed as mean±SD. ☐ Loss ☐ Restoration

Red digits represent the significant highest values from the raw state in different conditions.

In most of the conditions, iron content is mainly reduced by boiling, whereas in 24 hours and 15 days control preservation without preservative iron content is reduced by open pan dry roasting. In fresh condition, 14 days control preservation without preservative and 24 hours, 14 days KMS preservation, iron content is reduced by deep frying. In 24 hours, 48 hours, 15 days salt and turmeric preservation, iron content is reduced by shallow frying.

Retention of iron content occurs by open pan dry roasting mostly, but in 24 hours and 15 days salt and turmeric preservation, iron retention occurs by boiling, whereas in 24 hours, 48 hours control preservation without preservative, 14 days salt and turmeric preservation and 48 hours, 14 days KMS preservation, iron retention occurs by shallow frying. In 15 days control preservation without preservative and 15 days KMS preservation, iron retention occurs by deep frying.

The raw state, boiling and open pan dry roasting show the highest iron content in 14 days control preservation without preservative, whereas shallow frying shows the highest iron content in 24 hours control preservation without preservative. Deep frying shows the highest iron content in 15 days KMS preservation.

Boiling shows the increased iron content than the raw value in fresh condition, 24 hours control preservation without preservative, 15 days salt and turmeric preservation and 14 days KMS preservation. Open pan dry roasting shows the increased iron content than the raw value in fresh condition, 48 hours, 14 days control preservation without preservative and 24 hours, 14 days salt and turmeric preservation and 24 hours, 48 hours, 14 days, 15 days KMS preservation, whereas shallow frying shows the increased iron content than the raw state in 24 hours, 48 hours control preservation without preservative and 14 days salt and turmeric preservation and 24 hours, 48 hours, 14 days, 15 days KMS preservation. Deep frying shows the increased iron content than the raw value in 48 hours control preservation without preservative and 24 hours, 14 days, 15 days KMS preservation.

Molecular rearrangement during cooking and the addition of cooking oil during frying or the addition of the natural and synthetic preservatives may be the possible reason for the increased content of iron. Another possible reason may be the elimination of water during cooking[48] that concentrates the amount of iron, thus increasing the content of iron. The use of iron pan for cooking may be the additional possible reason due to iron absorption by prawn from the cooking pan.

Fig. 5.6.3.2 Graphical representation of Iron content of Prawn with respect to different conditions

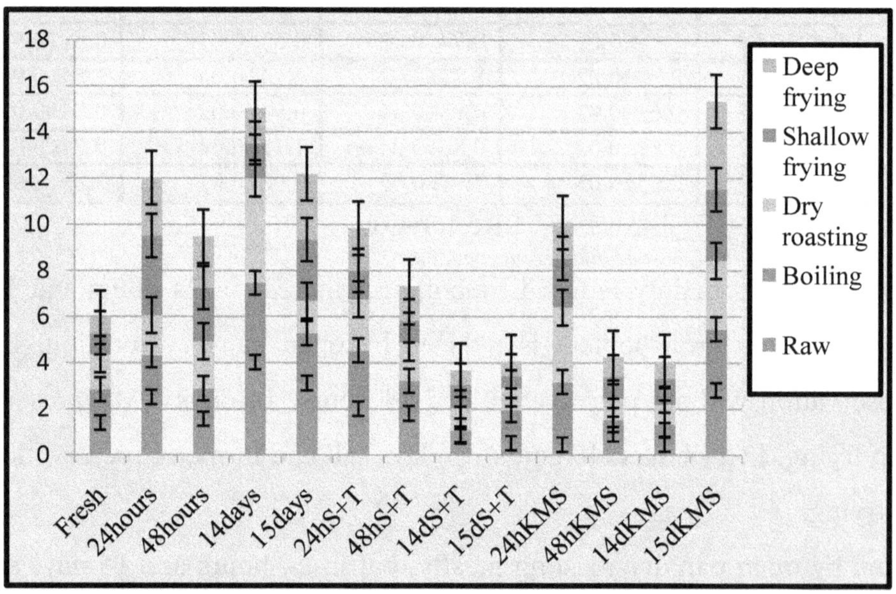

This graphical representation indicates that among all the preservation conditions, **15 days KMS preservation**[59] helps to increase the iron content in all the cooking methods. The possible reason may be the effectiveness of KMS that helps to restore the iron content as it is a very vulnerable mineral[39]. Here the graph shows that the control preservation without preservative and salt and turmeric also increase the iron content, but KMS preservative is more efficient here. Synthetic preservative possibly helps to modify the structure of iron, hence restoring the content.

Table no 5.6.3.3 ANOVA with regard to cooking conditions and preservation methods

Condition	Differences	Sum of Squares	df	Mean Square	F	Sig.
Fresh (control)	Between Groups	1.655	4	.414	411.086	.000(S)
	Within Groups	.010	10	.001		
	Total	1.665	14			
24 hours (control)	Between Groups	5.767	4	1.442	643.688	.000(S)
	Within Groups	.022	10	.002		
	Total	5.790	14			
48 hours (control)	Between Groups	2.226	4	.557	361.435	.000(S)
	Within Groups	.015	10	.002		
	Total	2.242	14			
14 days (control)	Between Groups	23.756	4	5.939	3.349E3	.000(S)
	Within Groups	.018	10	.002		
	Total	23.774	14			
15 days (control)	Between Groups	5.296	4	1.324	859.812	.000(S)
	Within Groups	.015	10	.002		
	Total	5.312	14			
24 hours (salt & turmeric)	Between Groups	4.885	4	1.221	1.138E3	.000(S)
	Within Groups	.011	10	.001		
	Total	4.896	14			
48 hours (salt & turmeric)	Between Groups	1.319	4	.330	453.761	.000(S)
	Within Groups	.007	10	.001		
	Total	1.326	14			
14 days (salt & turmeric)	Between Groups	1.111	4	.278	429.701	.000(S)
	Within Groups	.006	10	.001		
	Total	1.118	14			
15 days (salt & turmeric)	Between Groups	1.867	4	.467	985.894	.000(S)
	Within Groups	.005	10	.000		
	Total	1.871	14			
24 hours (KMS)	Between Groups	13.856	4	3.464	2.362E3	.000(S)
	Within Groups	.015	10	.001		
	Total	13.871	14			
48 hours (KMS)	Between Groups	.212	4	.053	47.036	.000(S)
	Within Groups	.011	10	.001		
	Total	.223	14			
14 days (KMS)	Between Groups	.667	4	.167	58.302	.000(S)
	Within Groups	.029	10	.003		
	Total	.696	14			
15 days (KMS)	Between Groups	2.441	4	.610	353.413	.000(S)
	Within Groups	.017	10	.002		
	Total	2.458	14			

$p<0.05$ S= Significant, NS= Non-significant. All abbreviations are on page so and so.

This statistical ANOVA table shows that all the values are significant, which means there is significant difference present in the values of iron content of prawn among different cooking methods and the raw state in respect to fresh condition along with different preservation methods.

Table no 5.6.3.4 Post hoc Duncan statistical analysis

Preservation	Duration	Raw state	Boiling	Dry roasting	Shallow frying	Deep frying
Control	Fresh	O,S,D^{a}	S,D^{b}	R,S,D^{c}	R,B,O,D^{d}	R,B,O,S^{e}
Control	24 hours	B,O,S^{f}	R,S,D^{c}	R,S,D^{c}	R,B,O,D^{d}	B,O,S^{f}
Control	48 hours	B,O,S,D^{g}	R,O,S,D^{h}	R,B,S,D^{i}	R,B,O,D^{d}	R,B,O,S^{e}
Control	14 days	B,O,S,D^{g}	R,O,S,D^{h}	R,B,S,D^{i}	R,B,O^{j}	R,B,O^{j}
Control	15 days	B,O,S,D^{g}	R,O,S,D^{h}	R,B,S,D^{i}	R,B,O,D^{d}	R,B,O,S^{e}
Salt &Turmeric	24 hours	B,O,S,D^{g}	R,O,S,D^{h}	R,B,S,D^{i}	R,B,O,D^{d}	R,B,O,S^{e}
Salt & Turmeric	48 hours	B,O,S,D^{g}	R,O,S,D^{h}	R,B,S,D^{i}	R,B,O,D^{d}	R,B,O,S^{e}
Salt & Turmeric	14 days	B,O,S,D^{g}	R,O,S,D^{h}	R,B,S,D^{i}	R,B,O,D^{d}	R,B,O,S^{e}
Salt & Turmeric	15 days	B,O,S^{f}	R,O,S,D^{h}	R,B,S,D^{i}	B,O,D^{k}	R,B,O,S^{e}
KMS	24 hours	B,O,S,D^{g}	R,O,S,D^{h}	R,B,S,D^{i}	R,B,O,D^{d}	R,B,O,S^{e}
KMS	48 hours	B,D^{l}	R,O,S,D^{h}	B,D^{l}	B,D^{l}	R,B,O,S^{e}
KMS	14 days	B,O,S,D^{g}	R,S^{m}	R,S^{m}	R,B,O,D^{d}	R,S^{m}
KMS	15 days	B,O,S,D^{g}	R,O,S,D^{h}	R,B,S,D^{i}	R,B,O,D^{d}	R,B,O,S^{e}

R= Raw state, B= Boiling, O= Open pan dry roasting, S= Shallow frying, D= Deep frying. The same uppercase alphabets represent that there is no significant difference present among the variables.

This table shows the significant difference among the different variables such as cooking methods and preservation conditions. The raw state significantly differs from boiling, open pan dry roasting, shallow frying and deep frying in all of the preservation conditions with preservatives and control preservation without preservative except in fresh condition, 24 hours control preservation, 15 days salt and turmeric preservation and 48 hours KMS preservation. Boiling significantly differs from the raw state, open pan dry roasting, shallow frying and deep frying in all the preservation conditions except in fresh conditions, 24 hours control preservation without preservative and 14 days KMS preservation. Open pan dry roasting significantly differs from the raw state, boiling, shallow frying and deep frying in all the preservation conditions except in fresh condition, 24 hours control preservation without preservative and 48 hours, 14 days KMS preservation. Shallow frying significantly differs from the raw state, boiling, open pan dry roasting and deep frying in all the preservation conditions except in 14 days control preservation without preservative, 15 days salt and turmeric preservation and 48 hours KMS preservation. Deep frying significantly differs from the raw state, boiling, open pan dry roasting and shallow frying in all the preservation conditions except in 24 hours, 14 days control preservation without preservative and 14 days KMS preservation.

The raw state significantly differs from open pan dry roasting, shallow frying and deep frying in fresh condition, whereas boiling significantly differs from shallow frying and deep frying in fresh condition. Open pan dry roasting significantly differs from the raw state, shallow frying and deep frying in fresh condition and 24 hours control preservation without preservative, and only boiling significantly differs from the raw state, shallow frying and deep frying in 24 hours control preservation without preservative.

The raw state and deep frying significantly differ from boiling, open pan dry roasting and shallow frying in 24 hours control preservation without preservative, and only the raw state significantly differs from boiling, open pan dry roasting and shallow frying in 15 days salt and turmeric preservation. Shallow frying and deep frying significantly differ from the raw state, boiling and open pan dry roasting in 14 days control preservation without preservative. Again shallow frying significantly differs from boiling, open pan dry roasting and deep frying in 15 days salt and turmeric preservation. The raw state, shallow frying and open pan dry roasting significantly differ from boiling and deep frying in 48 hours KMS preservation. Boiling, open pan dry roasting and deep frying significantly differ from the raw state and shallow frying in 14 days KMS preservation.

Table no 5.6.3.5 Gradation of cooking methods from higher to lower restoration with respect to preservation days

Preservation	Duration	Method 1	Method 2	Method 3	Method 4	Method 5
Control	Fresh	OPDR	B	R	SF	DF
Control	24 hours	SF	R	DF	B	OPDR
Control	48 hours	SF	DF	OPDR	R	B
Control	14 days	OPDR	R	B	SF	DF
Control	15 days	R	DF	SF	B	OPDR
Salt &Turmeric	24 hours	B	OPDR	DF	SF	R
Salt & Turmeric	48 hours	R	OPDR	DF	B	SF
Salt & Turmeric	14 days	SF	OPDR	R	DF	B
Salt &Turmeric	15 days	B	OPDR	DF	SF	R
KMS	24 hours	OPDR	B	SF	DF	R
KMS	48 hours	OPDR	SF	R	DF	B
KMS	14 days	SF	B	OPDR	DF	R
KMS	15 days	DF	SF	OPDR	R	B

R= Raw state, B= Boiling, OPDR= Open pan dry roasting, SF= Shallow frying, DF= Deep frying. Same colour represents the similar order.

In all the preservation techniques and fresh condition, iron retention occurs mainly by shallow frying than the other cooking methods. In fresh condition, retention occurs firstly in open pan dry roasting followed by boiling, raw state, shallow frying and deep frying. In 24 hours control preservation without preservative, retention occurs in the order of shallow frying followed by the raw state, deep frying, boiling and open pan dry roasting. In 48 hours control preservation without preservative, the order is shallow frying, deep frying, open pan dry roasting, raw state and boiling. In 14 days control preservation without preservative, the order is open pan dry roasting, raw state, boiling, shallow frying and deep frying. In 15 days control preservation without preservative, the order remains the raw state, deep frying, shallow frying, boiling and open pan dry roasting.

In 24 hours and 15 days salt and turmeric preservation, retention occurs firstly in boiling then open pan dry roasting, deep frying, shallow frying and the raw state. In 48 hours salt and turmeric preservation, it changes in the order of the raw state, open pan dry roasting, deep frying, boiling and shallow frying. In 14 days salt and turmeric preservation, the order becomes shallow frying, open pan dry roasting, raw state, deep frying and boiling.

In 24 hours KMS preservation, retention occurs firstly in open pan dry roasting followed by boiling, shallow frying, deep frying and the raw state. In 48 hours KMS preservation, the order becomes open pan dry roasting to shallow frying, raw state, deep frying and boiling. In 14 days KMS preservation, the order is shallow frying, boiling, open pan dry roasting deep frying and the raw state. In 15 days KMS preservation, the order remains deep frying, shallow frying, open pan dry roasting, raw state and boiling. The overall analysis of iron content of prawn is mostly restored by the gradation of methods as shallow frying>open pan dry roasting>deep frying> boiling> raw state.

Shallow frying can restore[66] iron rather than the other cooking methods possibly due to the protective covering of cooking oil and the other reason is the use of iron cooking pan for frying. Open pan dry roasting reduces the iron content due to the application of direct dry heat so that the iron may get charred, leading to reduction. Boiling can reduce some of the iron loss as iron pan is used and little amount iron is eliminated due to the higher solubility of iron in the cooking water, thus discarding the cooking water reduces iron content. Deep frying possibly causes the total dryness of prawn, hence eliminating iron. Thus among all the studied conventional cooking methods, **shallow frying** is the best method for prawn to restore iron content.

5.6.4 Lobster (*Macrobrachium rosenbergii*)

It has been reported that lobster contains 1.14 mg of iron per 100 gm[84] in the raw state. This value changes due to the application of different cooking methods and preservation conditions (vide Table no **5.6.4.1**).

Table no 5.6.4.1 Iron content of Lobster (mg/100gm)

Preservation	Duration	Raw state	Boiling	Dry roasting	Shallow frying	Deep frying
Control	Fresh	2.55±0.01	1.65±0.03	4.60±0.02	1.72±0.04	0.89±0.05
Control	24 hours	0.56±0.02	1.45±0.03	0.94 ±0.04	1.17±0.02	1.40±0.05
Control	48 hours	0.90±0.02	0.55±0.02	1.52±0.02	1.05±0.04	1.46±0.04
Control	14 days	0.61±0.06	1.63±0.05	0.56±0.04	0.70±0.05	1.07±0.02
Control	15 days	1.17±0.02	1.77±0.02	3.97±0.02	1.51±0.01	1.66±0.01
Salt & Turmeric	24 hours	0.87±0.02	0.74±0.04	3.19±0.55	3.53±0.02	1.02±0.02
Salt & Turmeric	48 hours	1.27±0.02	0.87±0.02	2.01±0.01	1.54±0.02	1.52±0.02
Salt & Turmeric	14 days	0.66±0.01	0.95±0.03	0.71±0.01	0.95±0.03	0.83±0.01
Salt & Turmeric	15 days	0.92±0.02	0.73±0.01	0.95±0.03	1.02±0.02	0.32±0.02
KMS	24 hours	0.62±0.02	0.67±0.02	1.37±0.02	1.22±0.02	1.52±0.02
KMS	48 hours	0.82±0.02	0.78±0.02	0.64±0.02	2.24±0.04	0.62±0.02
KMS	14 days	0.52±0.02	0.57±0.02	1.37±0.03	1.32±0.02	3.04±0.04
KMS	15 days	0.82±0.02	2.47±0.02	2.32±0.02	1.72±0.02	1.22±0.02

Values are expressed as mean±SD. ☐ Loss ▒ Restoration

Red digits represent the significant highest values from the raw state in different conditions.

In most of the conditions, iron content is mainly reduced by boiling, whereas in 24 hours, 14 days control preservation without preservative and 14 days salt and turmeric preservation, iron content is reduced by open pan dry roasting, whereas in 15 days control preservation without preservative, iron content is reduced by shallow frying. In fresh condition, 15 days control preservation without preservative and 48 hours, 15 days KMS preservation, iron content is reduced by deep frying.

Retention of iron content occurs by open pan dry roasting mostly, but in 24 hours, 14 days control preservation without preservative, 14 days salt and turmeric preservation and 15 days KMS preservation, iron retention occurs by boiling, whereas in 24 hours, 14 days, 15 days salt and turmeric preservation and

48 hours KMS preservation, iron retention occurs by shallow frying. In 24 hours and 14 days KMS preservation, iron retention occurs by deep frying.

The raw state and open pan dry roasting show the highest iron content in fresh condition, whereas shallow frying shows the highest iron content in 24 hours salt and turmeric preservation. Boiling and deep frying show the highest iron contents in 15 days and 14 days KMS preservation.

Boiling shows the increased iron content than the raw value in fresh condition, 24 hours, 14 days, 15 days control preservation without preservative, 14 days salt and turmeric preservation and 14 days, 15 days KMS preservation. Open pan dry roasting shows the increased iron content than the raw value in all the conditions except in 14 days control preservation without preservative and 48 hours KMS preservation, whereas shallow frying also shows the increased iron content than the raw value in all the preservation conditions except in fresh condition. Deep frying shows the increased iron content than the raw state in all the preservation conditions except fresh condition, 15 days salt and turmeric preservation and 48 hours KMS preservation.

The possible reason behind this increment of iron content may be due to the molecular rearrangement during cooking and the addition of cooking oil during frying or may be due to the addition of both the natural and synthetic preservatives. Additionally, it is also possible that the elimination of water during cooking[48] concentrates the amount of iron, increasing the content of iron. The use of iron pan for cooking can be a strong possible reason due to the absorption of iron by the lobster from the iron pan.

Fig. 5.6.4.2 Graphical representation of Iron content of Lobster with respect to different conditions

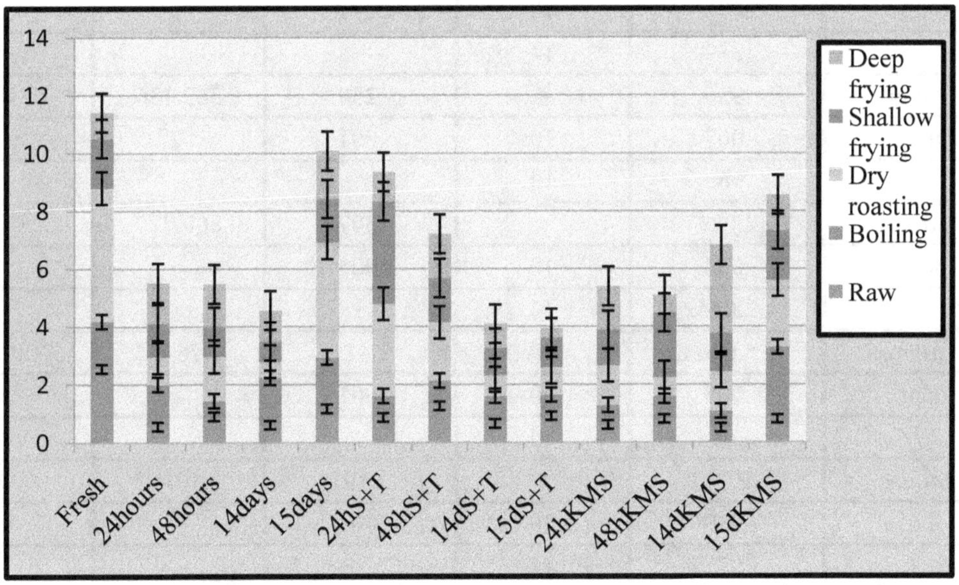

This graphical representation indicates that among all the preservation conditions, **fresh condition** helps to increase the iron content in all the cooking methods. The possible reason may be that the preservation can hamper the iron content as it is a very vulnerable mineral. Here the graph shows that the control preservation without preservative, salt-turmeric and KMS preservation also increase the iron content, but preservatives are not so effective here.

Table no 5.6.4.3 ANOVA with regard to cooking conditions and preservation methods

Condition	Differences	Sum of Squares	df	Mean Square	F	Sig.
Fresh (control)	Between Groups	24.457	4	6.114	2.075E3	.000(S)
	Within Groups	.029	10	.003		
	Total	24.486	14			
24 hours (control)	Between Groups	1.607	4	.402	295.348	.000(S)
	Within Groups	.014	10	.001		
	Total	1.620	14			
48 hours (control)	Between Groups	1.953	4	.488	466.513	.000(S)
	Within Groups	.010	10	.001		
	Total	1.964	14			
14 days (control)	Between Groups	2.410	4	.603	256.771	.000(S)
	Within Groups	.023	10	.002		
	Total	2.434	14			
15 days (control)	Between Groups	14.899	4	3.725	8.596E3	.000(S)
	Within Groups	.004	10	.000		
	Total	14.904	14			
24 hours (salt & turmeric)	Between Groups	23.759	4	5.940	309.689	.000(S)
	Within Groups	.192	10	.019		
	Total	23.951	14			
48 hours (salt & turmeric)	Between Groups	2.076	4	.519	1.162E3	.000(S)
	Within Groups	.004	10	.000		
	Total	2.080	14			
14 days (salt & turmeric)	Between Groups	.213	4	.053	84.016	.000(S)
	Within Groups	.006	10	.001		
	Total	.219	14			
15 days (salt & turmeric)	Between Groups	.956	4	.239	362.136	.000(S)
	Within Groups	.007	10	.001		
	Total	.963	14			
24 hours (KMS)	Between Groups	2.029	4	.507	800.779	.000(S)
	Within Groups	.006	10	.001		
	Total	2.035	14			
48 hours (KMS)	Between Groups	5.646	4	1.411	1.764E3	.000(S)
	Within Groups	.008	10	.001		
	Total	5.654	14			
14 days (KMS)	Between Groups	12.762	4	3.191	3.301E3	.000(S)
	Within Groups	.010	10	.001		
	Total	12.772	14			
15 days (KMS)	Between Groups	5.961	4	1.490	2.353E3	.000(S)
	Within Groups	.006	10	.001		
	Total	5.968	14			

$p<0.05$ S= Significant, NS= Non-significant. All abbreviations are on page so and so.

This statistical ANOVA table shows that all the values are significant, which means there is significant difference present in the values of iron content of lobster among different cooking methods and the raw state in respect to fresh condition along with different preservation methods.

Table no 5.6.4.4 Post hoc Duncan statistical analysis

Preservation	Duration	Raw state	Boiling	Dry roasting	Shallow frying	Deep frying
Control	Fresh	B,O,S,D^{a}	R,O,D^{b}	R,B,S,D^{c}	R,O,D^{b}	R,B,O,S^{d}
Control	24 hours	B,O,S,D^{a}	R,O,S^{e}	R,B,S,D^{c}	R,B,O,D^{f}	R,O,S^{e}
Control	48 hours	B,O,S,D^{a}	R,O,S,D^{g}	R,B,S^{h}	R,B,O,D^{f}	R,B,S^{h}
Control	14 days	B,D^{i}	R,O,S,D^{g}	B,S,D^{j}	B,O,D^{k}	R,B,O,S^{d}
Control	15 days	B,O,S,D^{a}	R,O,S,D^{g}	R,B,S,D^{c}	R,B,O,D^{f}	R,B,O,S^{d}
Salt &Turmeric	24 hours	O,S^{l}	O,S,D^{m}	R,B,D^{n}	R,B,D^{n}	B,O,S^{o}
Salt & Turmeric	48 hours	B,O,S,D^{a}	R,O,S,D^{g}	R,B,S,D^{c}	R,B,O^{p}	R,B,O^{p}
Salt & Turmeric	14 days	B,O,S,D^{a}	R,O,D^{b}	R,B,S,D^{c}	R,O,D^{b}	R,B,O,S^{d}
Salt & Turmeric	15 days	B,S,D^{j}	R,O,S,D^{g}	B,S,D^{j}	R,B,O,D^{f}	R,B,O,S^{d}
KMS	24 hours	B,O,S,D^{a}	R,O,S,D^{g}	R,B,S,D^{c}	R,B,O,D^{f}	R,B,O,S^{d}
KMS	48 hours	B,O,S,D^{a}	R,O,S,D^{g}	R,B,S^{h}	R,B,O,D^{f}	R,B,S^{h}
KMS	14 days	O,S,D^{m}	O,S,D^{m}	R,B,S,D^{c}	R,B,O,D^{f}	R,B,O,S^{d}
KMS	15 days	B,O,S,D^{a}	R,O,S,D^{g}	R,B,S,D^{c}	R,B,O,D^{f}	R,B,O,S^{d}

R= Raw state, B= Boiling, O= Open pan dry roasting, S= Shallow frying, D= Deep frying. The same uppercase alphabets signify that there is no significant difference present among the variables.

This table shows the significant difference among the different variables such as cooking methods and preservation conditions. The raw state significantly differs from boiling, open pan dry roasting, shallow frying and deep frying in all of the preservation conditions with preservatives and control preservation without preservative except in 14 days control preservation without preservative, 24 hours, 15 days salt and turmeric preservation and 14 days KMS preservation. Boiling significantly differs from the raw state, open pan dry roasting, shallow frying and deep frying in all the preservation conditions except in fresh condition, 24 hours control preservation without preservative, 24 hours, 14 days salt and turmeric preservation and 14 days KMS preservation. Open pan dry roasting significantly differs from the raw state, boiling, shallow frying and deep frying in all the preservation conditions except in 48 hours, 14 days control preservation without preservative, 24 hours, 15 days salt and turmeric preservation and 48 hours KMS preservation. Shallow frying significantly differs from the raw state, boiling, open pan dry roasting and deep frying in all the preservation conditions except in fresh condition, 14 days control preservation without preservative and 24 hours, 48 hours, 14 days salt and turmeric preservation. Deep frying significantly differs from the raw state, boiling, open pan dry roasting and shallow frying in all of the preservation conditions except in 24 hours, 48 hours control preservation without preservative, 24 hours, 48 hours salt and turmeric preservation and 48 hours KMS preservation.

Boiling and shallow frying significantly differ from the raw state, open pan dry roasting and deep frying in fresh condition and 14 days salt and turmeric preservation, whereas boiling and deep frying significantly differ from the raw state, open pan dry roasting and shallow frying in 24 hours control preservation without preservative. Open pan dry roasting and deep frying significantly differ from the raw state, boiling, shallow frying in 48 hours control preservation without preservative and 48 hours KMS preservation, and only the raw state significantly differs from boiling and deep frying in 14 days control preservation without preservative.

Open pan dry roasting significantly differs from boiling, shallow frying and deep frying in 14 days control preservation without preservative and 15 days salt and turmeric preservation. Shallow frying significantly differs from boiling, open pan dry roasting and deep frying in 14 days control preservation without preservative. The raw state and boiling significantly differs from open pan dry roasting, shallow frying and deep frying in 14 days KMS preservation, and only the raw state significantly differs from open pan dry roasting and shallow frying in 24 hours salt and turmeric preservation, whereas only boiling significantly differs from open pan dry roasting, shallow frying and deep frying in 24 hours salt and turmeric preservation.

Shallow frying and open pan dry roasting significantly differ from the raw state, boiling and deep frying in 24 hours salt and turmeric preservation. Again deep frying significantly differs from boiling, open pan dry roasting and shallow frying in 24 hours salt and turmeric preservation. Shallow frying and deep frying significantly differ from the raw state, boiling and open pan dry roasting in 48 hours salt and turmeric preservation.

Table no 5.6.4.5 Gradation of cooking methods from higher to lower restoration with respect to preservation days

Preservation	Duration	Method 1	Method 2	Method 3	Method 4	Method 5
Control	Fresh	OPDR	R	SF	B	DF
Control	24 hours	B	DF	SF	OPDR	R
Control	48 hours	OPDR	DF	SF	R	B
Control	14 days	B	DF	SF	R	OPDR
Control	15 days	OPDR	B	DF	SF	R
Salt & Turmeric	24 hours	SF	OPDR	DF	R	B
Salt & Turmeric	48 hours	OPDR	SF	DF	R	B
Salt & Turmeric	14 days	SF	B	DF	OPDR	R
Salt &Turmeric	15 days	SF	OPDR	R	B	DF
KMS	24 hours	DF	OPDR	SF	B	R
KMS	48 hours	SF	R	B	OPDR	DF
KMS	14 days	DF	OPDR	SF	B	R
KMS	15 days	B	OPDR	SF	DF	R

R= Raw state, B= Boiling, OPDR= Open pan dry roasting, SF= Shallow frying, DF= Deep frying. Same colour represents the similar order.

In all the preservation methods and fresh condition, iron retention occurs mainly in open pan dry roasting than the other cooking methods. In fresh condition, retention occurs firstly in open pan dry roasting then the raw state, shallow frying, boiling and deep frying. In 24 hours control preservation without preservative, retention occurs in the order of boiling followed by deep frying, shallow frying, open pan dry roasting and the raw state. In 48 hours control preservation without preservative, the order is open pan dry roasting, deep frying, shallow frying, raw state and boiling. In 14 days control preservation without preservative, the order remains boiling, deep frying, shallow frying, raw state and open pan dry roasting.

In 15 days control preservation without preservative, the order becomes open pan dry roasting then boiling, deep frying, shallow frying and the raw state.

In 24 hours salt and turmeric preservation, retention occurs firstly in shallow frying followed by open pan dry roasting, deep frying, raw state and boiling. In 48 hours salt and turmeric preservation, it changes in the following order: open pan dry roasting, shallow frying, deep frying, raw state and boiling. In 14 days salt and turmeric preservation, the order is shallow frying, boiling, deep frying, open pan dry roasting and the raw state. In 15 days salt and turmeric preservation, the order remains shallow frying then open pan dry roasting, raw state, boiling and deep frying.

In 24 hours, 14 days KMS preservation retention occurs firstly in deep frying then open pan dry roasting, shallow frying, boiling and the raw state. In 48 hours KMS preservation, the order is shallow frying, raw state, boiling, open pan dry roasting and deep frying. In 15 days KMS preservation, the order changes from boiling to open pan dry roasting, shallow frying, deep frying and the raw state.

The overall analysis of iron content of lobster is mostly restored by the gradation of methods as open pan dry roasting>deep frying>shallow frying> boiling> raw state.

Open pan dry roasting can restore iron more than the other cooking methods as the flesh of lobster is quite hard so the iron probably cannot be eliminated from the flesh. It may also be possible that the use of iron pan can increase the total iron content. As the flesh gets hard due to direct heat, it may possibly create a barrier to eliminate iron from the flesh. Deep frying causes the total dryness of lobster and thus iron gets eliminated. Shallow frying possibly can create a protective covering of cooking oil. Boiling can reduce some of the iron loss as iron pan is used and a little amount of iron is eliminated due to the solubility of iron in the cooking water, thus discarding this water reduces the iron content. Thus among all the studied conventional cooking methods, **open pan dry roasting** is the best method for lobster to restore iron content.

5.6.5 Pomfret (*Pampus argenteus*)

It has been reported that pomfret contains 0.9 mg of iron per 100 gm[84] in the raw state. This value changes due to the application of different cooking methods and preservation conditions (vide Table no **5.6.5.1**).

Table no 5.6.5.1 Iron content of Pomfret (mg/100gm)

Preservation	Duration	Raw state	Boiling	Dry roasting	Shallow frying	Deep frying
Control	Fresh	2.84±0.00	1.56±0.02	2.04±0.07	1.07±0.05	4.53±0.03
Control	24 hours	4.92±0.06	4.29±0.03	5.40±0.03	4.54±0.04	4.14±0.03
Control	48 hours	2.47±0.02	3.44±0.04	3.65±0.04	4.53±0.04	4.65±0.04
Control	14 days	3.56±0.01	3.05±0.03	1.85±0.03	2.91±0.08	2.92±0.06
Control	15 days	0.03±0.01	0.75±0.03	1.43±0.02	0.47±0.02	0.32±0.02
Salt & Turmeric	24 hours	1.12±0.02	1.12±0.02	1.02±0.02	1.02±0.02	0.47±0.02
Salt & Turmeric	48 hours	1.35±0.03	1.82±0.02	1.02±0.02	1.02±0.02	1.15±0.03
Salt & Turmeric	14 days	0.97±0.02	1.22±0.02	0.75±0.02	0.87±0.02	1.12±0.02
Salt & Turmeric	15 days	3.52±0.02	2.21±0.01	1.12±0.02	1.02±0.02	1.72±0.02
KMS	24 hours	0.92±0.02	0.81±0.02	1.52±0.02	0.82±0.02	0.74±0.04
KMS	48 hours	4.42±0.02	1.82±0.02	1.32±0.02	1.52±0.02	1.95±0.03
KMS	14 days	0.77±0.02	1.42±0.02	0.57±0.02	1.17±0.02	0.66±0.05
KMS	15 days	1.17±0.01	1.47±0.02	1.43±0.04	2.34±0.04	2.02±0.02

Values are expressed as mean±SD. ☐ Loss ▨ Restoration

Red digits represent the significant highest values from the raw state in different conditions.

In most of the conditions, iron content is mainly reduced by open pan dry roasting, whereas in 48 hours control preservation without preservative, iron content is reduced by boiling, whereas in fresh condition, 48 hours, 15 days salt and turmeric preservation, iron content is reduced by shallow frying. In 24 hours control preservation without preservative and 24 hours salt and turmeric preservation and 24 hours KMS preservation, iron content is reduced by deep frying.

Retention of iron content occurs by boiling mostly, but in 24 hours control preservation without preservative and 24 hours KMS preservation, iron retention occurs by open pan dry roasting, whereas in 15 days KMS preservation, iron retention occurs by shallow frying. In fresh condition, 48 hours control preservation without preservative and 48 hours KMS preservation, iron retention occurs by deep frying.

The raw state, boiling, open pan dry roasting and shallow frying show the highest iron content in 24 hours control preservation without preservative, whereas deep frying shows the highest iron content in 48 hours control preservation without preservative.

Deep frying shows the increased iron content than the raw value in fresh condition, 48 hours, 15 days control preservation without preservative and 48 hours, 14 days salt and turmeric preservation and 14 days, 15 days KMS preservation. Open pan dry roasting shows the increased iron content than the raw state in 24 hours, 48 hours, 15 days control preservation without preservative and 24 hours, 15 days KMS preservation, whereas shallow frying also shows the increased iron content than the raw value in 48 hours, 15 days control preservation without preservative, 14 days, 15 days KMS preservation. Deep frying shows the increased iron content than the raw value in fresh condition, 48 hours, 15 days control preservation without preservative and 15 days KMS preservation.

The molecular rearrangement during cooking and the addition of cooking oil during frying may be the possible cause. It is also possible that elimination of water during cooking[48] makes the iron content to become more concentrated, thus increasing its content. Additionally, iron pan is used for cooking which enhances the iron absorption by pomfret, increasing the content.

Fig. 5.6.5.2 Graphical representation of Iron content of Pomfret with respect to different conditions

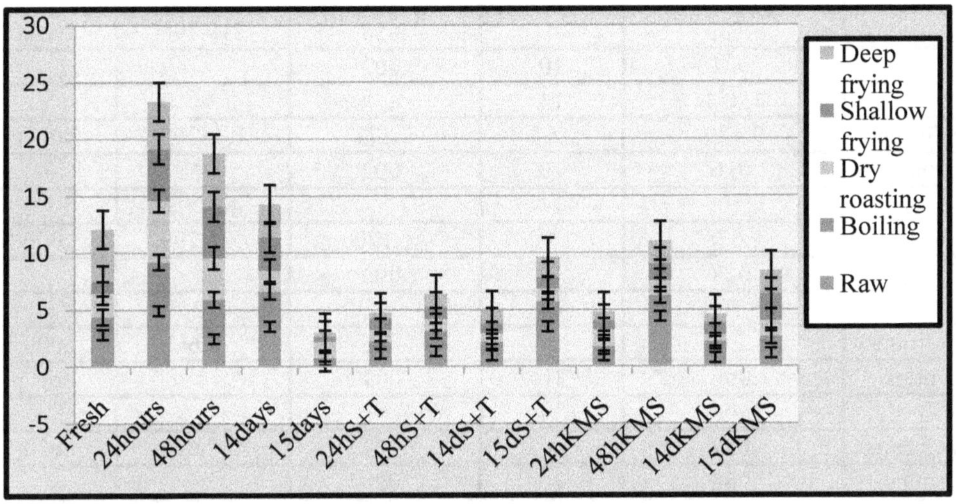

This graphical representation indicates that among all the preservation conditions, **24 hours control preservation without preservative** helps to increase the iron content in all the cooking methods. The possible reason may be that the preservation can hamper the iron content as it is very vulnerable mineral. Here the graph shows that the control preservation without preservative is more effective than salt-turmeric and KMS preservation.

Table no 5.6.5.3 ANOVA with regard to cooking conditions and preservation methods

Condition	Differences	Sum of Squares	df	Mean Square	F	Sig.
Fresh (control)	Between Groups	21.957	4	5.489	2.772E3	.000(S)
	Within Groups	.020	10	.002		
	Total	21.977	14			
24 hours (control)	Between Groups	1.833	4	.458	218.190	.000(S)
	Within Groups	.021	10	.002		
	Total	1.854	14			
48 hours (control)	Between Groups	9.489	4	2.372	1.452E3	.000(S)
	Within Groups	.016	10	.002		
	Total	9.505	14			
14 days (control)	Between Groups	4.678	4	1.170	425.799	.000(S)
	Within Groups	.027	10	.003		
	Total	4.706	14			
15 days (control)	Between Groups	3.384	4	.846	1.426E3	.000(S)
	Within Groups	.006	10	.001		
	Total	3.390	14			
24 hours (salt & turmeric)	Between Groups	.887	4	.222	443.620	.000(S)
	Within Groups	.005	10	.000		
	Total	.892	14			
48 hours (salt & turmeric)	Between Groups	1.346	4	.336	454.649	.000(S)
	Within Groups	.007	10	.001		
	Total	1.353	14			
14 days (salt & turmeric)	Between Groups	.417	4	.104	223.407	.000(S)
	Within Groups	.005	10	.000		
	Total	.422	14			
15 days (salt & turmeric)	Between Groups	12.412	4	3.103	6.465E3	.000(S)
	Within Groups	.005	10	.000		
	Total	12.417	14			
24 hours (KMS)	Between Groups	1.153	4	.288	393.145	.000(S)
	Within Groups	.007	10	.001		
	Total	1.161	14			
48 hours (KMS)	Between Groups	19.121	4	4.780	6.961E3	.000(S)
	Within Groups	.007	10	.001		
	Total	19.128	14			
14 days (KMS)	Between Groups	1.550	4	.388	375.006	.000(S)
	Within Groups	.010	10	.001		
	Total	1.560	14			
15 days (KMS)	Between Groups	2.732	4	.683	640.297	.000(S)
	Within Groups	.011	10	.001		
	Total	2.743	14			

$p<0.05$ S= Significant, NS= Non-significant. All abbreviations are on page so and so.

This statistical ANOVA table shows that all the values are significant, which means there is significant difference present in the values of iron content of pomfret among different cooking methods and the raw state in respect to fresh condition along with different preservation methods.

Table no 5.6.5.4 Post hoc Duncan statistical analysis

Preservation	Duration	Raw state	Boiling	Dry roasting	Shallow frying	Deep frying
Control	Fresh	B,O,S,D^{a}	R,O,S,D^{b}	R,B,S,D^{c}	R,B,O,D^{d}	R,B,O,S^{e}
Control	24 hours	B,O,S,D^{a}	R,O,S,D^{b}	R,B,S,D^{c}	R,B,O,D^{d}	R,B,O,S^{e}
Control	48 hours	B,O,S,D^{a}	R,O,S,D^{b}	R,B,S,D^{c}	R,B,O,D^{d}	R,B,O,S^{e}
Control	14 days	B,O,S,D^{a}	R,O,S,D^{b}	R,B,S,D^{c}	R,B,O^{f}	R,B,O^{f}
Control	15 days	B,O,S,D^{a}	R,O,S,D^{b}	R,B,S,D^{c}	R,B,O,D^{d}	R,B,O,S^{e}
Salt &Turmeric	24 hours	O,S,D^{g}	O,S,D^{g}	R,B,D^{h}	R,B,D^{h}	R,B,O,S^{e}
Salt & Turmeric	48 hours	B,O,S,D^{a}	R,O,S,D^{b}	R,B,D^{h}	R,B,D^{h}	R,B,O,S^{e}
Salt & Turmeric	14 days	B,O,S,D^{a}	R,O,S,D^{b}	R,B,S,D^{c}	R,B,O,D^{d}	R,B,O,S^{e}
Salt & Turmeric	15 days	B,O,S,D^{a}	R,O,S,D^{b}	R,B,S,D^{c}	R,B,O,D^{d}	R,B,O,S^{e}
KMS	24 hours	B,O,S,D^{a}	R,O,D^{i}	R,B,S,D^{c}	R,O,D^{i}	R,B,O,S^{e}
KMS	48 hours	B,O,S,D^{a}	R,O,S,D^{b}	R,B,S,D^{c}	R,B,O,D^{d}	R,B,O,S^{e}
KMS	14 days	B,O,S,D^{a}	R,O,S,D^{b}	R,B,S,D^{c}	R,B,O,D^{d}	R,B,O,S^{e}
KMS	15 days	B,O,S,D^{a}	R,S,D^{j}	R,S,D^{j}	R,B,O,D^{d}	R,B,O,S^{e}

R= Raw state, B= Boiling, O= Open pan dry roasting, S= Shallow frying, D= Deep frying. The same uppercase alphabets signify that there is no significant difference present among the variables.

This table shows the significant difference among the different variables such as cooking methods and preservation conditions. The raw state significantly differs from boiling, open pan dry roasting, shallow frying and deep frying in all of the preservation conditions with preservatives and control preservation without preservative except in 24 hours salt and turmeric preservation. Boiling significantly differs from the raw state, open pan dry roasting, shallow frying and deep frying in all the preservation conditions except in 24 hours salt and turmeric preservation as well as in 24 hours KMS preservation. Open pan dry roasting significantly differs from the raw state, boiling, shallow frying and deep frying in all the preservation conditions except in 24 hours, 48 hours salt and turmeric preservation and 15 days KMS preservation. Shallow frying significantly differs from the raw state, boiling, open pan dry roasting and deep frying in all of the preservation conditions except in fresh condition, 14 days control preservation and 24 hours, 48 hours salt and turmeric preservation and 24 hours KMS preservation. Deep frying significantly differs from the raw state, boiling, open pan dry roasting and shallow frying in all the preservation conditions except in 14 days control preservation without preservative.

Deep frying and shallow frying significantly differ from the raw state, boiling and open pan dry roasting in 14 days control preservation without preservative, whereas the raw state and boiling significantly differ from open pan dry roasting, shallow frying and deep frying in 24 hours salt and turmeric preservation. Open pan dry roasting and shallow frying significantly differ from the raw state, boiling and deep frying in 24 hours, 48 hours salt and turmeric preservation. Boiling and shallow frying significantly differ from the raw state, open pan dry roasting and deep frying in 24 hours KMS preservation. Boiling and open pan dry roasting significantly differ from the raw state, shallow frying and deep frying in 15 days KMS preservation.

Table no 5.6.5.5 Gradation of cooking methods from higher to lower restoration with respect to preservation days

Preservation	Duration	Method 1	Method 2	Method 3	Method 4	Method 5
Control	Fresh	DF	R	OPDR	B	SF
Control	24 hours	OPDR	R	SF	B	DF
Control	48 hours	DF	SF	OPDR	B	R
Control	14 days	R	B	DF	SF	OPDR
Control	15 days	OPDR	B	SF	DF	R
Salt &Turmeric	24 hours	B	R	SF	OPDR	DF
Salt & Turmeric	48 hours	B	R	DF	SF	OPDR
Salt & Turmeric	14 days	B	DF	R	SF	OPDR
Salt &Turmeric	15 days	R	B	DF	OPDR	SF
KMS	24 hours	OPDR	R	SF	B	DF
KMS	48 hours	R	DF	B	SF	OPDR
KMS	14 days	B	SF	R	DF	OPDR
KMS	15 days	SF	DF	B	OPDR	R

R= Raw state, B= Boiling, OPDR= Open pan dry roasting, SF= Shallow frying, DF= Deep frying. Same colour represents the similar order.

In all the preservation methods and fresh condition, iron retention occurs mainly in boiling than the other cooking methods. In fresh condition, retention occurs firstly in deep frying then the raw state, open pan dry roasting, boiling and shallow frying. In 24 hours control preservation without preservative and 24 hours KMS preservation, retention occurs in the order of open pan dry roasting followed by the raw state, shallow frying, boiling and deep frying. In 48 hours control preservation without preservative, the order of retention is deep frying, shallow frying, open pan dry roasting, boiling and the raw state. In 14 days control preservation without preservative, the order becomes the raw state, boiling, deep frying, shallow frying and open pan dry roasting. In 15 days control preservation without preservative, the order remains open pan dry roasting, boiling, shallow frying, deep frying and the raw state.

In 24 hours salt and turmeric preservation, retention occurs firstly in boiling then the raw state, shallow frying, open pan dry roasting and deep frying. In 48 hours salt and turmeric preservation, the order of retention becomes boiling, raw state, deep frying, shallow frying and open pan dry roasting. In 14 days salt and turmeric preservation, the order changes from boiling to deep frying, raw state, shallow frying and open pan dry roasting. In 15 days salt and turmeric preservation, the order remains the raw state, boiling, deep frying, open pan dry roasting and shallow frying.

In 48 hours KMS preservation, retention occurs firstly in the raw state followed by deep frying, boiling, shallow frying and open pan dry roasting. In 14 days KMS preservation, the order of retention becomes boiling, shallow frying, raw state, deep frying and open pan dry roasting. In 15 days KMS preservation, the order is shallow frying, deep frying, boiling, open pan dry roasting and the raw state.

The overall analysis of iron content of pomfret is mostly restored by the gradation of methods as boiling>raw state>deep frying>shallow frying> open pan dry roasting.

Boiling can restore some of the iron for using the iron pan as well as little amount of iron is eliminated due to the low solubility of iron in the cooking water, as the fatty tissues of pomfret possibly creates a barrier, so the iron cannot be eliminated[50]. Deep frying and shallow frying possibly cause the total dryness of pomfret as the fatty tissues get eliminated, reducing the iron content. Open pan dry roasting reduces iron more than the other cooking methods as the direct heat melts fatty tissues of pomfret and fats get eliminated along with iron. Thus among all the studied conventional cooking methods, **boiling** is the best method for pomfret to restore iron content.

5.6.6 *Hilsa* (*Tenualosa Ilisha*)

It has been reported that *hilsa* contains 2.1 mg of iron per 100 gm[84] in the raw state. This value changes due to the application of different cooking methods and preservation conditions (vide Table no **5.6.6.1**).

Table no 5.6.6.1 Iron content of *Hilsa* (mg/100gm)

Preservation	Duration	Raw state	Boiling	Dry roasting	Shallow frying	Deep frying
Control	Fresh	3.28±0.01	1.27±0.02	2.38±0.02	1.65±0.03	1.82±0.05
Control	24 hours	3.24±0.04	1.74±0.04	3.22±0.02	2.98±0.03	3.48±0.02
Control	48 hours	1.85±0.02	1.72±0.02	0.87±0.02	1.78±0.02	1.95±0.03
Control	14 days	1.55±0.04	2.55±0.03	2.06±0.04	2.11±0.03	1.52±0.03
Control	15 days	1.56±0.03	2.55±0.03	3.52±0.02	2.56±0.03	2.54±0.04
Salt & Turmeric	24 hours	1.62±0.02	1.57±0.01	1.92±0.02	1.92±0.02	2.42±0.02
Salt & Turmeric	48 hours	1.72±0.02	0.84±0.04	0.92±0.02	1.12±0.02	0.52±0.02
Salt & Turmeric	14 days	1.24±0.04	1.34±0.04	2.22±0.02	0.92±0.02	1.02±0.02
Salt & Turmeric	15 days	1.02±0.02	1.27±0.02	1.02±0.02	1.82±0.02	1.02±0.02
KMS	24 hours	0.77±0.02	1.17±0.02	1.31±0.03	1.43±0.04	1.52±0.02
KMS	48 hours	1.32±0.02	1.67±0.02	1.32±0.02	0.93±0.04	0.73±0.04
KMS	14 days	1.82±0.02	1.22±0.02	0.77±0.02	2.14±0.04	0.73±0.04
KMS	15 days	1.22±0.02	1.04±0.04	1.67±0.02	2.34±0.04	1.08±0.02

Values are expressed as mean±SD. Loss Restoration
Red digits represent the significant highest values from the raw state in different conditions.

In most of the conditions, iron content is mainly reduced by boiling, whereas in 14 days, 15 days control preservation without preservative, 48 hours, 15 days salt and turmeric preservation and 14 days KMS preservation, iron content is reduced by deep frying and in 48 hours control preservation without preservative and 15 days salt and turmeric preservation, iron content is reduced by open pan dry roasting. In 14 days salt and turmeric preservation, iron content is reduced by shallow frying.

Retention of iron content occurs by deep frying[66] mostly, but in 14 days control preservation without preservative and 48 hours KMS preservation, iron retention occurs by boiling, whereas in fresh condition, 15 days control preservation without preservative and 14 days salt and turmeric preservation, iron retention occurs by open pan dry roasting. In 48 hours, 15 days salt and turmeric preservation and 14 days, 15 days KMS preservation, iron retention occurs by shallow frying.

Boiling, open pan dry roasting and shallow frying show the highest iron content in 15 days control preservation without preservative, whereas deep frying shows the highest iron content in 24 hours control preservation without preservative and the raw state shows the highest iron content in fresh condition.

Boiling shows the increased iron content than the raw value in fresh condition, 14 days, 15 days control preservation without preservative and 14 days, 15 days salt and turmeric preservation and 24 hours, 48 hours KMS preservation. Open pan dry roasting shows the increased iron content than the raw state in 14 days, 15 days control preservation without preservative and 24 hours, 14 days salt and turmeric preservation as well as 24 hours, 15 days KMS preservation, whereas shallow frying also shows the increased iron content than the raw value in 14 days, 15 days control preservation without preservative, 24 hours, 15 days salt and turmeric preservation and 24 hours, 14 days, 15 days KMS preservation. Deep frying shows the increased iron content than the raw state in 24 hours, 48 hours, 15 days control preservation without preservative and 24 hours salt and turmeric preservation as well as 24 hours KMS preservation.

The possible reason may be due to the molecular rearrangement during cooking and the addition of cooking oil during frying. It may also be possible that the elimination of water during cooking[48] concentrates the iron content. Another possible reason for increasing iron content is due to the use of iron pan for cooking as iron absorption occurs by *hilsa* from the iron pan.

Fig. 5.6.6.2 Graphical representation of Iron content of *Hilsa* with respect to different conditions

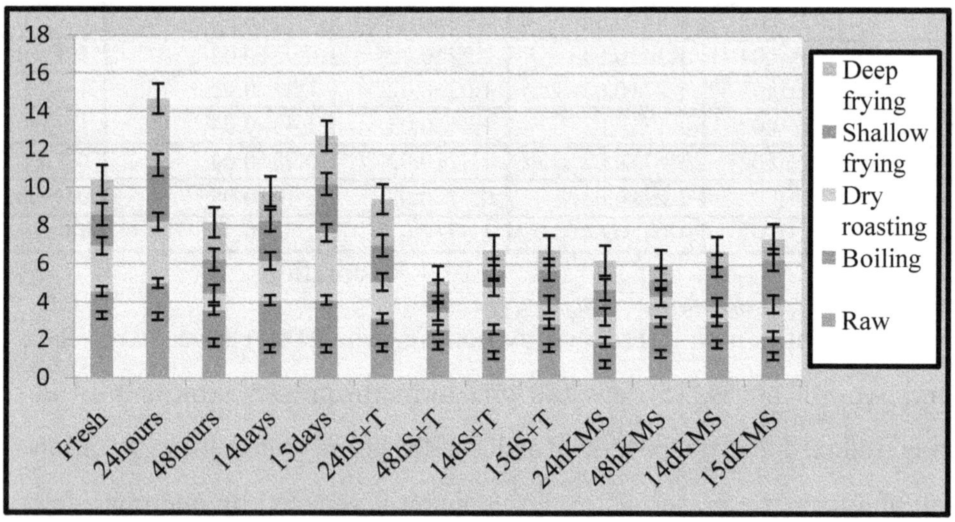

This graphical representation indicates that among all the preservation conditions, **24 hours control preservation without preservative** helps to increase the iron content in all the cooking methods. The possible reason may be that the preservation can hamper the iron content as it is very vulnerable mineral. Here the graph shows that the control preservation without preservative is more effective as compared to the salt-turmeric and KMS preservation.

Table no 5.6.6.3 ANOVA with regard to cooking conditions and preservation methods

Condition	Differences	Sum of Squares	df	Mean Square	F	Sig.
Fresh (control)	Between Groups	7.266	4	1.817	1.662E3	.000(S)
	Within Groups	.011	10	.001		
	Total	7.277	14			
24 hours (control)	Between Groups	5.717	4	1.429	1.056E3	.000(S)
	Within Groups	.014	10	.001		
	Total	5.731	14			
48 hours (control)	Between Groups	2.301	4	.575	837.680	.000(S)
	Within Groups	.007	10	.001		
	Total	2.308	14			
14 days (control)	Between Groups	2.213	4	.553	397.069	.000(S)
	Within Groups	.014	10	.001		
	Total	2.227	14			
15 days (control)	Between Groups	5.783	4	1.446	1.218E3	.000(S)
	Within Groups	.012	10	.001		
	Total	5.795	14			
24 hours (salt & turmeric)	Between Groups	1.491	4	.373	673.422	.000(S)
	Within Groups	.006	10	.001		
	Total	1.496	14			
48 hours (salt & turmeric)	Between Groups	2.385	4	.596	805.797	.000(S)
	Within Groups	.007	10	.001		
	Total	2.393	14			
14 days (salt & turmeric)	Between Groups	3.189	4	.797	771.445	.000(S)
	Within Groups	.010	10	.001		
	Total	3.199	14			
15 days (salt & turmeric)	Between Groups	1.447	4	.362	571.116	.000(S)
	Within Groups	.006	10	.001		
	Total	1.453	14			
24 hours (KMS)	Between Groups	1.023	4	.256	259.331	.000(S)
	Within Groups	.010	10	.001		
	Total	1.033	14			
48 hours (KMS)	Between Groups	1.640	4	.410	381.873	.000(S)
	Within Groups	.011	10	.001		
	Total	1.650	14			
14 days (KMS)	Between Groups	4.734	4	1.183	1.124E3	.000(S)
	Within Groups	.011	10	.001		
	Total	4.744	14			
15 days (KMS)	Between Groups	3.601	4	.900	860.127	.000(S)
	Within Groups	.010	10	.001		
	Total	3.612	14			

$p<0.05$ S= Significant, NS= Non-significant. All abbreviations are on page so and so.

This statistical ANOVA table shows that all the values are significant, which means there is significant difference present in the values of iron content of *hilsa* among different cooking methods and the raw state in respect to fresh condition along with different preservation methods.

Table no 5.6.6.4 Post hoc Duncan statistical analysis

Preservation	Duration	Raw state	Boiling	Dry roasting	Shallow frying	Deep frying
Control	Fresh	B,O,S,D^{a}	R,O,S,D^{b}	R,B,S,D^{c}	R,B,O,D^{d}	R,B,O,S^{e}
Control	24 hours	B,S,D^{f}	R,O,S,D^{b}	B,S,D^{f}	R,B,O,D^{d}	R,B,O,S^{e}
Control	48 hours	B,O,S,D^{a}	R,O,S,D^{b}	R,B,S,D^{c}	R,B,O,D^{d}	R,B,O,S^{e}
Control	14 days	B,O,S^{g}	R,O,S,D^{b}	R,B,D^{h}	R,B,D^{h}	B,O,S^{g}
Control	15 days	B,O,S,D^{a}	R,O^{i}	R,B,S,D^{c}	R,O^{i}	R,O^{i}
Salt & Turmeric	24 hours	B,O,S,D^{a}	R,O,S,D^{b}	R,B,D^{h}	R,B,D^{h}	R,B,O,S^{e}
Salt & Turmeric	48 hours	B,O,S,D^{a}	R,O,S,D^{b}	R,B,S,D^{c}	R,B,O,D^{d}	R,B,O,S^{e}
Salt & Turmeric	14 days	B,O,S,D^{a}	R,O,S,D^{b}	R,B,S,D^{c}	R,B,O,D^{d}	R,B,O,S^{e}
Salt & Turmeric	15 days	B,S^{j}	R,O,S,D^{b}	B,S^{j}	R,B,O,D^{d}	B,S^{j}
KMS	24 hours	B,O,S,D^{a}	R,O,S,D^{b}	R,B,S,D^{c}	R,B,O,D^{d}	R,B,O,S^{e}
KMS	48 hours	B,S,D^{f}	R,O,S,D^{b}	B,S,D^{f}	R,B,O,D^{d}	R,B,O,S^{e}
KMS	14 days	B,O,S,D^{a}	R,O,S,D^{b}	R,B,S^{k}	R,B,O,D^{d}	R,B,S^{k}
KMS	15 days	B,O,S,D^{a}	R,O,S^{l}	R,B,S,D^{c}	R,B,O,D^{d}	R,O,S^{l}

R= Raw state, B= Boiling, O= Open pan dry roasting, S= Shallow frying, D= Deep frying. The same uppercase alphabets signify that there is no significant difference present among the variables.

This table shows the significant difference among the different variables such as cooking methods and preservation conditions. The raw state significantly differs from boiling, open pan dry roasting, shallow frying and deep frying in all of the preservation conditions with preservatives and control preservation without preservative except in 24 hours, 14 days control preservation without preservative, 15 days salt and turmeric preservation as well as 48 hours KMS preservation. Boiling significantly differs from the raw state, open pan dry roasting, shallow frying and deep frying in all of the preservation conditions except in 15 days control preservation without preservative as well as 15 days KMS preservation. Open pan dry roasting significantly differs from the raw state, boiling, shallow frying and deep frying in all the preservation conditions except in 24 hours, 14 days control preservation without preservative, 24 hours, 15 days salt and turmeric preservation and 48 hours, 14 days KMS preservation. Shallow frying significantly differs from the raw state, boiling, open pan dry roasting and deep frying in all of the preservation conditions except in fresh condition, 14 days, 15 days control preservation without preservative and 24 hours salt and turmeric preservation. Deep frying significantly differs from the raw state, boiling, open pan dry roasting and shallow frying in all of the preservation conditions except in 14 days, 15 days control preservation without preservative, 15 days salt and turmeric preservation and 14 days KMS preservation.

The raw state and open pan dry roasting significantly differ from boiling, shallow frying and deep frying in 24 hours control preservation without preservative. Deep frying and the raw state significantly differ from boiling, open pan dry roasting and shallow frying in 14 days control preservation without preservative, whereas open pan dry roasting and shallow frying significantly differ from the raw state, boiling and deep frying in 14 days control preservation without preservative and 24 hours salt and turmeric preservation. Boiling, shallow frying and deep frying significantly differ from the raw state, open pan dry roasting in 15 days control preservation without preservative. The raw state, open pan dry roasting and deep frying significantly differ from boiling and shallow frying in 15 days salt and turmeric preservation. Deep frying and open pan dry roasting significantly differ from the raw state, boiling and shallow frying in 14 days

KMS preservation. Boiling and deep frying significantly differ from the raw state, open pan dry roasting and shallow frying in 15 days KMS preservation.

Table no 5.6.6.5 Gradation of cooking methods from higher to lower restoration with respect to preservation days

Preservation	Duration	Method 1	Method 2	Method 3	Method 4	Method 5
Control	Fresh	R	OPDR	DF	SF	B
Control	24 hours	DF	R	OPDR	SF	B
Control	48 hours	DF	R	SF	B	OPDR
Control	14 days	B	SF	OPDR	R	DF
Control	15 days	OPDR	SF	B	DF	R
Salt & Turmeric	24 hours	DF	SF	OPDR	R	B
Salt & Turmeric	48 hours	R	SF	OPDR	B	DF
Salt & Turmeric	14 days	OPDR	B	R	DF	SF
Salt &Turmeric	15 days	SF	B	DF	OPDR	R
KMS	24 hours	DF	SF	OPDR	B	R
KMS	48 hours	B	OPDR	R	SF	DF
KMS	14 days	SF	R	B	OPDR	DF
KMS	15 days	SF	OPDR	R	DF	B

R= Raw state, B= Boiling, OPDR= Open pan dry roasting, SF= Shallow frying, DF= Deep frying.

In all the preservation methods and fresh condition, iron retention occurs mainly by deep frying than the other cooking methods. In fresh condition, retention occurs firstly in the raw state followed by open pan dry roasting, deep frying, shallow frying and boiling. In 24 hours control preservation without preservative, the order of retention is deep frying, raw state, open pan dry roasting, shallow frying and boiling. In 48 hours control preservation without preservative, the order is deep frying, raw state, shallow frying, boiling and open pan dry roasting. In 14 days control preservation without preservative, the order becomes boiling, shallow frying, open pan dry roasting, raw state and deep frying. In 15 days control preservation without preservative, retention changes in the order of open pan dry roasting, shallow frying, boiling, deep frying and the raw state.

In 24 hours salt and turmeric preservation, retention occurs firstly in deep frying followed by shallow frying, open pan dry roasting, the raw state and boiling. In 48 hours salt and turmeric preservation, the order is boiling followed by the raw state, shallow frying, open pan dry roasting, boiling and deep frying. In 14 days salt and turmeric preservation, retention occurs in the order of open pan dry roasting, boiling, raw state, deep frying and shallow frying. In 15 days salt and turmeric preservation, the order becomes shallow frying, boiling, deep frying, open pan dry roasting and the raw state.

In 24 hours KMS preservation, retention occurs firstly in deep frying then shallow frying, open pan dry roasting, boiling and the raw state. In 48 hours KMS preservation, the order is boiling, open pan dry roasting, raw state, shallow frying, and deep frying. In 14 days KMS preservation, the order becomes shallow frying, raw state, boiling, open pan dry roasting and deep frying. In 15 days KMS preservation, the order of retention changes from shallow frying to open pan dry roasting, raw state, deep frying, boiling.

The overall analysis of iron content of *hilsa* is mostly restored by the gradation of methods as deep frying>shallow frying> open pan dry roasting>raw state>boiling.

Deep frying and shallow frying[66] possibly create a layer of fat surrounding *hilsa* and it also contains more fatty tissues than pomfret, thus iron possibly cannot be eliminated and content can be restored[50]. Open pan dry roasting reduces iron content as the direct heat possibly melts fatty tissues of *hilsa* and fats get eliminated along with iron. Boiling can reduce some of the iron as it is soluble in the cooking water and can be eliminated if the cooking water is discarded. Thus among all the studied conventional cooking methods, **deep frying** is the best method for *hilsa* to restore iron content.

5.7 Calcium content

It has been reported that generally fish contains 47.3-650 mg of calcium[86] in the raw state. This experiment is carried out to estimate the percentage of calcium content and also the changes of it in different cooking and preservation methods among different fish and edible aquatic species. Calcium content is estimated by AOAC method[71].

5.7.1 *Rohu* (*Labeo rohita*)

It has been reported that *rohu* contains 650 mg of calcium per 100 gm[84] in the raw condition. This value changes due to the application of different cooking methods and preservation conditions (vide Table no **5.7.1.1**).

Table no 5.7.1.1 Calcium content of *Rohu* (mg/100gm)

Preservation	Duration	Raw state	Boiling	Dry roasting	Shallow frying	Deep frying
Control	Fresh	161.02±1.00	172.03±2.51	271.06±1.00	202.09±2.64	434.12±4.04
Control	24 hours	186.10±1.52	131.02±1.00	152.15.±2.51	149.22±1.04	202.05±2.64
Control	48 hours	223.04±2.08	106.06±1.52	121.10±1.00	352.15±2.64	431.26±2.08
Control	14 days	121.01±1.00	231.03±1.00	216.09±1.52	182.29±1.52	232.18±2.00
Control	15 days	402.82±2.64	296.15±2.64	242.17±3.05	305.09±4.00	401.10±1.52
Salt & Turmeric	24 hours	123.34±4.16	156.45±1.52	267.87±2.51	67.46±2.51	217.66±2.51
Salt &Turmeric	48 hours	182.10±2.51	98.29±2.64	152.10±2.00	122.47±2.00	62.97±2.57
Salt & Turmeric	14 days	52.09±2.51	233.18±4.10	55.10±3.00	42.15±2.00	242.24±2.51
Salt & Turmeric	15 days	35.37±2.51	55.08±2.64	55.08±2.64	57.09±2.51	44.10±1.00
KMS	24 hours	42.18±2.00	434.28±2.00	45.38±2.08	552.10±2.00	804.10±4.04
KMS	48 hours	214.27±4.04	56.19±1.52	195.25±3.00	51.87±1.00	38.32±1.52
KMS	14 days	332.18±2.51	227.22±2.51	104.44±4.16	302.56±2.51	151.98±1.52
KMS	15 days	29.35±2.08	35.78±2.08	26.10±1.52	442.54±2.51	332.34±2.51

Values are expressed as mean±SD. ☐ Loss ☐ Restoration

Red digits represent the significant highest values from the raw state in different conditions.

In most of the conditions, calcium content is mainly reduced by open pan dry roasting, whereas in fresh condition, 24 hours, 48 hours control preservation without preservative, calcium content is reduced by boiling. In 14 days control preservation without preservative and 24 hours, 14 days salt and turmeric preservation, calcium content is reduced by shallow frying. In 48 hours, 15 days salt and turmeric preservation as well as 48 hours preservation, calcium content is reduced by deep frying.

Retention of calcium content occurs by deep frying mostly, but in 24 hours, 48 hours salt and turmeric preservation and 48 hours KMS preservation, calcium retention occurs by open pan dry roasting, whereas in 15 days salt and turmeric preservation and 14 days, 15 days KMS preservation, calcium retention occurs by shallow frying.

Boiling, shallow frying and deep frying show the highest calcium content in 24 hours KMS preservation, whereas open pan dry roasting shows the highest calcium content in fresh condition and the raw state shows the highest iron content in 15 days control preservation without preservative.

Boiling shows the increased calcium content than the raw value in fresh condition, 14 days control preservation without preservative and 24 hours, 14 days, 15 days salt and turmeric preservation and 24 hours, 15 days KMS preservation. Open pan dry roasting shows the increased calcium content than the raw value in fresh condition, 14 days control preservation without preservative and 24 hours, 14 days, 15 days salt and turmeric preservation and 24 hours KMS preservation, whereas shallow frying also shows the increased calcium content than the raw state in fresh condition, 48 hours, 14 days control preservation without preservative and 15 days salt and turmeric preservation as well as 24 hours, 15 days KMS preservation. Deep frying shows the increased calcium content than the raw value in all the preservation conditions except in 15 days control preservation without preservative and 48 hours salt and turmeric preservation as well as 48 hours, 14 days KMS preservation.

This may occur due to the molecular rearrangement during cooking and the addition of cooking oil during frying. Another possible reason may be the elimination of water during cooking[48] that concentrates the amount of calcium. Another possible reason for increasing calcium content is due to the elimination of anti-nutritional factors due to cooking. Addition of both the natural and synthetic preservatives possibly helps to modify the calcium content.

Fig. 5.7.1.2 Graphical representation of Calcium content of *Rohu* with respect to different conditions

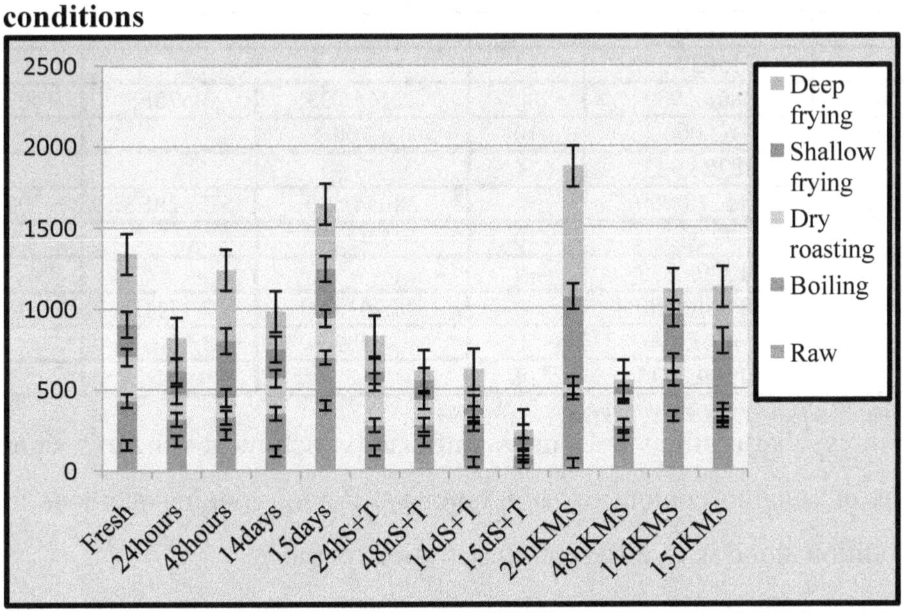

This graphical representation indicates that among all the preservation conditions, **24 hours KMS preservation** helps to increase the calcium content in all the cooking methods. The possible reason may be the effectiveness of KMS to restore the calcium content. Here the graph shows that the control preservation without preservative is also effective, but salt and turmeric preservation is not very much effective to restore calcium content in *rohu*. It is also possible that KMS can modify the molecular structure of calcium, increasing the calcium content. The possible reason may be the synthetic preservative helps to modify the structure of calcium, restoring the content.

Table no 5.7.1.3 ANOVA with regard to cooking conditions and preservation methods

Condition	Differences	Sum of Squares	df	Mean Square	F	Sig.
Fresh (control)	Between Groups	130498.400	4	32624.600	5.151E3	.000(S)
	Within Groups	63.333	10	6.333		
	Total	130561.733	14			
24 hours (control)	Between Groups	10199.600	4	2549.900	721.670	.000(S)
	Within Groups	35.333	10	3.533		
	Total	10234.933	14			
48 hours (control)	Between Groups	250410.000	4	62602.500	1.647E4	.000(S)
	Within Groups	38.000	10	3.800		
	Total	250448.000	14			
14 days (control)	Between Groups	26322.000	4	6580.500	3.085E3	.000(S)
	Within Groups	21.333	10	2.133		
	Total	26343.333	14			
15 days (control)	Between Groups	59180.400	4	14795.100	1.775E3	.000(S)
	Within Groups	83.333	10	8.333		
	Total	59263.733	14			
24 hours (salt & turmeric)	Between Groups	73762.400	4	18440.600	2.385E3	.000(S)
	Within Groups	77.333	10	7.733		
	Total	73839.733	14			
48 hours (salt & turmeric)	Between Groups	26002.000	4	6500.500	1.175E3	.000(S)
	Within Groups	55.333	10	5.533		
	Total	26057.333	14			
14 days (salt & turmeric)	Between Groups	127718.000	4	31929.500	3.713E3	.000(S)
	Within Groups	86.000	10	8.600		
	Total	127804.000	14			
15 days (salt & turmeric)	Between Groups	1074.267	4	268.567	48.536	.000(S)
	Within Groups	55.333	10	5.533		
	Total	1129.600	14			
24 hours (KMS)	Between Groups	1315571.333	4	328892.833	4.983E4	.000(S)
	Within Groups	66.000	10	6.600		
	Total	1315637.333	14			
48 hours (KMS)	Between Groups	88662.933	4	22165.733	3.575E3	.000(S)
	Within Groups	62.000	10	6.200		
	Total	88724.933	14			
14 days (KMS)	Between Groups	112218.000	4	28054.500	3.628E3	.000(S)
	Within Groups	77.333	10	7.733		
	Total	112295.333	14			
15 days (KMS)	Between Groups	411046.400	4	102761.600	2.171E4	.000(S)
	Within Groups	47.333	10	4.733		
	Total	411093.733	14			

$p<0.05$ S= Significant, NS= Non-significant. All abbreviations are on page so and so.

This statistical ANOVA table shows that all the values are significant, which means there is significant difference present in the values of calcium content of *rohu* among different cooking methods and the raw state in respect to fresh condition along with different preservation methods.

Table no 5.7.1.4 Post hoc Duncan statistical analysis

Preservation	Duration	Raw state	Boiling	Dry roasting	Shallow frying	Deep frying
Control	Fresh	B,O,S,D^{a}	R,S,D^{b}	R,S,D^{b}	R,B,O,D^{c}	R,B,O,S^{d}
Control	24 hours	B,O,S,D^{a}	R,O,S,D^{e}	R,B,S,D^{f}	R,B,O,D^{c}	R,B,O,S^{d}
Control	48 hours	B,O,S,D^{a}	R,O,S,D^{e}	R,B,S,D^{f}	R,B,O,D^{c}	R,B,O,S^{d}
Control	14 days	B,O,S,D^{a}	R,O,S^{g}	R,B,S,D^{f}	R,B,O,D^{c}	R,O,S^{g}
Control	15 days	B,O,S^{h}	R,O,S,D^{e}	R,B,S,D^{f}	R,B,O,D^{c}	B,O,S^{h}
Salt & Turmeric	24 hours	B,O,S,D^{a}	R,O,S,D^{e}	R,B,S,D^{f}	R,B,O,D^{c}	R,B,O,S^{d}
Salt & Turmeric	48 hours	B,O,S,D^{a}	R,O,S,D^{e}	R,B,S,D^{f}	R,B,O,D^{c}	R,B,O,S^{d}
Salt & Turmeric	14 days	B,S,D^{i}	R,O,S,D^{e}	B,S,D^{i}	R,B,O,D^{c}	R,B,O,S^{d}
Salt & Turmeric	15days	B,O,S,D^{a}	R,D^{j}	R,D^{j}	R,D^{j}	R,B,O,S^{d}
KMS	24 hours	B,S,D^{i}	R,O,S,D^{e}	B,S,D^{i}	R,B,O,D^{c}	R,B,O,S^{d}
KMS	48 hours	B,O,S,D^{a}	R,O,S,D^{e}	R,B,S,D^{f}	R,B,O,D^{c}	R,B,O,S^{d}
KMS	14days	B,O,S,D^{a}	R,O,S,D^{e}	R,B,S,D^{f}	R,B,O,D^{c}	R,B,O,S^{d}
KMS	15days	B,O,S,D^{a}	R,O,S,D^{e}	R,B,S,D^{f}	R,B,O,D^{c}	R,B,O,S^{d}

R= Raw state, B= Boiling, O= Open pan dry roasting, S= Shallow frying, D= Deep frying. The same uppercase alphabets represent that there is no significant difference present among the variables.

This table shows the significant difference among the different variables such as cooking methods and preservation conditions. The raw state significantly differs from boiling, open pan dry roasting, shallow frying and deep frying in all of the preservation conditions with preservatives and control preservation without preservative except in 15 days control preservation without preservative, 14 days salt and turmeric preservation and 24 hours KMS preservation. Boiling significantly differs from the raw state, open pan dry roasting, shallow frying and deep frying in all the preservation conditions except in fresh condition, 14 days control preservation without preservative as well as 15 days salt and turmeric preservation. Open pan dry roasting significantly differs from the raw state, boiling, shallow frying and deep frying in all the preservation conditions except in fresh condition, 14 days, 15 days salt and turmeric preservation. Shallow frying significantly differs from the raw state, boiling, open pan dry roasting and deep frying in all the preservation conditions except in 15 days salt and turmeric preservation. Deep frying significantly differs from the raw state, boiling, open pan dry roasting and shallow frying in all the preservation conditions except in 14 days, 15 days control preservation without preservative.

Boiling and open pan dry roasting significantly differ from the raw state, shallow frying and deep frying in fresh condition. Deep frying and boiling significantly differs from the raw state, open pan dry roasting and shallow frying in 14 days control preservation without preservative, whereas the raw state and deep frying significantly differ from boiling, open pan dry roasting and shallow frying in 15 days control preservation without preservative. The raw state and open pan dry roasting significantly differ from boiling, shallow frying and deep frying in 14 days salt and turmeric preservation and 24 hours KMS preservation. Boiling, open pan dry roasting and shallow frying significantly differ from the raw state and deep frying in 15 days salt and turmeric preservation.

Table no 5.7.1.5 Gradation of cooking methods from higher to lower restoration with respect to preservation days

Preservation	Duration	Method 1	Method 2	Method 3	Method 4	Method 5
Control	Fresh	DF	B	OPDR	SF	R
Control	24 hours	DF	R	OPDR	SF	B
Control	48 hours	DF	SF	R	OPDR	B
Control	14 days	DF	B	OPDR	SF	R
Control	15 days	R	DF	SF	B	OPDR
Salt & Turmeric	24 hours	OPDR	DF	B	R	SF
Salt & Turmeric	48 hours	R	OPDR	SF	B	DF
Salt & Turmeric	14 days	DF	B	OPDR	R	SF
Salt &Turmeric	15 days	SF	OPDR	B	DF	R
KMS	24 hours	DF	SF	B	OPDR	R
KMS	48 hours	R	OPDR	B	SF	DF
KMS	14 days	R	SF	B	DF	OPDR
KMS	15 days	SF	DF	R	B	OPDR

R= Raw state, B= Boiling, OPDR= Open pan dry roasting, SF= Shallow frying, DF= Deep frying. Same colour represents the similar order.

In all the preservation techniques and fresh condition, calcium retention occurs mainly by deep frying than the other cooking methods. In fresh condition and 14 days control preservation without preservative, retention occurs firstly in deep frying followed by boiling, open pan dry roasting, shallow frying and the raw state. In 24 hours control preservation without preservative, retention occurs in the order of deep frying, raw state, open pan dry roasting, shallow frying and boiling. In 48 hours control preservation without preservative, the order of retention is deep frying, shallow frying, raw state, open pan dry roasting, boiling. In 15 days control preservation without preservative, the order changes from the raw state to deep frying, shallow frying, boiling and open pan dry roasting.

In 24 hours salt and turmeric preservation, retention occurs firstly in open pan dry roasting followed by deep frying, boiling, raw state and shallow frying. In 48 hours salt and turmeric preservation, the order of retention is the raw state, open pan dry roasting, shallow frying, boiling and deep frying. In 14 days salt and turmeric preservation, the order becomes deep frying, boiling, open pan dry roasting, raw state and shallow frying. In 15 days salt and turmeric preservation, the order changes from shallow frying to open pan dry roasting, boiling, deep frying and the raw state.

In 24 hours KMS preservation, retention occurs firstly in deep frying then shallow frying, boiling, open pan dry roasting and the raw state. In 48 hours KMS preservation, retention occurs in the order of the raw state, open pan dry roasting, boiling, shallow frying and deep frying. In 14 days KMS preservation, the order becomes the raw state, shallow frying, boiling, deep frying and open pan dry roasting. In 15 days KMS preservation, the order is shallow frying, deep frying, raw state, boiling and open pan dry roasting.

The overall analysis of calcium content of *rohu* is mostly restored by the gradation of methods as deep frying> boiling> open pan dry roasting>shallow frying>raw state.

Deep frying possibly creates a fatty layer surrounding *rohu*, thus calcium cannot be eliminated and its content can be restored[66]. Boiling can reduce some of the calcium possibly as it is soluble in the cooking water and can be eliminated if the water is discarded. Open pan dry roasting reduces calcium content possibly as the direct heat melts fatty tissues of the fish and fats get eliminated along with calcium. Shallow frying reduces calcium content possibly as frying oil is unable to cover the surface area of the fish flesh, so the protective layer becomes very weak, eliminating calcium from the fish. Thus among all the studied conventional cooking methods, **deep frying** is the best method for *rohu* to restore calcium content.

5.7.2 *Katla* (*Catla catla*)

It has been reported that *katla* contains 530 mg of calcium per 100 gm[84] in the raw state. This value changes due to the application of different cooking methods and preservation conditions (vide Table no **5.7.2.1**).

Table no 5.7.2.1 Calcium content of *Katla* (mg/100gm)

Preservation	Duration	Raw state	Boiling	Dry roasting	Shallow frying	Deep frying
Control	Fresh	152.11±2.51	62.22±2.51	152.43±2.64	145.29±4.61	152.35±2.00
Control	24 hours	96.09±1.52	127.10±2.08	122.10±2.51	72.35±2.51	136.16±1.52
Control	48 hours	322.07±2.51	278.04±2.64	288.10±2.64	272.11±2.51	362.13±2.51
Control	14 days	52.26±2.51	301.17±1.00	66.16±1.52	203.28±3.21	531.13±1.00
Control	15 days	171.28±1.00	136.37±1.52	203.56±3.21	602.78±2.51	402.97±2.64
Salt & Turmeric	24 hours	172.24±2.51	165.22±3.00	382.67±2.51	151.93±1.52	92.26±2.00
Salt &Turmeric	48 hours	105.19±4.04	111.22±1.00	132.34±2.51	251.45±1.52	142.46±1.52
Salt & Turmeric	14 days	182.66±2.51	432.24±2.51	122.36±2.51	481.16±1.57	235.22±3.00
Salt & Turmeric	15 days	252.36±2.51	207.27±1.00	44.93±1.00	492.44±2.50	62.04±2.08
KMS	24 hours	142.67±2.00	192.03±2.51	342.05±2.51	182.17±2.00	162.49±2.00
KMS	48 hours	352.22±2.52	652.44±2.00	182.77±2.00	102.86±2.00	122.57±2.00
KMS	14 days	152.22±2.00	195.46±3.00	117.03±2.08	106.28±1.52	112.14±2.00
KMS	15 days	451.03±1.52	202.05±2.00	276.16±1.52	201.38±1.52	115.11±0.57

Values are expressed as mean±SD. ☐ Loss ▨ Restoration

Red digits represent the significant highest values from the raw state in different conditions.

In most of the conditions, calcium content is mainly reduced by shallow frying, whereas in fresh condition, 15 days control preservation without preservative and 48 hours salt and turmeric preservation, calcium content is reduced by boiling. In 14 days control preservation without preservative and 14 days, 15 days salt and turmeric preservation, calcium content is reduced by open pan dry roasting. In 24 hours salt and turmeric preservation, calcium content is reduced by deep frying.

Retention of calcium content occurs by deep frying mostly, but in 48 hours, 14 days KMS preservation, calcium retention occurs by boiling, whereas in fresh condition, 24 hours salt and turmeric preservation and 24 hours, 15 days KMS preservation, calcium retention occurs by open pan dry roasting. In 15 days control preservation without preservative and 48 hours, 14 days, 15 days salt and turmeric preservation, calcium retention occurs by shallow frying.

The raw state and boiling show the highest calcium content in 48 hours KMS preservation, whereas open pan dry roasting shows the highest calcium content in 24 hours KMS preservation. Shallow frying and deep frying show the highest calcium content in 15 days control preservation without preservative and 14 days control preservation without preservative respectively.

Boiling shows the increased calcium content than the raw state in 24 hours, 14 days control preservation without preservative and 48 hours, 14 days salt and turmeric preservation and 24 hours, 48 hours, 14 days KMS preservation. Open pan dry roasting shows the increased calcium content than the raw state in fresh condition, 24 hours, 14 days, 15 days control preservation without preservative and 24 hours, 48 hours salt and turmeric preservation and 24 hours KMS preservation, whereas shallow frying also shows the increased calcium content than the raw state in 14 days, 15 days control preservation without preservative and 48 hours, 14 days, 15 days salt and turmeric preservation and 24 hours KMS preservation. Deep frying shows the increased calcium content than the raw state in all of the preservation conditions except in 24 hours, 15 days salt and turmeric preservation as well as 48 hours, 14 days, 15 days KMS preservation.

This may occur due to the molecular rearrangement during cooking and the addition of cooking oil during frying. Another possible reason may be the elimination of water during cooking[48] that concentrates the calcium content. Additionally the calcium content is increased possibly due to the elimination of anti-nutritional factors during cooking. Addition of both the natural and synthetic preservatives can also be a possible cause for the modification of calcium content.

Fig. 5.7.2.2 Graphical representation of Calcium content of *Katla* with respect to different conditions

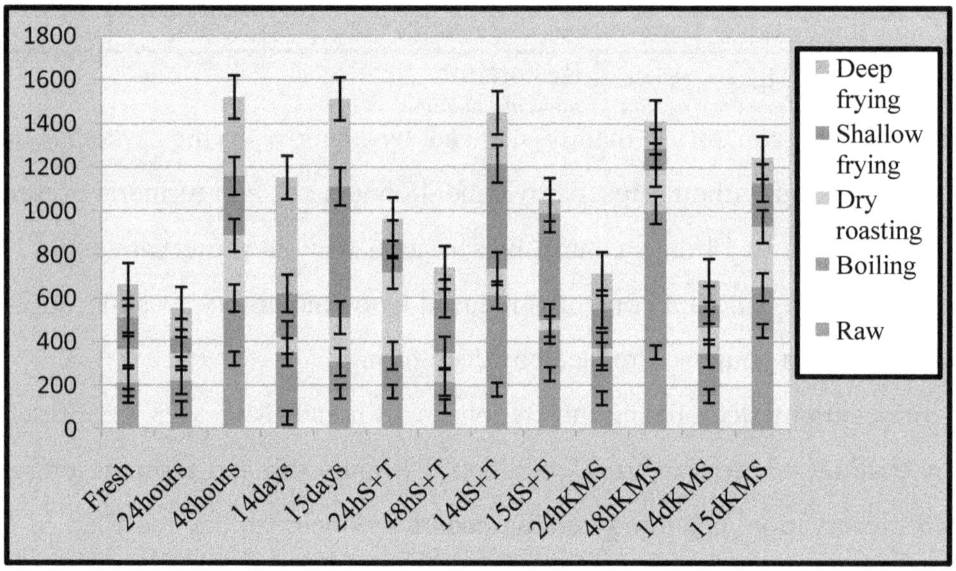

This graphical representation indicates that among all the preservation conditions, **48 hours and 15 days control preservation** without preservative help to increase the calcium content in all the cooking methods. Here the graph shows that the control preservation without preservative is effective, but salt-turmeric and KMS preservations are not very much effective to restore calcium content in *katla*. As calcium is vulnerable mineral, thus the content reduced due to the preservation with preservatives.

Table no 5.7.2.3 ANOVA with regard to cooking conditions and preservation methods

Condition	Differences	Sum of Squares	df	Mean Square	F	Sig.
Fresh (control)	Between Groups	18724.400	4	4681.100	520.122	.000(S)
	Within Groups	90.000	10	9.000		
	Total	18814.400	14			
24 hours (control)	Between Groups	8212.667	4	2053.167	473.808	.000(S)
	Within Groups	43.333	10	4.333		
	Total	8256.000	14			
48 hours (control)	Between Groups	17015.600	4	4253.900	644.530	.000(S)
	Within Groups	66.000	10	6.600		
	Total	17081.600	14			
14 days (control)	Between Groups	464051.733	4	116012.933	2.762E4	.000(S)
	Within Groups	42.000	10	4.200		
	Total	464093.733	14			
15 days (control)	Between Groups	464009.733	4	116002.433	2.148E4	.000(S)
	Within Groups	54.000	10	5.400		
	Total	464063.733	14			
24 hours (salt & turmeric)	Between Groups	146901.333	4	36725.333	6.558E3	.000(S)
	Within Groups	56.000	10	5.600		
	Total	146957.333	14			
48 hours (salt & turmeric)	Between Groups	42550.933	4	10637.733	1.645E3	.000(S)
	Within Groups	64.667	10	6.467		
	Total	42615.600	14			
14 days (salt & turmeric)	Between Groups	299164.267	4	74791.067	1.233E4	.000(S)
	Within Groups	60.667	10	6.067		
	Total	299224.933	14			
15 days (salt & turmeric)	Between Groups	386146.933	4	96536.733	2.540E4	.000(S)
	Within Groups	38.000	10	3.800		
	Total	386184.933	14			
24 hours (KMS)	Between Groups	76092.400	4	19023.100	3.856E3	.000(S)
	Within Groups	49.333	10	4.933		
	Total	76141.733	14			
48 hours (KMS)	Between Groups	629540.267	4	157385.067	3.524E4	.000(S)
	Within Groups	44.667	10	4.467		
	Total	629584.933	14			
14 days (KMS)	Between Groups	75700.400	4	18925.100	3.998E3	.000(S)
	Within Groups	47.333	10	4.733		
	Total	75747.733	14			
15 days (KMS)	Between Groups	192141.067	4	48035.267	2.119E4	.000(S)
	Within Groups	22.667	10	2.267		
	Total	192163.733	14			

$p<0.05$ S= Significant, NS= Non-significant. All abbreviations are on page so and so.

This statistical ANOVA table shows that all the values are significant, which means there is significant difference present in the values of calcium content of *katla* among different cooking methods and the raw state in respect to fresh condition along with different preservation methods.

Table no 5.7.2.4 Post hoc Duncan statistical analysis

Preservation	Duration	Raw state	Boiling	Dry roasting	Shallow frying	Deep frying
Control	Fresh	B,S[a]	R,O,S,D[b]	B,S[a]	R,B,O,D[c]	B,S[a]
Control	24 hours	B,O,S,D[d]	R,O,S,D[b]	R,B,S,D[e]	R,B,O,D[c]	R,B,O,S[f]
Control	48 hours	B,O,S,D[d]	R,O,S,D[b]	R,B,S,D[e]	R,B,O,D[c]	R,B,O,S[f]
Control	14 days	B,O,S,D[d]	R,O,S,D[b]	R,B,S,D[e]	R,B,O,D[c]	R,B,O,S[f]
Control	15 days	B,O,S,D[d]	R,O,S,D[b]	R,B,S,D[e]	R,B,O,D[c]	R,B,O,S[f]
Salt &Turmeric	24 hours	B,O,S,D[d]	R,O,S,D[b]	R,B,S,D[e]	R,B,O,D[c]	R,B,O,S[f]
Salt & Turmeric	48 hours	B,O,S,D[d]	R,O,S,D[b]	R,B,S,D[e]	R,B,O,D[c]	R,B,O,S[f]
Salt & Turmeric	14 days	B,O,S,D[d]	R,O,S,D[b]	R,B,S,D[e]	R,B,O,D[c]	R,B,O,S[f]
Salt & Turmeric	15 days	B,O,S,D[d]	R,O,S,D[b]	R,B,S,D[e]	R,B,O,D[c]	R,B,O,S[f]
KMS	24 hours	B,O,S,D[d]	R,O,S,D[b]	R,B,S,D[e]	R,B,O,D[c]	R,B,O,S[f]
KMS	48 hours	B,O,S,D[d]	R,O,S,D[b]	R,B,S,D[e]	R,B,O,D[c]	R,B,O,S[f]
KMS	14 days	B,O,S,D[d]	R,O,S,D[b]	R,B,S,D[e]	R,B,O,D[c]	R,B,O,S[f]
KMS	15 days	B,O,S,D[d]	R,O,D[g]	R,B,S,D[e]	R,O,D[g]	R,B,O,S[f]

R= Raw state, B= Boiling, O= Open pan dry roasting, S= Shallow frying, D= Deep frying. The same uppercase alphabets signify that there is no significant difference present among the variables.

This table shows the significant difference among the different variables such as cooking methods and preservation conditions. The raw state significantly differs from boiling, open pan dry roasting, shallow frying and deep frying in all of the preservation conditions with preservatives and control preservation without preservative except in fresh condition. Boiling significantly differs from raw state, open pan dry roasting, shallow frying and deep frying in all the preservation conditions except in 15 days KMS preservation. Open pan dry roasting significantly differs from the raw state, boiling, shallow frying and deep frying in all the preservation conditions except in fresh condition. Shallow frying significantly differs from the raw state, boiling, open pan dry roasting and deep frying in all the preservation conditions except in 15 days KMS preservation. Deep frying significantly differs from the raw state, boiling, open pan dry roasting and shallow frying in all the preservation conditions except in fresh condition.

The raw state, open pan dry roasting and deep frying significantly differ from boiling and shallow frying in fresh condition. Boiling and shallow frying significantly differ from the raw state, open pan dry roasting and deep frying in 15 days KMS preservation.

Table no 5.7.2.5 Gradation of cooking methods from higher to lower with respect to preservation days

Preservation	Duration	Method 1	Method 2	Method 3	Method 4	Method 5
Control	Fresh	R	DF	OPDR	SF	B
Control	24 hours	DF	B	OPDR	R	SF
Control	48 hours	DF	R	OPDR	B	SF
Control	14 days	DF	B	SF	OPDR	R
Control	15 days	SF	DF	OPDR	R	B
Salt &Turmeric	24 hours	OPDR	R	B	SF	DF
Salt & Turmeric	48 hours	SF	DF	OPDR	B	R
Salt & Turmeric	14 days	SF	B	DF	R	OPDR
Salt &Turmeric	15 days	SF	R	B	DF	OPDR
KMS	24 hours	OPDR	B	SF	DF	R
KMS	48 hours	B	R	OPDR	DF	SF
KMS	14 days	B	R	OPDR	DF	SF
KMS	15 days	R	OPDR	B	SF	DF

R= Raw state, B= Boiling, OPDR= Open pan dry roasting, SF= Shallow frying, DF= Deep frying. Same colour represents the similar order.

In all the preservation methods and fresh condition, calcium retention occurs mainly in shallow frying than the other cooking methods. In fresh condition, retention occurs firstly in the raw state then deep frying, open pan dry roasting, shallow frying and boiling. In 24 hours control preservation without preservative, the order of retention is deep frying followed by boiling, open pan dry roasting, raw state and shallow frying. In 48 hours control preservation without preservative, the order is deep frying, raw state, open pan dry roasting, boiling and shallow frying. In 14 days control preservation without preservative, the order becomes deep frying, boiling, shallow frying, open pan dry roasting and the raw state. In 15 days control preservation without preservative, the order changes from shallow frying to deep frying, open pan dry roasting, raw state and boiling.

In 24 hours salt and turmeric preservation, retention occurs firstly in open pan dry roasting followed by the raw state, boiling, shallow frying and deep frying. In 48 hours salt and turmeric preservation the order of retention is shallow frying, deep frying, open pan dry roasting, boiling and the raw state. In 14 days salt and turmeric preservation, the order becomes shallow frying, boiling, deep frying, raw state and open pan dry roasting. In 15 days salt and turmeric preservation, the order remains shallow frying, raw state, boiling, deep frying and open pan dry roasting.

In 24 hours KMS preservation, retention occurs firstly in open pan dry roasting, boiling, shallow frying, deep frying and the raw state. In 48 hours and 14 days KMS preservation, the order is boiling, raw state, open pan dry roasting, deep frying and shallow frying. In 15 days KMS preservation, the order remains the raw state, open pan dry roasting, boiling, shallow frying and deep frying.

The overall analysis of iron content of *katla* is mostly restored by the gradation of methods as shallow frying> boiling> open pan dry roasting>deep frying>raw state.

Shallow frying possibly creates a fatty layer surrounding *katla*, thus calcium cannot be eliminated and content can be restored[66]. Boiling can reduce some of the calcium possibly as it is soluble in the cooking water and can be eliminated if the cooking water is discarded. Open pan dry roasting reduces calcium content possibly as the direct heat melts the fatty tissues of the fish and fats get eliminated along with calcium. Deep frying reduces calcium content as frying oil is possibly unable to cover the surface area of the fish flesh, so the protective layer becomes very weak, eliminating the calcium from the fish. Thus among all the studied conventional cooking methods, **shallow frying** is the best method for *katla* to restore calcium content.

5.7.3 Prawn (*Fenneropenaeus indicus*)

It has been reported that prawn contains 323 mg of calcium per 100 gm[84] in the raw state. This value changes due to the application of different cooking methods and preservation conditions (vide Table no **5.7.3.1**).

Table no 5.7.3.1 Calcium content of Prawn (mg/100gm)

Preservation	Duration	Raw state	Boiling	Dry roasting	Shallow frying	Deep frying
Control	Fresh	177.23±2.08	302.10±2.00	251.12±2.00	50.04±1.00	40.18±1.52
Control	24 hours	216.13±1.52	248.22±2.64	131.10±1.00	201.14±208	126.27±1.52
Control	48 hours	176.04±1.52	106.28±1.52	336.08±1.00	501.10±2.08	201.11±1.52
Control	14 days	136.10±1.52	136.34±1.52	227.33±2.51	202.65±2.64	162.39±2.00
Control	15 days	185.10±3.00	180.45±2.00	152.37±2.51	142.44±2.51	201.60±2.08
Salt & Turmeric	24 hours	42.11±2.00	46.35±1.00	32.33±2.51	152.38±2.00	25.04±1.52
Salt &Turmeric	48 hours	72.16±2.00	112.30±2.00	117.40±2.00	192.44±2.00	137.47±2.51
Salt & Turmeric	14 days	136.11±1.52	136.39±1.52	227.04±2.51	202.13±2.64	162.04±2.00
Salt & Turmeric	15 days	185.18±3.00	180.39±2.00	152.94±2.51	142.87±2.51	201.07±2.08
KMS	24 hours	192.05±2.00	151.28±1.52	137.47±2.08	116.45±1.52	152.03±2.51
KMS	48 hours	161.39±1.52	151.30±1.52	275.48±3.00	143.74±1.52	145.49±1.00
KMS	14 days	143.36±1.52	202.03±2.00	216.38±1.52	182.37±2.00	252.48±2.00
KMS	15 days	182.44±2.00	137.38±2.08	175.94±3.00	236.64±1.52	382.27±2.00

Values are expressed as mean±SD. ☐ Loss ☐ Restoration

Red digits represent the significant highest values from the raw state in different conditions.

In most of the conditions, calcium content is mainly reduced by shallow frying, whereas in 48 hours, 14 days control preservation without preservative and 48 hours, 14 days salt and turmeric preservation and 15 days KMS preservation, calcium content is reduced by boiling. In fresh condition, 24 hours control preservation without preservative and 24 hours salt and turmeric preservation, calcium content is reduced by deep frying.

Retention of calcium content occurs by deep frying mostly, but in fresh condition, 24 hours control preservation without preservative, calcium retention occurs by boiling, whereas in 14 days control preservation without preservative, 14 days salt and turmeric preservation and 48 hours KMS preservation, calcium retention occurs by open pan dry roasting. In 48 hours control preservation without preservative and 24 hours, 48 hours salt and turmeric preservation, calcium retention occurs by shallow frying.

Open pan dry roasting and shallow frying show the highest calcium content in 48 hours control preservation without preservative, whereas the raw state shows the highest calcium content in 24 hours control preservation without preservative. Boiling and deep frying shows the highest calcium content in fresh condition and 15 days KMS preservation respectively.

Boiling shows the increased calcium content than the raw state in fresh condition, 24 hours control preservation without preservative and 24 hours, 48 hours, 14 days salt and turmeric preservation and 14 days KMS preservation. Open pan dry roasting shows the increased calcium content than the raw state in fresh condition, 48 hours, 14 days control preservation without preservative and 48 hours, 14 days salt and turmeric preservation and 48 hours, 14 days KMS preservation, whereas shallow frying also shows the increased calcium content than the raw value in 48 hours, 14 days control preservation without preservative and 24 hours, 48 hours, 14 days salt and turmeric preservation and 14 days, 15 days KMS preservation. Deep frying shows the increased calcium content than the raw value in 48 hours, 14 days, 15 days control preservation without preservative, 48 hours, 14 days, 15 days salt and turmeric preservation as well as 14 days, 15 days KMS preservation.

This may be due to the molecular rearrangement during cooking and the addition of cooking oil during frying. Additionally, the elimination of water during cooking[48] causes the increased concentration of the calcium. Another possible reason for increasing calcium content is due to the elimination of anti-nutritional factor during cooking. Additions of both the natural and synthetic preservatives help in the modification of calcium content.

Fig. 5.7.3.2 Graphical representation of Calcium content of Prawn with respect to different conditions

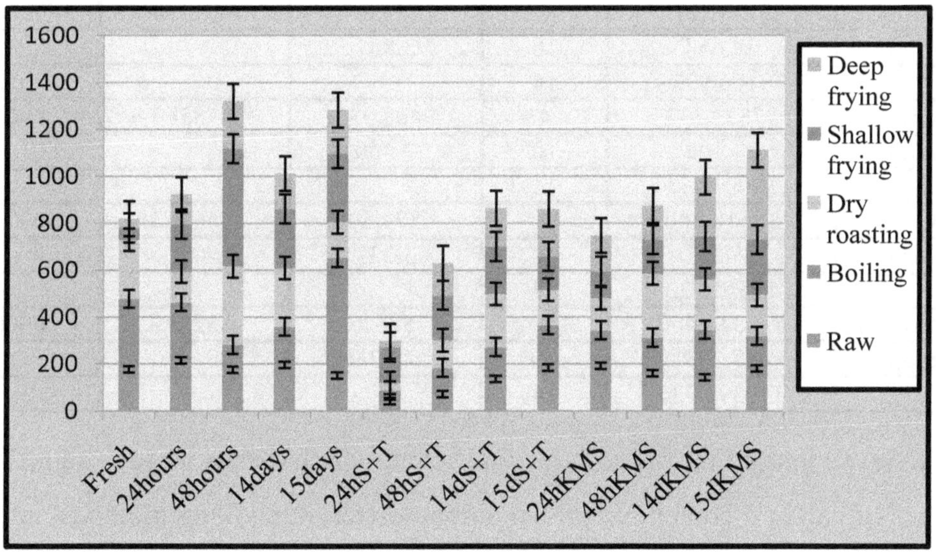

This graphical representation indicates that among all the preservation conditions, **48 hours control preservation without preservative** helps to increase the calcium content in all the cooking methods. Here the graph shows that the control preservation without preservative is more effective than salt and turmeric preservation and KMS preservation to restore calcium content in prawn.

Table no 5.7.3.3 ANOVA with regard to cooking conditions and preservation methods

Condition	Differences	Sum of Squares	df	Mean Square	F	Sig.
Fresh (control)	Between Groups	165240.400	4	41310.100	1.631E4	.000(S)
	Within Groups	25.333	10	2.533		
	Total	165265.733	14			
24 hours (control)	Between Groups	34640.933	4	8660.233	2.547E3	.000(S)
	Within Groups	34.000	10	3.400		
	Total	34674.933	14			
48 hours (control)	Between Groups	223404.933	4	55851.233	2.264E4	.000(S)
	Within Groups	24.667	10	2.467		
	Total	223429.600	14			
14 days (control)	Between Groups	27071.067	4	6767.767	2.986E3	.000(S)
	Within Groups	22.667	10	2.267		
	Total	27093.733	14			
15 days (control)	Between Groups	265162.000	4	66290.500	4.323E4	.000(S)
	Within Groups	15.333	10	1.533		
	Total	265177.333	14			
24 hours (salt & turmeric)	Between Groups	32850.400	4	8212.600	1.895E3	.000(S)
	Within Groups	43.333	10	4.333		
	Total	32893.733	14			
48 hours (salt & turmeric)	Between Groups	23055.067	4	5763.767	1.290E3	.000(S)
	Within Groups	44.667	10	4.467		
	Total	23099.733	14			
14 days (salt & turmeric)	Between Groups	19917.733	4	4979.433	1.132E3	.000(S)
	Within Groups	44.000	10	4.400		
	Total	19961.733	14			
15 days (salt & turmeric)	Between Groups	7187.733	4	1796.933	230.376	.000(S)
	Within Groups	78.000	10	7.800		
	Total	7265.733	14			
24 hours (KMS)	Between Groups	9128.267	4	2282.067	590.190	.000(S)
	Within Groups	38.667	10	3.867		
	Total	9166.933	14			
48 hours (KMS)	Between Groups	37873.333	4	9468.333	2.785E3	.000(S)
	Within Groups	34.000	10	3.400		
	Total	37907.333	14			
14 days (KMS)	Between Groups	19518.400	4	4879.600	1.464E3	.000(S)
	Within Groups	33.333	10	3.333		
	Total	19551.733	14			
15 days (KMS)	Between Groups	110344.400	4	27586.100	5.828E3	.000(S)
	Within Groups	47.333	10	4.733		
	Total	110391.733	14			

$p<0.05$ S= Significant, NS= Non-significant. All abbreviations are on page so and so.

This statistical ANOVA table shows that all the values are significant, which means there is significant difference present in the values of calcium content of prawn among different cooking methods and the raw state in respect to fresh condition along with different preservation methods.

Table no 5.7.3.4 Post hoc Duncan statistical analysis

Preservation	Duration	Raw state	Boiling	Dry roasting	Shallow frying	Deep frying
Control	Fresh	B,O,S,D^{a}	R,O,S,D^{b}	R,B,S,D^{c}	R,B,O,D^{d}	R,B,O,S^{e}
Control	24 hours	B,O,S,D^{a}	R,O,S,D^{b}	R,B,S,D^{c}	R,B,O,D^{d}	R,B,O,S^{e}
Control	48 hours	B,O,S,D^{a}	R,O,S,D^{b}	R,B,S,D^{c}	R,B,O,D^{d}	R,B,O,S^{e}
Control	14 days	B,O,S,D^{a}	R,O,S,D^{b}	R,B,D^{f}	R,B,D^{f}	R,B,O,S^{e}
Control	15 days	B,S,D^{g}	R,O,S,D^{b}	B,S,D^{g}	R,B,O,D^{d}	R,B,O,S^{e}
Salt & Turmeric	24 hours	B,O,S,D^{a}	R,O,S,D^{b}	R,B,S,D^{c}	R,B,O,D^{d}	R,B,O,S^{e}
Salt & Turmeric	48 hours	B,O,S,D^{a}	R,O,S,D^{b}	R,B,S,D^{c}	R,B,O,D^{d}	R,B,O,S^{e}
Salt & Turmeric	14 days	O,S,D^{h}	O,S,D^{h}	R,B,S,D^{c}	R,B,O,D^{d}	R,B,O,S^{e}
Salt & Turmeric	15 days	O,S,D^{h}	O,S,D^{h}	R,B,S,D^{c}	R,B,O,D^{d}	R,B,O,S^{e}
KMS	24 hours	B,O,S,D^{a}	R,O,S^{i}	R,B,S,D^{c}	R,B,O,D^{d}	R,O,S^{i}
KMS	48 hours	B,O,S,D^{a}	R,O,S,D^{b}	R,B,S,D^{c}	R,B,O^{j}	R,B,O^{j}
KMS	14 days	B,O,S,D^{a}	R,O,S,D^{b}	R,B,S,D^{c}	R,B,O,D^{d}	R,B,O,S^{e}
KMS	15 days	B,O,S,D^{a}	R,O,S,D^{b}	R,B,S,D^{c}	R,B,O,D^{d}	R,B,O,S^{e}

R= Raw state, B= Boiling, O= Open pan dry roasting, S= Shallow frying, D= Deep frying. The same uppercase alphabets represent that there is no significant difference present among the variables.

This table shows the significant difference among the different variables such as cooking methods and preservation conditions. The raw state significantly differs from boiling, open pan dry roasting, shallow frying and deep frying in all of the preservation conditions with preservatives and control preservation without preservative except in 15 days control preservation without preservative and 14 days, 15 days salt and turmeric preservation. Boiling significantly differs from the raw state, open pan dry roasting, shallow and deep frying in all the preservation conditions except in 14 days, 15 days salt and turmeric preservation and 24 hours KMS preservation. Open pan dry roasting significantly differs from the raw state, boiling, shallow frying and deep frying in all the preservation conditions except in 14 days, 15 days control preservation without preservative. Shallow frying significantly differs from the raw state, boiling, open pan dry roasting and deep frying in all the preservation conditions except in 14 days control preservation without preservative, 48 hours KMS preservation. Deep frying significantly differs from the raw state, boiling, open pan dry roasting and shallow frying in all the preservation conditions except in 24 hours, 48 hours KMS preservation.

Open pan dry roasting and shallow frying significantly differ from the raw state, boiling and deep frying in 14 days control preservation without preservative. The raw state and open pan dry roasting significantly differ from boiling, shallow frying and deep frying in 15 days control preservation without preservative. The raw state and boiling significantly differ from open pan dry roasting, shallow frying and deep frying in 14 days, 15 days salt and turmeric preservation. Boiling and deep frying significantly differ from the raw state, open pan dry roasting, shallow frying in 24 hours KMS preservation. Shallow frying and deep frying significantly differ from the raw state, boiling and open pan dry roasting in 48 hours KMS preservation.

Table no 5.7.3.5 Gradation of cooking methods from higher to lower restoration with respect to preservation days

Preservation	Duration	Method 1	Method 2	Method 3	Method 4	Method 5
Control	Fresh	B	OPDR	R	SF	DF
Control	24 hours	B	R	SF	OPDR	DF
Control	48 hours	SF	OPDR	B	DF	R
Control	14 days	SF	OPDR	R	B	DF
Control	15 days	B	SF	DF	OPDR	R
Salt &Turmeric	24 hours	SF	B	R	OPDR	DF
Salt & Turmeric	48 hours	SF	DF	OPDR	B	R
Salt & Turmeric	14 days	OPDR	SF	DF	B	R
Salt &Turmeric	15 days	DF	R	B	OPDR	SF
KMS	24 hours	R	DF	B	OPDR	SF
KMS	48 hours	OPDR	R	B	DF	SF
KMS	14 days	DF	OPDR	B	SF	R
KMS	15 days	DF	SF	R	OPDR	B

R= Raw state, B= Boiling, OPDR= Open pan dry roasting, SF= Shallow frying, DF= Deep frying.

In all the preservation methods and fresh condition, calcium retention occurs mainly in shallow frying than the other cooking methods. In fresh condition, retention occurs firstly in boiling followed by open pan dry roasting, raw state, shallow frying and deep frying. In 24 hours control preservation without preservative, the order is boiling, raw state, shallow frying, open pan dry roasting and deep frying. In 48 hours control preservation without preservative, the order of retention changes from shallow frying to open pan dry roasting, boiling, deep frying and the raw state. In 14 days control preservation without preservative, the order remains shallow frying, open pan dry roasting, raw state, boiling and deep frying. In 15 days control preservation without preservative, the order becomes boiling, shallow frying, deep frying, open pan dry roasting and the raw state.

In 24 hours salt and turmeric preservation, retention occurs firstly in shallow frying followed by boiling, raw state, open pan dry roasting and deep frying. In 48 hours salt and turmeric preservation, retention occurs in the order of shallow frying, deep frying, open pan dry roasting, boiling and the raw state. In 14 days salt and turmeric preservation, the order remains open pan dry roasting, shallow frying, deep frying, boiling and the raw state. In 15 days salt and turmeric preservation, the order is deep frying, raw state, boiling, open pan dry roasting and shallow frying.

In 24 hours KMS preservation, retention occurs firstly in the raw state then deep frying, boiling, open pan dry roasting and shallow frying. In 48 hours KMS preservation, the order of retention occurs firstly in open pan dry roasting followed by the raw state, boiling, deep frying and shallow frying. In 14 days KMS preservation, the order becomes deep frying then open pan dry roasting, boiling, shallow frying and the raw state. In 15 days KMS preservation, the order is deep frying, shallow frying, raw state, open pan dry roasting and boiling.

The overall analysis of calcium content of prawn is mostly restored by the gradation of methods as shallow frying> deep frying> boiling> open pan dry roasting> raw state.

Shallow frying and deep frying possibly create a fatty layer surrounding prawn, thus the calcium cannot be eliminated and content can be restored[66]. Boiling can reduce some of the calcium as it is possibly soluble in the cooking water and can be eliminated if the cooking water is discarded. Open pan dry roasting reduces calcium content as the direct heat possibly melts the tissues of the prawn, eliminating the calcium. Thus among all the studied conventional cooking methods, **shallow frying** is the best method for prawn to restore calcium content.

5.7.4 Lobster (*Macrobrachium rosenbergii*)

It has been reported that lobster contains 610 mg of calcium per 100 gm[84] in the raw state. This value changes due to the application of different cooking methods and preservation conditions (vide Table no **5.7.4.1**).

Table no 5.7.4.1 Calcium content of Lobster (mg/100gm)

Preservation	Duration	Raw state	Boiling	Dry roasting	Shallow frying	Deep frying
Control	Fresh	241.34±1.52	271.35±1.52	241.44±1.00	201.37±1.52	151.44±1.52
Control	24 hours	201.25±1.52	260.24±2.00	161.33±1.52	123.33±2.52	151.36±1.52
Control	48 hours	167.37±3.78	212.94±2.64	166.23±2.52	125.27±2.08	125.06±2.08
Control	14 days	351.95±1.00	501.65±1.00	281.88±1.00	265.32±2.08	151.36±1.52
Control	15 days	133.47±1.52	153.37±1.52	152.25±2.08	141.10±1.52	136.56±2.08
Salt & Turmeric	24 hours	204.23±4.00	395.88±3.00	52.46±2.51	64.22±4.04	66.07±1.52
Salt &Turmeric	48 hours	302.93±2.51	132.23±2.51	132.33±2.51	86.43±1.52	75.33±2.00
Salt & Turmeric	14 days	46.12±1.52	76.05±1.00	50.25±1.52	102.03±2.51	175.40±3.00
Salt & Turmeric	15 days	207.25±2.51	186.55±2.51	192.27±2.51	177.04±2.51	222.48±2.00
KMS	24 hours	70.44±1.52	72.26±2.00	64.84±2.00	94.05±2.00	185.57±1.52
KMS	48 hours	43.25±2.08	302.05±2.00	252.23±2.00	246.14±1.52	45.36±2.08
KMS	14 days	205.25±2.08	423.33±2.64	242.54±2.51	140.23±2.00	152.33±2.00
KMS	15 days	272.92±2.51	423.38±2.64	315.12±2.08	342.35±2.51	502.56±2.00

Values are expressed as mean±SD. ☐ Loss ☐ Restoration
Red digits represent the significant highest values from the raw state in different conditions.

In most of the conditions, calcium content is mainly reduced by deep frying, whereas in 24 hours, 14 days salt and turmeric preservation and 24 hours, 15 days KMS preservation, calcium content is reduced by open pan dry roasting. In 24 hours control preservation without preservative and 48 hours, 15 days salt and turmeric preservation and 14 days KMS preservation, calcium content is reduced by shallow frying.

Retention of calcium content occurs by boiling mostly, but in 48 hours salt and turmeric preservation, calcium retention occurs by open pan dry roasting, whereas in 14 days, 15 days salt and turmeric preservation and 24 hours, 15 days KMS preservation, calcium retention occurs by deep frying.

Open pan dry roasting, shallow frying and deep frying show the highest calcium content in 15 days KMS preservation, whereas the raw state and boiling show the highest calcium content in 14 days control preservation without preservative.

Boiling shows the increased calcium content than the raw value in all the preservation conditions including fresh condition except in 48 hours, 15 days salt and turmeric preservation. Open pan dry roasting shows the increased calcium content than the raw state in fresh condition, 48 hours, 15 days control preservation without preservative and 14 days salt and turmeric preservation and 48 hours, 14 days, 15 days KMS preservation, whereas shallow frying also shows the increased calcium content than the raw value in 14 days salt and turmeric preservation and 24 hours, 48 hours, 15 days KMS preservation. Deep frying shows the increased calcium content than the raw value in 14 days, 15 days salt and turmeric preservation as well as 24 hours, 48 hours, 15 days KMS preservation.

This may occur due to the addition of cooking oil during frying and the molecular rearrangement during cooking. Another possible reason may be the elimination of water during cooking[48]concentrates the calcium content. Addition of both the natural and synthetic preservatives may be a possible cause of modification of calcium content. Additionally, the calcium content is increased due to the elimination of anti-nutritional factors during cooking.

Fig. 5.7.4.2 Graphical representation of Calcium content of Lobster with respect to different conditions

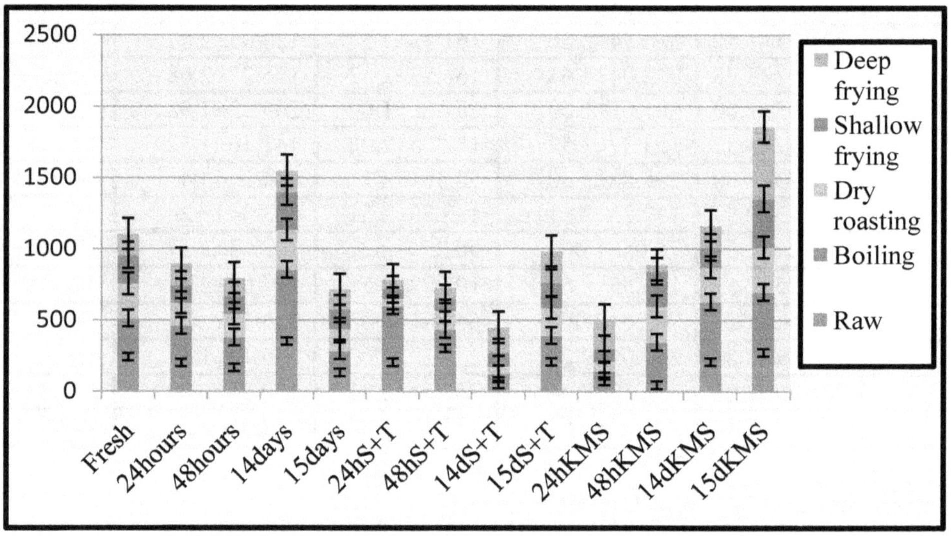

This graphical representation indicates that among all the preservation conditions, **15 days KMS preservation**[59] helps to increase the calcium content in all the cooking methods. Here the graph shows that the control preservation without preservative and salt and turmeric preservation also help to restore the calcium content, but KMS is more effective among the other preservation methods[39]. The possible reason may be that the synthetic preservative helps to modify the structure of calcium, restoring the content.

Table no 5.7.4.3 ANOVA with regard to cooking conditions and preservation methods

Condition	Differences	Sum of Squares	df	Mean Square	F	Sig.
Fresh (control)	Between Groups	25720.933	4	6430.233	3.111E3	.000(S)
	Within Groups	20.667	10	2.067		
	Total	25741.600	14			
24 hours (control)	Between Groups	34474.267	4	8618.567	3.232E3	.000(S)
	Within Groups	26.667	10	2.667		
	Total	34500.933	14			
48 hours (control)	Between Groups	11770.267	4	2942.567	455.036	.000(S)
	Within Groups	64.667	10	6.467		
	Total	11834.933	14			
14 days (control)	Between Groups	248753.600	4	62188.400	3.217E4	.000(S)
	Within Groups	19.333	10	1.933		
	Total	248772.933	14			
15 days (control)	Between Groups	38262.267	4	9565.567	3.053E3	.000()
	Within Groups	31.333	10	3.133		
	Total	38293.600	14			
24 hours (salt & turmeric)	Between Groups	259841.600	4	64960.400	6.496E3	.000(S)
	Within Groups	100.000	10	10.000		
	Total	259941.600	14			
48 hours (salt & turmeric)	Between Groups	100242.667	4	25060.667	4.946E3	.000(S)
	Within Groups	50.667	10	5.067		
	Total	100293.333	14			
14 days (salt & turmeric)	Between Groups	33160.000	4	8290.000	1.974E3	.000(S)
	Within Groups	42.000	10	4.200		
	Total	33202.000	14			
15 days (salt & turmeric)	Between Groups	3743.733	4	935.933	184.724	.000(S)
	Within Groups	50.667	10	5.067		
	Total	3794.400	14			
24 hours (KMS)	Between Groups	30710.400	4	7677.600	2.303E3	.000(S)
	Within Groups	33.333	10	3.333		
	Total	30743.733	14			
48 hours (KMS)	Between Groups	183236.933	4	45809.233	1.206E4	.000(S)
	Within Groups	38.000	10	3.800		
	Total	183274.933	14			
14 days (KMS)	Between Groups	132070.267	4	33017.567	6.432E3	.000(S)
	Within Groups	51.333	10	5.133		
	Total	132121.600	14			
15 days (KMS)	Between Groups	100450.933	4	25112.733	4.484E3	.000(S)
	Within Groups	56.000	10	5.600		
	Total	100506.933	14			

$p<0.05$ S= Significant, NS= Non-significant. All abbreviations are on page so and so.

This statistical ANOVA table shows that all the values are significant, which means there is significant difference present in the values of calcium content of lobster among different cooking methods and the raw state in respect to fresh condition along with different preservation methods.

Table no 5.7.4.4 Post hoc Duncan statistical analysis

Preservation	Duration	Raw state	Boiling	Dry roasting	Shallow frying	Deep frying
Control	Fresh	B,S,D[a]	R,O,S,D[b]	BS,D[a]	R,B,O,D[c]	R,B,O,S[d]
Control	24 hours	B,O,S,D[e]	R,O,S,D[b]	R,B,S,D[f]	R,B,O,D[c]	R,B,O,S[d]
Control	48 hours	B,S,D[a]	R,O,S,D[b]	B,S,D[a]	R,B,O,D[c]	R,B,O,S[d]
Control	14 days	B,O,S,D[e]	R,O,S,D[b]	R,B,S,D[f]	R,B,O,D[c]	R,B,O,S[d]
Control	15 days	B,O,S,D[e]	R,O,S,D[b]	R,B,S,D[f]	R,B,O,D[c]	R,B,O,S[d]
Salt & Turmeric	24 hours	B,O,S,D[e]	R,O,S,D[b]	R,B,S,D[f]	R,B,O[g]	R,B,O[g]
Salt & Turmeric	48 hours	B,O,S,D[e]	R,S,D[h]	R,S,D[h]	R,B,O,D[c]	R,B,O,S[d]
Salt & Turmeric	14 days	B,O,S,D[e]	R,O,S,D[b]	R,B,S,D[f]	R,B,O,D[c]	R,B,O,S[d]
Salt & Turmeric	15 days	B,O,S,D[e]	R,O,S,D[b]	R,B,S,D[f]	R,B,O,D[c]	R,B,O,S[d]
KMS	24 hours	O,S,D[i]	O,S,D[i]	R,B,S,D[f]	R,B,O,D[c]	R,B,O,S[d]
KMS	48 hours	B,O,S[j]	R,O,S,D[b]	R,B,S,D[f]	R,B,O,D[c]	B,O,S[j]
KMS	14 days	B,O,S,D[e]	R,O,S,D[b]	R,B,S,D[f]	R,B,O,D[c]	R,B,O,S[d]
KMS	15 days	B,O,S,D[e]	R,O,S,D[b]	R,B,S,D[f]	R,B,O,D[c]	R,B,O,S[d]

R= Raw state, B= Boiling, O= Open pan dry roasting, S= Shallow frying, D= Deep frying. The same uppercase alphabets represent that there is no significant difference present among the variables.

This table shows the significant difference among the different variables such as cooking methods and preservation conditions. The raw state significantly differs from boiling, open pan dry roasting, shallow frying and deep frying in all of the preservation conditions with preservatives and control preservation without preservative except in fresh condition, 48 hours control preservation without preservative and 24 hours, 48 hours KMS preservation. Boiling significantly differs from the raw state, open pan dry roasting, shallow frying and deep frying in all the preservation condition except in 48 hours salt and turmeric preservation and 24 hours KMS preservation. Open pan dry roasting significantly differs from the raw state, boiling, shallow frying and deep frying in all the preservation conditions except in fresh condition, 48 hours control preservation without preservative and 48 hours salt and turmeric preservation. Shallow frying significantly differs from the raw state, boiling, open pan dry roasting and deep frying in all the preservation conditions except in 24 hours salt and turmeric preservation. Deep frying significantly differs from the raw state, boiling, open pan dry roasting and shallow frying in all the preservation conditions except in 24 hours salt and turmeric preservation and 48 hours KMS preservation.

Open pan dry roasting and the raw state significantly differ from boiling, shallow frying and deep frying in fresh condition and 48 hours control preservation without preservative. Shallow frying and deep frying significantly differ from the raw state, boiling and open pan dry roasting in 24 hours salt and turmeric preservation. Boiling and open pan dry roasting significantly differ from the raw state, shallow frying and deep frying in 48 hours salt and turmeric preservation. Boiling and the raw state significantly differ from open pan dry roasting, shallow frying and deep frying in 24 hours KMS preservation. The raw state and deep frying significantly differ from boiling, open pan dry roasting and shallow frying in 48 hours KMS preservation.

Table no 5.7.4.5 Gradation of cooking methods from higher to lower restoration with respect to preservation days

Preservation	Duration	Method 1	Method 2	Method 3	Method 4	Method 5
Control	Fresh	B	R	OPDR	SF	DF
Control	24 hours	B	R	OPDR	DF	SF
Control	48 hours	B	R	OPDR	DF	SF
Control	14 days	B	R	OPDR	SF	DF
Control	15 days	OPDR	DF	B	SF	R
Salt & Turmeric	24 hours	B	R	DF	SF	OPDR
Salt & Turmeric	48 hours	R	OPDR	B	SF	DF
Salt & Turmeric	14 days	DF	SF	B	OPDR	R
Salt &Turmeric	15 days	DF	R	OPDR	B	SF
KMS	24 hours	DF	SF	B	R	OPDR
KMS	48 hours	B	OPDR	SF	DF	R
KMS	14 days	B	DF	OPDR	R	SF
KMS	15 days	DF	B	SF	OPDR	R

R= Raw state, B= Boiling, OPDR= Open pan dry roasting, SF= Shallow frying, DF= Deep frying. Same colours represent the similar order.

In all the preservation techniques and fresh condition, calcium retention occurs mainly in boiling than the other cooking methods. In fresh condition and 14 days control preservation without preservative, retention occurs firstly in boiling followed by the raw state, open pan dry roasting, shallow frying and deep frying. In 24 hours and 48 hours control preservation without preservative, the retention occurs in the order of boiling, raw state, open pan dry roasting, deep frying and shallow frying. In 15 days control preservation without preservative, the order is open pan dry roasting, deep frying, boiling, shallow frying and the raw state.

In 24 hours salt and turmeric preservation, retention occurs firstly in boiling then the raw state, deep frying, shallow frying and open pan dry roasting. In 48 hours salt and turmeric preservation, the order is the raw state, open pan dry roasting, boiling, shallow frying and deep frying. In 14 days salt and turmeric preservation, the order remains deep frying, shallow frying, open pan dry roasting, boiling and the raw state. In 15 days salt and turmeric preservation, the order changes from deep frying, raw state, open pan dry roasting, boiling and shallow frying.

In 24 hours KMS preservation, retention occurs firstly in deep frying followed by shallow frying, boiling, raw state and open pan dry roasting. In 48 hours KMS preservation, the order is boiling, open pan dry roasting, shallow frying, deep frying and the raw state. In 14 days KMS preservation, the order remains boiling, deep frying, open pan dry roasting, raw state and shallow frying. In 15 days KMS preservation, the order of retention occurs from deep frying to boiling, shallow frying, open pan dry roasting and the raw state.

The overall analysis of calcium content of lobster is mostly restored by the gradation of methods as boiling> raw state> open pan dry roasting> shallow frying>deep frying.

Boiling can restore calcium content possibly as the flesh of lobster becomes very hard when heat is applied, preventing the calcium to become soluble in the cooking water. Open pan dry roasting reduces calcium content as the direct heat possibly chars the tissues, eliminating the calcium. Shallow frying and deep frying possibly cause total dryness of the flesh and it becomes tough, thus the calcium can be eliminated and content can be reduced. Thus among all the studied conventional cooking methods, **boiling** is the best method for lobster to restore calcium content.

5.7.5 Pomfret (*Pampus argenteus*)

It has been reported that pomfret contains 200 mg of calcium per 100 gm[84] in the raw state. This value changes due to the application of different cooking methods and preservation conditions (vide Table no **5.7.5.1**).

Table no 5.7.5.1 Calcium content of Pomfret (mg/100gm)

Preservation	Duration	Raw state	Boiling	Dry roasting	Shallow frying	Deep frying
Control	Fresh	151.04±1.52	151.23±1.52	156.33±1.52	86.24±1.52	246.39±1.52
Control	24 hours	642.59±2.51	302.25±2.00	302.28±0.57	402.04±2.00	182.05±2.00
Control	48 hours	382.35±2.51	202.05±2.51	127.37±2.08	136.05±1.52	175.29±3.00
Control	14 days	195.24±3.00	297.45±2.08	417.94±2.51	185.47±3.00	243.37±3.60
Control	15 days	166.25±1.52	362.37±2.51	282.38±2.00	213.06±3.21	208.04±3.21
Salt & Turmeric	24 hours	101.05±2.08	372.55±2.51	252.33±2.00	104.10±4.04	102.27±2.51
Salt &Turmeric	48 hours	292.22±2.51	97.95±2.08	302.06±2.51	63.33±2.64	252.33±2.51
Salt & Turmeric	14 days	352.15±2.00	82.56±2.51	115.49±3.00	402.04±3.05	342.28±2.51
Salt & Turmeric	15 days	284.15±2.00	64.23±2.00	68.33±1.52	42.16±2.00	64.66±3.05
KMS	24 hours	183.11±1.52	202.35±2.00	725.29±3.00	152.33±2.00	134.04±2.08
KMS	48 hours	22.56±2.51	62.45±2.51	552.37±2.00	104.33±4.00	42.08±3.05
KMS	14 days	176.78±1.52	502.05±2.51	652.04±2.00	506.38±2.00	502.40±3.05
KMS	15 days	872.97±2.51	702.37±2.51	502.55±3.05	304.04±4.04	297.47±2.51

Values are expressed as mean±SD. ☐ Loss ☐ Restoration

Red digits represent the significant highest values from the raw state in different conditions.

In most of the conditions calcium content is mainly reduced by deep frying, whereas in 14 days salt and turmeric preservation and 14 days KMS preservation, calcium content is reduced by boiling. In 48 hours control preservation without preservative, calcium content is reduced by open pan dry roasting. In fresh condition, 14 days control preservation without preservative, 48 hours, 15 days salt and turmeric preservation calcium content is reduced by shallow frying.

Retention of calcium content occurs by open pan dry roasting mostly, but in 48 hours, 14 days, 15 days control preservation without preservative, 24 hours salt and turmeric preservation and 15 days KMS preservation, calcium retention occurs by boiling, whereas in 24 hours control preservation without preservative and in 14 days salt and turmeric preservation, calcium retention occurs by shallow frying. In fresh condition calcium retention occurs by deep frying.

Boiling, shallow frying and deep frying show the highest calcium content in 14 days KMS preservation, whereas the raw state and open pan dry roasting show the highest calcium content in 24 hours control preservation without preservative and 24 hours KMS preservation respectively.

Boiling shows the increased calcium content than the raw state in 14 days, 15 days control preservation without preservative, 24 hours salt and turmeric preservation and 24 hours, 48 hours, 14 days KMS preservation. Open pan dry roasting shows the increased calcium content than the raw state value in all the preservation conditions including fresh condition except in 24 hours 48 hours control preservation without preservative and 14 days, 15 days salt and turmeric preservation and 15 days KMS preservation, whereas shallow frying also shows the increased calcium content than the raw state in all the preservation conditions including fresh condition except in 24 hours, 48 hours, 14 days control preservation without preservative, 48 hours, 15 days salt and turmeric preservative and 24 hours, 15 days KMS preservation. Deep frying shows the increased calcium content than the raw state in fresh condition, 14 days, 15 days control preservation without preservative, 24 hours salt and turmeric preservation as well as 48 hours, 14 days KMS preservation.

This may occur due to the molecular rearrangement during cooking and the addition of cooking oil during frying. Another possible reason may be the elimination of water during cooking, [48] which concentrates calcium, increasing the content. Addition of both the natural and synthetic preservative may be a possible cause of modification of calcium content. Another possible reason for increasing calcium content is due to the elimination of anti nutritional factor during cooking.

Fig. 5.7.5.2 Graphical representation of calcium content of Pomfret with respect to different conditions

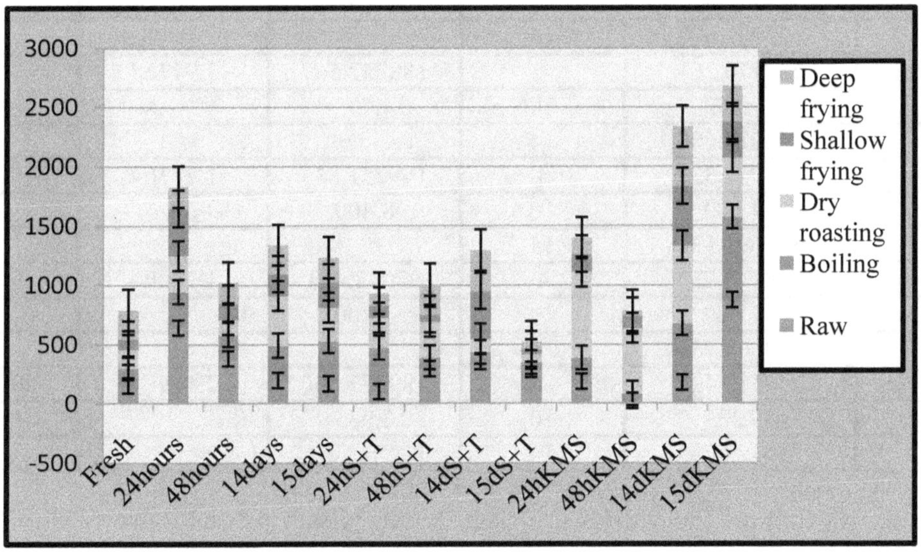

This graphical representation indicates that among all the preservation conditions **15 days KMS preservation** helps to increase the calcium content in all the cooking methods. Here the graph shows that control preservation without preservative and salt and turmeric preservation also help to restore calcium content, but KMS is more effective among the other preservation methods. Additionally, synthetic preservative may help to modify the structure of calcium, restoring the content.

Table no 5.7.5.3 ANOVA with regard to cooking conditions and preservation methods

Condition	Differences	Sum of Squares	df	Mean Square	F	Sig.
Fresh (control)	Between Groups	39108.400	4	9777.100	4.190E3	.000(S)
	Within Groups	23.333	10	2.333		
	Total	39131.733	14			
24 hours (control)	Between Groups	358857.067	4	89714.267	2.403E4	.000(S)
	Within Groups	37.333	10	3.733		
	Total	358894.400	14			
48 hours (control)	Between Groups	129166.267	4	32291.567	5.699E3	.000(S)
	Within Groups	56.667	10	5.667		
	Total	129222.933	14			
14 days (control)	Between Groups	105333.600	4	26333.400	1.837E3	.000(S)
	Within Groups	143.333	10	14.333		
	Total	105476.933	14			
15 days (control)	Between Groups	70895.067	4	17723.767	2.439E3	.000(S)
	Within Groups	72.667	10	7.267		
	Total	70967.733	14			
24 hours (salt & turmeric)	Between Groups	179569.067	4	44892.267	6.012E3	.000(S)
	Within Groups	74.667	10	7.467		
	Total	179643.733	14			
48 hours (salt & turmeric)	Between Groups	153105.067	4	38276.267	6.309E3	.000(S)
	Within Groups	60.667	10	6.067		
	Total	153165.733	14			
14 days (salt & turmeric)	Between Groups	264541.733	4	66135.433	9.448E3	.000(S)
	Within Groups	70.000	10	7.000		
	Total	264611.733	14			
15 days (salt & turmeric)	Between Groups	121984.267	4	30496.067	6.443E3	.000(S)
	Within Groups	47.333	10	4.733		
	Total	122031.600	14			
24 hours (KMS)	Between Groups	752970.267	4	188242.567	3.977E4	.000(S)
	Within Groups	47.333	10	4.733		
	Total	753017.600	14			
48 hours (KMS)	Between Groups	597007.333	4	149251.833	1.777E4	.000(S)
	Within Groups	84.000	10	8.400		
	Total	597091.333	14			
14 days (KMS)	Between Groups	368249.733	4	92062.433	1.770E4	.000(S)
	Within Groups	52.000	10	5.200		
	Total	368301.733	14			
15 days (KMS)	Between Groups	757110.400	4	189277.600	2.119E4	.000(S)
	Within Groups	89.333	10	8.933		
	Total	757199.733	14			

$p<0.05$ S= significant, NS= Non-significant. All abbreviations are on page so and so.

This statistical ANOVA table shows that all the values are significant, which means there is significant difference present in the values of calcium content of pomfret among different cooking methods and the raw state in respect to fresh condition along with different preservation methods.

Table no 5.7.5.4 Post hoc Duncan statistical analysis

Preservation	Duration	Raw state	Boiling	Dry roasting	Shallow frying	Deep frying
Control	Fresh	O,S,D[a]	O,S,D[a]	R,B,S,D[b]	R,B,O,D[c]	R,B,O,S[d]
Control	24 hours	B,O,S,D[e]	R,S,D[f]	R,S,D[f]	R,B,O,D[c]	R,B,O,S[d]
Control	48 hours	B,O,S,D[e]	R,O,S,D[g]	R,B,S,D[b]	R,B,O,D[c]	R,B,O,S[d]
Control	14 days	B,O,S,D[e]	R,O,S,D[g]	R,B,S,D[b]	R,B,O,D[c]	R,B,O,S[d]
Control	15 days	B,O,S,D[e]	R,O,S,D[g]	R,B,S,D[b]	R,B,O,D[c]	R,B,O,S[d]
Salt &Turmeric	24 hours	B,O[h]	R,O,S,D[g]	R,B,S,D[b]	B,O[h]	B,O[h]
Salt & Turmeric	48 hours	B,O,S,D[e]	R,O,S,D[g]	R,B,S,D[b]	R,B,O,D[c]	R,B,O,S[d]
Salt & Turmeric	14 days	B,O,S,D[e]	R,O,S,D[g]	R,B,S,D[b]	R,B,O,D[c]	R,B,O,S[d]
Salt & Turmeric	15 days	B,O,S,D[e]	R,O,S[i]	R,B,S[j]	R,B,O,D[c]	R,S[k]
KMS	24 hours	B,O,S,D[e]	R,O,S,D[g]	R,B,S,D[b]	R,B,O,D[c]	R,B,O,S[d]
KMS	48 hours	B,O,S,D[e]	R,O,S,D[g]	R,B,S,D[b]	R,B,O,D[c]	R,B,O,S[d]
KMS	14 days	B,O,S,D[e]	R,O[l]	R,B,S,D[b]	R,O[l]	R,O[l]
KMS	15 days	B,O,S,D[e]	R,O,S,D[g]	R,B,S,D[b]	R,B,O,D[c]	R,B,O,S[d]

R= Raw state, B= Boiling, O= open pan dry roasting, S= Shallow frying, D= Deep frying. The same uppercase alphabets represent that there is no significant difference present among the variables.

This table shows the significant difference among the different variables such as cooking methods and preservation conditions. The raw state significantly differs from boiling, open pan dry roasting, shallow frying and deep frying in all of the preservation conditions with preservatives and control preservation without preservative except in fresh condition, 24 hours salt and turmeric preservation. Boiling significantly differs from the raw state, open pan dry roasting, shallow frying and deep frying in all the preservation condition except in fresh condition, 24 hours control preservation without preservative, 15 days salt and turmeric preservation and 14 days KMS preservation. Open pan dry roasting significantly differs from the raw state, boiling, shallow frying and deep frying in all the preservation condition except in 24 hours control preservation without preservative and 15 days salt and turmeric preservation. Shallow frying significantly differs from the raw state, boiling, open pan dry roasting and deep frying in all the preservation conditions except in 24 hours salt and turmeric preservation and 14 days KMS preservation. Deep frying significantly differs from the raw state, boiling, open pan dry roasting and shallow frying in all of the preservation conditions except in 24 hours, 15 days salt and turmeric preservation and 14 days KMS preservation.

Boiling and raw state significantly differ from open pan dry roasting, shallow frying and deep frying in fresh condition. Both boiling and open pan dry roasting significantly differ from the raw state, shallow frying and deep frying in 24 hours control preservation without preservative. The raw state, shallow frying and deep frying significantly differ from boiling and open pan dry roasting in 24 hours salt and turmeric preservation. Boiling significantly differs from the raw state, open pan dry roasting and shallow frying in 15 days salt and turmeric preservation. Deep frying significantly differs from the raw state, shallow frying in 15 days salt and turmeric preservation. Boiling, shallow frying and deep frying significantly differ from the raw state and open pan dry roasting in 14 days KMS preservation.

Table no 5.7.5.5 Gradation of cooking methods from higher to lower with respect to preservation days

Preservation	Duration	Method 1	Method 2	Method 3	Method 4	Method 5
Control	Fresh	DF	OPDR	R	B	SF
Control	24 hours	R	SF	OPDR	B	DF
Control	48 hours	R	B	DF	SF	OPDR
Control	14 days	OPDR	B	DF	R	SF
Control	15 days	B	OPDR	SF	DF	R
Salt & Turmeric	24 hours	B	OPDR	SF	DF	R
Salt & Turmeric	48 hours	OPDR	R	DF	B	SF
Salt & Turmeric	14 days	SF	R	DF	OPDR	B
Salt &Turmeric	15 days	R	OPDR	DF	B	SF
KMS	24 hours	OPDR	B	R	SF	DF
KMS	48 hours	OPDR	SF	B	DF	R
KMS	14 days	OPDR	SF	DF	B	R
KMS	15 days	R	B	OPDR	SF	DF

R= Raw state, B= Boiling, OPDR= open pan dry roasting, SF= Shallow frying, DF= Deep frying. Same colour represents the similar order.

In all the preservation and fresh condition calcium retention occurs mainly in open pan dry roasting than the other cooking methods. In fresh condition retention occurs firstly in deep frying then open pan dry roasting, raw state, boiling and shallow frying. In 24 hours control preservation without preservative, retention occurs in the order of raw state, shallow frying, open pan dry roasting, boiling and deep frying. In 48 hours control preservation without preservative, retention occurs in the manner of the raw state, boiling, deep frying, shallow frying and open pan dry roasting. In 14 days control preservation without preservative, the order is open pan dry roasting then boiling, deep frying, raw state and shallow frying. In 15 days control preservation without preservative and 24 hours salt and turmeric preservation, the order is boiling, open pan dry roasting, shallow frying, deep frying and the raw state.

In 48 hours salt and turmeric preservation, retention occurs firstly in open pan dry roasting followed by the raw state, deep frying, boiling and shallow frying. In 14 days salt and turmeric preservation, the order of retention occurs in shallow frying, raw state, deep frying, open pan dry roasting and boiling. In 15 days salt and turmeric preservation, the order is the raw state, open pan dry roasting, deep frying, boiling and shallow frying.

In 24 hours KMS preservation, retention occurs firstly in open pan dry roasting then boiling, raw state, shallow frying and deep frying. In 48 hours KMS preservation, the order changes in the order of open pan dry roasting, shallow frying, boiling, deep frying and the raw state. In 14 days KMS preservation, the order is open pan dry roasting, shallow frying, deep frying, boiling and the raw state. In 15 days KMS retention, the order changes from the raw state to boiling, open pan dry roasting, shallow frying and deep frying.

The overall analysis of calcium content of pomfret is mostly restored by the gradation of methods as open pan dry roasting>raw state>deep frying>boiling>shallow frying.

Open pan dry roasting restores the calcium content as pomfret is fatty fish, thus the fatty layer possibly helps to restore the calcium content[50]. Deep frying possibly causes total dryness of fish and the fatty layers melts and calcium is also eliminated. Boiling can reduce the calcium content possibly due to the solubility of calcium in the cooking water, thus discarding the cooking water reduces the calcium content. Shallow frying reduces the calcium content as cooking oil possibly cannot cover the total surface of the fish, hence calcium can be eliminated and content can be reduced. Thus among the entire studied conventional cooking methods, **open pan dry roasting** is the best method for pomfret to restore calcium content.

5.7.6 *Hilsa* (*Tenualosa Ilisha*)

It has been reported that *hilsa* contains 180 mg of calcium per 100 gm[84] in the raw state. This value changes due to the application of different cooking methods and preservation conditions (vide Table no **5.7.6.1**).

Table no 5.7.6.1 Calcium content of *Hilsa* (mg/100gm)

Preservation	Duration	Raw state	Boiling	Dry roasting	Shallow frying	Deep frying
Control	Fresh	201.03±1.52	277.37±2.08	301.34±1.00	351.04±2.00	151.47±1.52
Control	24 hours	221.26±1.52	196.05±1.52	161.04±1.52	292.19±2.00	501.88±2.08
Control	48 hours	222.03±2.00	201.19±1.52	218.45±1.52	402.33±2.00	194.54±5.03
Control	14 day	232.27±2.00	301.33±2.08	332.34±2.00	352.05±2.00	201.45±2.08
Control	15 days	202.84±2.00	227.35±2.08	501.55±1.52	242.37±2.51	251.65±1.52
Salt & Turmeric	24 hours	752.27±2.51	422.46±2.64	104.38±4.04	653.05±4.16	504.94±4.16
Salt &Turmeric	48 hours	447.22±2.51	324.04±4.04	452.11±2.00	351.17±1.00	105.05±3.00
Salt & Turmeric	14 days	337.34±2.51	552.27±2.00	504.38±4.16	337.39±2.51	351.±1.00
Salt & Turmeric	15 days	602.48±2.51	342.44±2.51	652.04±2.00	403.22±4.16	375.29±3.00
KMS	24 hours	652.58±3.05	252.34±2.00	402.10±2.51	654.35±4.16	401.33±2.08
KMS	48 hours	45.27±2.64	302.87±2.00	252.78±2.00	244.11±4.04	45.54±2.08
KMS	14 days	205.05±2.08	424.06±4.04	242.05±3.05	142.05±2.51	252.19±2.00
KMS	15 days	272.22±2.00	425.34±2.08	315.35±3.00	342.22±2.51	502.07±2.00

Values are expressed as mean±SD. ☐ Loss ☐ Restoration

Red digits represent the significant highest values from the raw state in different conditions.

In most of the conditions, calcium content is mainly reduced by deep frying, whereas in 15 days control preservation without preservative and 15 days salt and turmeric preservation and 24 hours KMS preservation, calcium content is reduced by boiling. In 24 hours control preservation, 24 hours salt and turmeric preservation and 15 days KMS preservation, calcium content is reduced by open pan dry roasting. In 14 days KMS preservation, calcium content is reduced by shallow frying.

Retention of calcium content occurs by shallow frying mostly, but in 14 days salt and turmeric preservation and 48 hours, 14 days KMS preservation, the calcium retention occurs by boiling, whereas in 15 days control preservation without preservative, 48 hours, 15 days salt and turmeric preservation, calcium retention occurs by shallow frying. In 24 hours control preservation without preservative and 15 days KMS preservation, calcium retention occurs by deep frying.

The raw state shows the highest calcium content in 24 hours salt and turmeric preservation, whereas boiling and open pan dry roasting show the highest calcium content in 14 days and 15 days salt and turmeric preservation respectively. Shallow frying and deep frying show the highest calcium content in 24 hours and 15 days KMS preservation respectively.

Boiling shows the increased calcium content than the raw value in fresh condition, 14 days, 15 days control preservation without preservative, 14 days salt and turmeric preservation and 48 hours, 14 days, 15 days KMS preservation. Open pan dry roasting shows the increased calcium content than the raw state in all the preservation conditions including fresh condition except in 24 hours control preservation without preservative and 24 hours salt and turmeric preservation and 24 hours KMS preservation, whereas shallow frying also shows the increased calcium content than the raw value in all the preservation methods including fresh condition except in 24 hours, 48 hours, 15 days salt and turmeric preservation and 14 days KMS preservation. Deep frying shows the increased calcium content than the raw value in 24 hours, 15 days control preservation without preservative, 14 days salt and turmeric preservation as well as 48 hours, 14 days, 15 days KMS preservation.

This may occur due to the molecular rearrangement during cooking and the addition of cooking oil during frying. Another possible reason may be the elimination of water during cooking, [48] which concentrates the calcium, increasing the content. Addition of both the natural and synthetic preservative may be a possible cause of modification of calcium content. Another possible reason for increasing calcium content is due to the elimination of antinutritional factor during cooking.

Fig. 5.7.6.2 Graphical representation of Calcium content of *Hilsa* with respect to different conditions

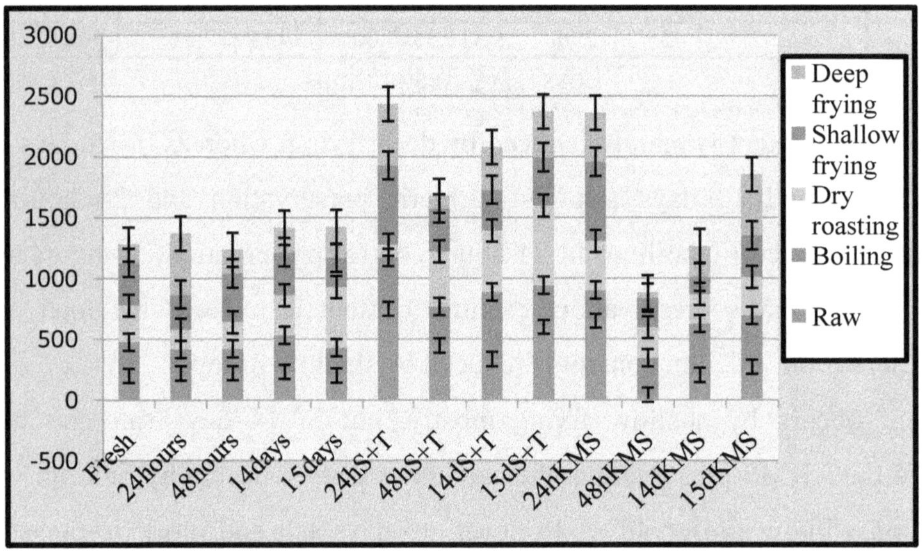

This graphical representation indicates that among all the preservation conditions **24 hours salt and turmeric preservation**[55] helps to increase the calcium content in all the cooking methods[52]. Here the graph shows that the control preservation without preservative and KMS preservation also help to restore the calcium content, but salt and turmeric preservation is more effective among the other preservation methods. The possible reason may be the natural preservative helps to modify the structure of calcium, thus the content is restored.

Table no 5.7.6.3 ANOVA with regard to cooking conditions and preservation methods

Condition	Differences	Sum of Squares	df	Mean Square	F	Sig.
Fresh (control)	Between Groups	76703.333	4	19175.833	6.849E3	.000(S)
	Within Groups	28.000	10	2.800		
	Total	76731.333	14			
24 hours (control)	Between Groups	220580.667	4	55145.167	1.798E4	.000(S)
	Within Groups	30.667	10	3.067		
	Total	220611.333	14			
48 hours (control)	Between Groups	90822.933	4	22705.733	2.988E3	.000(S)
	Within Groups	76.000	10	7.600		
	Total	90898.933	14			
14 days (control)	Between Groups	50168.400	4	12542.100	3.034E3	.000(S)
	Within Groups	41.333	10	4.133		
	Total	50209.733	14			
15 days (control)	Between Groups	680038.267	4	170009.567	4.397E4	.000(S)
	Within Groups	38.667	10	3.867		
	Total	680076.933	14			
24 hours (salt & turmeric)	Between Groups	747116.667	4	186779.167	1.452E4	.000(S)
	Within Groups	128.667	10	12.867		
	Total	747245.333	14			
48 hours (salt & turmeric)	Between Groups	238942.667	4	59735.667	8.146E3	.000(S)
	Within Groups	73.333	10	7.333		
	Total	239016.000	14			
14 days (salt & turmeric)	Between Groups	128559.600	4	32139.900	4.591E3	.000(S)
	Within Groups	70.000	10	7.000		
	Total	128629.600	14			
15 days (salt & turmeric)	Between Groups	240838.000	4	60209.500	7.001E3	.000(S)
	Within Groups	86.000	10	8.600		
	Total	240924.000	14			
24 hours (KMS)	Between Groups	372616.667	4	93154.167	1.127E4	.000(S)
	Within Groups	82.667	10	8.267		
	Total	372699.333	14			
48 hours (KMS)	Between Groups	181359.067	4	45339.767	6.356E3	.000(S)
	Within Groups	71.333	10	7.133		
	Total	181430.400	14			
14 days (KMS)	Between Groups	131848.933	4	32962.233	4.086E3	.000(S)
	Within Groups	80.667	10	8.067		
	Total	131929.600	14			
15 days (KMS)	Between Groups	101722.267	4	25430.567	4.596E3	.000(S)
	Within Groups	55.333	10	5.533		
	Total	101777.600	14			

$p<0.05$ S= significant, NS= Non-significant. All abbreviations are on page so and so.

This statistical ANOVA table shows that all the values are significant, which means there is significant difference present in the values of calcium content of *hilsa* among different cooking methods and the raw state in respect to fresh condition along with different preservation methods.

Table no 5.7.6.4 Post hoc Duncan statistical analysis

Preservation	Duration	Raw state	Boiling	Dry roasting	Shallow frying	Deep frying
Control	Fresh	B,O,S,D^{a}	R,O,S,D^{b}	R,B,S,D^{c}	R,B,O,D^{d}	R,B,O,S^{e}
Control	24 hours	B,O,S,D^{a}	R,O,S,D^{b}	R,B,S,D^{c}	R,B,O,D^{d}	R,B,O,S^{e}
Control	48 hours	B,S,D^{f}	R,O,S,D^{b}	B,S,D^{f}	R,B,O,D^{d}	R,B,O,S^{e}
Control	14 days	B,O,S,D^{a}	R,O,S,D^{b}	R,B,S,D^{c}	R,B,O,D^{d}	R,B,O,S^{e}
Control	15 days	B,O,S,D^{a}	R,O,S,D^{b}	R,B,S,D^{c}	R,B,O,D^{d}	R,B,O,S^{e}
Salt & Turmeric	24 hours	B,O,S,D^{a}	R,O,S,D^{b}	R,B,S,D^{c}	R,B,O,D^{d}	R,B,O,S^{e}
Salt & Turmeric	48 hours	B,S,D^{f}	R,O,S,D^{b}	B,S,D^{f}	R,B,O,D^{d}	R,B,O,S^{e}
Salt & Turmeric	14 days	B,O,D^{g}	R,O,S,D^{b}	R,B,S,D^{c}	B,O,D^{g}	R,B,O,S^{e}
Salt & Turmeric	15 days	B,O,S,D^{a}	R,O,S,D^{b}	R,B,S,D^{c}	R,B,O,D^{d}	R,B,O,S^{e}
KMS	24 hours	B,O,D^{g}	R,O,S,D^{b}	R,B,S^{h}	B,O,D^{g}	R,B,S^{h}
KMS	48 hours	B,O,S^{i}	R,O,S,D^{b}	R,B,S,D^{c}	R,B,O,D^{d}	B,O,S^{i}
KMS	14 days	B,O,S,D^{a}	R,O,S,D^{b}	R,B,S,D^{c}	R,B,O,D^{d}	R,B,O,S^{e}
KMS	15 days	B,O,S,D^{a}	R,O,S,D^{b}	R,B,S,D^{c}	R,B,O,D^{d}	R,B,O,S^{e}

R= Raw state, B= Boiling, O= open pan dry roasting, S= Shallow frying, D= Deep frying. The same uppercase alphabets represent that there is no significant difference present among the variables.

This table shows the significant difference among the different variables such as cooking methods and preservation conditions. The raw state significantly differs from boiling, open pan dry roasting, shallow frying and deep frying in all of the preservation conditions with preservatives and control preservation without preservative except in 48 hours control preservation, 48 hours, 14 days salt and turmeric preservation and 24 hours, 48 hours KMS preservation. Boiling significantly differs from the raw state, open pan dry roasting, shallow frying and deep frying in all the preservation conditions. Open pan dry roasting significantly differs from the raw state, boiling, shallow frying and deep frying in all the preservation conditions except in 48 hours control preservation without preservative and 48 hours salt and turmeric preservation and 24 hours KMS preservation. Shallow frying significantly differs from the raw state, boiling, open pan dry roasting and deep frying in all the preservation conditions except in 14 days salt and turmeric preservation and 24 hours KMS preservation. Deep frying significantly differs from the raw state, boiling, open pan dry roasting and shallow frying in all of the preservation conditions except in 24 hours, 48 hours KMS preservation.

Open pan dry roasting and the raw state significantly differ from boiling, shallow frying and deep frying in 48 hours control preservation without preservative and 48 hours salt and turmeric preservation. The raw state and shallow frying significantly differ from boiling, open pan dry roasting and deep frying in 14 days salt and turmeric preservation and 24 hours KMS preservation. Boiling and deep frying significantly differ from the raw state, open pan dry roasting and shallow frying in 24 hours KMS preservation. The raw state and deep frying significantly differ from boiling, open pan dry roasting and shallow frying in 48 hours KMS preservation.

Table no 5.7.6.5 Gradation of cooking methods from higher to lower restoration with respect to preservation days

Preservation	Duration	Method 1	Method 2	Method 3	Method 4	Method 5
Control	Fresh	SF	OPDR	B	R	DF
Control	24 hours	DF	SF	R	B	OPDR
Control	48 hours	SF	R	OPDR	B	DF
Control	14 days	SF	OPDR	B	R	DF
Control	15 days	DF	OPDR	SF	B	R
Salt & Turmeric	24 hours	R	SF	DF	B	OPDR
Salt & Turmeric	48 hours	OPDR	R	SF	B	DF
Salt & Turmeric	14 days	B	OPDR	DF	SF	R
Salt &Turmeric	15 days	OPDR	R	SF	DF	B
KMS	24 hours	SF	R	OPDR	DF	B
KMS	48 hours	B	OPDR	SF	DF	R
KMS	14 days	B	DF	OPDR	R	SF
KMS	15 days	DF	B	SF	OPDR	R

R= Raw state, B= Boiling, OPDR= open pan dry roasting, SF= Shallow frying, DF= Deep frying. Same colour represents the similar order.

In all the preservation and fresh condition, calcium retention occurs mainly in shallow frying than the other cooking methods. In fresh condition and 14 days control preservation without preservative, retention occurs firstly in shallow frying followed by open pan dry roasting, boiling, raw state and deep frying. In 24 hours control preservation without preservative, the order changes from deep frying, shallow frying, raw state, boiling and open pan dry roasting. In 48 hours control preservation without preservative, the order is shallow frying, raw state, open pan dry roasting, boiling and deep frying. In 15 days control preservation without preservative, the order changes from deep frying to open pan dry roasting, shallow frying, boiling and the raw state.

In 24 hours salt and turmeric preservation, retention occurs firstly in the raw state then shallow frying, deep frying, boiling and open pan dry roasting. In 48 hours salt and turmeric preservation, the order is open pan dry roasting, raw state, shallow frying, boiling and deep frying. In 14 days salt and turmeric preservation, the order changes from boiling to open pan dry roasting, deep frying, shallow frying and the raw state. In 15 days salt and turmeric preservation, it changes in the order of open pan dry roasting followed by the raw state, shallow frying, deep frying and boiling.

In 24 hours KMS preservation, retention occurs firstly in shallow frying followed by the raw state, open pan dry roasting, deep frying and boiling. In 48 hours KMS preservation, the order changes from boiling to open pan dry roasting, shallow frying, deep frying and the raw state. In 14 days KMS preservation, the order is boiling, deep frying, open pan dry roasting, raw state and shallow frying. In 15 days KMS preservation, the order of retention becomes deep frying then boiling, shallow frying, open pan dry roasting and the raw state.

The overall analysis of calcium content of *hilsa* is mostly restored by the gradation of methods as shallow frying> open pan dry roasting >deep frying>boiling>raw state.

Shallow frying restores[66] the calcium content as cooking oil possibly cover the total surface of the fish, thus calcium cannot be eliminated. Open pan dry roasting restores calcium content as *hilsa* is fatty fish, thus the fatty layer probably helps to restore the calcium content[50]. Deep frying causes total dryness of fish and the fatty layers possibly melts and calcium is also eliminated. Boiling can reduce calcium content possibly due to the solubility of calcium in the cooking water, thus discarding the cooking water reduces the calcium content. Thus among all the studied conventional cooking methods, **shallow frying** is the best method for *hilsa* to restore calcium content.

5.8 Energy Content

It has been reported that generally fish contains 72-349 kcal of energy[84] in the raw state. This experiment is carried out to estimate the percentage of energy content along with its changes in different cooking and preservation methods among different fish and edible aquatic species. Energy content is estimated by energy conversion factor[73].

5.8.1 *Rohu* (*Labeo rohita*)

It has been reported that *rohu* contains 97 kcal of energy per 100 gm[83] in the raw condition. This value changes due to the application of different cooking methods and preservation conditions (vide Table no **5.8.1.1**).

Table no 5.8.1.1 Energy content of *Rohu* (kcal/100gm)

Preservation	Duration	Raw state	Boiling	Dry roasting	Shallow frying	Deep frying
Control	Fresh	128.30±1.47	55.66±0.52	51.67±0.42	133.66±1.01	92.81±0.88
Control	24 hours	93.45±1.94	81.82±0.36	86.49±0.30	121.13±1.50	119.88±0.84
Control	48 hours	160.67±2.21	56.55±0.19	62.98±0.80	94.02±0.34	87.42±0.60
Control	14 days	58.54±1.37	43.89±2.04	48.04±2.22	102.33±2.27	67.38±2.50
Control	15 days	63.69±0.88	77.23±1.00	124.65±1.62	114.21±1.96	86.76±1.07
Salt & Turmeric	24 hours	140.67±0.78	73.06±0.87	109.15±0.16	167.68±0.81	166.68±2.14
Salt & Turmeric	48 hours	163.49±0.84	91.67±0.43	89.68±0.49	136.44±1.28	122.06±0.66
Salt & Turmeric	14 days	162.76±0.47	55.83±0.42	99.93±0.52	171.48±0.24	119.37±0.53
Salt & Turmeric	15 days	140.39±1.19	50.93±1.28	74.62±0.71	131.92±1.02	98.63±0.21
KMS	24 hours	123.08±1.22	67.05±0.53	82.94±0.73	89.52±1.25	94.19±0.63
KMS	48 hours	78.27±0.55	44.64±0.70	34.99±0.78	102.47±0.47	93.58±1.04
KMS	14 days	129.30±1.48	81.76±0.54	57.97±0.68	109.83±0.64	114.83±4.49
KMS	15 days	105.89±1.17	73.86±0.09	84.33±0.79	99.61±0.97	96.89±0.37

Values are expressed as mean±SD. ☐ Loss ☐ Restoration

Red digits represent the significant highest values from the raw state in different conditions.

In most of the conditions, calcium content is mainly reduced by boiling, whereas in fresh condition, 48 hours salt and turmeric preservation and 48 hours, 14 days KMS preservation, energy content is reduced by open pan dry roasting.

Retention of energy content occurs by shallow frying mostly, but in 15 days control preservation without preservative, energy retention occurs by open pan dry roasting, whereas in 24 hours, 14 days KMS preservation energy retention occurred by deep frying.

Boiling and open pan dry roasting show the highest energy content in 15 days control preservation without preservative, whereas shallow frying and deep frying show the highest energy content in 14 days and 24 hours salt and turmeric preservation respectively. The raw state shows the highest calcium content in 48 hours salt and turmeric preservation.

Boiling and open pan dry roasting show the increased energy content than the raw value in 15 days control preservation without preservative. Shallow frying also shows the increased energy content than the raw state in all the preservation conditions except in fresh condition, 24 hours, 14 days, 15 days control preservation without preservative, 24 hours, 14 days salt and turmeric preservation and 48 hours KMS preservation. Deep frying shows the increased energy content than the raw state in 24 hours, 14 days, 15 days control preservation without preservative, 24 hours salt and turmeric preservation as well as 48 hours KMS preservation.

This may occur due to the molecular rearrangement during cooking and the addition of cooking oil during frying. Another possible reason may be the elimination of water during cooking[48] that concentrates the macronutrient, increasing the energy content. Addition of both the natural and synthetic preservative may be a possible cause for the modification of macronutrient content.

Fig. 5.8.1.2 Graphical representation of Energy content of *Rohu* with respect to different conditions

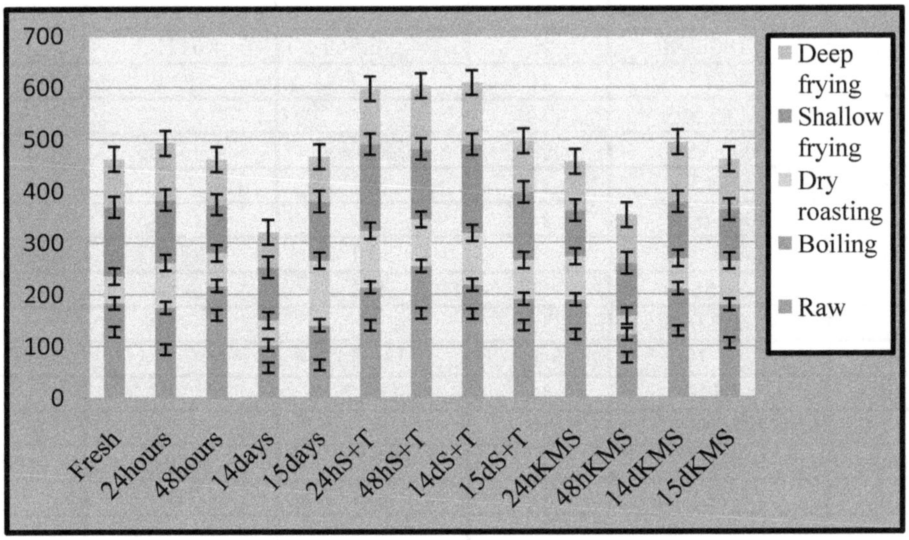

This graphical representation indicates that among all the preservation conditions, **14 days salt and turmeric preservation**[55] helps to increase the energy content in all the cooking methods[52]. Here the graph shows that control preservation without preservative and KMS preservation also help to restore energy content, but salt and turmeric preservation is more effective among the other preservation methods[34]. The possible reason may be that the natural preservative helps to modify the structure of macronutrients, thus the content is restored.

Table no 5.8.1.3 ANOVA with regard to cooking conditions and preservation methods

Condition	Differences	Sum of Squares	df	Mean Square	F	Sig.
Fresh (control)	Between Groups	17997.280	4	4499.320	5.067E3	.000(S)
	Within Groups	8.880	10	.888		
	Total	18006.161	14			
24 hours (control)	Between Groups	4188.928	4	1047.232	754.929	.000(S)
	Within Groups	13.872	10	1.387		
	Total	4202.800	14			
48 hours (control)	Between Groups	20548.947	4	5137.237	4.448E3	.000(S)
	Within Groups	11.549	10	1.155		
	Total	20560.496	14			
14 days (control)	Between Groups	6509.059	4	1627.265	363.210	.000(S)
	Within Groups	44.802	10	4.480		
	Total	6553.862	14			
15 days (control)	Between Groups	7792.238	4	1948.059	1.037E3	.000(S)
	Within Groups	18.780	10	1.878		
	Total	7811.017	14			
24 hours (salt & turmeric)	Between Groups	19706.471	4	4926.618	4.095E3	.000(S)
	Within Groups	12.031	10	1.203		
	Total	19718.502	14			
48 hours (salt & turmeric)	Between Groups	11656.740	4	2914.185	4.533E3	.000(S)
	Within Groups	6.429	10	.643		
	Total	11663.169	14			
14 days (salt & turmeric)	Between Groups	26945.286	4	6736.322	3.353E4	.000(S)
	Within Groups	2.009	10	.201		
	Total	26947.295	14			
15 days (salt & turmeric)	Between Groups	17106.278	4	4276.569	4.611E3	.000(S)
	Within Groups	9.275	10	.927		
	Total	17115.553	14			
24 hours (KMS)	Between Groups	5037.996	4	1259.499	1.462E3	.000(S)
	Within Groups	8.615	10	.862		
	Total	5046.611	14			
48 hours (KMS)	Between Groups	10632.597	4	2658.149	4.870E3	.000(S)
	Within Groups	5.458	10	.546		
	Total	10638.055	14			
14days (KMS)	Between Groups	9797.790	4	2449.447	519.838	.000(S)
	Within Groups	47.119	10	4.712		
	Total	9844.909	14			
15 days (KMS)	Between Groups	1987.152	4	496.788	799.912	.000(S)
	Within Groups	6.211	10	.621		
	Total	1993.363	14			

$p<0.05$ S= significant, NS= Non-significant. All abbreviations are on page so and so.

This statistical ANOVA table shows that all the values are significant, which means there is significant difference present in the values of energy content of *rohu* among different cooking methods and the raw state in respect to fresh condition along with different preservation methods.

Table no 5.8.1.4 Post hoc Duncan statistical analysis

Preservation	Duration	Raw state	Boiling	Dry roasting	Shallow frying	Deep frying
Control	Fresh	B,O,S,D[a]	R,O,S,D[b]	R,B,S,D[c]	R,B,O,D[d]	R,B,O,S[e]
Control	24 hours	B,O,S,D[a]	R,O,S,D[b]	R,B,S,D[c]	R,B,O[f]	R,B,O[f]
Control	48 hours	B,O,S,D[a]	R,O,S,D[b]	R,B,S,D[c]	R,B,O,D[d]	R,B,O,S[e]
Control	14 days	B,O,S,D[a]	R,O,S,D[b]	R,B,S,D[c]	R,B,O,D[d]	R,B,O,S[e]
Control	15 days	B,O,S,D[a]	R,O,S,D[b]	R,B,S,D[c]	R,B,O,D[d]	R,B,O,S[e]
Salt &Turmeric	24 hours	B,O,S,D[a]	R,O,S,D[b]	R,B,S,D[c]	R,B,O[f]	R,B,O[f]
Salt & Turmeric	48 hours	B,O,S,D[a]	R,O,S,D[b]	R,B,S,D[c]	R,B,O,D[d]	R,B,O,S[e]
Salt & Turmeric	14 days	B,O,S,D[a]	R,O,S,D[b]	R,B,S,D[c]	R,B,O,D[d]	R,B,O,S[e]
Salt & Turmeric	15 days	B,O,S,D[a]	R,O,S,D[b]	R,B,S,D[c]	R,B,O,D[d]	R,B,O,S[e]
KMS	24 hours	B,O,S,D[a]	R,O,S,D[b]	R,B,S,D[c]	R,B,O,D[d]	R,B,O,S[e]
KMS	48 hours	B,O,S,D[a]	R,O,S,D[b]	R,B,S,D[c]	R,B,O,D[d]	R,B,O,S[e]
KMS	14 days	B,O,S,D[a]	R,O,S,D[b]	R,B,S,D[c]	R,B,O,D[d]	R,B,O,S[e]
KMS	15 days	B,O,S,D[a]	R,O,S,D[b]	R,B,S,D[c]	R,B,O,D[d]	R,B,O,S[e]

R= Raw state, B= Boiling, O= open pan dry roasting, S= Shallow frying, D= Deep frying. The same uppercase alphabets represent that there is no significant difference present among the variables.

This table shows the significant difference among the different variables such as cooking methods and preservation conditions. The raw state significantly differs from boiling, open pan dry roasting, shallow frying and deep frying in all of the preservation conditions with preservatives and control preservation without preservative. Boiling significantly differs from the raw state, open pan dry roasting, shallow frying and deep frying in all of the preservation conditions. Open pan dry roasting significantly differs from the raw state, boiling, shallow frying and deep frying in all the preservation conditions. Shallow frying significantly differs from the raw state, boiling, open pan dry roasting and deep frying in all the preservation conditions except in 24 hours control preservation without preservative and 24 hours salt and turmeric preservation. Deep frying significantly differs from the raw state, boiling, open pan dry roasting and shallow frying in all the preservation conditions except in 24 hours control preservation without preservative and 24 hours salt and turmeric preservation.

Shallow frying and deep frying significantly differ from the raw state, boiling, open pan dry roasting in 24 hours control preservation without preservative and 24 hours salt and turmeric preservation.

Table no 5.8.1.5 Gradation of cooking methods from higher to lower restoration with respect to preservation days

Preservation	Duration	Method 1	Method 2	Method 3	Method 4	Method 5
Control	Fresh	SF	R	DF	B	OPDR
Control	24 hours	SF	DF	R	OPDR	B
Control	48 hours	R	SF	DF	OPDR	B
Control	14 days	SF	DF	R	OPDR	B
Control	15 days	OPDR	SF	DF	B	R
Salt &Turmeric	24 hours	SF	DF	R	OPDR	B
Salt & Turmeric	48 hours	R	SF	DF	B	OPDR
Salt & Turmeric	14 days	SF	R	DF	OPDR	B
Salt &Turmeric	15 days	R	SF	DF	OPDR	B
KMS	24 hours	R	DF	SF	OPDR	B
KMS	48 hours	SF	DF	R	B	OPDR
KMS	14 days	R	DF	SF	B	OPDR
KMS	15 days	R	SF	DF	OPDR	B

R= Raw state, B= Boiling, OPDR= open pan dry roasting, SF= Shallow frying, DF= Deep frying. Same colours represent the similar order.

In all the preservation methods and fresh condition, energy retention occurs mainly by shallow frying than the other cooking methods. In fresh condition, energy retention occurs firstly in shallow frying then the raw state, deep frying, boiling and open pan dry roasting. In 24 hours, 14 days control preservation without preservative and 24 hours salt and turmeric preservation, retention occurs in the order of shallow frying, deep frying, raw state, open pan dry roasting and boiling. In 48 hours control preservation, 15 days salt and turmeric preservation and 15 days KMS preservation, the order changes from the raw state to shallow frying, deep frying, open pan dry roasting and boiling. In 15 days control preservation without preservative, the order is open pan dry roasting then shallow frying, deep frying, boiling and the raw state.

In 48 hours salt and turmeric preservation, retention occurs firstly in the raw state followed by shallow frying, deep frying, boiling and open pan dry roasting. In 14 days salt and turmeric preservation, the order becomes shallow frying, raw state, deep frying, open pan dry roasting and boiling.

In 24 hours KMS preservation, retention occurs firstly in the raw state then deep frying, shallow frying, open pan dry roasting and boiling. In 48 hours KMS preservation, the order remains shallow frying, deep frying, raw state, boiling and open pan dry roasting. In 14 days KMS preservation, the order becomes the raw state, deep frying, shallow frying, boiling and open pan dry roasting.

The overall analysis of energy content of *rohu* is mostly restored by the gradation of methods as shallow frying>deep frying>raw state> open pan dry roasting>boiling.

Shallow frying and deep frying restore[66] the energy content possibly as cooking oil is absorbed by the fish. Open pan dry roasting reduces the energy content as fatty tissues of fish possibly melts by the application of dry heat. Boiling can reduce the energy content probably due to the higher solubility of macro nutrients in the cooking water, thus discarding the cooking water reduces the calorie value. Thus among all the studied conventional cooking methods, **shallow frying** is the best method for *rohu to* restore energy content.

5.8.2 *Katla* (*Catla catla*)

It has been reported that *katla* contains 111 kcal of energy per 100 gm[84] in the raw condition. This value changes due to the application of different cooking methods and preservation conditions (vide Table no **5.8.2.1**).

Table no 5.8.2.1 Energy content of *Katla* (kcal/100gm)

Preservation	Duration	Raw state	Boiling	Dry roasting	Shallow frying	Deep frying
Control	Fresh	185.02±1.70	96.05±0.23	68.05±0.86	141.02±0.50	114.05±1.25
Control	24 hours	147.02±2.88	106.05±0.49	121.02±0.89	149.08±0.37	100.02±0.96
Control	48 hours	167.02±2.61	103.82±0.68	83.05±0.85	126.00±1.03	111.05±0.63
Control	14 days	183.03±4.03	120.05±0.53	59.00±1.32	86.30±0.83	116.54±2.64
Control	15 days	157.38±1.28	85.72±0.11	109.63±0.97	108.22±0.64	76.85±0.26
Salt & Turmeric	24 hours	185.52±2.23	120.10±1.19	94.52±1.13	132.42±1.62	116.20±1.06
Salt & Turmeric	48 hours	261.32±1.51	113.68±1.07	107.12±0.66	167.63±1.11	134.64±1.03
Salt & Turmeric	14 days	152.69±2.40	118.75±0.74	74.59±1.00	93.22±0.92	119.63±0.54
Salt & Turmeric	15 days	137.13±0.72	71.78±1.37	120.46±0.59	136.52±0.61	139.06±1.12
KMS	24 hours	146.75±1.36	85.93±1.07	74.99±1.68	154.64±1.05	146.31±2.56
KMS	48 hours	233.42±1.21	86.72±1.60	88.03±1.71	136.31±1.19	131.33±2.37
KMS	14 days	146.33±0.65	139.33±1.25	74.41±0.95	90.70±1.68	126.11±1.70
KMS	15 days	102.87±2.00	98.51±0.78	66.83±2.22	92.90±0.99	106.43±1.70

Values are expressed as mean±SD. ☐ Loss ☐ Restoration

Red digits represent the significant highest values from the raw state in different conditions.

In most of the conditions, energy content is mainly reduced by open pan dry roasting, whereas in 48 hours, 15 days salt and turmeric preservation and 48 hours KMS preservation, energy content is reduced by boiling. In 24 hours, 15 days control preservation without preservative, energy content is reduced by deep frying.

Retention of energy content occurs by shallow frying mostly, but in 14 days control preservation without preservative and 14 days KMS energy retention occurs by boiling, whereas in 15 days control preservation without preservative, energy retention occurs by open pan dry roasting. In 48 hours, 14 days, 15 days salt and turmeric preservation and 15 days KMS preservation, energy retention occurs by deep frying.

The raw state and boiling show the highest energy content in 48 hours and 14 days KMS preservation, whereas shallow frying and deep frying show the highest energy content in 24 hours KMS preservation and 15 days salt and turmeric preservation respectively. Open pan dry roasting shows the highest energy content in 24 hours control preservation without preservative.

Shallow frying shows the increased energy content than the raw value in all the preservation conditions except in fresh condition, 24 hours control preservation without preservative and 24 hours KMS preservation. Deep frying shows the increased energy content than the raw state in 15 days salt and turmeric preservation.

This may occur due to the addition of cooking oil during frying and the molecular rearrangement during cooking. Another possible reason may be the elimination of water during cooking[48] that concentrates the macronutrient content, increasing the energy content. Addition of both the natural and synthetic preservative may be a possible cause for the modification of macronutrient content.

Fig. 5.8.2.2 Graphical representation of Energy content of *Katla* with respect to different conditions

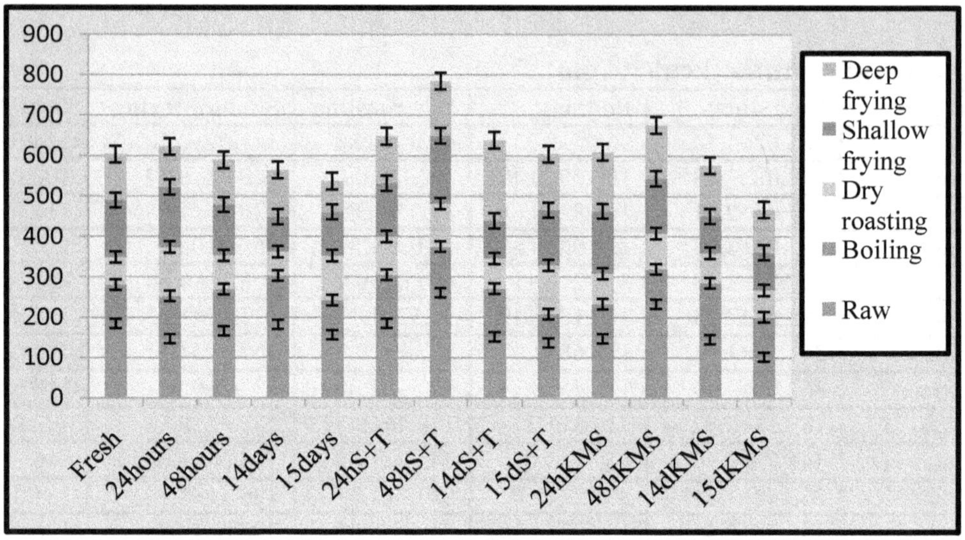

This graphical representation indicates that among all the preservation conditions, **48 hours salt and turmeric preservation**[55] helps to increase the energy content in all the cooking methods[52]. Here the graph shows that control preservation without preservative and KMS preservation also help to restore energy content, but salt and turmeric preservation is more effective among the other preservation methods. The possible reason may be that the natural preservative helps to modify the structure of macronutrients, thus the content is restored.

Table no 5.8.2.3 ANOVA with regard to cooking conditions and preservation methods

Condition	Differences	Sum of Squares	df	Mean Square	F	Sig.
Fresh (control)	Between Groups	23919.712	4	5979.928	5.412E3	.000(S)
	Within Groups	11.049	10	1.105		
	Total	23930.761	14			
24 hours (control)	Between Groups	6200.248	4	1550.062	743.782	.000(S)
	Within Groups	20.840	10	2.084		
	Total	6221.088	14			
48 hours (control)	Between Groups	11628.124	4	2907.031	620.011	.000(S)
	Within Groups	46.887	10	4.689		
	Total	11675.010	14			
14 days (control)	Between Groups	25983.942	4	6495.986	1.249E3	.000(S)
	Within Groups	51.998	10	5.200		
	Total	26035.940	14			
15 days (control)	Between Groups	11719.968	4	2929.992	4.795E3	.000(S)
	Within Groups	6.110	10	.611		
	Total	11726.078	14			
24 hours (salt & turmeric)	Between Groups	13906.735	4	3476.684	1.496E3	.000(S)
	Within Groups	23.232	10	2.323		
	Total	13929.967	14			
48 hours (salt & turmeric)	Between Groups	47579.061	4	11894.765	9.676E3	.000(S)
	Within Groups	12.292	10	1.229		
	Total	47591.354	14			
14 days (salt & turmeric)	Between Groups	10533.536	4	2633.384	1.560E3	.000(S)
	Within Groups	16.881	10	1.688		
	Total	10550.417	14			
15 days (salt & turmeric)	Between Groups	9749.298	4	2437.324	2.780E3	.000(S)
	Within Groups	8.767	10	.877		
	Total	9758.065	14			
24 hours (KMS)	Between Groups	17214.923	4	4303.731	1.586E3	.000(S)
	Within Groups	27.140	10	2.714		
	Total	17242.062	14			
48 hours (KMS)	Between Groups	42716.202	4	10679.051	3.802E3	.000(S)
	Within Groups	28.090	10	2.809		
	Total	42744.292	14			
14 days (KMS)	Between Groups	11799.120	4	2949.780	1.707E3	.000(S)
	Within Groups	17.282	10	1.728		
	Total	11816.402	14			
15 days (KMS)	Between Groups	2810.490	4	702.623	238.163	.000(S)
	Within Groups	26.552	9	2.950		
	Total	2837.042	13			

$p<0.05$ S= significant, NS= Non-significant. All abbreviations are on page so and so.

This statistical ANOVA table shows that all the values are significant, which means there is significant difference present in the values of energy content of *katla* among different cooking methods and the raw state in respect to fresh condition along with different preservation methods.

Table no 5.8.2.4 Post hoc Duncan statistical analysis

Preservation	Duration	Raw state	Boiling	Dry roasting	Shallow frying	Deep frying
Control	Fresh	B,O,S,D^{a}	R,O,S,D^{b}	R,B,S,D^{c}	R,B,O,D^{d}	R,B,O,S^{e}
Control	24 hours	B,O,D^{f}	R,O,S,D^{b}	R,B,S,D^{c}	B,O,D^{f}	R,B,O,S^{e}
Control	48 hours	B,O,S,D^{a}	R,O,S,D^{b}	R,B,S,D^{c}	R,B,O,D^{d}	R,B,O,S^{e}
Control	14 days	B,O,S,D^{a}	R,O,S^{g}	R,B,S,D^{c}	R,B,O,D^{d}	R,O,S^{g}
Control	15 days	B,O,S,D^{a}	R,O,S,D^{b}	R,B,D^{h}	R,B,D^{h}	R,B,O,S^{e}
Salt & Turmeric	24 hours	B,O,S,D^{a}	R,O,S,D^{b}	R,B,S,D^{c}	R,B,O,D^{d}	R,B,O,S^{e}
Salt & Turmeric	48 hours	B,O,S,D^{a}	R,O,S,D^{b}	R,B,S,D^{c}	R,B,O,D^{d}	R,B,O,S^{e}
Salt & Turmeric	14 days	B,O,S,D^{a}	R,O,S^{g}	R,B,S,D^{c}	R,B,O,D^{d}	R,O,S^{g}
Salt & Turmeric	15 days	B,O,D^{f}	R,O,S,D^{b}	R,B,S,D^{c}	B,O,D^{f}	R,B,O,S^{e}
KMS	24 hours	B,O,S^{i}	R,O,S,D^{b}	R,B,S,D^{c}	R,B,O,D^{d}	B,O,S^{i}
KMS	48 hours	B,O,S,D^{a}	R,S,D^{j}	R,S,D^{j}	R,B,O,D^{d}	R,B,O,S^{e}
KMS	14 days	B,O,S,D^{a}	R,O,S,D^{b}	R,B,S,D^{c}	R,B,O,D^{d}	R,B,O,S^{e}
KMS	15 days	B,O,S,D^{a}	R,O,S,D^{b}	R,B,S,D^{c}	R,B,O,D^{d}	R,B,O,S^{e}

R= Raw state, B= Boiling, O= open pan dry roasting, S= Shallow frying, D= Deep frying. The same uppercase alphabets represent that there is no significant difference present among the variables.

This table shows the significant difference among the different variables such as cooking methods and preservation conditions. The raw state significantly differs from boiling, open pan dry roasting, shallow frying and deep frying in all of the preservation conditions with preservatives and control preservation without preservative except in 24 hours control preservation without preservative, 15 days salt and turmeric preservation and 24 hours KMS preservation. Boiling significantly differs from the raw state, open pan dry roasting, shallow frying and deep frying in all of the preservation conditions. Open pan dry roasting significantly differs from the raw state, boiling, shallow frying and deep frying in all the preservation conditions except in 14 days control preservation without preservative, 14 days salt and turmeric preservation and 48 hours KMS preservation. Shallow frying significantly differs from the raw state, boiling, open pan dry roasting and deep frying in all the preservation conditions except in 24 hours, 15 days control preservation without preservative and 15 days salt and turmeric preservation. Deep frying significantly differs from the raw state, boiling, open pan dry roasting and shallow frying in all the preservation conditions except in 14 days control preservation without preservative and 14 days salt and turmeric preservation and 24 hours KMS preservation.

Shallow frying and the raw state significantly differs from boiling, open pan dry roasting, deep frying in 24 hours control preservation without preservative and 15 days salt and turmeric preservation. Boiling and deep frying significantly differs from the raw state, open pan dry roasting and shallow frying in 14 days control preservation without preservative and 14 days salt and turmeric preservation. Open pan dry roasting and shallow frying significantly differs from the raw state, boiling and deep frying in 15 days control preservation without preservative. The raw state and deep frying significantly differ from boiling, open pan dry roasting and shallow frying in 24 hours KMS preservation. Boiling and open pan dry roasting significantly differ from the raw state, shallow frying and deep frying in 48 hours KMS preservation.

Table no 5.8.2.5 Gradation of cooking methods from higher to lower restoration with respect to preservation days

Preservation	Duration	Method 1	Method 2	Method 3	Method 4	Method 5
Control	Fresh	R	SF	DF	B	OPDR
Control	24 hours	SF	R	OPDR	B	DF
Control	48 hours	R	SF	DF	B	OPDR
Control	14 days	R	B	DF	SF	OPDR
Control	15 days	R	OPDR	SF	B	DF
Salt &Turmeric	24 hours	R	SF	B	DF	OPDR
Salt & Turmeric	48 hours	R	SF	DF	B	OPDR
Salt & Turmeric	14 days	R	B	DF	SF	OPDR
Salt &Turmeric	15 days	DF	R	SF	OPDR	B
KMS	24 hours	SF	R	DF	B	OPDR
KMS	48 hours	R	SF	DF	OPDR	B
KMS	14 days	R	B	DF	SF	OPDR
KMS	15 days	DF	R	B	SF	OPDR

R= Raw state, B= Boiling, OPDR= open pan dry roasting, SF= Shallow frying, DF= Deep frying. Same colours represent the similar order.

In all the preservation techniques and fresh condition, energy retention occurs mainly in the raw state than the other cooking methods. In fresh condition, 48 hours control preservation without preservative and 48 hours salt and turmeric preservation, energy retention occurs firstly in the raw state followed by shallow frying, deep frying, boiling and open pan dry roasting. In 24 hours control preservation without preservative, retention occurs in the order of shallow frying, raw state, open pan dry roasting, boiling and deep frying. In 14 days control preservation without preservative, 14 days salt and turmeric preservation and 14 days KMS preservation, the order changes from the raw state to boiling, deep frying, shallow frying and open pan dry roasting. In 15 days control preservation without preservative, the order remains the raw state then open pan dry roasting, shallow frying, boiling and deep frying.

In 24 hours salt and turmeric preservation, retention occurs firstly in the raw state then shallow frying, boiling, deep frying and open pan dry roasting. In 15 days salt and turmeric preservation, the order becomes deep frying, raw state, shallow frying, open pan dry roasting and boiling.

In 24 hours KMS preservation, retention occurs firstly in shallow frying followed by the raw state, deep frying, boiling and open pan dry roasting. In 48 hours KMS preservation, the order changes from the raw state to shallow frying, deep frying, open pan dry roasting and boiling. In 15 days KMS preservation, the order is deep frying, raw state, boiling, shallow frying and open pan dry roasting.

The overall analysis of energy content of *katla* is mostly restored by the gradation of methods as the raw state>shallow frying>deep frying>boiling> open pan dry roasting.

Shallow frying and deep frying restore[66] the energy content possibly as cooking oil is absorbed by the fish. Boiling can reduce the energy content probably due to the solubility of macro nutrients in the cooking water, thus discarding the cooking water reduces the calorie value. Open pan dry roasting reduces the energy content as fatty tissues of fish probably melts by the application of dry heat. Thus among all the studied conventional cooking methods, **shallow frying** is the best method for *katla* to restore energy content.

5.8.3 Prawn (*Fenneropenaeus indicus*)

It has been reported that prawn contains 89 kcal of energy per 100 gm[84] in the raw condition. This value changes due to the application of different cooking methods and preservation conditions (vide Table no **5.8.3.1**).

Table no 5.8.3.1 Energy content of Prawn (kcal/100gm)

Preservation	Duration	Raw state	Boiling	Dry roasting	Shallow frying	Deep frying
Control	Fresh	96.61±1.74	41.26±0.61	58.36±0.29	89.55±0.24	87.01±0.72
Control	24 hours	77.54±1.30	34.86±0.56	48.22±1.24	124.48±0.25	171.13±0.85
Control	48 hours	62.88±0.11	23.53±0.61	38.70±0.58	47.04±0.33	63.79±0.56
Control	14 days	86.02±1.92	39.65±1.79	66.46±0.28	89.42±1.14	85.04±1.19
Control	15 day	75.25±0.50	48.41±1.80	41.59±3.07	105.95±2.00	93.19±0.74
Salt & Turmeric	24 hours	79.88±0.35	39.19±1.62	54.37±2.03	71.54±0.47	89.35±2.67
Salt &Turmeric	48 hours	81.28±0.27	39.75±3.43	55.50±1.85	96.93±0.90	99.60±0.77
Salt & Turmeric	14 days	79.44±2.19	58.77±2.79	56.29±0.35	99.37±0.42	88.17±0.97
Salt & Turmeric	15 days	86.08±4.08	52.77±1.12	72.93±1.89	105.78±2.60	125.35±1.93
KMS	24 hours	94.00±0.70	93.45±2.65	93.12±2.86	91.11±2.23	92.62±0.69
KMS	48 hours	55.70±1.04	63.68±2.07	39.89±0.94	78.01±2.26	89.96±0.97
KMS	14 days	96.74±1.45	58.10±0.13	95.12±2.71	108.12±1.38	105.46±1.89
KMS	15 days	88.29±0.62	34.33±1.21	78.53±2.21	94.15±1.27	98.69±2.69

Values are expressed as mean±SD. ☐ Loss ☐ Restoration
Red digits represent the significant highest values from the raw state in different conditions.

In most of the conditions, energy content is mainly reduced by boiling, whereas in 15 days control preservation without preservative, 14 days salt and turmeric preservation and 48 hours KMS preservation, energy content is reduced by open pan dry roasting. In 24 hours KMS preservation, energy content is reduced by shallow frying. Retention of energy content occurs by deep frying mostly, but in 24 hours KMS preservation energy retention occurs by boiling, whereas in fresh condition, 14 days, 15 days control preservation without preservative, 14 days salt and turmeric preservation and 14 days KMS preservation, energy retention occurs by shallow frying.

The raw state and open pan dry roasting show the highest energy content in 14 days KMS preservation, whereas shallow frying and deep frying show the highest energy content in 24 hours control preservation without preservative. Boiling shows the highest energy content in 48 hours KMS preservation.

Boiling shows the increased energy content than the raw state in all the preservation conditions except in fresh 48 hours KMS preservation. Shallow frying shows the increased energy content than the raw value in all the preservation conditions except in fresh condition, 48 hours control preservation without preservative, 24 hours salt and turmeric preservation and 24 hours KMS preservation. Deep frying shows the increased energy content than the raw value in all the preservation conditions except in fresh condition, 14 days control preservation without preservative and 24 hours KMS preservation.

This may occur due to the molecular rearrangement during cooking and the addition of cooking oil during frying. It is also possible that the elimination of water during cooking[48]concentrates the macronutrient content, increasing the energy content. Another possible reason may be the addition of both the natural and synthetic preservatives which can cause modification of macronutrient content.

Fig. 5.8.3.2 Graphical representation of Energy content of Prawn with respect to different conditions

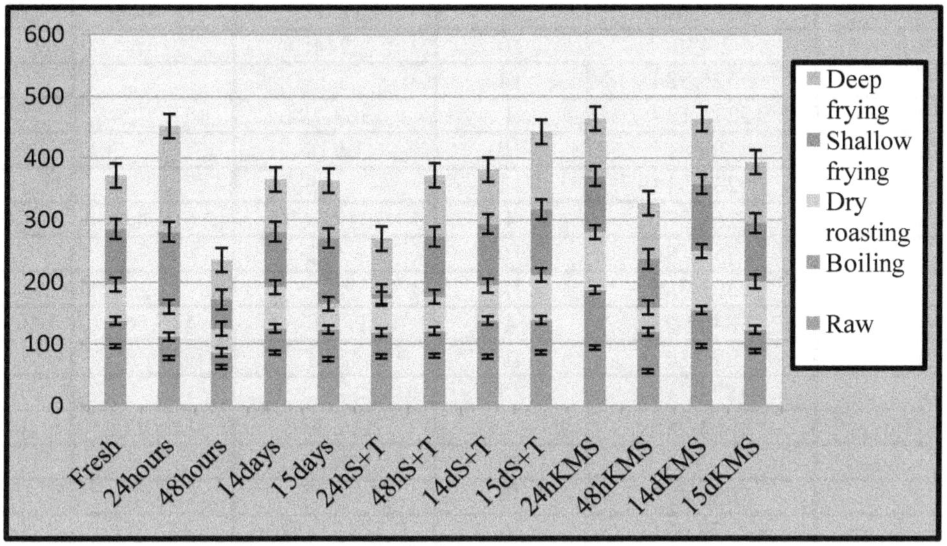

This graphical representation indicates that among all the preservation conditions, **14 days KMS preservation**[59] helps to increase the energy content in all the cooking methods. Here the graph shows that control preservation without preservative and salt and turmeric preservation also help to restore energy content, but KMS preservation is more effective among the other preservation methods[39]. The possible reason may be that the synthetic preservative helps to modify the structure of macronutrients, restoring the content.

Table no 5.8.3.3 ANOVA with regard to cooking conditions and preservation methods

Condition	Differences	Sum of Squares	df	Mean Square	F	Sig.
Fresh (control)	Between Groups	6711.930	4	1677.983	2.055E3	.000(S)
	Within Groups	8.166	10	.817		
	Total	6720.096	14			
24 hours (control)	Between Groups	18212.286	4	4553.072	5.356E3	.000(S)
	Within Groups	8.501	10	.850		
	Total	18220.787	14			
48 hours (control)	Between Groups	3524.147	4	881.037	3.614E3	.000(S)
	Within Groups	2.438	10	.244		
	Total	3526.584	14			
14 days (control)	Between Groups	5215.137	4	1303.784	672.724	.000(S)
	Within Groups	19.381	10	1.938		
	Total	5234.518	14			
15 days (control)	Between Groups	9268.271	4	2317.068	659.801	.000(S)
	Within Groups	35.118	10	3.512		
	Total	9303.389	14			
24 hours (salt & turmeric)	Between Groups	4845.903	4	1211.476	435.566	.000(S)
	Within Groups	27.814	10	2.781		
	Total	4873.716	14			
48 hours (salt & turmeric)	Between Groups	8023.785	4	2005.946	586.987	.000(S)
	Within Groups	34.174	10	3.417		
	Total	8057.959	14			
14 days (salt & turmeric)	Between Groups	4172.001	4	1043.000	377.617	.000(S)
	Within Groups	27.621	10	2.762		
	Total	4199.622	14			
15 days (salt & turmeric)	Between Groups	9365.815	4	2341.454	366.468	.000(S)
	Within Groups	63.892	10	6.389		
	Total	9429.708	14			
24 hours (KMS)	Between Groups	32.564	4	8.141	1.419	.297(NS)
	Within Groups	57.390	10	5.739		
	Total	89.954	14			
48 hours (KMS)	Between Groups	4529.476	4	1132.369	458.907	.000(S)
	Within Groups	24.675	10	2.468		
	Total	4554.151	14			
14 days (KMS)	Between Groups	4858.880	4	1214.720	404.807	.000(S)
	Within Groups	30.007	10	3.001		
	Total	4888.888	14			
15 days (KMS)	Between Groups	8096.263	4	2024.066	647.139	.000(S)
	Within Groups	31.277	10	3.128		
	Total	8127.540	14			

$p<0.05$ S= significant, NS= Non-significant. All abbreviations are on page so and so.

This statistical ANOVA table shows that all the values are significant, which means there is significant difference present in the values of energy content of prawn among different cooking methods and the raw state in respect to fresh condition along with different preservation methods.

Table no 5.8.3.4 Post hoc Duncan statistical analysis

Preservation	Duration	Raw state	Boiling	Dry roasting	Shallow frying	Deep frying
Control	Fresh	B,O,S,D[a]	R,O,S,D[b]	R,B,S,D[c]	R,B,O,D[d]	R,B,O,S[e]
Control	24 hours	B,O,S,D[a]	R,O,S,D[b]	R,B,S,D[c]	R,B,O,D[d]	R,B,O,S[e]
Control	48 hours	B,O,S,D[a]	R,O,S,D[b]	R,B,S,D[c]	R,B,O,D[d]	R,B,O,S[e]
Control	14 days	B,O,S[f]	R,O,S,D[b]	R,B,S,D[c]	R,B,O,D[d]	B,O,S[f]
Control	15 days	B,O,S,D[a]	R,O,S,D[b]	R,B,S,D[c]	R,B,O,D[d]	R,B,O,S[e]
Salt &Turmeric	24 hours	B,O,S,D[a]	R,O,S,D[b]	R,B,S,D[c]	R,B,O,D[d]	R,B,O,S[e]
Salt & Turmeric	48 hours	B,O,S,D[a]	R,O,S,D[b]	R,B,S,D[c]	R,B,O[g]	R,B,O[g]
Salt & Turmeric	14 days	B,O,S,D[a]	R,S,D[h]	R,S,D[h]	R,B,O,D[d]	R,B,O,S[e]
Salt & Turmeric	15 days	B,O,S,D[a]	R,O,S,D[b]	R,B,S,D[c]	R,B,O,D[d]	R,B,O,S[e]
KMS	24 hours	---	---	---	---	---
KMS	48 hours	B,O,S,D[a]	R,O,S,D[b]	R,B,S,D[c]	R,B,O,D[d]	R,B,O,S[e]
KMS	14 days	B,S,D[i]	R,O,S,D[b]	B,S,D[i]	R,B,O[j]	R,B,O[j]
KMS	15 days	B,O,S,D[a]	R,O,S,D[b]	R,B,S,D[c]	R,B,O,D[d]	R,B,O,S[e]

R= Raw state, B= Boiling, O= open pan dry roasting, S= Shallow frying, D= Deep frying. The same uppercase alphabets represent that there is no significant difference present among the variables.

This table shows the significant difference among the different variables such as cooking methods and preservation conditions. The raw state significantly differs from boiling, open pan dry roasting, shallow frying and deep frying in all of the preservation conditions with preservatives and control preservation without preservative except in 14 days control preservation without preservative and 14 days KMS preservation. Boiling significantly differs from the raw state, open pan dry roasting, shallow frying and deep frying in all the preservation conditions except in 14 days salt and turmeric preservation. Open pan dry roasting significantly differs from the raw state, boiling, shallow frying and deep frying in all the preservation conditions except in 14 days salt and turmeric preservation and 14 days KMS preservation. Shallow frying significantly differs from the raw state, boiling, open pan dry roasting and deep frying in all the preservation conditions except in 48 hours salt and turmeric preservation and 14 days KMS preservation. Deep frying significantly differs from the raw state, boiling, open pan dry roasting and shallow frying in all the preservation conditions except in 14 days control preservation without preservative and 48 hours salt and turmeric preservation and 14 days KMS preservation.

The raw state and deep frying significantly differ from boiling, open pan dry roasting and shallow frying in 14 days control preservation without preservative. Shallow frying and deep frying significantly differ from the raw state, boiling, open pan dry roasting in 48 hours salt and turmeric preservation and 14 days KMS preservation. Open pan dry roasting and boiling significantly differ from the raw state, shallow frying and deep frying in 14 days salt and turmeric preservation. The raw state and open pan dry roasting significantly differs from boiling, shallow frying and deep frying in 14 days KMS preservation. Boiling and open pan dry roasting significantly differs from the raw state, shallow frying and deep frying in 14 days KMS preservation.

Table no 5.8.3.5 Gradation of cooking methods from higher to lower restoration with respect to preservation days

Preservation	Duration	Method 1	Method 2	Method 3	Method 4	Method 5
Control	Fresh	R	SF	DF	OPDR	B
Control	24 hours	SF	DF	R	OPDR	B
Control	48 hours	DF	R	SF	OPDR	B
Control	14 days	SF	R	DF	OPDR	B
Control	15 days	SF	DF	R	B	OPDR
Salt &Turmeric	24 hours	DF	R	SF	OPDR	B
Salt & Turmeric	48 hours	DF	SF	R	OPDR	B
Salt & Turmeric	14 days	SF	DF	R	B	OPDR
Salt &Turmeric	15 days	DF	SF	R	OPDR	B
KMS	24 hours	R	B	OPDR	DF	SF
KMS	48 hours	DF	SF	B	R	OPDR
KMS	14 days	SF	DF	R	OPDR	B
KMS	15 days	DF	SF	R	OPDR	B

R= Raw state, B= Boiling, OPDR= open pan dry roasting, SF= Shallow frying, DF= Deep frying. Same colours represent the similar order.

In all the preservation methods and fresh condition, calcium retention occurs mainly in shallow frying than the other cooking methods. In fresh condition, energy retention occurs firstly in the raw state followed by shallow frying, deep frying, open pan dry roasting and boiling. In 24 hours control preservation without preservative and 14 days KMS preservation, the order changes from shallow frying, deep frying, raw state, open pan dry roasting and boiling. In 48 hours control preservation without preservative and 24 hours salt and turmeric preservation, the order is deep frying, raw state, shallow frying, open pan dry roasting and boiling. In 14 days control preservation without preservative, the order remains shallow frying, raw state, deep frying, open pan dry roasting and boiling. In 15 days control preservation without preservative and 14 days salt and turmeric preservation, the order becomes shallow frying then deep frying, raw state, boiling and open pan dry roasting.

In 48 hours, 15 days salt and turmeric preservation, retention occurs firstly in deep frying then shallow frying, raw state, open pan dry roasting, boiling.

In 24 hours KMS preservation, retention occurs firstly in the raw state followed by boiling, open pan dry roasting, deep frying and shallow frying. In 48 hours KMS preservation, the order changes from deep frying to shallow frying, boiling, raw state and then open pan dry roasting. In 15 days KMS preservation, the order is deep frying, shallow frying, raw state, open pan dry roasting and boiling.

The overall analysis of energy content of prawn is mostly restored by the gradation of methods as shallow frying>deep frying>raw state>open pan dry roasting>boiling.

Shallow frying and deep frying restore[66] the energy content probably as the cooking oil is absorbed by the prawn. Open pan dry roasting reduces the energy content possibly due to the elimination of macronutrient content by the application of dry heat. Boiling can reduce the energy content possibly due to the higher solubility of macro nutrients in the cooking water, thus discarding the cooking water reduces the calorie value. Thus among all the studied conventional cooking methods, **shallow frying** is the best method for prawn to restore energy content.

5.8.4 Lobster (*Macrobrachium rosenbergii*)

It has been reported that lobster contains 90 kcal of energy per 100 gm[84] in the raw condition. This value changes due to the application of different cooking methods and preservation conditions (vide Table no **5.8.4.1**).

Table no 5.8.4.1 Energy content of Lobster (kcal/100gm)

Preservation	Duration	Raw state	Boiling	Dry roasting	Shallow frying	Deep frying
Control	Fresh	106.87±0.53	67.37±0.35	56.71±0.94	110.87±0.91	117.54±1.28
Control	24 hours	78.82±0.31	38.25±0.49	38.60±0.40	76.16±0.41	79.04±0.34
Control	48 hours	61.91±2.19	39.35±0.62	30.66±2.13	82.03±0.27	97.90±0.54
Control	14 days	87.22±0.47	41.59±2.18	54.76±2.65	85.06±2.98	97.70±1.78
Control	15 days	83.30±1.98	64.31±2.61	47.24±2.36	110.28±2.21	101.96±2.44
Salt & Turmeric	24 hours	100.13±4.42	84.89±1.29	51.83±1.31	87.07±0.80	99.93±2.13
Salt &Turmeric	48 hours	111.35±1.18	34.97±2.30	93.36±0.98	82.61±1.20	104.99±3.27
Salt & Turmeric	14 days	97.61±0.90	65.34±1.18	62.74±1.13	89.61±1.85	55.47±1.67
Salt & Turmeric	15 days	109.93±3.16	69.58±4.69	60.20±1.67	112.83±1.17	116.41±1.34
KMS	24 hours	77.27±1.18	41.78±1.50	54.95±2.25	58.94±1.19	70.13±1.30
KMS	48 hours	82.70±1.86	60.50±3.07	79.49±1.12	125.48±0.90	79.46±1.68
KMS	14 days	93.68±2.85	74.38±1.47	92.79±3.57	122.77±1.19	88.72±2.10
KMS	15 days	100.32±1.57	47.98±1.99	97.38±1.43	83.10±1.11	137.38±3.15

Values are expressed as mean±SD. Loss Restoration

Red digits represent the significant highest values from the raw state in different conditions.

In most of the conditions, energy content is mainly reduced by boiling, whereas in fresh condition, 48 hours, 15 days control preservation without preservative and 24 hours, 15 days salt and turmeric preservation, energy content is reduced by open pan dry roasting. In 14 days salt and turmeric preservation, energy content is reduced by deep frying.

Retention of energy content occurs by deep frying mostly, but in 15 days control preservation without preservative, 48 hours salt and turmeric preservation and 48 hours, 14 days KMS preservation, energy retention occurs by shallow frying.

Deep frying and open pan dry roasting show the highest energy content in 15 days KMS preservation, whereas shallow frying and boiling show the highest energy content in 48 hours KMS preservation and 15 days salt and turmeric preservation respectively. The raw state shows the highest energy content in 48 hours salt and turmeric preservation.

Shallow frying shows the increased energy content than the raw value in fresh condition, 48 hours, 15 days control preservation without preservative, 15 days salt and turmeric preservation and 48 hours, 14 days KMS preservation. Deep frying shows the increased energy content than the raw state in fresh condition, 24 hours, 48 hours, 14 days, 15 days control preservation without preservative and 15 days salt and turmeric preservation and 15 days KMS preservation.

This may occur due to the molecular rearrangement during cooking and the addition of cooking oil during frying. Another possible reason may be the elimination of water during cooking[48] that concentrates the macronutrients content, increasing the energy content. Addition of both the natural and synthetic preservatives may be a possible cause for the modification of macronutrients content.

Fig. 5.8.4.2 Graphical representation of Energy content of Lobster with respect to different conditions

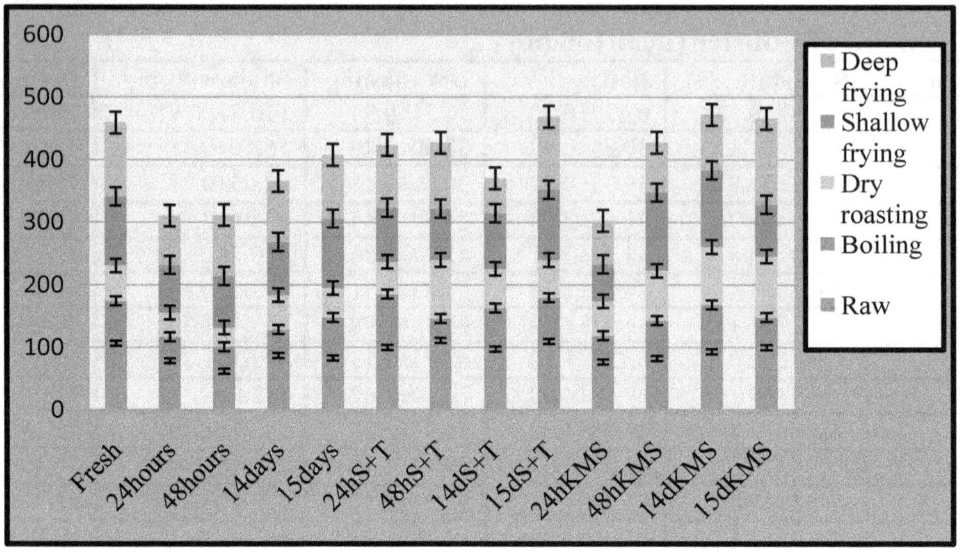

This graphical representation indicates that among all the preservation conditions, **14 days and 15 days KMS preservation** help to increase the energy content in all the cooking methods. Here the graph shows that control preservation without preservative and salt and turmeric preservation also help to restore energy content, but KMS preservation is more effective among the other preservation methods[39]. It may be possible due to the synthetic preservative, which helps to modify the structure of macronutrients, restoring the content.

Table no 5.8.4.3 ANOVA with regard to cooking conditions and preservation methods

Condition	Differences	Sum of Squares	df	Mean Square	F	Sig.
Fresh (control)	Between Groups	9250.083	4	2312.521	3.081E3	.000(S)
	Within Groups	7.505	10	.751		
	Total	9257.588	14			
24 hours (control)	Between Groups	5655.699	4	1413.925	9.027E3	.000(S)
	Within Groups	1.566	10	.157		
	Total	5657.265	14			
48 hours (control)	Between Groups	9552.621	4	2388.155	1.186E3	.000(S)
	Within Groups	20.137	10	2.014		
	Total	9572.758	14			
14 days (control)	Between Groups	7122.104	4	1780.526	312.148	.000(S)
	Within Groups	57.041	10	5.704		
	Total	7179.146	14			
15 days (control)	Between Groups	8142.717	4	2035.679	371.626	.000(S)
	Within Groups	54.778	10	5.478		
	Total	8197.495	14			
24 hours (salt & turmeric)	Between Groups	4667.344	4	1166.836	206.901	.000(S)
	Within Groups	56.396	10	5.640		
	Total	4723.739	14			
48 hours (salt & turmeric)	Between Groups	11014.457	4	2753.614	696.201	.000(S)
	Within Groups	39.552	10	3.955		
	Total	11054.009	14			
14 days (salt & turmeric)	Between Groups	4038.603	4	1009.651	522.480	.000(S)
	Within Groups	19.324	10	1.932		
	Total	4057.927	14			
15 days (salt & turmeric)	Between Groups	8547.849	4	2136.962	281.516	.000(S)
	Within Groups	75.909	10	7.591		
	Total	8623.758	14			
24 hours (KMS)	Between Groups	2272.991	4	568.248	239.570	.000(S)
	Within Groups	23.719	10	2.372		
	Total	2296.711	14			
48 hours (KMS)	Between Groups	6910.039	4	1727.510	490.825	.000(S)
	Within Groups	35.196	10	3.520		
	Total	6945.235	14			
14 days (KMS)	Between Groups	3722.752	4	930.688	160.582	.000(S)
	Within Groups	57.957	10	5.796		
	Total	3780.710	14			
15 days (KMS)	Between Groups	12497.640	4	3124.410	791.770	.000(S)
	Within Groups	39.461	10	3.946		
	Total	12537.101	14			

$p<0.05$ S= significant, NS= Non-significant. All abbreviations are on page so and so.

This statistical ANOVA table shows that all the values are significant, which means there is significant difference present in the values of energy content of lobster among different cooking methods and the raw state in respect to fresh condition along with different preservation methods.

Table no 5.8.4.4 Post hoc Duncan statistical analysis

Preservation	Duration	Raw state	Boiling	Dry roasting	Shallow frying	Deep frying
Control	Fresh	B,O,S,D^{a}	R,O,S,D^{b}	R,B,S,D^{c}	R,B,O,D^{d}	R,B,O,S^{e}
Control	24 hours	B,O,S^{f}	R,S,D^{g}	R,S,D^{g}	R,B,O,D^{d}	B,O,S^{f}
Control	48 hours	B,O,S,D^{a}	R,O,S,D^{b}	R,B,S,D^{c}	R,B,O,D^{d}	R,B,O,S^{e}
Control	14 days	B,O,D^{h}	R,O,S,D^{b}	R,B,S,D^{c}	B,O,D^{h}	R,B,O,S^{e}
Control	15 days	B,O,S,D^{a}	R,O,S,D^{b}	R,B,S,D^{c}	R,B,O,D^{d}	R,B,O,S^{e}
Salt & Turmeric	24 hours	B,O,S^{f}	R,O,D^{i}	R,B,S,D^{c}	R,O,D^{i}	B,O,S^{f}
Salt & Turmeric	48 hours	B,O,S,D^{a}	R,O,S,D^{b}	R,B,S,D^{c}	R,B,O,D^{d}	R,B,O,S^{e}
Salt & Turmeric	14 days	B,O,S,D^{a}	R,O,S,D^{b}	R,B,S,D^{c}	R,B,O,D^{d}	R,B,O,S^{e}
Salt & Turmeric	15 days	B,O,D^{h}	R,O,S,D^{b}	R,B,S,D^{c}	B,O^{j}	R,B,O^{k}
KMS	24 hours	B,O,S,D^{a}	R,O,S,D^{b}	RB,S,D^{c}	R,B,O,D^{d}	R,B,O,S^{e}
KMS	48 hours	B,S^{l}	R,O,S,D^{b}	B,S^{l}	R,B,O,D^{d}	B,S^{l}
KMS	14 days	B,S,D^{m}	R,O,S,D^{b}	B,S^{l}	R,B,O,D^{d}	R,B,S^{n}
KMS	15 days	B,S,D^{m}	R,O,S,D^{b}	B,S,D^{m}	R,B,O,D^{d}	R,B,O,S^{e}

R= Raw state, B= Boiling, O= open pan dry roasting, S= Shallow frying, D= Deep frying. The same uppercase alphabets represent that there is no significant difference present among the variables.

This table shows the significant difference among the different variables such as cooking methods and preservation conditions. The raw state significantly differs from boiling, open pan dry roasting, shallow frying and deep frying in all of the preservation conditions with preservatives and control preservation without preservative except in 24 hours, 14 days control preservation without preservative and 24 hours, 15 days salt and turmeric preservation and 48 hours, 14 days, 15 days KMS preservation. Boiling significantly differs from the raw state, open pan dry roasting, shallow frying and deep frying in all the preservation conditions except in 24 hours control preservation without preservative and 24 hours salt and turmeric preservation. Open pan dry roasting significantly differs from the raw state, boiling, shallow frying and deep frying in all the preservation conditions except in 24 hours control preservation without preservative and 48 hours, 14 days, 15 days KMS preservation. Shallow frying significantly differs from the raw state, boiling, open pan dry roasting and deep frying in all the preservation conditions except in 14 days control preservation without preservative, 24 hours, 15 days salt and turmeric preservation. Deep frying significantly differs from the raw state, boiling, open pan dry roasting and shallow frying in all the preservation conditions except in 24 hours control preservation without preservative and 24 hours, 15 days salt and turmeric preservation and 48 hours, 14 days KMS preservation.

The raw state and deep frying significantly differ from boiling, open pan dry roasting, shallow frying in 24 hours control preservation without preservative and 24 hours salt and turmeric preservation. Open pan dry roasting and boiling significantly differ from the raw state, shallow frying, deep frying in 24 hours control preservation without preservative. The raw state and shallow frying significantly differ from boiling, open pan dry roasting, deep frying in 14 days control preservation without preservative. The raw state significantly differs from boiling, open pan dry roasting and deep frying in 15 days salt and turmeric preservation.

Boiling significantly differs from boiling and open pan dry roasting in 15 days salt and turmeric preservation. Boiling and shallow frying significantly differ from the raw state, open pan dry roasting and deep frying in 24 hours salt and turmeric preservation. Deep frying significantly differs from the raw state, boiling and open pan dry roasting in 15 days salt and turmeric preservation. The raw state, open pan dry roasting and deep frying significantly differ from boiling and shallow frying in 48 hours KMS preservation. The raw state significantly differs from boiling, shallow frying and deep frying in 14 days and 15 days KMS preservation. Open pan dry roasting significantly differs from boiling and shallow frying in 14 days KMS preservation, whereas deep frying significantly differs from the raw state, boiling and shallow frying in 14 days KMS preservation. Again open pan dry roasting significantly differs from boiling, shallow frying and deep frying in 15 days KMS preservation.

Table no 5.8.4.5 Gradation of cooking methods from higher to lower restoration with respect to preservation days

Preservation	Duration	Method 1	Method 2	Method 3	Method 4	Method 5
Control	Fresh	DF	SF	R	B	OPDR
Control	24 hours	DF	R	SF	OPDR	B
Control	48 hours	DF	SF	R	B	OPDR
Control	14 days	DF	SF	R	OPDR	B
Control	15 days	SF	DF	R	B	OPDR
Salt &Turmeric	24 hours	R	DF	SF	B	OPDR
Salt & Turmeric	48 hours	R	DF	OPDR	SF	B
Salt & Turmeric	14 days	R	SF	B	OPDR	DF
Salt &Turmeric	15 days	DF	SF	R	B	OPDR
KMS	24 hours	R	DF	SF	OPDR	B
KMS	48 hours	SF	R	OPDR	DF	B
KMS	14 days	SF	R	OPDR	DF	B
KMS	15 days	DF	R	OPDR	SF	B

R= Raw state, B= Boiling, OPDR= open pan dry roasting, SF= Shallow frying, DF= Deep frying. Same colours represent the similar order.

In all the preservation methods and fresh condition, energy retention occurs mainly in deep frying than the other cooking methods. In fresh condition, 48 hours control preservation without preservative and 15 days salt and turmeric preservation, energy retention occurs firstly in deep frying followed by shallow frying, raw state, boiling and open pan dry roasting. In 24 hours control preservation without preservative, the order changes from deep frying to the raw state, shallow frying, open pan dry roasting and boiling. In 14 days control preservation without preservative, the order becomes deep frying, shallow frying, raw state, open pan dry roasting and boiling. In 15 days control preservation without preservative, the order remains shallow frying, deep frying, raw state, boiling and open pan dry roasting. In 24 hours salt and turmeric preservation, retention occurs firstly in the raw state followed by deep frying, shallow frying, boiling and open pan dry roasting. In 48 hours salt and turmeric preservation, the order is the raw state, deep frying, open pan dry roasting, shallow frying and boiling. In 14 days salt and turmeric preservation, the order becomes the raw state, shallow frying, boiling, open pan dry roasting and deep frying.

In 24 hours KMS preservation, retention occurs firstly in the raw state followed by deep frying, shallow frying, open pan dry roasting and boiling. In 48 hours, 14 days KMS preservation, the order changes from shallow frying to the raw state, open pan dry roasting, deep frying and boiling. In 15 days KMS preservation, the order is deep frying, raw state, open pan dry roasting, shallow frying and boiling.

The overall analysis of energy content of lobster is mostly restored by the gradation of methods as deep frying> shallow frying>raw state>open pan dry roasting>boiling.

Shallow frying and deep frying restore[66] the energy content as the cooking oil is absorbed by the lobster. Open pan dry roasting reduces the energy content due to the elimination of macronutrients content by the application of dry heat. Boiling can reduce the energy content due to the higher solubility of macro nutrients in the cooking water, thus discarding this water reduces the calorie value. Thus among all the studied conventional cooking methods, **deep frying** is the best method for Lobster to restore energy content.

5.8.5 Pomfret (*Pampus argenteus*)

It has been reported that pomfret contains 87 kcal of energy per 100 gm[84] in the raw condition. This value changes due to the application of different cooking methods and preservation conditions (vide Table no **5.8.5.1**).

Table no 5.8.5.1 Energy content of Pomfret (kcal/100gm)

Preservation	Duration	Raw state	Boiling	Dry roasting	Shallow frying	Deep frying
Control	Fresh	89.22±0.23	48.45±0.17	85.72±0.95	85.38±0.76	81.85±0.49
Control	24 hours	118.56±0.96	75.39±1.07	50.265±1.04	107.98±0.29	84.98±0.95
Control	48 hours	202.80±0.68	181.31±0.79	24.49±0.86	193.63±1.18	121.93±0.54
Control	14 days	182.50±2.50	148.21±1.31	99.94±3.87	74.12±1.40	105.94±2.13
Control	15 days	162.00±0.30	114.14±1.90	163.96±2.04	169.24±1.43	125.99±2.18
Salt & Turmeric	24 hours	226.82±1.34	222.57±1.54	168.52±1.26	196.14±1.81	219.77±1.19
Salt & Turmeric	48 hours	221.65±0.81	149.76±1.27	179.96±1.05	194.99±1.75	168.44±1.67
Salt & Turmeric	14 days	104.41±1.08	205.31±1.50	161.32±2.08	113.62±1.54	138.78±3.05
Salt & Turmeric	15 days	250.97±1.30	111.79±1.76	171.05±2.79	184.46±2.18	128.08±1.01
KMS	24 hours	286.32±1.96	154.62±2.34	219.16±1.44	398.65±1.81	190.26±1.66
KMS	48 hours	253.29±0.24	130.97±2.57	156.70±2.28	252.83±1.84	190.94±1.92
KMS	14 days	227.97±1.01	188.20±1.80	143.18±2.78	135.27±2.13	160.03±2.14
KMS	15 days	245±1.11	130.83±2.86	190.10±1.55	197.81±1.80	154.22±2.86

Values are expressed as mean±SD. ☐ Loss ☐ Restoration

Red digits represent the significant highest values from the raw state in different conditions.

In most of the conditions, energy content is mainly reduced by boiling, whereas in 24 hours, 48 hours control preservation without preservative and 24 hours salt and turmeric preservation, energy content is reduced by open pan dry roasting. In 14 days salt and turmeric preservation and 14 days KMS preservation, energy content is reduced by shallow frying.

Retention of energy content occurs by shallow frying mostly, but in 24 hours, 14 days salt and turmeric preservation, energy retention occurs by boiling. In fresh condition, energy retention occurs by open pan dry roasting. In 14 days control preservation without preservative energy retention occurs by deep frying.

Shallow frying, open pan dry roasting and the raw state show the highest energy content in 24 hours KMS preservation, whereas deep frying and boiling show the highest energy content in 24 hours and 14 days salt and turmeric preservation respectively.

Boiling, open pan dry roasting and deep frying show the increased energy content than the raw state in 14 days salt and turmeric preservation. Shallow frying shows the increased energy content than the raw value in 15 days control preservation without preservative, 14 days salt and turmeric preservation and 24 hours KMS preservation.

This may occur due to the molecular rearrangement during cooking and the addition of cooking oil during frying. Another possible reason may be the elimination of water during[48] cooking that concentrates the macronutrients, increasing the energy content. Addition of both the natural and synthetic preservatives may be a possible cause for the modification of macronutrients content.

Fig. 5.8.5.5 Graphical representation of Energy content of Pomfret with respect to different conditions

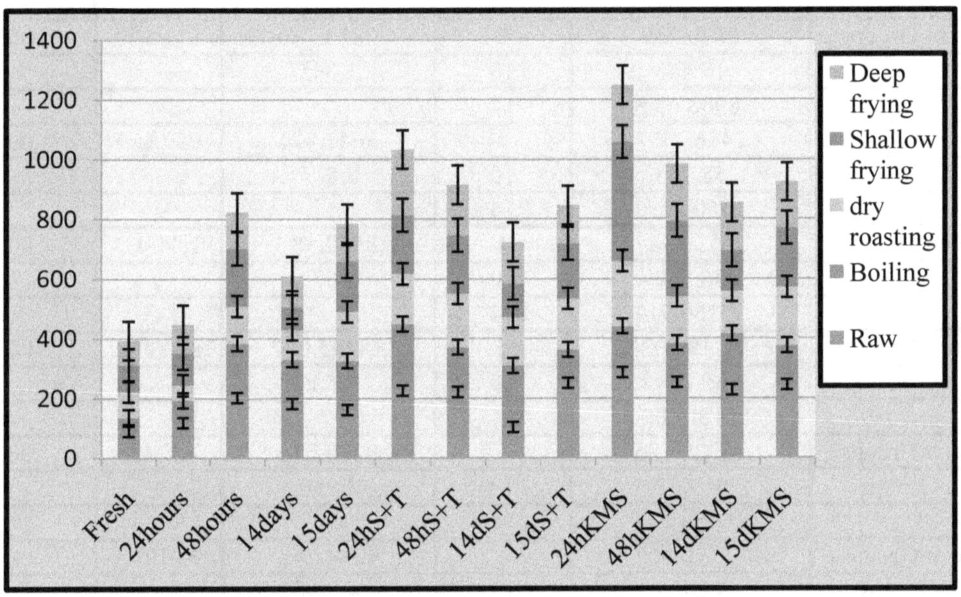

This graphical representation indicates that among all the preservation conditions, **24 hours KMS preservation** helps to increase the energy content in all the cooking methods. Here the graph shows that control preservation without preservative and salt and turmeric preservation also help to restore energy content, but KMS preservation is more effective among the other preservation methods. The possible reason may be that the synthetic preservative helps to modify the structure of macronutrients, restoring the content.

Table no 5.8.5.3 ANOVA with regard to cooking conditions and preservation methods

Condition	Differences	Sum of Squares	df	Mean Square	F	Sig.
Fresh (control)	Between Groups	3386.139	4	846.535	2.390E3	.000(S)
	Within Groups	3.542	10	.354		
	Total	3389.681	14			
24 hours (control)	Between Groups	8773.364	4	2193.341	2.660E3	.000(S)
	Within Groups	8.244	10	.824		
	Total	8781.608	14			
48 hours (control)	Between Groups	18030.953	4	4507.738	6.432E3	.000(S)
	Within Groups	7.009	10	.701		
	Total	18037.962	14			
14 days (control)	Between Groups	22153.293	4	5538.323	928.705	.000(S)
	Within Groups	59.635	10	5.963		
	Total	22212.928	14			
15 days (control)	Between Groups	7586.247	4	1896.562	648.475	.000(S)
	Within Groups	29.246	10	2.925		
	Total	7615.493	14			
24 hours (salt & turmeric)	Between Groups	7190.822	4	1797.706	863.236	.000(S)
	Within Groups	20.825	10	2.083		
	Total	7211.648	14			
48 hours (salt & turmeric)	Between Groups	8890.239	4	2222.560	1.205E3	.000(S)
	Within Groups	18.448	10	1.845		
	Total	8908.687	14			
14 days (salt & turmeric)	Between Groups	14565.497	4	3641.374	939.627	.000(S)
	Within Groups	38.753	10	3.875		
	Total	14604.250	14			
15 days (salt & turmeric)	Between Groups	35730.347	4	8932.587	2.443E3	.000(S)
	Within Groups	36.567	10	3.657		
	Total	35766.914	14			
24 hours (KMS)	Between Groups	113180.026	4	28295.007	8.070E3	.000(S)
	Within Groups	35.064	10	3.506		
	Total	113215.090	14			
48 hours (KMS)	Between Groups	36920.186	4	9230.046	2.430E3	.000(S)
	Within Groups	37.992	10	3.799		
	Total	36958.177	14			
14 days (KMS)	Between Groups	17136.968	4	4284.242	1.010E3	.000(S)
	Within Groups	42.438	10	4.244		
	Total	17179.405	14			
15 days (KMS)	Between Groups	23015.648	4	5753.912	1.234E3	.000(S)
	Within Groups	46.635	10	4.664		
	Total	23062.283	14			

$p<0.05$ S= significant, NS= Non-significant. All abbreviations are on page so and so.

This statistical ANOVA table shows that all the values are significant, which means there is significant difference present in the values of energy content of pomfret among different cooking methods and the raw state in respect to fresh condition along with different preservation methods.

Table no 5.8.5.4 Post hoc Duncan statistical analysis

Preservation	Duration	Raw state	Boiling	Dry roasting	Shallow frying	Deep frying
Control	Fresh	B,O,S,D[a]	R,O,S,D[b]	R,B,D[c]	R,B,D[c]	R,B,O,S[f]
Control	24 hours	B,O,S,D[a]	R,O,S,D[b]	R,B,S,D[d]	R,B,O,D[e]	R,B,O,S[f]
Control	48 hours	B,O,S,D[a]	R,O,S,D[b]	R,B,S,D[d]	R,B,O,D[e]	R,B,O,S[f]
Control	14 days	B,O,S,D[a]	R,O,S,D[b]	R,B,S,D[d]	R,B,O,D[e]	R,B,O,S[f]
Control	15 days	B,S,D[g]	R,O,S,D[b]	B,S,D[g]	R,B,O,D[e]	R,B,O,S[f]
Salt &Turmeric	24 hours	B,O,S,D[a]	R,O,S,D[b]	R,B,S,D[d]	R,B,O,D[e]	R,B,O,S[f]
Salt & Turmeric	48 hours	B,O,S,D[a]	R,O,S,D[b]	R,B,S,D[d]	R,B,O,D[e]	R,B,O,S[f]
Salt & Turmeric	14 days	B,O,S,D[a]	R,O,S,D[b]	R,B,S,D[d]	R,B,O,D[e]	R,B,O,S[f]
Salt & Turmeric	15 days	B,O,S,D[a]	R,O,S,D[b]	R,B,S,D[d]	R,B,O,D[e]	R,B,O,S[f]
KMS	24 hours	B,O,S,D[a]	R,O,S,D[b]	R,B,S,D[d]	R,B,O,D[e]	R,B,O,S[f]
KMS	48 hours	B,O,D[h]	R,O,S,D[b]	R,B,S,D[d]	B,O,D[h]	R,B,O,S[f]
KMS	14 days	B,O,S,D[a]	R,O,S,D[b]	R,B,S,D[d]	R,B,O,D[e]	R,B,O,S[f]
KMS	15 days	B,O,S,D[a]	R,O,S,D[b]	R,B,S,D[d]	R,B,O,D[e]	R,B,O,S[f]

R= Raw state, B= Boiling, O= open pan dry roasting, S= Shallow frying, D= Deep frying. The same uppercase alphabets represent that there is no significant difference present among the variables.

This table shows the significant difference among the different variables such as cooking methods and preservation conditions. The raw state significantly differs from boiling, open pan dry roasting, shallow frying and deep frying in all of the preservation conditions with preservatives and control preservation without preservative except in 15 days control preservation without preservative and 48 hours KMS preservation. Boiling significantly differs from the raw state, open pan dry roasting, shallow frying and deep frying in all the preservation conditions. Open pan dry roasting significantly differs from the raw state, boiling, shallow frying and deep frying in all the preservation conditions except in fresh condition and 15 days control preservation without preservative. Shallow frying significantly differs from the raw state, boiling, open pan dry roasting and deep frying in all the preservation conditions except in fresh condition and 48 hours KMS preservation. Deep frying significantly differs from the raw state, boiling, open pan dry roasting and shallow frying in all the preservation conditions.

Open pan dry roasting and shallow frying significantly differ from the raw state, boiling and deep frying in fresh condition. The raw state and open pan dry roasting significantly differ from boiling, shallow frying and deep frying in 15 days control preservation without preservative. The raw state and shallow frying significantly differ from boiling, open pan dry roasting and deep frying in 48 hours KMS preservation.

Table no 5.8.5.5 Gradation of cooking methods from higher to lower restoration with respect to preservation days

Preservation	Duration	Method 1	Method 2	Method 3	Method 4	Method 5
Control	Fresh	R	OPDR	SF	DF	B
Control	24 hours	R	SF	DF	B	OPDR
Control	48 hours	R	SF	B	OPDR	DF
Control	14 days	R	B	DF	OPDR	SF
Control	15 days	SF	OPDR	R	DF	B
Salt & Turmeric	24 hours	R	DF	B	SF	OPDR
Salt & Turmeric	48 hours	R	SF	OPDR	DF	B
Salt & Turmeric	14 days	B	R	OPDR	DF	SF
Salt &Turmeric	15 days	R	SF	OPDR	DF	B
KMS	24 hours	SF	R	OPDR	DF	B
KMS	48 hours	R	SF	DF	OPDR	B
KMS	14 days	R	B	DF	OPDR	SF
KMS	15 days	R	SF	OPDR	DF	B

R= Raw state, B= Boiling, OPDR= open pan dry roasting, SF= Shallow frying, DF= Deep frying. Same colours represent the similar order.

In all the preservation and fresh condition, energy retention occurs mainly in the raw state than the other cooking methods. In fresh condition, energy retention occurs firstly in the raw state then open pan dry roasting, shallow frying, deep frying and boiling. In 24 hours control preservation without preservative, the order changes from the raw state to shallow frying, deep frying, boiling and open pan dry roasting. In 48 hours control preservation without preservative, the order changes from the raw state to shallow frying, boiling, open pan dry roasting and deep frying and. In 14 days control preservation without preservative and 14 days KMS preservation, the order becomes the raw state, boiling, deep frying, open pan dry roasting and shallow frying. In 15 days control preservation without preservative, the order remains shallow frying, open pan dry roasting, raw state, deep frying and boiling.

In 24 hours salt and turmeric preservation, retention occurs firstly in the raw state, deep frying, boiling, shallow frying and open pan dry roasting. In 48 hours, 15 days salt and turmeric preservation, the order becomes the raw state, shallow frying, open pan dry roasting, deep frying and boiling. In 14 days salt and turmeric preservation, the order becomes boiling, raw state, open pan dry roasting, deep frying and shallow frying.

In 24 hours KMS preservation, retention occurs firstly in shallow frying followed by the raw state, open pan dry roasting, deep frying and boiling. In 48 hours KMS preservation, the order remains the raw state, shallow frying, deep frying, open pan dry roasting and boiling. In 15 days KMS preservation, the order becomes the raw state, shallow frying, open pan dry roasting, deep frying and boiling.

The overall analysis of energy content of pomfret is mostly restored by the gradation of methods as the raw state> shallow frying>open pan dry roasting>deep frying>boiling.

Shallow frying probably restores[66] the energy content as cooking oil is absorbed by the pomfret. Open pan dry roasting reduces the energy content probably due to the elimination of macronutrients content by the application of dry heat. Deep frying possibly melts the fatty layer of pomfret, thus macronutrient especially fat content is reduced along with the total energy content. Boiling can reduce the energy content possibly due to the solubility of macro nutrients in the cooking water, thus discarding the cooking water reduces the calorie value. Thus among all the studied conventional cooking methods, **shallow frying** is the best method for pomfret to restore energy content.

5.8.6 *Hilsa* (*Tenualosa Ilisha*)

It has been reported that *hilsa* contains 273 kcal of energy per 100gm[83] in the raw condition. This value changes due to the application of different cooking methods and preservation conditions (vide Table no **5.8.6.1**).

Table no 5.8.6.1 Energy content of *Hilsa* (kcal/100gm)

Preservation	Duration	Raw state	Boiling	Dry roasting	Shallow frying	Deep frying
Control	Fresh	233.90±0.14	161.15±5.41	103.83±0.60	109.28±0.50	94.63±0.38
Control	24 hour	336.60±2.50	133.11±0.96	88.19±1.00	107.37±1.06	86.32±0.50
Control	48 hours	348.20±0.76	139.88±0.70	137.57±0.88	116.11±0.60	134.52±0.48
Control	14 day	325.63±0.60	201.10±2.13	141.38±1.17	184.00±1.44	143.17±2.05
Control	15 days	323.16±3.71	219.94±1.43	159.95±1.09	142.66±1.35	114.25±2.73
Salt & Turmeric	24 hours	274.76±1.51	229.43±3.73	99.43±1.73	191.28±1.30	134.16±2.55
Salt & Turmeric	48 hours	306.36±0.95	269.94±2.22	142.57±1.26	142.54±2.62	147.63±1.92
Salt & Turmeric	14 days	284.94±2.60	267.02±2.09	138.72±1.13	152.20±2.33	98.96±2.11
Salt & Turmeric	15days	238.42±1.19	203.27±1.65	154.48±1.57	170.16±1.42	125.03±1.98
KMS	24 hours	294.65±0.97	259.70±0.72	132.05±1.31	111.45±1.18	122.06±2.39
KMS	48 hours	329±0.78	287.36±1.61	115.75±2.00	161.61±1.87	193.83±0.60
KMS	14days	318.14±0.55	258.47±1.63	151.61±1.61	179.47±1.52	146.61±2.78
KMS	15days	305.60±0.16	320.00±1.23	241.16±0.98	161.87±3.41	181.63±3.01

Values are expressed as mean±SD. ☐ Loss ☐ Restoration
Red digit represents the significant highest values from the raw state in a single condition.

In most of the conditions, energy content is reduced mainly by deep frying, whereas in 14 days control preservation without preservative and 24 hours salt and turmeric preservation and 48 hours KMS preservation, energy content is reduced by open pan dry roasting. In 48 hours control preservation without preservative and 24 hours, 15 days KMS preservation, energy content is reduced by shallow frying. Retention of energy content occurs by boiling in all the preservation conditions.

Boiling and open pan dry roasting show the highest energy content in 15 days KMS preservation, whereas both shallow frying and deep frying show the highest energy content in 24 hours salt and turmeric preservation and 48 hours KMS preservation respectively.

Boiling shows the increased energy content than the raw value in 15 days KMS preservation. This may occur due to the molecular rearrangement during cooking and the addition of cooking oil during frying. Another possible reason may be the elimination of water during cooking[48] that concentrates the macronutrients, increasing the of energy content. Addition of both the natural and synthetic preservatives may be a possible cause for the modification of macronutrients content.

Fig. 5.8.6.2 Graphical representation of Energy content of *Hilsa* with respect to different conditions

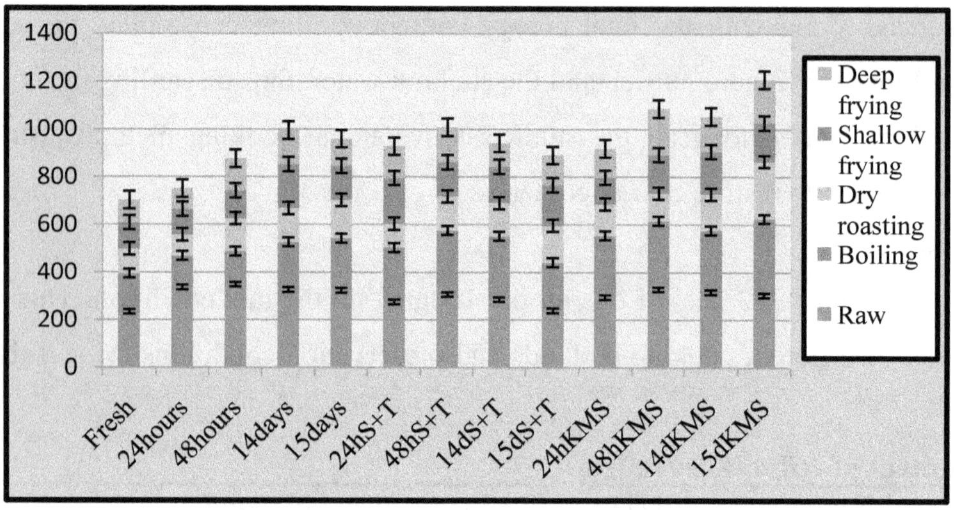

This graphical representation indicates that among all the preservation conditions, **15 days KMS preservation** helps to increase the energy content in all the cooking methods. Here the graph shows that control preservation without preservative and salt and turmeric preservation also help to restore energy content, but KMS preservation is more effective among the other preservation methods. The possible reason may be the synthetic preservative helps to modify the structure of macronutrients, restoring the content.

Table no 5.8.6.3 ANOVA with regard to cooking conditions and preservation methods

Condition	Differences	Sum of Squares	df	Mean Square	F	Sig.
Fresh (control)	Between Groups	40149.680	4	10037.420	1.018E4	.000(S)
	Within Groups	9.858	10	.986		
	Total	40159.537	14			
24 hours (control)	Between Groups	133548.539	4	33387.135	1.748E4	.000(S)
	Within Groups	19.101	10	1.910		
	Total	133567.640	14			
48 hours (control)	Between Groups	113208.341	4	28302.085	5.979E4	.000(S)
	Within Groups	4.733	10	.473		
	Total	113213.075	14			
14 days (control)	Between Groups	68105.115	4	17026.279	5.554E3	.000(S)
	Within Groups	30.655	10	3.066		
	Total	68135.770	14			
15 days (control)	Between Groups	83102.329	4	20775.582	3.272E3	.000(S)
	Within Groups	63.500	10	6.350		
	Total	83165.829	14			
24 hours (salt & turmeric)	Between Groups	59920.831	4	14980.208	2.735E3	.000(S)
	Within Groups	54.775	10	5.478		
	Total	59975.606	14			
48 hours (salt & turmeric)	Between Groups	76589.260	4	19147.315	5.331E3	.000(S)
	Within Groups	35.919	10	3.592		
	Total	76625.179	14			
14 days (salt & turmeric)	Between Groups	81836.951	4	20459.238	4.580E3	.000(S)
	Within Groups	44.672	10	4.467		
	Total	81881.623	14			
15 days (salt & turmeric)	Between Groups	23133.144	4	5783.286	2.316E3	.000(S)
	Within Groups	24.975	10	2.498		
	Total	23158.119	14			
24 hours (KMS)	Between Groups	89319.290	4	22329.823	1.081E4	.000(S)
	Within Groups	20.662	10	2.066		
	Total	89339.952	14			
48 hours (KMS)	Between Groups	94677.113	4	23669.278	1.064E4	.000(S)
	Within Groups	22.250	10	2.225		
	Total	94699.362	14			
14 days (KMS)	Between Groups	67199.103	4	16799.776	5.352E3	.000(S)
	Within Groups	31.389	10	3.139		
	Total	67230.492	14			
15 days (KMS)	Between Groups	60579.771	4	15144.943	3.248E3	.000(S)
	Within Groups	46.627	10	4.663		
	Total	60626.398	14			

$p<0.05$ S= significant, NS= Non-significant. All abbreviations are on page so and so.

This statistical ANOVA table shows that all the values are significant, which means there is significant difference present in the values of energy content of *hilsa* among different cooking methods and the raw state in respect to fresh condition along with different preservation methods.

Table no 5.8.6.4 Post hoc Duncan statistical analysis

Preservation	Duration	Raw state	Boiling	Dry roasting	Shallow frying	Deep frying
Control	Fresh	B,O,S,D^a	R,O,S,D^b	R,B,S,D^c	R,B,O,D^d	R,B,O,S^e
Control	24 hours	B,O,S,D^a	R,O,S,D^b	R,B,S^f	R,B,O,D^d	R,B,S^f
Control	48 hours	B,O,S,D^a	R,O,S,D^b	R,B,S,D^c	R,B,O,D^d	R,B,O,S^e
Control	14 days	B,O,S,D^a	R,O,S,D^b	R,B,S^f	R,B,O,D^d	R,B,S^f
Control	15 days	B,O,S,D^a	R,O,S,D^b	R,B,S,D^c	R,B,O,D^d	R,B,O,S^e
Salt &Turmeric	24 hours	B,O,S,D^a	R,O,S,D^b	R,B,S,D^c	R,B,O,D^d	R,B,O,S^e
Salt & Turmeric	48 hours	B,O,S,D^a	R,O,S,D^b	R,B,D^g	R,B,D^g	R,B,O,S^e
Salt & Turmeric	14 days	B,O,S,D^a	R,O,S,D^b	R,B,S,D^c	R,B,O,D^d	R,B,O,S^e
Salt & Turmeric	15days	B,O,S,D^a	R,O,S,D^b	R,B,S,D^c	R,B,O,D^d	R,B,O,S^e
KMS	24 hours	B,O,S,D^a	R,O,S,D^b	R,B,S,D^c	R,B,O,D^d	R,B,O,S^e
KMS	48 hours	B,O,S,D^a	R,O,S,D^b	R,B,S,D^c	R,B,O,D^d	R,B,O,S^e
KMS	14days	B,O,S,D^a	R,O,S,D^b	R,B,S,D^c	R,B,O,D^d	R,B,O,S^e
KMS	15days	B,O,S,D^a	R,O,S,D^b	R,B,S,D^c	R,B,O,D^d	R,B,O,S^e

R= Raw state, B= Boiling, O= open pan dry roasting, S= Shallow frying, D= Deep frying. The same uppercase alphabets represent that there is no significant difference present among the variables.

This table shows the significant difference among the different variables such as cooking methods and preservation conditions. The raw state significantly differs from boiling, open pan dry roasting, shallow frying and deep frying in all of the preservation conditions with preservatives and control preservation without preservative. Boiling significantly differs from the raw state, open pan dry roasting, shallow frying and deep frying in all the preservation conditions. Open pan dry roasting significantly differs from the raw state, boiling, shallow frying and deep frying in all the preservation conditions except in 24 hours, 14 days control preservation without preservative and 48 hours salt and turmeric preservation. Shallow frying significantly differs from the raw state, boiling, open pan dry roasting and deep frying in all the preservation conditions except in 48 hours salt and turmeric preservation. Deep frying significantly differs from the raw state, boiling, open pan dry roasting and shallow frying in all the preservation conditions except in 24 hours, 14 days control preservation without preservative.

Open pan dry roasting and deep frying significantly differ from the raw state, boiling, shallow frying in 24 hours and 14 days control preservation without preservative. Open pan dry roasting and shallow frying significantly differs from the raw state, boiling and deep frying in 48 hours salt and turmeric preservation.

Table no 5.8.6.5 Gradation of cooking method from higher to lower restoration with respect to preservation days

Preservation	Duration	Method 1	Method 2	Method 3	Method 4	Method 5
Control	Fresh	R	B	SF	OPDR	DF
Control	24 hours	R	B	SF	OPDR	DF
Control	48 hours	R	B	OPDR	DF	SF
Control	14 days	R	B	SF	DF	OPDR
Control	15 days	R	B	OPDR	SF	DF
Salt &Turmeric	24 hours	R	B	SF	DF	OPDR
Salt & Turmeric	48 hours	R	B	DF	OPDR	SF
Salt & Turmeric	14 days	R	B	SF	OPDR	DF
Salt &Turmeric	15days	R	B	SF	OPDR	DF
KMS	24 hours	R	B	OPDR	DF	SF
KMS	48 hours	R	B	DF	SF	OPDR
KMS	14days	R	B	SF	OPDR	DF
KMS	15days	R	B	OPDR	DF	SF

R= Raw state, B= Boiling, OPDR= open pan dry roasting, SF= Shallow frying, DF= Deep frying. Same colours represent the similar order.

In all the preservation methods and fresh condition, energy retention occurs mainly in the raw state than the other cooking methods. In fresh condition, 24 hours control preservation without preservative and 14 days, 15 days salt and turmeric preservation and 14 days KMS preservation, energy retention occurs firstly in the raw state followed by boiling, shallow frying, open pan dry roasting and deep frying. In 48 hours control preservation without preservative and 24 hours, 15 days KMS preservation, the order changes from the raw state to boiling, open pan dry roasting, deep frying and shallow frying. In 14 days control preservation without preservative and 24 hours salt and turmeric preservation, the order remains the raw state, boiling, shallow frying, deep frying and open pan dry roasting. In 15 days control preservation without preservative, the order becomes the raw state, boiling, open pan dry roasting, shallow frying and deep frying.

In 48 hours salt and turmeric preservation, retention occurs firstly in the raw state followed by boiling, deep frying, open pan dry roasting and shallow frying.

In 48 hours KMS preservation retention occurs firstly in the raw state then boiling, deep frying, shallow frying and open pan dry roasting.

The overall analysis of energy content of *hilsa* is mostly restored by the gradation of methods as the raw state>boiling> shallow frying>open pan dry roasting>deep frying.

Boiling can restore the energy content possibly due to the high fat content of *hilsa* that reduces solubility of macronutrients in the cooking water, restoring the calorie value. Shallow frying restores the energy content as cooking oil is possibly absorbed by *hilsa*. Open pan dry roasting reduces the energy content probably due to the elimination of macronutrients content by the application of dry heat. Deep frying possibly melts the fatty layer of *hilsa*, thus macronutrients especially fat content is reduced along with the total energy content. Thus among all the studied conventional cooking methods, **boiling** is the best method for *hilsa* to restore energy content.

5.9 Paired t test between the raw samples and cooking conditions

This statistical test is carried out to evaluate any significant deviation between the raw and cooked fish and other edible aquatic species with respect to different nutritional parameters (carbohydrate, protein, fat, moisture, ash, calcium, iron and energy) under different preservation methods. Significant level is checked at 5% level, meaning if the p value is less than 0.05 then it is significant.

Table no 5.9.1 Carbohydrate content (WOP= Without preservative, **ST**= Salt & Turmeric, **KMS**= Potassium metabisulphite)

Raw vs.		WOP					ST				KMS			
		FRESH	**24Hr**	**48Hr**	**14D**	**15D**	**24Hr**	**48Hr**	**14D**	**15D**	**24Hr**	**48Hr**	**14D**	**15D**
Rohu	B	0.003	0.001	0.000	0.004	0.000	0.001	0.202(NS)	0.000	0.006	0.001	0.000	0.024	0.013
	DR	0.001	0.001	0.008	0.222(NS)	0.008	0.000	0.022	0.002	0.088(NS)	0.006	0.000	0.150(NS)	0.141(NS)
	SF	0.001	0.002	0.005	0.271(NS)	0.024	0.002	0.052(NS)	0.039	0.004	0.004	0.000	0.003	0.007
	DF	0.002	0.008	0.020	0.053(NS)	0.004	0.120(NS)	0.006	0.006	0.040	0.000	0.001	0.004	0.065(NS)
Katla	B	0.010	0.001	0.026	0.001	0.001	0.005	0.016	0.000	0.149(NS)	0.002	0.000	0.000	0.001
	DR	0.043	0.005	0.020	0.001	0.035	0.003	0.002	0.005	0.005	0.004	0.001	0.000	0.001
	SF	0.152(NS)	0.157(NS)	0.009	0.000	0.004	0.007	0.000	0.021	0.004	0.005	0.000	0.001	0.004
	DF	0.082(NS)	0.024	0.008	0.001	0.006	0.008	0.000	0.000	0.028	0.013	0.004	0.000	0.009
Prawn	B	0.062(NS)	0.013	0.041	0.001	0.000	0.020	0.007	0.000	0.004	0.011	0.042	0.035	0.001
	DR	0.199(NS)	0.038	0.873(NS)	0.082(NS)	0.000	0.027	0.038	0.001	0.047	0.003	0.007	0.009	0.009
	SF	0.250(NS)	0.467(NS)	0.205(NS)	0.023	0.000	0.010	0.001	0.936(NS)	0.002	0.001	0.018	0.199(NS)	0.007
	DF	0.014	0.032	0.601(NS)	0.108(NS)	0.084(NS)	0.002	0.000	0.042	0.002	0.031	0.001	0.022	0.003
Lobster	B	0.000	0.404(NS)	0.004	0.002	0.002	0.000	0.001	0.000	0.001	0.002	0.000	0.000	0.001
	DR	0.005	0.005	0.001	0.010	0.003	0.001	0.000	0.000	0.000	0.000	0.000	0.000	0.002
	SF	0.197(NS)	0.723(NS)	0.874(NS)	0.069(NS)	0.004	0.003	0.002	0.000	0.001	0.001	0.000	0.000	0.002
	DF	0.006	0.037	0.005	0.046	0.004	0.000	0.002	0.000	0.017	0.001	0.000	0.000	0.023
Pomfret	B	0.013	0.046	0.016	0.013	0.011	0.001	0.001	0.000	0.000	0.000	0.002	0.001	0.005
	DR	0.006	0.079(NS)	0.004	0.011	0.481(NS)	0.000	0.013	0.000	0.001	0.001	0.000	0.000	0.085(NS)
	SF	0.078(NS)	0.196(NS)	0.042	0.001	0.430(NS)	0.000	0.635(NS)	0.002	0.000	0.000	0.001	0.000	0.002
	DF	0.847(NS)	0.155(NS)	0.590(NS)	0.002	0.000	0.001	0.005	0.000	0.001	0.001	0.001	0.001	0.015
Hilsa	B	0.002	0.057(NS)	0.089(NS)	0.001	0.001	0.004	0.003	0.000	0.000	0.004	0.060(NS)	0.000	0.001
	DR	0.000	0.028	0.015	0.003	0.016	0.002	0.005	0.001	0.001	0.003	0.000	0.000	0.017
	SF	0.011	0.095(NS)	0.013	0.004	0.002	0.002	0.007	0.022	0.000	0.023	0.042	0.001	0.001
	DF	0.080(NS)	0.018	0.001	0.000	0.000	0.011	0.022	0.006	0.025	0.000	0.017	0.000	0.000

NS= non-significant values that mean there is no significant difference present between the raw and cooked sample. R= Raw, B= Boiling, DR= Dry roasting, SF= Shallow frying, DF= Deep frying.

This table shows the p value of the carbohydrate content between the raw and cooked samples for all the fish and crustaceans. In 14 days control preservation without preservative, *rohu* shows non-significant p value for open pan dry roasting, shallow frying and deep frying with respect to the raw condition. 48 hours salt and turmeric preservation shows non-significant p value for boiling and shallow frying, whereas 24 hours salt and turmeric preservation shows non-significant p value for deep frying, and 15 days salt and turmeric preservation shows non-significant p value for open pan dry roasting with respect to the raw condition. 14 days KMS preservation shows non-significant p value for open pan dry roasting and 15 days KMS preservation shows non-significant p value for open pan dry roasting and deep frying with respect to the raw condition. Rest of the values are significant which means there is significant difference present among the raw and cooked samples in all of the preservation methods.

In fresh condition, *katla* shows non-significant p value for shallow frying and deep frying, and in 24 hours control preservation without preservative, p value is non-significant for shallow frying with respect to the raw condition. Rest of the values are significant which means there is significant difference present among the raw and cooked samples in all the preservation methods.

In fresh condition, prawn shows non-significant p value for boiling, open pan dry roasting and shallow frying, and in 24 hours control preservation without preservative, p value is non-significant for shallow frying, whereas in 48 hours control preservation without preservative, p value is non-significant for open pan dry roasting, shallow frying and deep frying with respect to the raw condition. In 14 days control preservation without preservative, p value is also non-significant for open pan dry roasting and deep frying, whereas only 15 days control preservation without preservative shows non-significant p value for deep frying with respect to the raw condition. Both salt and turmeric preservation and KMS preservation show non-significant p value for shallow frying in 14 days preservation. Rest of the values are significant which means there is significant difference present among the raw and cooked samples in all the preservation methods.

In fresh condition, 48 hours and 14 days control preservation without preservative, lobster show non-significant p value for shallow frying, whereas in 24 hours control preservation without preservative, p value is non-significant for boiling and shallow frying with respect to the raw condition. Rest of the values are significant which means there is significant difference present among the raw and cooked samples in all the preservation methods.

In fresh condition, pomfret shows non-significant p value for shallow frying and deep frying, and in 24 hours control preservation without preservative, p value is non-significant for open pan dry roasting, shallow frying and deep frying, whereas in 48 hours control preservation without preservative, p value is non-significant for deep frying with respect to the raw condition. In 15 days control preservation without preservative, p value is also non-significant for open pan dry roasting and shallow frying with respect to the raw condition. 48 hours salt and turmeric preservation shows non-significant p value for shallow frying, and 15 days KMS preservation shows non-significant p value for open pan dry roasting. Rest of the values are significant which means there is significant difference present among the raw and cooked samples in all the preservation methods.

In fresh condition, *hilsa* shows non-significant p value for deep frying, and in 24 hours control preservation without preservative, p value is non-significant for boiling and shallow frying, whereas in 48 hours control preservation without preservative, p value is non-significant for boiling with respect to the raw condition. KMS preservation shows non-significant p value for boiling in 48 hours. Rest of the values are significant which means there is significant difference present among the raw state and cooked samples in all of the preservation methods.

Overall analysis indicates that there is statistically significant difference present between the raw and cooked values for all the fish and other edible aquatic species with respect to the carbohydrate content, which means the carbohydrate contents vary in different cooking methods from the raw condition.

Table no 5.9.2 Protein content (WOP= Without preservative, **ST=** Salt & Turmeric, **KMS=** Potassium metabisulphite)

Raw vs.		WOP					ST				KMS			
		FRESH	24Hr	48Hr	14D	15D	24Hr	48Hr	14D	15D	24Hr	48Hr	14D	15D
Rohu	B	0.000	0.000	0.001	0.000	0.031	0.000	0.000	0.000	0.000	0.000	0.000	0.000	0.000
	DR	0.001	0.000	0.002	0.010	0.029	0.000	0.000	0.000	0.000	0.003	0.001	0.000	0.000
	SF	0.001	0.000	0.001	0.068(NS)	0.145(NS)	0.001	0.000	0.000	0.000	0.000	0.000	0.000	0.000
	DF	0.001	0.001	0.001	0.002	0.037	0.011	0.000	0.000	0.005	0.000	0.000	0.000	0.000
Katla	B	0.000	0.001	0.000	0.015	0.000	0.000	0.000	0.001	0.000	0.000	0.000	0.000	0.012
	DR	0.000	0.002	0.001	0.015	0.000	0.000	0.000	0.001	0.001	0.000	0.001	0.000	0.012
	SF	0.000	0.001	0.000	0.005	0.000	0.000	0.000	0.006	0.002	0.002	0.000	0.003	0.001
	DF	0.000	0.001	0.000	0.046	0.000	0.000	0.000	0.037	0.010	0.013	0.307(NS)	0.001	0.027
Prawn	B	0.000	0.000	0.000	0.003	0.000	0.000	0.000	0.007	0.009	0.001	0.004	0.000	0.001
	DR	0.000	0.000	0.001	0.003	0.002	0.004	0.001	0.007	0.232(NS)	0.018	0.013	0.002	0.061(NS)
	SF	0.000	0.000	0.001	0.000	0.000	0.001	0.000	0.002	0.004	0.000	0.004	0.000	0.016
	DF	0.001	0.000	0.001	0.001	0.019	0.002	0.000	0.009	0.093NS)	0.000	0.001	0.001	0.050(NS)
Lobster	B	0.000	0.000	0.002	0.000	0.032	0.011	0.000	0.002	0.008	0.000	0.000	0.002	0.000
	DR	0.000	0.000	0.003	0.010	0.002	0.028	0.004	0.004	0.003	0.003	0.110(NS)	0.690(NS)	0.273(NS)
	SF	0.000	0.000	0.004	0.001	0.001	0.006	0.000	0.001	0.011	0.006	0.003	0.007	0.002
	DF	0.000	0.000	0.003	0.004	0.007	0.019	0.001	0.001	0.029	0.010	0.004	0.010	0.005
Pomfret	B	0.000	0.000	0.000	0.024	0.041	0.020	0.003	0.001	0.008	0.010	0.010	0.006	0.008
	DR	0.000	0.000	0.000	0.699(NS)	0.016	0.044	0.019	0.003	0.262(NS)	0.127(NS)	0.149(NS)	0.117(NS)	0.156(NS)
	SF	0.000	0.000	0.001	0.548(NS)	0.005	0.020	0.166(NS)	0.043	0.065(NS)	0.061(NS)	0.101(NS)	0.001	0.006
	DF	0.001	0.000	0.001	0.013	0.012	0.023	0.069(NS)	0.041	0.792(NS)	0.020	0.022	0.223(NS)	0.001
Hilsa	B	0.000	0.000	0.000	0.002	0.002	0.001	0.003	0.001	0.007	0.000	0.000	0.003	0.007
	DR	0.000	0.000	0.000	0.001	0.005	0.001	0.000	0.001	0.011	0.000	0.001	0.005	0.012
	SF	0.000	0.000	0.000	0.000	0.002	0.001	0.000	0.002	0.037	0.001	0.000	0.007	0.077(NS)
	DF	0.000	0.000	0.000	0.004	0.008	0.004	0.005	0.001	0.044	0.001	0.000	0.198(NS)	0.052(NS)

NS= non-significant values that mean there is no significant difference present between the raw and cooked samples. R= Raw, B= Boiling, DR = Dry roasting, SF= Shallow frying, DF= Deep frying.

This table shows the p value of the protein content between the raw state and cooked samples for all the fish and crustaceans. In 14 days and 15 days control preservation without preservative, *rohu* shows non-significant p value for shallow frying with respect to the raw condition. Rest of the values are significant which means there is significant difference present among the raw and cooked samples in all the preservation methods.

In 48 hours KMS preservation, *katla* shows non-significant p value for deep frying with respect to the raw condition. Rest of the values are significant which means there is significant difference present among the raw state and cooked samples in all the preservation methods.

Both 15 days salt and turmeric preservation and KMS preservation, prawn shows non-significant p value for open pan dry roasting and deep frying with respect to the raw condition. Rest of the values are significant, which means there is significant difference present among the raw and cooked samples in all of the preservation methods.

In 48 hours, 14 days and 15 days KMS preservation, lobster shows non-significant p value for open pan dry roasting with respect to the raw condition. Rest of the values are significant, which means there is significant difference present among the raw state and cooked samples in all the preservation methods.

In 14 days control preservation without preservative, pomfret shows non-significant p value for open pan dry roasting and shallow frying, whereas in 48 hours salt and turmeric preservation, p value is non-significant for shallow frying and deep frying. In 15 days salt and turmeric preservation, p value is non-significant for open pan dry roasting, shallow frying and deep frying with respect to the raw condition. In 24 hours, 48 hours KMS preservation, p value is also non-significant for open pan dry roasting and shallow frying with respect to the raw condition. 14 days KMS preservation shows non-significant p value for open pan dry roasting and deep frying, and 15 days KMS preservation shows non-significant p value for open pan dry roasting with respect to the raw condition. Rest of the values are significant, which means there is significant difference present among the raw state and cooked samples in all of the preservation methods.

In 14 days KMS preservation, *hilsa* shows non-significant p value for deep frying, and in 15 days KMS preservation, p value is non-significant for shallow frying and deep frying with respect to the raw condition. Rest of the values are significant, which means there is significant difference present among the raw state and cooked samples in all of the preservation methods.

Overall analysis indicates that there is statistically significant difference present between the raw and cooked values for all the fish and other edible aquatic species in respect to the protein content, which means the protein contents vary in different cooking methods from the raw condition.

Table no 5.9.3 Fat content (**WOP**= Without preservative, **ST**= Salt & Turmeric, **KMS**= Potassium metabisulphite)

Raw vs.		WOP					ST				KMS			
		FRESH	24Hr	48Hr	14D	15D	24Hr	48Hr	14D	15D	24Hr	48Hr	14D	15D
Rohu	B	0.007	0.000	0.000	0.029	0.000	0.000	0.000	0.000	0.000	0.001	0.010	0.000	0.001
	DR	0.000	0.000	0.000	0.077(NS)	0.000	0.002	0.000	0.000	0.000	0.002	0.000	0.000	0.243(NS)
	SF	0.000	0.000	0.000	0.000	0.000	0.000	0.001	0.000	0.001	0.000	0.000	0.005	0.000
	DF	0.002	0.000	0.000	0.771(NS)	0.000	0.000	0.000	0.000	0.000	0.000	0.000	0.001	0.006
Katla	B	0.002	0.000	0.001	0.000	0.000	0.004	0.000	0.000	0.000	0.000	0.000	0.000	0.000
	DR	0.000	0.001	0.000	0.000	0.002	0.000	0.000	0.000	0.742(NS)	0.000	0.000	0.000	0.001
	SF	0.181(NS)	0.000	0.053(NS)	0.000	0.000	0.002	0.000	0.000	0.002	0.000	0.000	0.000	0.000
	DF	0.009	0.008	0.000	0.000	0.000	0.000	0.000	0.000	0.002	0.002	0.000	0.006	0.002
Prawn	B	0.005	0.000	0.000	0.109(NS)	0.065(NS)	0.128(NS)	0.130(NS)	0.000	0.009	0.000	0.000	0.001	0.000
	DR	0.007	0.050	0.000	0.034	0.115(NS)	0.004	0.003	0.003	0.004	0.001	0.017	0.000	0.000
	SF	0.000	0.000	0.000	0.000	0.000	0.000	0.000	0.000	0.000	0.000	0.000	0.000	0.002
	DF	0.001	0.000	0.000	0.000	0.002	0.000	0.000	0.000	0.000	0.000	0.000	0.000	0.423(NS)
Lobster	B	0.000	0.006	0.007	0.001	0.089(NS)	0.000	0.001	0.001	0.000	0.069(NS)	0.000	0.001	0.020
	DR	0.331(NS)	0.004	0.003	0.001	0.731(NS)	0.000	0.002	0.002	0.009	0.005	0.002	0.001	0.005
	SF	0.000	0.000	0.000	0.000	0.000	0.000	0.000	0.000	0.001	0.002	0.000	0.000	0.003
	DF	0.000	0.000	0.000	0.000	0.000	0.000	0.000	0.185(NS)	0.000	0.002	0.000	0.000	0.001
Pomfret	B	0.002	0.011	0.000	0.000	0.000	0.000	0.000	0.000	0.000	0.000	0.000	0.000	0.000
	DR	0.000	0.000	0.000	0.000	0.001	0.000	0.000	0.000	0.000	0.000	0.000	0.000	0.000
	SF	0.000	0.001	0.000	0.000	0.000	0.000	0.000	0.000	0.000	0.000	0.001	0.000	0.000
	DF	0.000	0.017	0.000	0.000	0.000	0.009	0.000	0.000	0.000	0.000	0.000	0.000	0.000
Hilsa	B	0.570(NS)	0.000	0.000	0.000	0.000	0.003	0.001	0.000	0.001	0.000	0.000	0.000	0.000
	DR	0.000	0.000	0.000	0.000	0.000	0.000	0.000	0.000	0.000	0.000	0.000	0.000	0.000
	SF	0.000	0.000	0.000	0.000	0.000	0.000	0.000	0.000	0.000	0.000	0.000	0.000	0.000
	DF	0.000	0.000	0.000	0.000	0.000	0.000	0.000	0.000	0.000	0.000	0.000	0.000	0.000

NS= non-significant values that mean there is no significant difference present between the raw and cooked samples. R= Raw, B= Boiling, DR = Dry roasting, SF= Shallow frying, DF= Deep frying.

This table shows the p value of the fat content between the raw state and cooked samples for all the fish and crustaceans. In 14 days control preservation without preservative, *rohu* shows non-significant p value for open pan dry roasting and shallow frying with respect to the raw condition. In 15 days salt and turmeric preservation p value is non-significant for open pan dry roasting with respect to the raw condition. Rest of the values are significant, which means there is significant difference present among the raw and cooked samples in all the preservation methods.

In fresh condition and 48 hours control preservation without preservative, *katla* shows non-significant p value for shallow frying, whereas in 15 days salt and turmeric preservation, p value is non-significant for open pan dry roasting with respect to the raw condition. Rest of the values are significant which means there is significant difference present among the raw and cooked samples in all the preservation methods.

In 14 days control preservation without preservative, prawn shows non-significant p value for boiling and in 15 days control preservation without preservative p value is non-significant for boiling and open pan dry roasting, whereas in 24 hours, 48 hours salt and turmeric preservation, p value is non-significant for boiling with respect to the raw condition. Rest of the values are significant which means there is significant difference present among the raw and cooked samples in all the preservation methods.

In fresh condition, lobster shows non-significant p value for open pan dry roasting, and in 15 days control preservation without preservative, p value is non-significant for boiling and open pan dry roasting with respect to the raw condition. In 14 days salt and turmeric preservation, p value is also non-significant for deep frying, and 24 hours KMS preservation shows non-significant p value for boiling with respect to the raw condition. Rest of the values are significant, which means there is significant difference present among the raw and cooked samples in all of the preservation methods.

In all preservation conditions including fresh condition, pomfret shows all the values are significant, which means there is significant difference present among the raw and cooked samples in all the preservation methods.

In 24 hours control preservation without preservative, *hilsa* shows non-significant p value for boiling with respect to the raw condition. Rest of the values are significant, which means there is significant difference present among the raw and cooked samples in all of the preservation methods.

Overall analysis indicates that there is statistically significant difference present between the raw and cooked values for all the fish and other edible aquatic species in respect to the fat content which means the fat contents vary in different cooking methods from the raw condition.

Table no 5.9.4 Moisture content (WOP= Without preservative, **ST**= Salt & Turmeric, **KMS**= Potassium metabisulphite)

Raw vs.		WOP					ST				KMS			
		FRESH	24Hr	48Hr	14D	15D	24Hr	48Hr	14D	15D	24Hr	48Hr	14D	15D
Rohu	B	0.003	0.002	0.087(NS)	0.000	0.010	0.012	0.000	0.003	0.028	0.006	0.000	0.000	0.000
	DR	0.000	0.007	0.002	0.002	0.009	0.000	0.000	0.001	0.003	0.001	0.001	0.000	0.000
	SF	0.000	0.002	0.001	0.008	0.001	0.001	0.001	0.003	0.001	0.002	0.000	0.000	0.002
	DF	0.000	0.002	0.000	0.001	0.000	0.000	0.000	0.000	0.001	0.001	0.000	0.000	0.000
Katla	B	0.008	0.001	0.000	0.000	0.010	0.006	0.000	0.003	0.011	0.002	0.008	0.000	0.004
	DR	0.001	0.004	0.003	0.000	0.009	0.006	0.000	0.001	0.001	0.001	0.000	0.001	0.001
	SF	0.000	0.007	0.003	0.000	0.009	0.000	0.000	0.002	0.000	0.000	0.001	0.000	0.000
	DF	0.002	0.004	0.001	0.000	0.001	0.000	0.000	0.000	0.000	0.000	0.000	0.000	0.000
Prawn	B	0.000	0.000	0.000	0.000	0.001	0.000	0.007	0.009	0.001	0.000	0.000	0.002	0.000
	DR	0.001	0.000	0.000	0.000	0.000	0.000	0.001	0.001	0.001	0.000	0.000	0.000	0.001
	SF	0.001	0.000	0.000	0.000	0.000	0.000	0.002	0.000	0.000	0.000	0.000	0.000	0.001
	DF	0.000	0.000	0.000	0.000	0.000	0.000	0.000	0.000	0.000	0.000	0.000	0.000	0.000
Lobster	B	0.006	0.001	0.000	0.002	0.000	0.005	0.000	0.001	0.001	0.000	0.002	0.001	0.003
	DR	0.000	0.000	0.000	0.000	0.000	0.000	0.000	0.000	0.002	0.000	0.000	0.000	0.000
	SF	0.000	0.000	0.000	0.000	0.000	0.000	0.000	0.000	0.001	0.000	0.001	0.000	0.000
	DF	0.001	0.000	0.000	0.001	0.002	0.001	0.001	0.000	0.001	0.000	0.000	0.000	0.000
Pomfret	B	0.002	0.002	0.000	0.000	0.000	0.000	0.001	0.000	0.000	0.000	0.000	0.000	0.000
	DR	0.000	0.003	0.000	0.000	0.000	0.001	0.001	0.000	0.000	0.000	0.000	0.000	0.000
	SF	0.001	0.001	0.000	0.000	0.000	0.000	0.002	0.000	0.000	0.000	0.007	0.000	0.000
	DF	0.000	0.000	0.000	0.000	0.000	0.001	0.000	0.000	0.000	0.000	0.000	0.000	0.000
Hilsa	B	0.000	0.000	0.000	0.000	0.068NS)	0.243(NS)	0.000	0.001	0.017	0.018	0.007	0.001	0.001
	DR	0.000	0.000	0.000	0.000	0.004	0.000	0.000	0.001	0.000	0.000	0.000	0.000	0.000
	SF	0.000	0.000	0.000	0.000	0.004	0.000	0.000	0.000	0.000	0.000	0.000	0.000	0.000
	DF	0.000	0.000	0.000	0.000	0.004	0.000	0.000	0.000	0.000	0.000	0.000	0.000	0.000

NS= non-significant values that mean there is no significant difference present between the raw and cooked samples. R= Raw, B= Boiling, DR = Dry roasting, SF= Shallow frying, DF= Deep frying.

This table shows the p value of the moisture content between the raw state and cooked samples for all the fish and crustaceans. In 48 hours control preservation without preservative, *rohu* shows non-significant p value for boiling with respect to the raw condition. Rest of the values are significant, which means there is significant difference present among the raw state and cooked samples in all of the preservation methods.

All the values are significant for *Katla*, prawn, lobster, pomfret, which means there is significant difference present among the raw state and cooked samples in all of the preservation methods.

In 24 hours, 48 hours preservation with salt and turmeric preservation, *hilsa* shows non-significant p value for boiling with respect to the raw condition. Rest of the values are significant which means there is significant difference present among the raw state and cooked samples in all of the preservation methods.

Overall analysis indicates that there is statistically significant difference present between the raw and cooked values for all the fish and other edible aquatic species in respect to the moisture content, which means the moisture contents vary in different cooking methods from the raw condition.

Table no 5.9.5 Ash content (**WOP**= Without preservative, **ST**= Salt & Turmeric, **KMS**= Potassium metabisulphite)

Raw vs.		WOP					ST				KMS			
		FRESH	24Hr	48Hr	14D	15D	24Hr	48Hr	14D	15D	24Hr	48Hr	14D	15D
Rohu	B	0.001	0.010	0.017	0.002	0.000	0.001	0.000	0.000	0.006	0.000	0.000	0.006	0.093(NS)
	DR	0.001	0.002	0.013	0.005	0.000	0.000	0.000	0.000	0.000	0.001	0.000	0.002	0.004
	SF	0.001	0.004	0.003	0.002	0.001	0.000	0.000	0.000	0.024	0.000	0.013	0.002	0.016
	DF	0.001	0.000	0.000	0.005	0.000	0.000	0.000	0.000	0.001	0.000	0.005	0.001	0.001
Katla	B	0.001	0.042	0.000	0.000	0.000	0.067(NS)	0.001	0.000	0.001	0.029	0.000	0.000	0.001
	DR	0.000	0.006	0.000	0.000	0.000	0.001	0.002	0.001	0.000	0.004	0.007	0.001	0.004
	SF	0.020	0.001	0.000	0.002	0.001	0.001	0.021	0.003	0.000	0.115(NS)	0.014	0.000	0.000
	DF	0.000	0.006	0.000	0.000	0.000	0.005	0.000	0.002	0.000	0.362(NS)	0.126(NS)	0.013	0.000
Prawn	B	0.000	0.006	0.000	0.002	0.005	0.000	0.002	0.000	0.010	0.000	0.003	0.012	0.000
	DR	0.000	0.016	0.001	0.423(NS)	0.000	0.000	0.007	0.000	0.130(NS)	0.000	0.007	0.000	0.000
	SF	0.001	0.022	0.000	0.005	0.001	0.000	0.023	0.000	0.001	0.000	0.030	0.001	0.000
	DF	0.001	0.004	0.000	0.000	0.000	0.000	0.000	0.000	0.926(NS)	0.000	0.209(NS)	0.000	0.000
Lobster	B	0.002	0.004	0.006	0.001	0.089(NS)	0.000	0.000	0.000	0.000	0.001	0.001	0.000	0.004
	DR	0.095(NS)	0.007	0.005	0.001	0.731(NS)	0.000	0.000	0.000	0.002	0.007	0.001	0.000	0.001
	SF	0.000	0.000	0.000	0.000	0.000	0.000	0.000	0.001	0.004	0.001	0.000	0.000	0.000
	DF	0.000	0.000	0.000	0.000	0.000	0.000	0.000	0.000	0.000	0.002	0.000	0.000	0.000
Pomfret	B	0.000	0.000	0.005	0.062(NS)	0.001	0.014	0.000	0.000	0.001	0.000	0.001	0.003	0.001
	DR	0.000	0.000	0.003	0.001	0.001	0.000	0.001	0.000	0.000	0.000	0.008	0.038	0.001
	SF	0.000	0.001	0.001	0.002	0.019	0.001	0.002	0.000	0.002	0.000	0.020	0.001	0.001
	DF	0.000	0.245(NS)	0.050	0.000	0.001	0.000	0.002	0.000	0.000	0.000	0.003	0.001	0.000
Hilsa	B	0.000	0.000	0.002	0.023	0.024	0.000	0.001	0.029	0.005	0.000	0.001	0.371(NS)	0.025
	DR	0.000	0.000	0.001	0.001	0.004	0.000	0.001	0.000	0.002	0.001	0.001	0.001	0.423(NS)
	SF	0.001	0.000	0.001	0.129(NS)	0.002	0.025	0.000	0.000	0.002	0.000	0.001	0.069(NS)	0.002
	DF	0.000	0.000	0.009	0.000	0.029	0.000	0.000	0.000	0.010	0.224(NS)	0.000	0.001	0.000

NS= non-significant values that mean there is no significant difference present between the raw and cooked samples. R= Raw, B= Boiling, DR = Dry roasting, SF= Shallow frying, DF= Deep frying.

This table shows the p value of the ash content between the raw state and cooked samples for all the fish and crustaceans. In 15 days KMS preservation, *rohu* shows non-significant p value for boiling with respect to the raw condition. Rest of the values are significant, which means there is significant difference present among the raw state and cooked samples in all the preservation methods.

In 24 hours salt and turmeric preservation, *katla* shows non-significant p value for boiling, whereas in 24 hours KMS preservation without preservative, p value is non-significant for shallow frying and deep frying, and in 48 hours KMS preservation, p value is non-significant for deep frying with respect to the raw condition. Rest of the values are significant, that means there is significant difference present among the raw state and cooked samples in all of the preservation methods.

In 14 days control preservation without preservative, prawn shows non-significant p value for open pan dry roasting, and 15 days salt and turmeric preservation, shows non-significant p value for deep frying and open pan dry roasting, whereas in 48 hours KMS preservation, p value is non-significant for deep frying with respect to the raw condition. Rest of the values are significant that means there is significant difference present among the raw state and cooked samples in all of the preservation methods.

In fresh condition, lobster shows non-significant p value for open pan dry roasting, and in 15 days control preservation without preservative, p value is non-significant for boiling and open pan dry roasting with respect to the raw condition. Rest of the values are significant, which means there is significant difference present among the raw state and cooked samples in all the preservation methods.

In 24 hours control preservation without preservative, pomfret shows non-significant p value for deep frying, and in 14 days control preservation without preservative, p value is non-significant for boiling with respect to the raw condition. Rest of the values are significant, which means there is significant difference present among the raw sample and cooked samples in all of the preservation methods.

In 14 days control preservation without preservative, *hilsa* shows non-significant p value for shallow frying, and in 24 hours KMS preservation, p value is non-significant for deep frying, whereas in 14 days KMS preservation, p value is non-significant for boiling and shallow frying with respect to the raw condition. In 15 days KMS preservation, p value is non-significant for open pan dry roasting with respect to the raw condition. Rest of the values are significant that means there is significant difference present among the raw state and cooked samples in all of the preservation methods.

Overall analysis indicates that there is statistically significant difference present between the raw and cooked values for all the fish and other edible aquatic species in respect to the ash content, which means the ash contents vary in different cooking methods from the raw condition.

Table no 5.9.6 Calcium content (**WOP**= Without preservative, **ST**= Salt & Turmeric, **KMS**= Potassium metabisulphite)

Raw vs.		WOP					ST				KMS			
		FRESH	24Hr	48Hr	14D	15D	24Hr	48Hr	14D	15D	24Hr	48Hr	14D	15D
Rohu	B	0.000	0.000	0.000	0.000	0.001	0.006	0.000	0.000	0.002	0.000	0.000	0.000	0.000
	DR	0.000	0.005	0.000	0.000	0.000	0.000	0.000	0.120(NS)	0.000	0.187(NS)	0.029	0.000	0.000
	SF	0.001	0.001	0.000	0.000	0.000	0.000	0.000	0.005	0.000	0.000	0.000	0.002	0.000
	DF	0.000	0.009	0.000	0.000	0.742(NS)	0.000	0.000	0.000	0.001	0.000	0.000	0.000	0.004
Katla	B	0.000	0.000	0.000	0.000	0.001	0.123(NS)	0.177(NS)	0.000	0.000	0.000	0.000	0.000	0.000
	DR	0.423(NS)	0.001	0.000	0.006	0.002	0.000	0.004	0.000	0.000	0.000	0.000	0.001	0.000
	SF	0.056(NS)	0.001	0.000	0.000	0.000	0.013	0.000	0.000	0.000	0.000	0.000	0.000	0.000
	DF	0.423(NS)	0.000	0.000	0.000	0.000	0.000	0.008	0.003	0.000	0.002	0.000	0.001	0.000
Prawn	B	0.000	0.001	0.000	0.000	0.000	0.035	0.000	0.423(NS)	0.013	0.000	0.004	0.000	0.000
	DR	0.001	0.000	0.000	0.000	0.423(NS)	0.012	0.000	0.000	0.007	0.000	0.000	0.000	0.076(NS)
	SF	0.000	0.002	0.000	0.000	0.000	0.000	0.000	0.001	0.002	0.000	0.003	0.002	0.000
	DF	0.000	0.000	0.001	0.001	0.000	0.013	0.000	0.004	0.026	0.004	0.000	0.000	0.000
Lobster	B	0.001	0.000	0.001	0.000	0.000	0.000	0.000	0.000	0.001	0.074(NS)	0.000	0.000	0.000
	DR	0.184(NS)	0.000	0.580(NS)	0.000	0.000	0.000	0.000	0.074(NS)	0.005	0.019	0.000	0.004	0.002
	SF	0.000	0.000	0.002	0.000	0.035	0.000	0.000	0.001	0.002	0.001	0.000	0.000	0.000
	DF	0.000	0.000	0.035	0.000	0.000	0.000	0.000	0.000	0.006	0.000	0.074(NS)	0.000	0.000
Pomfret	B	0.742(NS)	0.000	0.000	0.000	0.000	0.000	0.000	0.000	0.000	0.008	0.001	0.000	0.000
	DR	0.005	0.000	0.000	0.000	0.000	0.000	0.001	0.000	0.000	0.000	0.000	0.000	0.000
	SF	0.000	0.000	0.000	0.001	0.001	0.549(NS)	0.000	0.000	0.000	0.002	0.001	0.000	0.000
	DF	0.000	0.000	0.000	0.005	0.001	0.667(NS)	0.000	0.065(NS)	0.000	0.000	0.010	0.000	0.000
Hilsa	B	0.000	0.001	0.002	0.000	0.000	0.000	0.001	0.000	0.000	0.000	0.000	0.000	0.000
	DR	0.000	0.000	0.118(NS)	0.000	0.000	0.000	0.082(NS)	0.000	0.001	0.000	0.000	0.005	0.003
	SF	0.000	0.000	0.000	0.000	0.000	0.000	0.000	0.423(NS)	0.000	0.423(NS)	0.000	0.001	0.000
	DF	0.001	0.000	0.011	0.003	0.000	0.000	0.000	0.007	0.000	0.000	0.774(NS)	0.002	0.000

NS= non-significant values that mean there is no significant difference present between the raw and cooked samples. R= Raw, B= Boiling, DR = Dry roasting, SF= Shallow frying, DF= Deep frying.

This table shows the p value of the calcium content between the raw state and cooked samples for all the fish and crustaceans. In 15 days control preservation without preservative, *rohu* shows non-significant p value for deep frying, and in 14 days salt and turmeric preservation and 24 hours KMS preservation, p value is non-significant for open pan dry roasting with respect to the raw condition. Rest of the values are significant, which means there is significant difference present among the raw state and cooked samples in all the preservation methods.

In fresh condition, *katla* shows non-significant p value for open pan dry roasting, shallow frying and deep frying, whereas in 24 hours salt and turmeric preservation, p value is non-significant for boiling with respect to the raw condition. Rest of the values are significant, which means there is significant difference present among the raw state and cooked samples in all of the preservation methods.

In 15 days control preservation without preservative and 15 days KMS preservation, prawn shows non-significant p value for open pan dry roasting, and 14 days salt and turmeric preservation shows that for boiling with respect to the raw condition. Rest of the values are significant that means there is significant difference present among the raw state and cooked samples in all the preservation methods.

In fresh condition, 48 hours control preservation without preservative and 14 days salt and turmeric preservation, lobster shows non-significant p value for open pan dry roasting, and in 24 hours and 48 hours KMS preservation, p value is non-significant for boiling and deep frying respectively in comparison to the raw condition. Rest of the values are significant, which means there is significant difference present among the raw state and cooked samples in all the preservation methods.

In fresh condition, pomfret shows non-significant p value for boiling, and in 24 hours salt and turmeric preservation, p value is non-significant for shallow frying and deep frying, whereas in 14 days salt and turmeric preservation, p value is non-significant for deep frying with respect to the raw condition. Rest of the values are significant, which means there is significant difference present among the raw and cooked samples in all the preservation methods.

In 48 hours control preservation without preservative and 48 hours salt and turmeric preservation, *hilsa* shows non-significant p value for open pan dry roasting, and in 14 days salt and turmeric preservation as well as 24 hours KMS preservation, p value is non-significant for shallow frying, whereas in 48 hours KMS preservation p value is non-significant for deep frying with respect to the raw condition. Rest of the values are significant, which means there is significant difference present among the raw state and cooked samples in all the preservation methods.

Overall analysis indicates that there is statistically significant difference present between the raw and cooked values for all the fish and other edible aquatic species in respect to the calcium content, which means the calcium contents vary in different cooking methods from the raw condition.

Table no 5.9.7 Iron content (**WOP**= Without preservative, **ST**= Salt & Turmeric, **KMS**= Potassium metabisulphite)

Raw vs.		WOP					ST				KMS			
		FRESH	24Hr	48Hr	14D	15D	24Hr	48Hr	14D	15D	24Hr	48Hr	14D	15D
Rohu	B	0.015	0.000	0.001	0.006	0.000	0.000	0.000	0.000	0.000	0.000	0.363(NS)	0.003	0.000
	DR	0.001	0.000	0.001	0.014	0.000	0.001	0.000	0.000	0.023	0.001	0.426(NS)	0.000	0.000
	SF	0.000	0.001	0.000	0.000	0.004	0.002	0.001	0.000	0.000	0.000	0.003	0.018	0.001
	DF	0.000	0.000	0.000	0.423(NS)	0.002	0.009	0.004	0.000	0.001	0.020	0.113(NS)	0.005	0.000
Katla	B	0.001	0.083(NS)	0.003	0.001	0.001	0.000	0.002	0.103(NS)	0.025	0.001	0.000	0.013	0.598(NS)
	DR	0.000	0.045	0.001	0.015	0.006	0.000	0.004	0.007	0.000	0.001	0.000	0.001	0.015
	SF	0.027	0.001	0.000	0.270(NS)	0.000	0.002	0.002	0.005	0.002	0.000	0.000	0.006	0.003
	DF	0.000	0.001	0.001	0.000	0.003	0.017	0.000	0.042	0.001	0.001	0.000	0.001	0.003
Prawn	B	0.038	0.007	0.029	0.010	0.001	0.000	0.001	0.000	0.001	0.000	0.004	0.000	0.024
	DR	0.007	0.000	0.002	0.005	0.000	0.000	0.010	0.013	0.003	0.000	0.897(NS)	0.001	0.001
	SF	0.000	0.000	0.002	0.000	0.001	0.023	0.001	0.015	0.199(NS)	0.000	0.857(NS)	0.000	0.045
	DF	0.002	0.184(NS)	0.001	0.000	0.012	0.002	0.002	0.003	0.013	0.002	0.028	0.003	0.000
Lobster	B	0.001	0.000	0.000	0.002	0.000	0.056(NS)	0.000	0.003	0.005	0.065(NS)	0.226(NS)	0.004	0.000
	DR	0.000	0.007	0.001	0.185(NS)	0.000	0.020	0.000	0.026	0.122(NS)	0.000	0.002	0.000	0.000
	SF	0.001	0.001	0.045	0.126(NS)	0.001	0.000	0.000	0.003	0.004	0.000	0.000	0.000	0.001
	DF	0.000	0.000	0.003	0.004	0.000	0.002	0.001	0.010	0.000	0.000	0.003	0.000	0.003
Pomfret	B	0.000	0.007	0.000	0.001	0.001	0.423(NS)	0.004	0.002	0.000	0.074(NS)	0.000	0.000	0.001
	DR	0.003	0.161(NS)	0.001	0.000	0.000	0.020	0.002	0.004	0.000	0.002	0.000	0.004	0.000
	SF	0.000	0.001	0.000	0.004	0.001	0.021	0.002	0.011	0.000	0.074(NS)	0.000	0.001	0.001
	DF	0.000	0.005	0.000	0.002	0.001	0.000	0.029	0.013	0.000	0.036	0.000	0.114(NS)	0.002
Hilsa	B	0.000	0.000	0.031	0.000	0.001	0.003	0.001	0.074(NS)	0.010	0.004	0.000	0.001	0.036
	DR	0.000	0.582(NS)	0.000	0.001	0.000	0.007	0.000	0.000	0.423(NS)	0.004	0.423(NS)	0.000	0.000
	SF	0.000	0.030	0.054(NS)	0.000	0.001	0.007	0.001	0.006	0.000	0.000	0.001	0.003	0.001
	DF	0.000	0.029	0.018	0.562(NS)	0.000	0.000	0.000	0.006	0.423(NS)	0.002	0.000	0.001	0.002

NS= non-significant values that mean there is no significant difference present between the raw and cooked samples. R= Raw, B= Boiling, DR = Dry roasting, SF= Shallow frying, DF= Deep frying.

This table shows the p value of the iron content between the raw state and cooked samples for all the fish and crustaceans. In 14 days control preservation without preservative, *rohu* shows non-significant p value for deep frying, whereas in 48 hours KMS preservation, p value is non-significant for boiling, open pan dry roasting and deep frying with respect to the raw condition. Rest of the values are significant, which means there is significant difference present among the raw state and cooked samples in all the preservation methods.

In 24 hours control preservation without preservative, 14 days salt and turmeric preservation and 15 days KMS preservation, *katla* shows non-significant p value for boiling, whereas in 14 days control preservation without preservative, p value is non-significant for shallow frying with respect to the raw condition. Rest of the values are significant, which means there is significant difference present among the raw state and cooked samples in all of the preservation methods.

In 24 hours control preservation without preservative, prawn shows non-significant p value for deep frying, and in 15 days salt and turmeric preservation, p value is non-significant for shallow frying, whereas in 48 hours KMS preservation, p value is non-significant for shallow frying and open pan dry roasting with respect to the raw condition. Rest of the values are significant, which means there is significant difference present among the raw state and cooked samples in all the preservation methods.

In 14 days control preservation without preservative, lobster shows non-significant p value for open pan dry roasting and shallow frying, whereas in 24 hours salt and turmeric preservation and 24 hours, 48 hours KMS preservation p value is non-significant for boiling with respect to the raw condition. In 15 days salt and turmeric preservation, p value is non-significant for open pan dry roasting. Rest of the values are significant, which means there is significant difference present among the raw and cooked samples in all of the preservation methods.

In 24 hours control preservation without preservative, pomfret shows non-significant p value for open pan dry roasting, whereas in 24 hours salt and turmeric preservation, p value is non-significant for boiling with respect to the raw condition. In 24 hours KMS preservation, p value is non-significant for boiling and shallow frying with respect to the raw condition. In 14 days KMS preservation p value is also non-significant for deep frying with respect to the raw condition. Rest of the values are significant, which means there is significant difference present among the raw state and cooked samples in all of the preservation methods.

In 24 hours, 48 hours and 14 days control preservation, *hilsa* shows non-significant p value for open pan dry roasting, shallow frying and deep frying respectively, and in 14 days salt and turmeric preservation, p value is non-significant for boiling with respect to the raw condition. In 15 days salt and turmeric preservation, p value is non-significant for open pan dry roasting and deep frying, whereas in 48 hours KMS preservation, p value is non-significant for open pan dry roasting with respect to the raw condition.

Rest of the values are significant, which means there is significant difference present among the raw state and cooked samples in all of the preservation methods.

Overall analysis indicates that there is statistically significant difference present between the raw and cooked values for all the fish and other edible aquatic species in respect to the iron content, which means the iron contents vary in different cooking methods from the raw condition.

Table no 5.9.8 Energy content (**WOP**= Without preservative, **ST**= Salt & Turmeric, **KMS**= Potassium metabisulphite)

Raw vs.		WOP					ST				KMS			
		FRESH	24Hr	48Hr	14D	15D	24Hr	48Hr	14D	15D	24Hr	48Hr	14D	15D
Rohu	B	0.000	0.011	0.000	0.001	0.005	0.000	0.000	0.000	0.000	0.000	0.000	0.000	0.000
	DR	0.000	0.021	0.000	0.035	0.000	0.000	0.000	0.000	0.000	0.001	0.000	0.000	0.001
	SF	0.015	0.003	0.000	0.001	0.000	0.001	0.002	0.001	0.002	0.002	0.000	0.004	0.033
	DF	0.001	0.003	0.000	0.009	0.000	0.001	0.000	0.000	0.000	0.000	0.003	0.017	0.010
Katla	B	0.000	0.001	0.001	0.002	0.000	0.000	0.000	0.001	0.000	0.000	0.000	0.002	0.086(NS)
	DR	0.000	0.002	0.001	0.001	0.000	0.000	0.000	0.000	0.002	0.000	0.000	0.000	0.003
	SF	0.001	0.352(NS)	0.001	0.000	0.000	0.000	0.000	0.001	0.399(NS)	0.022	0.000	0.000	0.007
	DF	0.000	0.001	0.001	0.003	0.000	0.000	0.000	0.001	0.071(NS)	0.805(NS)	0.000	0.001	0.041
Prawn	B	0.000	0.000	0.000	0.001	0.001	0.001	0.002	0.019	0.006	0.683(NS)	0.007	0.000	0.000
	DR	0.001	0.000	0.000	0.003	0.002	0.002	0.002	0.003	0.083(NS)	0.709(NS)	0.003	0.181(NS)	0.009
	SF	0.016	0.000	0.000	0.063(NS)	0.001	0.003	0.001	0.003	0.010	0.122(NS)	0.006	0.003	0.022
	DF	0.012	0.000	0.095(NS)	0.236(NS)	0.000	0.030	0.000	0.040	0.001	0.013	0.001	0.021	0.030
Lobster	B	0.000	0.000	0.003	0.001	0.018	0.044	0.000	0.001	0.003	0.000	0.002	0.002	0.000
	DR	0.000	0.000	0.004	0.002	0.004	0.005	0.005	0.001	0.001	0.001	0.115(NS)	0.807(NS)	0.232(NS)
	SF	0.007	0.018	0.005	0.295(NS)	0.001	0.031	0.000	0.012	0.140(NS)	0.003	0.001	0.006	0.008
	DF	0.003	0.511(NS)	0.001	0.006	0.005	0.963(NS)	0.040	0.001	0.043	0.033	0.227(NS)	0.202(NS)	0.005
Pomfret	B	0.000	0.001	0.001	0.004	0.000	0.117(NS)	0.000	0.000	0.000	0.000	0.000	0.000	0.000
	DR	0.015	0.000	0.000	0.002	0.284(NS)	0.000	0.000	0.008	0.001	0.000	0.000	0.000	0.000
	SF	0.013	0.003	0.012	0.000	0.014	0.001	0.001	0.000	0.000	0.000	0.725(NS)	0.000	0.001
	DF	0.001	0.000	0.000	0.000	0.001	0.037	0.001	0.004	0.000	0.000	0.000	0.000	0.000
Hilsa	B	0.002	0.000	0.000	0.000	0.000	0.001	0.000	0.006	0.001	0.001	0.000	0.000	0.003
	DR	0.000	0.000	0.000	0.000	0.000	0.000	0.000	0.000	0.000	0.000	0.000	0.000	0.000
	SF	0.000	0.000	0.000	0.000	0.000	0.000	0.000	0.000	0.000	0.000	0.000	0.000	0.000
	DF	0.000	0.000	0.000	0.000	0.000	0.000	0.000	0.000	0.000	0.000	0.000	0.000	0.000

NS= non-significant values that mean there is no significant difference present between the raw and cooked samples. R= Raw, B= Boiling, DR = Dry roasting, SF= Shallow frying, DF= Deep frying.

This table shows the p value of the energy content between the raw state and cooked samples for all the fish and crustaceans. All the values are significant for *rohu* that means there is significant difference present among the raw state and cooked samples in all the preservation methods.

In 24 hours control preservation without preservative, *katla* shows non-significant p value for shallow frying, whereas in 15 days salt and turmeric preservation, p value is non-significant for shallow frying and deep frying, whereas in 24 hours and 15 days KMS preservation, p value is non-significant for deep frying and boiling respectively in comparison to the raw condition. Rest of the values are significant, which means there is significant difference present among the raw state and cooked samples in all the preservation methods.

In 48 hours control preservation without preservative, prawn shows non-significant p value for deep frying, and in 14 days control preservation without preservative, p value is non-significant for shallow frying and deep frying, whereas in 15 days salt and turmeric preservation, p value is non-significant for open pan dry roasting with respect to the raw condition. In 24 hours KMS preservation, p value is non-significant for boiling, open pan dry roasting and shallow frying, whereas in 14 days KMS preservation, p value is non-significant for open pan dry roasting. Rest of the values are significant, which means there is significant difference present among the raw state and cooked samples in all of the preservation methods.

In 24 hours and 14 days control preservation without preservative, lobster shows non-significant p value for deep frying and shallow frying respectively, whereas in 24 hours and 15 days salt and turmeric preservation, p value is non-significant for deep frying and shallow frying respectively with respect to the raw condition. In 48 hours and 14 days KMS preservation, p value is non-significant for deep frying with respect to the raw condition. Rest of the values are significant, which means there is significant difference present among the raw state and cooked samples in all the preservation methods.

In 15 days control preservation without preservative, pomfret shows non-significant p value for open pan dry roasting, whereas in 24 hours salt and turmeric preservation, p value is non-significant for boiling with respect to the raw condition. In 48 hours KMS preservation, p value is non-significant for shallow frying with respect to the raw condition. Rest of the values are significant, which means there is significant difference present among the raw state and cooked samples in all the preservation methods.

All the values are significant for *hilsa*, which means there is significant difference present among the raw state and cooked samples in all the preservation methods.

Overall analysis indicates that there is statistically significant difference present between the raw and cooked values for all the fish and other edible aquatic species in respect to the energy content, which means the energy contents vary in different cooking methods from the raw condition.

5.10 Student t test among carp, crustaceans and salt water samples

This statistical test is carried out to evaluate any significant deviation among the three groups i.e. carp, crustaceans and salt water fish with respect to different nutritional parameters (carbohydrate, protein, fat, moisture, ash, calcium, iron and energy) under the raw and cooked conditions and different preservation methods. Significant level is checked at 5% level, meaning if the p value is less than 0.05 then it is significant.

Table no 5.10.1 Carbohydrate content (**WOP**= Without preservative, **ST**= Salt & Turmeric, **KMS**= Potassium metabisulphite)

Raw vs.		WOP					ST				KMS			
		FRESH	24Hr	48Hr	14D	15D	24Hr	48Hr	14D	15D	24Hr	48Hr	14D	15D
CARP	B	0.002	0.001	0.006	0.000	0.001	0.003	0.301(NS)	0.000	0.000	0.000	0.000	0.011	0.005
	DR	0.008	0.001	0.008	0.008	0.009	0.001	0.005	0.001	0.007	0.002	0.000	0.226(NS)	0.014
	SF	0.011	0.009	0.005	0.005	0.002	0.004	0.004	0.021	0.120(NS)	0.001	0.000	0.008	0.003
	DF	0.002	0.009	0.002	0.003	0.001	0.004	0.001	0.002	0.003	0.001	0.002	0.018	0.488(NS)
CRUSTACEAN	B	0.012	0.078(NS)	0.020	0.001	0.001	0.000	0.001	0.000	0.000	0.000	0.001	0.001	0.001
	DR	0.009	0.008	0.065(NS)	0.000	0.001	0.000	0.007	0.000	0.000	0.000	0.000	0.001	0.001
	SF	0.224(NS)	0.554(NS)	0.273(NS)	0.021	0.001	0.046	0.001	0.001	0.408(NS)	0.018	0.002	0.000	0.007
	DF	0.008	0.011	0.014	0.039	0.009	0.009	0.019	0.001	0.182(NS)	0.000	0.034	0.001	0.007
SALT WATER FISH	B	0.002	0.035	0.012	0.000	0.036	0.000	0.002	0.000	0.000	0.001	0.003	0.000	0.000
	DR	0.000	0.044	0.007	0.005	0.044	0.000	0.009	0.000	0.001	0.001	0.000	0.000	0.003
	SF	0.008	0.114(NS)	0.015	0.013	0.016	0.000	0.015	0.001	0.000	0.001	0.002	0.000	0.000
	DF	0.108(NS)	0.704(NS)	0.006	0.001	0.000	0.000	0.010	0.706(NS)	0.002	0.011	0.001	0.000	0.009

NS = Non- significant values that mean there is no significant difference present among the three categories of samples with respect to the raw and cooked conditions. R= Raw, B= Boiling, DR = Dry roasting, SF= Shallow frying, DF= Deep frying.

This table shows the p value of the carbohydrate content among the three categories of samples with respect to the raw and cooked conditions. In 48 hours and 15 days salt and turmeric preservation, carp shows non-significant p value for boiling and shallow frying respectively, whereas in 14 days and 15 days KMS preservation, p value is non-significant for open pan dry roasting and deep frying respectively with respect to the raw condition. Rest of the values are significant that means there is significant difference present among the raw state and cooked samples in all of the preservation methods.

In fresh condition, crustaceans show non-significant p value for shallow frying, whereas in 24 hours control preservation without preservative, p value is non-significant for boiling and shallow frying, and in 14 days control preservation without preservative, p value is non-significant for open pan dry roasting and shallow frying with respect to the raw condition. In 15 days salt and turmeric preservation, p value is non-significant for shallow frying and deep frying. Rest of the values are significant, which means there is significant difference present among the raw state and cooked samples in all of the preservation methods.

In fresh condition, salt water fish shows non-significant p value for deep frying, whereas in 24 hours control preservation without preservative, p value is non-significant for shallow frying and deep frying, and in 14 days salt and turmeric preservation, p value is non-significant for deep frying with respect to the raw condition. Rest of the values are significant, which means there is significant difference present among the raw state and cooked samples in all the preservation methods.

Overall analysis indicates that there is statistically significant difference present among the three groups i.e. carp, crustaceans and salt water fish with respect to the raw and cooked values regarding the carbohydrate content, which means the carbohydrate contents vary among the three groups of sample.

Table no 5.10.2 Protein content (WOP= Without preservative, **ST**= Salt & Turmeric, **KMS**= Potassium metabisulphite)

Raw vs.		WOP					ST				KMS			
		FRESH	24Hr	48Hr	14D	15D	24Hr	48Hr	14D	15D	24Hr	48Hr	14D	15D
CARP	B	0.000	0.000	0.000	0.008	0.002	0.000	0.000	0.000	0.000	0.000	0.000	0.000	0.001
	DR	0.000	0.000	0.000	0.010	0.000	0.000	0.000	0.000	0.000	0.001	0.001	0.000	0.002
	SF	0.000	0.000	0.000	0.007	0.001	0.000	0.000	0.000	0.000	0.000	0.000	0.000	0.000
	DF	0.000	0.000	0.000	0.168(NS)	0.001	0.000	0.000	0.002	0.001	0.000	0.003	0.000	0.001
CRUSTACEANS	B	0.000	0.000	0.001	0.002	0.005	0.002	0.000	0.004	0.001	0.000	0.000	0.001	0.000
	DR	0.000	0.000	0.001	0.001	0.002	0.012	0.001	0.005	0.007	0.010	0.020	0.044	0.002
	SF	0.000	0.000	0.001	0.000	0.000	0.001	0.000	0.000	0.001	0.000	0.002	0.001	0.001
	DF	0.000	0.000	0.002	0.002	0.303(NS)	0.002	0.000	0.001	0.003	0.002	0.001	0.002	0.009
SALT WATER FISH	B	0.000	0.000	0.000	0.002	0.002	0.001	0.002	0.001	0.007	0.002	0.001	0.000	0.001
	DR	0.000	0.000	0.000	0.007	0.060(NS)	0.007	0.000	0.001	0.170(NS)	0.002	0.004	0.021	0.328(NS)
	SF	0.000	0.000	0.000	0.008	0.010	0.002	0.000	0.001	0.005	0.003	0.002	0.004	0.008
	DF	0.000	0.000	0.000	0.009	0.019	0.037	0.002	0.014	0.126(NS)	0.003	0.004	0.121(NS)	0.002

□ *NS = Non- significant values that mean there is no significant difference present among the three categories of samples with respect to the raw and cooked conditions. R= Raw, B= Boiling, DR = Dry roasting, SF= Shallow frying, DF= Deep frying.*

This table shows the p value of the protein content among the three categories of samples with respect to the raw and cooked conditions. In 14 days control preservation without preservative, carp shows non-significant p value for deep frying with respect to the raw condition. Rest of the values are significant which means there is significant difference present among the raw state and cooked samples in all the preservation methods.

In 15 days control preservation without preservative, crustaceans show non-significant p value for deep frying with respect to the raw condition. Rest of the values are significant, which means there is significant difference present among the raw state and cooked samples in all the preservation methods.

In 15 days control preservation without preservative, salt water fish shows non-significant p value for open pan dry roasting, and in 15 days salt and turmeric preservation, p value is non-significant for open pan dry roasting and deep frying, whereas in 14 days and 15 days KMS preservation p value is non-significant for deep frying and open pan dry roasting with respect to the raw condition. Rest of the values are significant which means there is significant difference present among the raw state and cooked samples in all of the preservation methods.

Overall analysis indicates that there is statistically significant difference present among the three groups i.e. carp, crustaceans and salt water fish with respect to the raw and cooked values regarding the protein content, which means the protein contents vary among the three groups of sample.

Table no 5.10.3 Fat content (WOP= Without preservative, **ST=** Salt & Turmeric, **KMS=** Potassium metabisulphite)

Raw vs.		WOP					ST				KMS			
		FRESH	24Hr	48Hr	14D	15D	24Hr	48Hr	14D	15D	24Hr	48Hr	14D	15D
CARP	B	0.004	0.000	0.000	0.001	0.000	0.000	0.000	0.000	0.000	0.000	0.000	0.006	0.075(NS)
	DR	0.000	0.000	0.000	0.000	0.000	0.000	0.000	0.000	0.000	0.000	0.000	0.000	0.013
	SF	0.000	0.000	0.001	0.114(NS)	0.000	0.000	0.001	0.628(NS)	0.001	0.000	0.000	0.000	0.000
	DF	0.000	0.000	0.000	0.000	0.000	0.004	0.000	0.000	0.001	0.001	0.000	0.002	0.003
CRUSTACEANS	B	0.002	0.002	0.014	0.024	0.881(NS)	0.000	0.001	0.000	0.001	0.001	0.000	0.001	0.000
	DR	0.033	0.012	0.032	0.009	0.327(NS)	0.000	0.002	0.002	0.000	0.007	0.003	0.000	0.002
	SF	0.000	0.000	0.000	0.000	0.000	0.000	0.000	0.000	0.000	0.000	0.000	0.000	0.002
	DF	0.000	0.000	0.000	0.000	0.000	0.000	0.000	0.000	0.000	0.001	0.000	0.000	0.001
SALT WATER FISH	B	0.023	0.000	0.000	0.000	0.000	0.004	0.000	0.000	0.000	0.000	0.000	0.000	0.000
	DR	0.003	0.000	0.000	0.000	0.000	0.000	0.000	0.000	0.000	0.000	0.000	0.000	0.000
	SF	0.001	0.000	0.000	0.000	0.000	0.000	0.000	0.000	0.000	0.000	0.000	0.000	0.000
	DF	0.000	0.000	0.000	0.000	0.000	0.000	0.000	0.000	0.000	0.000	0.000	0.000	0.000

NS = Non- significant values that mean there is no significant difference present among the three categories of samples with respect to the raw and cooked conditions. R= Raw, B= Boiling, DR = Dry roasting, SF= Shallow frying, DF= Deep frying.

This table shows the p value of the fat content among the three categories of samples with respect to the raw and cooked conditions. In 14 days control preservation without preservative, carp shows non-significant p value for shallow frying, whereas in 14 days salt and turmeric preservation and 15 days KMS preservation, p value is non-significant for shallow frying and boiling respectively in comparison to the raw condition. Rest of the values are significant which means there is significant difference present among the raw state and cooked samples in all the preservation methods.

In 15 days control preservation without preservative, crustaceans show non-significant p value for boiling and open pan dry roasting with respect to the raw condition. Rest of the values are significant which means there is significant difference present among the raw and cooked samples in all the preservation methods.

All the values are significant for salt water fish, which means there is significant difference present among the raw state and cooked samples in all the preservation methods.

Overall analysis indicates that there is statistically significant difference present among the three groups i.e. carp, crustaceans and salt water fish with respect to the raw and cooked values regarding the fat content, which means the fat contents vary among the three groups of sample.

Table no 5.10.4 Moisture content (**WOP**= Without preservative, **ST**= Salt & Turmeric, **KMS**= Potassium metabisulphite)

Raw vs.		WOP					ST				KMS			
		FRESH	24Hr	48Hr	14D	15D	24Hr	48Hr	14D	15D	24Hr	48Hr	14D	15D
CARP	B	0.002	0.000	0.014	0.000	0.007	0.003	0.001	0.000	0.018	0.001	0.001	0.000	0.002
	DR	0.000	0.001	0.002	0.001	0.005	0.000	0.001	0.000	0.001	0.001	0.000	0.000	0.000
	SF	0.000	0.002	0.000	0.004	0.002	0.000	0.323(NS)	0.001	0.000	0.001	0.000	0.000	0.001
	DF	0.001	0.002	0.000	0.000	0.000	0.000	0.000	0.000	0.000	0.000	0.000	0.000	0.000
CRUSTACEANS	B	0.000	0.000	0.000	0.001	0.000	0.001	0.001	0.000	0.001	0.000	0.000	0.001	0.000
	DR	0.000	0.000	0.000	0.000	0.000	0.000	0.000	0.000	0.001	0.000	0.000	0.000	0.000
	SF	0.000	0.000	0.000	0.000	0.000	0.000	0.001	0.000	0.000	0.000	0.001	0.000	0.000
	DF	0.000	0.000	0.000	0.001	0.001	0.000	0.000	0.000	0.000	0.000	0.000	0.000	0.000
SALT WATER FISH	B	0.001	0.001	0.000	0.000	0.003	0.000	0.001	0.000	0.000	0.000	0.000	0.000	0.000
	DR	0.000	0.001	0.000	0.000	0.001	0.000	0.000	0.000	0.000	0.000	0.000	0.000	0.000
	SF	0.000	0.000	0.000	0.000	0.001	0.000	0.000	0.000	0.000	0.000	0.002	0.000	0.000
	DF	0.000	0.000	0.000	0.000	0.001	0.000	0.000	0.000	0.000	0.000	0.000	0.000	0.000

NS = Non- significant values that mean there is no significant difference present among the three categories of samples with respect to the raw and cooked conditions. R= Raw, B= Boiling, DR = Dry roasting, SF= Shallow frying, DF= Deep frying.

This table shows the p value of the moisture content among the three categories of samples with respect to the raw and cooked conditions. In 48 hours salt and turmeric preservation, carp shows non-significant p value for shallow frying in comparison to the raw condition. Rest of the values are significant, which means there is significant difference present among the raw state and cooked samples in all of the preservation methods.

All the values are significant for crustaceans and salt water fish, which mean there is significant difference present among the raw state and cooked samples in all the preservation methods.

Overall analysis indicates that there is statistically significant difference present among the three groups i.e. carp, crustaceans and salt water fish with respect to the raw and cooked values regarding the moisture content, which means the moisture contents vary among the three groups of sample.

Table no 5.10.5 Ash content (**WOP**= Without preservative, **ST**= Salt & Turmeric, **KMS**= Potassium metabisulphite)

Raw vs.		WOP					ST				KMS			
		FRESH	**24Hr**	**48Hr**	**14D**	**15D**	**24Hr**	**48Hr**	**14D**	**15D**	**24Hr**	**48Hr**	**14D**	**15D**
CARP	B	0.000	0.004	0.001	0.000	0.000	0.000	0.000	0.000	0.010	0.000	0.001	0.001	0.024
	DR	0.204(NS)	0.003	0.000	0.000	0.000	0.000	0.004	0.000	0.000	0.000	0.002	0.000	0.003
	SF	0.662(NS)	0.725(NS)	0.000	0.000	0.000	0.000	0.579(NS)	0.000	0.000	0.003	0.216(NS)	0.001	0.009
	DF	0.000	0.010	0.000	0.000	0.000	0.000	0.001	0.000	0.000	0.000	0.024	0.007	0.000
CRUSTACEANS	B	0.000	0.003	0.001	0.012	0.030	0.000	0.000	0.000	0.001	0.000	0.001	0.000	0.000
	DR	0.000	0.010	0.001	0.007	0.005	0.000	0.000	0.000	0.016	0.000	0.001	0.000	0.000
	SF	0.000	0.001	0.000	0.000	0.001	0.000	0.000	0.000	0.003	0.000	0.001	0.029	0.000
	DF	0.000	0.008	0.000	0.000	0.000	0.000	0.000	0.004	0.001	0.000	0.007	0.001	0.002
SALT WATER FISH	B	0.000	0.000	0.004	0.020	0.003	0.001	0.000	0.000	0.002	0.000	0.000	0.043	0.002
	DR	0.000	0.000	0.001	0.034	0.002	0.025	0.001	0.000	0.001	0.000	0.000	0.007	0.001
	SF	0.000	0.001	0.001	0.001	0.005	0.003	0.001	0.000	0.000	0.000	0.000	0.005	0.001
	DF	0.000	0.000	0.033	0.000	0.762(NS)	0.002	0.133(NS)	0.000	0.073(NS)	0.001	0.000	0.000	0.000

NS = Non-significant values that mean there is no significant difference present among the three categories of samples with respect to the raw and cooked conditions. R= Raw, B= Boiling, DR = Dry roasting, SF= Shallow frying, DF= Deep frying.

This table shows the p value of the ash content among the three categories of samples with respect to the raw and cooked conditions. In fresh condition, carp shows non-significant p value for open pan dry roasting and shallow frying, whereas in 24 hours control preservation without preservative, p value is non-significant for shallow frying in comparison to the raw condition. In 48 hours salt and turmeric preservation and 48 hours KMS preservation, p value is non-significant for shallow frying in comparison to the raw condition. Rest of the values are significant, which means there is significant difference present among the raw state and cooked samples in all the preservation methods.

All the values are significant for crustaceans, which mean there is significant difference present among the raw state and cooked samples in all preservation methods.

In 15 days control preservation without preservative, 48 hours and 15 days salt and turmeric preservation, salt water fish shows non-significant p value for deep frying in comparison to the raw condition. Rest of the values are significant, which means there is significant difference present among the raw state and cooked samples in all of the preservation methods.

Overall analysis indicates that there is statistically significant difference present among the three groups i.e. carp, crustaceans and salt water fish with respect to the raw and cooked values regarding the ash content, which means the ash contents vary among the three groups of sample.

Table no 5.10.6 Calcium content (**WOP**= Without preservative, **ST**= Salt & Turmeric, **KMS**= Potassium metabisulphite)

Raw vs.		WOP					ST				KMS			
		FRESH	24Hr	48Hr	14D	15D	24Hr	48Hr	14D	15D	24Hr	48Hr	14D	15D
CARP	B	0.001	0.001	0.000	0.000	0.000	0.041	0.002	0.000	0.001	0.000	0.000	0.002	0.000
	DR	0.000	0.074(NS)	0.000	0.000	0.000	0.000	0.187(NS)	0.000	0.000	0.000	0.000	0.000	0.000
	SF	0.004	0.000	0.000	0.000	0.000	0.002	0.001	0.000	0.000	0.000	0.000	0.000	0.000
	DF	0.000	0.001	0.000	0.000	0.000	0.012	0.002	0.000	0.000	0.000	0.000	0.000	0.000
CRUSTACEANS	B	0.000	0.000	0.001	0.000	0.000	0.000	0.000	0.000	0.001	0.000	0.000	0.000	0.000
	DR	0.000	0.000	0.000	0.005	0.000	0.000	0.000	0.001	0.003	0.000	0.000	0.001	0.011
	SF	0.000	0.000	0.000	0.000	0.000	0.006	0.000	0.001	0.000	0.001	0.000	0.003	0.000
	DF	0.000	0.000	0.107(NS)	0.000	0.000	0.000	0.000	0.000	0.011	0.001	0.003	0.000	0.000
SALT WATER FISH	B	0.000	0.000	0.000	0.000	0.000	0.005	0.000	0.000	0.000	0.000	0.000	0.000	0.012
	DR	0.000	0.000	0.000	0.000	0.000	0.000	0.008	0.003	0.000	0.000	0.000	0.000	0.000
	SF	0.000	0.000	0.000	0.000	0.000	0.000	0.000	0.001	0.000	0.007	0.000	0.000	0.000
	DF	0.001	0.000	0.000	0.010	0.000	0.000	0.000	0.483(NS)	0.000	0.000	0.000	0.000	0.000

NS = Non-significant values that mean there is no significant difference present among the three categories of samples with respect to the raw and cooked conditions. R= Raw, B= Boiling, DR = Dry roasting, SF= Shallow frying, DF= Deep frying.

This table shows the p value of the calcium content among the three categories of samples with respect to the raw and cooked conditions. In 24 hours control preservation without preservative and 48 hours salt and turmeric preservation, carp shows non-significant p value for open pan dry roasting with respect to the raw condition. Rest of the values are significant, which means there is significant difference present among the raw state and cooked samples in all of the preservation methods.

In 48 hours control preservation without preservative, crustaceans show non-significant p value for deep frying with respect to the raw condition. Rest of the values are significant, which means there is significant difference present among the raw state and cooked samples in all the preservation methods.

In 14 days salt and turmeric preservation, salt water fish shows non-significant p value for deep frying with respect to the raw condition. Rest of the values are significant, which means there is significant difference present among the raw state and cooked samples in all the preservation methods.

Overall analysis indicates that there is statistically significant difference present among the three groups i.e. carp, crustaceans and salt water fish with respect to the raw and cooked values regarding the calcium content, which means the calcium contents vary among the three groups of sample.

Table no 5.10.7 Iron content (**WOP**= Without preservative, **ST**= Salt & Turmeric, **KMS**= Potassium metabisulphite)

Raw vs.		WOP					ST				KMS			
		FRESH	24Hr	48Hr	14D	15D	24Hr	48Hr	14D	15D	24Hr	48Hr	14D	15D
CARP	B	0.005	0.006	0.006	0.001	0.001	0.000	0.003	0.000	0.007	0.002	0.004	0.007	0.000
	DR	0.001	0.001	0.001	0.919(NS)	0.018	0.000	0.001	0.001	0.000	0.011	0.004	0.000	0.000
	SF	0.002	0.001	0.000	0.000	0.001	0.001	0.001	0.001	0.360(NS)	0.000	0.000	0.003	0.001
	DF	0.000	0.001	0.000	0.000	0.006	0.691(NS)	0.002	0.000	0.001	0.420(NS)	0.004	0.005	0.000
CRUSTACEANS	B	0.002	0.112(NS)	0.005	0.044	0.007	0.001	0.000	0.002	0.002	0.000	0.007	0.000	0.000
	DR	0.000	0.016	0.001	0.018	0.000	0.008	0.003	0.003	0.002	0.000	0.017	0.000	0.000
	SF	0.000	0.000	0.000	0.001	0.004	0.000	0.001	0.004	0.014	0.000	0.001	0.000	0.002
	DF	0.001	0.001	0.001	0.001	0.016	0.001	0.085(NS)	0.525(NS)	0.001	0.000	0.008	0.000	0.000
SALT WATER FISH	B	0.000	0.001	0.001	0.000	0.001	0.012	0.020	0.003	0.001	0.017	0.000	0.123(NS)	0.135(NS)
	DR	0.001	0.429(NS)	0.005	0.000	0.000	0.024	0.001	0.001	0.000	0.001	0.000	0.000	0.000
	SF	0.000	0.008	0.000	0.125(NS)	0.001	0.025	0.001	0.002	0.000	0.002	0.000	0.000	0.001
	DF	0.007	0.027	0.000	0.001	0.000	0.001	0.001	0.083(NS)	0.000	0.000	0.000	0.001	0.003

NS = Non- significant values that mean there is no significant difference present among the three categories of samples with respect to the raw and cooked conditions. R= Raw, B= Boiling, DR = Dry roasting, SF= Shallow frying, DF= Deep frying.

This table shows the p value of the iron content among the three categories of samples with respect to the raw and cooked conditions. In 14 days control preservation without preservative, carp shows non-significant p value for open pan dry roasting with respect to the raw condition. In 24 hours and 15 days salt and turmeric preservation, p value is non-significant for deep frying and shallow frying with respect to the raw condition. Rest of the values are significant, which means there is significant difference present among the raw state and cooked samples in all the preservation methods.

In 24 hours control preservation without preservative, crustaceans show non-significant p value for boiling, whereas in 48 hours and 14 days salt and turmeric preservation, p value is non-significant for deep frying with respect to the raw condition. Rest of the values are significant, which means there is significant difference present among the raw state and cooked samples in all the preservation methods.

In 24 hours and 14 days control preservation without preservative, salt water fish shows non-significant p value for open pan dry roasting and shallow frying, whereas in 14 days salt and turmeric preservation, p value is non-significant for deep frying with respect to the raw condition. Rest of the values are significant, which means there is significant difference present among the raw state and cooked samples in all of the preservation methods.

Overall analysis indicates that there is statistically significant difference present among the three groups i.e. carp, crustaceans and salt water fish with respect to the raw and cooked values regarding the iron content, which means the iron contents vary among the three groups of sample.

Table no 5.10.8 Energy content (**WOP**= Without preservative, **ST**= Salt & Turmeric, **KMS**= Potassium metabisulphite)

Raw vs.		WOP					ST				KMS			
		FRESH	24Hr	48Hr	14D	15D	24Hr	48Hr	14D	15D	24Hr	48Hr	14D	15D
CARP	B	0.000	0.001	0.000	0.001	0.001	0.000	0.000	0.000	0.000	0.000	0.000	0.000	0.003
	DR	0.000	0.002	0.000	0.001	0.003	0.000	0.000	0.000	0.000	0.000	0.000	0.000	0.002
	SF	0.000	0.009	0.000	0.002	0.270(NS)	0.002	0.000	0.001	0.003	0.001	0.000	0.001	0.015
	DF	0.000	0.013	0.000	0.003	0.000	0.000	0.000	0.000	0.000	0.002	0.000	0.005	0.036
CRUSTACEANS	B	0.000	0.000	0.000	0.001	0.005	0.002	0.000	0.006	0.001	0.000	0.003	0.001	0.000
	DR	0.000	0.000	0.001	0.000	0.003	0.003	0.001	0.002	0.003	0.009	0.004	0.523(NS)	0.004
	SF	0.130(NS)	0.001	0.121(NS)	0.602(NS)	0.000	0.008	0.003	0.008	0.002	0.001	0.001	0.002	0.027
	DF	0.557(NS)	0.000	0.001	0.016	0.002	0.062(NS)	0.015	0.008	0.000	0.019	0.005	0.124(NS)	0.008
SALT WATR FISH	B	0.001	0.000	0.000	0.000	0.000	0.003	0.000	0.007	0.000	0.000	0.000	0.000	0.000
	DR	0.000	0.000	0.000	0.000	0.001	0.000	0.000	0.000	0.000	0.000	0.000	0.000	0.000
	SF	0.000	0.000	0.000	0.000	0.000	0.000	0.000	0.000	0.000	0.002	0.000	0.000	0.000
	DF	0.000	0.000	0.000	0.000	0.000	0.000	0.000	0.000	0.000	0.000	0.000	0.000	0.000

NS = Non-significant values that mean there is no significant difference present among the three categories of samples with respect to the raw and cooked conditions. R= Raw, B= Boiling, DR = Dry roasting, SF= Shallow frying, DF= Deep frying.

This table shows the p value of the energy content among the three categories of samples with respect to the raw and cooked conditions. In 15 days control preservation without preservative, carp shows non-significant p value for shallow frying with respect to the raw condition. Rest of the values are significant, which means there is significant difference present among the raw state and cooked samples in all of the preservation methods.

In fresh condition, crustaceans show non-significant p value for shallow frying and deep frying, whereas in 48 hours and 14 days control preservation without preservative, p value is non-significant for shallow frying with respect to the raw condition. In 24 hours salt and turmeric preservation and 14 days KMS preservation, p value is non-significant for deep frying with respect to the raw condition. Rest of the values are significant, which means there is significant difference present among the raw and cooked samples in all of the preservation methods.

All the values are significant for salt water fish, which means there is significant difference present among the raw and cooked samples in all the preservation methods.

Overall analysis indicates that there is statistically significant difference present among the three groups i.e. carp, crustaceans and salt water fish with respect to the raw and cooked values regarding the energy content, which means the energy contents vary among the three groups of sample.

5.11 Student t test between samples preserved with and without Preservatives

This statistical test is carried out to estimate any significant deviation among different fish and other edible aquatic species, preserved with and without preservatives under the raw and cooked conditions regarding different nutritional parameters (carbohydrate, protein, fat, moisture, ash, calcium, iron and energy). Significant level is checked at 5% level, which means if the p value is less than 0.05 then it is significant. This statistical analysis helps to reveal the effectiveness of the two preservatives i.e. combination of salt and turmeric (natural preservative) and potassium metabisulphite/KMS (artificial preservative) with respect to the control preservation without preservative.

Table no 5.11.1 Carbohydrate content (WOP= Without preservative, **ST=** Salt & Turmeric, **KMS=** Potassium metabisulphite)

		WOP vs. ST				WOP vs. KMS				ST vs. KMS			
		24Hr	48Hr	14D	15D	24Hr	48Hr	14D	15D	24Hr	48Hr	14D	15D
Rohu	R	0.019	0.128	0.001	0.013	0.423(NS)	0.130(NS)	0.040	0.001	0.017	0.249(NS)	0.001	0.013
	B	0.946	0.001	0.004	0.002	0.012	0.050	0.093(NS)	0.001	0.027	0.000	0.005	0.070(NS)
	OPDR	0.071	0.695	0.036	0.135	0.059(NS)	0.979(NS)	0.327(NS)	0.002	0.091(NS)	0.437(NS)	0.011	0.007
	SF	0.027	0.020	0.002	0.034	0.011	0.002	0.172(NS)	0.016	0.001	0.018	0.003	0.004
	DF	0.002	0.024	0.008	0.045	0.022	0.076(NS)	0.007	0.009	0.003	0.001	0.022	0.054(NS)
Katla	R	0.009	0.001	0.000	0.009	0.092(NS)	0.013	0.001	0.001	0.003	0.001	0.201(NS)	0.185(NS)
	B	0.208	0.006	0.019	0.019	0.020	0.560(NS)	0.017	0.051(NS)	0.082(NS)	0.000	0.184(NS)	0.009
	OPDR	0.003	0.392	0.003	0.002	0.103(NS)	0.191(NS)	0.011	0.001	0.004	0.092(NS)	0.626(NS)	0.423(NS)
	SF	0.127	0.023	0.059	0.004	0.001	0.906(NS)	0.210(NS)	0.004	0.004	0.002	0.132(NS)	0.833(NS)
	DF	0.001	0.001	0.001	0.000	0.103(NS)	0.012	0.000	0.003	0.004	0.464(NS)	0.678(NS)	0.188(NS)
Prawn	R	0.010	0.001	0.049	0.004	0.006	0.694(NS)	0.008	0.001	0.002	0.005	0.003	0.001
	B	0.004	0.002	0.177	0.015	0.007	0.016	0.040	0.128(NS)	0.233(NS)	0.006	0.019	0.002
	OPDR	0.005	0.000	0.006	0.000	0.001	0.021	0.092(NS)	0.006	0.000	0.000	0.002	0.003
	SF	0.001	0.005	0.606	0.000	0.000	0.006	0.002	0.018	0.007	0.019	0.008	0.001
	DF	0.001	0.000	0.597	0.007	0.012	0.001	0.247(NS)	0.074(NS)	0.000	0.006	0.170(NS)	0.005
Lobster	R	0.003	0.002	0.087	0.005	0.000	0.002	0.102(NS)	0.852(NS)	0.027	0.017	0.001	0.007
	B	0.003	0.469	0.093	0.045	0.004	0.086(NS)	0.156(NS)	0.002	0.001	0.061(NS)	0.42(NS)	0.001
	OPDR	0.423	0.010	0.000	0.423	0.008	0.010	0.001	0.065(NS)	0.005	0.054(NS)	0.184(NS)	0.011
	SF	0.001	0.023	0.011	0.022	0.038	0.368(NS)	0.028	0.730(NS)	0.199(NS)	0.011	0.240(NS)	0.004
	DF	0.007	0.001	0.001	0.020	0.011	0.000	0.001	0.008	0.980(NS)	0.010	0.004	0.003
Pomfret	R	0.000	0.003	0.001	0.002	0.003	0.003	0.003	0.012	0.000	0.423(NS)	0.000	0.000
	B	0.001	0.005	0.005	0.005	0.015	0.001	0.001	0.318(NS)	0.003	0.015	0.001	0.003
	OPDR	0.021	0.000	0.004	0.027	0.003	0.011	0.003	0.003	0.184(NS)	0.001	0.003	0.007
	SF	0.000	0.002	0.007	0.142	0.016	0.029	0.001	0.001	0.001	0.005	0.000	0.000
	DF	0.007	0.000	0.007	0.006	0.140(NS)	0.063(NS)	0.000	0.000	0.000	0.000	0.000	0.002
Hilsa	R	0.007	0.008	0.036	0.002	0.032	0.002	0.003	0.003	0.011	0.014	0.002	0.002
	B	0.020	0.000	0.000	0.002	0.096(NS)	0.006	0.000	0.002	0.074(NS)	0.003	0.002	0.013
	OPDR	0.099	0.076	0.001	0.013	0.894(NS)	0.002	0.001	0.008	0.029	0.038	0.004	0.035
	SF	0.635	0.010	0.002	0.009	0.073(NS)	0.003	0.118(NS)	0.002	0.019	0.026	0.000	0.001
	DF	0.003	0.002	0.025	0.051	0.000	0.270(NS)	0.000	0.004	0.000	0.002	0.000	0.009

NS= Non-Significant value that means there is no significant difference present among the samples, preserved with the combination of salt and turmeric, potassium metabisulphite and without preservative in respect to the raw and cooked conditions. R= Raw, B= Boiling, OPDR=Open Pan Dry roasting, SF= Shallow frying, DF= Deep frying.

This table shows the p values of the carbohydrate content among the preserved sample with and without preservatives. Preservation without preservative and combination of salt and turmeric preservation show that all the values are significant in case of all the samples, which means significant differences present among the samples preserved without preservative and preserved with the combination of salt and turmeric. It indicates that salt and turmeric preservation is effective to restore carbohydrate content than preservation without preservative for all the samples.

Rohu shows non-significant p values for the raw state, boiling, open pan dry roasting, shallow frying and deep frying in 24 hours, 48 hours and 14 days control preservation without preservative and KMS preservation. In the case of the raw state, boiling, open pan dry roasting and deep frying show non-significant p values in 24 hours, 48 hours and 15 days preservation with salt and turmeric and KMS. It indicates that there is no such significant difference present between the preservation without preservative and preservation with KMS, but on the other hand, there are significant differences present between salt and turmeric preservation and KMS preservation. Thus salt and turmeric preservation is effective here.

Katla shows non-significant p values for the raw state, boiling, open pan dry roasting, shallow frying and deep frying in 24 hours, 48 hours, 14 days and 15 days preservation both for control preservation without preservative and KMS preservation as well as preservation with salt and turmeric and KMS. It indicates that there is no such significant difference present between the preservation without preservative and preservation with KMS, and also for the salt-turmeric preservation and KMS preservation. Here KMS preservation is more effective than salt and turmeric preservation.

Prawn shows non-significant p values for the raw state, boiling, open pan dry roasting and deep frying in 48 hours, 14 days and 15 days preservation without preservative and KMS preservation. In the case of boiling and deep frying show non-significant p values in 24 hours and 14 days preservation with salt and turmeric and KMS. It indicates that there is no such significant difference present between the control preservation without preservative and with KMS preservation, but on the other hand, there are significant differences present between the salt and turmeric preservation and KMS preservation. Here salt and turmeric preservation is more effective than KMS preservation.

Lobster shows non-significant p values for the raw state, boiling, open pan dry roasting and shallow frying in 48 hours, 14 days and 15 days control preservation without preservative and KMS preservation, whereas boiling, open pan dry roasting, shallow frying and deep frying show non-significant p values in 24 hours, 48 hours and 14 days preservation with salt and turmeric and KMS. It indicates that there is no such significant difference present between the preservation without preservative and with KMS preservation as well as between salt-turmeric preservation and KMS preservation. Here the effects of both the preservatives are quite similar.

Pomfret shows non-significant p values for boiling and deep frying in 24 hours, 48 hours and 14 days control preservation without preservative and KMS preservation. In the case of the raw state and open pan dry roasting show non-significant p values in 24 hours and 48 hours preservation with salt and turmeric and KMS. It indicates that there are some significant differences present between the preservation without preservative and with KMS preservation as well as salt and turmeric preservation and KMS preservation. Here both the preservatives are effective.

Hilsa shows non-significant p values for boiling, open pan dry roasting, shallow frying and deep frying in 24 hours, 48 hours and 14 days control preservation without preservative and KMS preservation. In the case of boiling shows non-significant p value in 24 hours preservation with salt and turmeric and KMS. It indicates that there is some significant difference present between the preservation without preservative and with KMS preservation as well as between the salt and turmeric preservation and KMS preservation. Here salt and turmeric preservation is more effective than KMS preservation.

Overall analysis reveals that the salt and turmeric preservation is effective to restore carbohydrate content as compared to the preservation of samples without preservative, whereas it is also effective than KMS preservation for *rohu*, prawn and *hilsa.* KMS preservation is effective as compared to the salt and turmeric preservation for *katla*, and both the preservatives are similarly effective for lobster and pomfret preservation to restore carbohydrate content.

Table no 5.11.2 Protein content (WOP= Without preservative, **ST**= Salt & Turmeric, **KMS**= Potassium metabisulphite)

		WOP vs. ST				WOP vs. KMS				ST vs. KMS			
		24Hr	48Hr	14D	15D	24Hr	48Hr	14D	15D	24Hr	48Hr	14D	15D
Rohu	R	0.324	0.014	0.001	0.001	0.001	0.005	0.001	0.001	0.001	0.000	0.400(NS)	0.423(NS)
	B	0.001	0.000	0.213	0.080	0.002	0.000	0.200(NS)	0.097(NS)	0.001	0.000	0.423(NS)	0.362(NS)
	OPDR	0.000	0.001	0.002	0.012	0.327(NS)	0.006	0.002	0.010	0.003	0.000	0.423(NS)	0.384(NS)
	SF	0.000	0.000	0.166	0.039	0.003	0.000	0.191(NS)	0.023	0.000	0.000	0.742(NS)	0.477(NS)
	DF	0.000	0.000	0.032	0.003	0.001	0.000	0.028	0.006	0.000	0.000	0.423(NS)	0.499(NS)
Katla	R	0.128	0.051	0.338	0.001	0.006	0.004	0.222(NS)	0.003	0.000	0.001	0.689(NS)	0.015
	B	0.023	0.000	0.003	0.000	0.004	0.007	0.007	0.003	0.001	0.350(NS)	0.095(NS)	0.033
	OPDR	0.004	0.001	0.065	0.002	0.003	0.050	0.023	0.048	0.009	0.002	0.044	0.010
	SF	0.001	0.003	0.000	0.000	0.275(NS)	0.096(NS)	0.016	0.002	0.071(NS)	0.001	0.009	0.001
	DF	0.000	0.000	0.022	0.001	0.002	0.001	0.184(NS)	0.012	0.184(NS)	0.024	0.001	0.014
Prawn	R	0.014	0.001	0.118	0.270	0.005	0.024	0.004	0.007	0.009	0.001	0.010	0.086(NS)
	B	0.006	0.002	0.040	0.022	0.000	0.013	0.099(NS)	0.000	0.000	0.452(NS)	0.235(NS)	0.002
	OPDR	0.002	0.005	0.435	0.006	0.002	0.005	0.017	0.013	0.007	0.396(NS)	0.010	0.057(NS)
	SF	0.006	0.001	0.068	0.065	0.014	0.075(NS)	0.002	0.047	0.423(NS)	0.006	0.740(NS)	0.034
	DF	0.027	0.003	0.014	0.000	0.001	0.062(NS)	0.022	0.103(NS)	0.001	0.002	0.004	0.285(NS)
Lobster	R	0.431	0.005	0.003	0.015	0.003	0.078(NS)	0.038	0.000	0.063(NS)	0.009	0.225(NS)	0.222(NS)
	B	0.398	0.398	0.009	0.056	0.912(NS)	0.109(NS)	0.004	0.023	0.227(NS)	0.698(NS)	0.018	0.023
	OPDR	0.001	0.002	0.025	0.010	0.004	0.001	0.010	0.000	0.196(NS)	0.015	0.007	0.001
	SF	0.004	0.126	0.039	0.004	0.006	0.031	0.001	0.007	0.005	0.052(NS)	0.009	0.005
	DF	0.297	0.046	0.016	0.003	0.298(NS)	0.015	0.075(NS)	0.002	0.960(NS)	0.524(NS)	0.020	0.003
Pomfret	R	0.001	0.000	0.003	0.187	0.000	0.000	0.007	0.038	0.024	0.423(NS)	0.513(NS)	0.039
	B	0.748	0.340	0.012	0.010	0.494(NS)	0.385(NS)	0.008	0.001	0.561(NS)	0.189(NS)	0.184(NS)	0.382(NS)
	OPDR	0.013	0.153	0.423	0.014	0.071(NS)	0.648(NS)	0.032	0.015	0.686(NS)	0.581(NS)	0.020	0.128(NS)
	SF	0.054	0.064	0.002	0.000	0.029	0.030	0.004	0.094(NS)	0.254(NS)	0.423(NS)	0.038	0.038
	DF	0.111	0.188	0.015	0.040	0.034	0.039	0.002	0.021	0.031	0.680(NS)	0.023	0.002
Hilsa	R	0.001	0.001	0.035	0.009	0.000	0.001	0.005	0.005	0.107(NS)	0.010	0.001	0.004
	B	0.250	0.095	0.055	0.049	0.015	0.030	0.080(NS)	0.016	0.478(NS)	0.624(NS)	0.060(NS)	0.000
	OPDR	0.008	0.001	0.174	0.048	0.000	0.007	0.211(NS)	0.010	0.559(NS)	0.252(NS)	0.010	0.075(NS)
	SF	0.004	0.894	0.008	0.410	0.007	0.022	0.005	0.713(NS)	0.423(NS)	0.087(NS)	0.199(NS)	0.277(NS)
	DF	0.009	0.011	0.000	0.395	0.002	0.001	0.004	0.942(NS)	0.001	0.013	0.005	0.184(NS)

NS= Non-Significant values that mean there is no significant difference present among the samples, preserved with the combination of salt and turmeric, potassium metabisulphite and without preservative in respect to the raw and cooked conditions. R= Raw, B= Boiling, OPDR= Open Pan Dry roasting, SF= Shallow frying, DF= Deep frying.

This table shows the p values of the protein content among the preserved samples with and without preservatives. Preservation without preservative and combination of salt and turmeric preservation show that all the values are significant in case of all the samples, which means significant differences present among the samples preserved without preservative and preserved with the combination of salt and turmeric. It indicates that the salt and turmeric preservation is effective to restore protein content than preservation without preservative for all the samples.

Rohu shows non-significant p values for open pan dry roasting in 24 hours, boiling and shallow frying in 14 days, and boiling in 15 days control preservation without preservative and KMS preservation. In the case of the raw state, boiling, open pan dry roasting, shallow frying and deep frying show non-significant p values in 14 days and 15 days preservation with salt-turmeric and KMS. It indicates that there are some significant differences present between the preservation without preservative and with KMS preservation, but on the other hand, there is no such significant difference present between salt and turmeric preservation and KMS preservation in 14 days and 15 days preservation. The effect of KMS is prominent to restore protein content in *rohu.*

Katla shows non-significant p values for shallow frying in 24 hours and 48 hours, and for the raw state and deep frying in 14 days control preservation without preservative and KMS preservation. In the case of shallow frying and deep frying in 24 hours, boiling in 48 hours, and the raw state and boiling show non-significant p values in 14 days preservation with salt and turmeric and KMS. It indicates that there are some significant differences present between the preservation without preservative and KMS preservation as well as for the salt and turmeric preservation and KMS preservation. Thus here the effects of both the preservatives are quite similar to restore protein content in *katla.*

Prawn shows non-significant p values for shallow frying and deep frying in 48 hours, boiling in 14 days and deep frying in 15 days control preservation without preservative and KMS preservation. In the case of shallow frying in 24 hours, boiling and open pan dry roasting in 48 hours, boiling and shallow frying in 14 days, and the raw state and open pan dry roasting in 15 days show non-significant p values by preservation with salt and turmeric and KMS. It indicates that there is no such significant difference present between the preservation without preservative and KMS preservation, but on the other hand, there is significant differences present between the salt and turmeric preservation and KMS preservation. Thus the effect of KMS is prominent to restore protein content in prawn.

Lobster shows non-significant p values for boiling, deep frying in 24 hours, the raw state and boiling in 48 hours, and deep frying in 14 days control preservation without preservative and KMS preservation. In the case of the raw state, boiling, open pan dry roasting and deep frying in 24 hours, and boiling, shallow frying and deep frying in 48 hours, and the raw state in 14 days and 15 days show non-significant p values by preservation with salt and turmeric and KMS. It indicates that there are some significant differences present between the preservation without preservative and KMS preservation, but on the other hand, there is no such significant difference present between the salt and turmeric preservation and KMS preservation. Thus the effect of KMS is prominent to restore protein content in lobster.

Pomfret shows non-significant p values for boiling and open pan dry roasting in 24 hours, 48 hours, and shallow frying in 15 days control preservation without preservative and KMS preservation. In the case of boiling, open pan dry roasting, shallow frying in 24 hours, and the raw state, boiling, open pan dry roasting, shallow frying and deep frying in 48 hours, and the raw state and boiling in 14 days, and boiling and open pan dry roasting in 15 days show non-significant p values by preservation with salt and turmeric and KMS. It indicates that there are some significant differences present between the control preservation without preservative and KMS preservation. But no such significant difference present between the salt and turmeric preservation and KMS preservation. Here also KMS is effective.

Hilsa shows non-significant p value for boiling and open pan dry roasting in 14 days, and shallow frying and deep frying in 15 days preservation without preservative and KMS preservation. In the case of the raw state, boiling, open pan dry roasting and shallow frying in 24 hours, and boiling, open pan dry roasting and shallow frying in 48 hours, and boiling and shallow frying in 14 days, and open pan dry roasting, shallow frying and deep frying in 15 days show non-significant p values by the preservation with salt and turmeric and KMS. It indicates that there is some significant difference present between the preservation without preservative and KMS preservation. But no such significant difference present between the salt and turmeric preservation and KMS preservation. Here also KMS is effective.

Overall analysis reveals that the salt and turmeric preservation is effective to restore protein content as compared to the preservation of samples without preservative, whereas KMS is effective than salt and turmeric preservation for *rohu*, prawn, lobster, pomfret and *hilsa.* Both the preservatives are similarly effective for *katla* preservation to restore protein content.

Table no 5.11.3 Fat content (WOP= Without preservative, **ST**= Salt & Turmeric, **KMS**= Potassium metabisulphite)

		WOP vs. ST				WOP vs. KMS				ST vs. KMS			
		24Hr	48Hr	14D	15D	24Hr	48Hr	14D	15D	24Hr	48Hr	14D	15D
Rohu	R	0.000	0.000	0.000	0.000	0.000	0.000	0.000	0.000	0.002	0.000	0.001	0.008
	B	0.000	0.000	0.027	0.000	0.007	0.005	0.000	0.001	0.000	0.000	0.000	0.000
	OPDR	0.000	0.000	0.000	0.000	0.015	0.000	0.000	0.013	0.002	0.000	0.001	0.008
	SF	0.001	0.000	0.000	0.004	0.001	0.000	0.001	0.118(NS)	0.000	0.001	0.000	0.006
	DF	0.002	0.000	0.000	0.021	0.002	0.001	0.000	0.000	0.001	0.003	0.001	0.000
Katla	R	0.000	0.000	0.000	0.000	0.000	0.000	0.000	0.000	0.001	0.049	0.003	0.000
	B	0.002	0.014	0.000	0.002	0.000	0.000	0.000	0.000	0.000	0.003	0.000	0.000
	OPDR	0.000	0.002	0.001	0.002	0.000	0.003	0.001	0.000	0.001	0.001	0.001	0.000
	SF	0.001	0.000	0.001	0.001	0.003	0.006	0.002	0.003	0.000	0.001	0.001	0.001
	DF	0.000	0.184	0.232	0.000	0.000	0.001	0.000	0.000	0.000	0.000	0.002	0.000
Prawn	R	0.000	0.001	0.022	0.024	0.003	0.005	0.046	0.000	0.001	0.001	0.000	0.001
	B	0.001	0.011	0.000	0.002	0.000	0.000	0.000	0.009	0.000	0.000	0.016	0.004
	OPDR	0.000	0.001	0.000	0.017	0.001	0.000	0.000	0.002	0.000	0.042	0.000	0.000
	SF	0.000	0.000	0.002	0.001	0.000	0.000	0.001	0.000	0.001	0.108(NS)	0.002	0.001
	DF	0.000	0.006	0.000	0.000	0.000	0.000	0.000	0.002	0.009	0.001	0.073(NS)	0.000
Lobster	R	0.000	0.001	0.025	0.023	0.128(NS)	0.003	0.022	0.003	0.000	0.000	0.000	0.002
	B	0.000	0.033	0.001	0.016	0.018	0.000	0.000	0.009	0.000	0.000	0.019	0.041
	OPDR	0.031	0.000	0.004	0.021	0.033	0.001	0.000	0.957(NS)	0.009	0.000	0.001	0.003
	SF	0.001	0.034	0.044	0.001	0.001	0.000	0.000	0.000	0.000	0.000	0.000	0.003
	DF	0.000	0.000	0.000	0.000	0.012	0.000	0.005	0.000	0.001	0.000	0.000	0.000
Pomfret	R	0.000	0.000	0.678	0.000	0.000	0.000	0.000	0.000	0.000	0.000	0.000	0.001
	B	0.000	0.000	0.000	0.005	0.000	0.000	0.000	0.000	0.000	0.000	0.008	0.001
	OPDR	0.000	0.000	0.000	0.001	0.000	0.000	0.000	0.000	0.000	0.000	0.009	0.000
	SF	0.000	0.000	0.000	0.000	0.000	0.000	0.000	0.000	0.000	0.000	0.000	0.000
	DF	0.000	0.000	0.000	0.000	0.000	0.000	0.000	0.000	0.001	0.000	0.000	0.001
Hilsa	R	0.003	0.000	0.000	0.000	0.304(NS)	0.069(NS)	0.085(NS)	0.001	0.000	0.000	0.000	0.000
	B	0.000	0.000	0.000	0.105	0.000	0.000	0.000	0.000	0.000	0.015	0.000	0.000
	OPDR	0.000	0.001	0.012	0.099	0.000	0.001	0.004	0.000	0.000	0.001	0.000	0.000
	SF	0.000	0.000	0.001	0.000	0.003	0.000	0.005	0.001	0.000	0.002	0.000	0.017
	DF	0.000	0.026	0.000	0.005	0.000	0.000	0.423(NS)	0.000	0.000	0.000	0.000	0.000

NS= Non-Significant values that mean there is no significant difference present among the samples, preserved with the combination of salt and turmeric, potassium metabisulphite and without preservative in respect to the raw and cooked conditions. R= Raw, B= Boiling, DR= Dry roasting, SF= Shallow frying, DF= Deep frying.

This table shows the p values of the fat content among the preserved samples with and without preservatives. Preservation without preservative and combination of salt and turmeric preservation show that all the values are significant in case of all the samples, which means significant differences present among the samples preserved without preservative and preserved with the combination of salt and turmeric. It indicates that the salt and turmeric preservation is effective to restore fat content as compared to the preservation without preservative for all the samples.

Rohu shows non-significant p value for shallow frying in 15 days control preservation without preservative and KMS preservation, whereas all the values are significant in preservation with salt and turmeric and KMS. It indicates that there are some significant differences present between the preservation without preservative and KMS preservation, but overall significant difference present between the salt and turmeric preservation and KMS preservation. Thus the effect of salt and turmeric is prominent to restore fat content in *rohu.*

Katla shows significant p values for all the cooking methods with respect to all the preservation methods. It indicates that there is significant differences present between the preservation without preservative and KMS preservation, as well as for the salt and turmeric preservation and KMS preservation. Thus here the effects of both the preservatives are quite similar to restore fat content in *katla.*

Prawn shows significant p values for all cooking methods with respect to the preservation without preservative and KMS preservation. In the case of shallow frying in 48 hours, and deep frying in 14 days show non-significant p values by preservation with salt-turmeric and KMS. It indicates that there is significant difference present between the preservation without preservative and KMS preservation, but on the other hand, some significant differences present between the salt and turmeric preservation and KMS preservation. Thus the effect of KMS is prominent to restore fat content in prawn.

Lobster shows non-significant p values for the raw state in 24 hours, and open pan dry roasting in 15 days control preservation without preservative and KMS preservation, whereas all the values are significant by preservation with salt and turmeric and KMS. It indicates that there is significant differences present between the preservation without preservative and KMS preservation as well as between the salt and turmeric preservation and KMS preservation. Thus the effects of both the preservative are prominent to restore fat content in lobster.

Pomfret shows significant p values for all cooking methods with respect to the preservation methods. It indicates that there is significant difference present between the preservation without preservative and KMS preservation as well as between the salt and turmeric preservation and KMS preservation. Here also both the preservatives are effective to restore fat content.

Hilsa shows non-significant p values for the raw state in 24 hours, 48 hours, and the raw state and deep frying in 14 days control preservation without preservative and KMS preservation, whereas all the values are significant by the preservation with salt and turmeric and KMS. It indicates that there are some significant differences present between the preservation without preservative and KMS preservation, but overall significant difference present between the salt and turmeric preservation and KMS preservation. Here salt and turmeric preservation is effective to restore fat content.

Overall analysis reveals that the salt and turmeric preservation is effective to restore fat content as compared to the preservation of samples without preservative, whereas it is also effective than KMS preservation for *rohu* and *hilsa.* KMS is more effective than salt and turmeric preservation for prawn. Both the preservatives are similarly effective for *katla*, lobster and pomfret preservation to restore fat content.

Table no 5.11.4 Moisture content (WOP= Without preservative, **ST**= Salt & Turmeric, **KMS**= Potassium metabisulphite)

		WOP vs. ST				WOP vs. KMS				ST vs. KMS			
		24Hr	48Hr	14D	15D	24Hr	48Hr	14D	15D	24Hr	48Hr	14D	15D
Rohu	R	0.085	0.037	0.357	0.162	0.583(NS)	0.144(NS)	0.586(NS)	0.157(NS)	0.353(NS)	0.141(NS)	0.057(NS)	0.298(NS)
	B	0.050	0.202	0.045	0.038	0.044	0.497(NS)	0.028	0.137(NS)	0.252(NS)	0.022	0.154(NS)	0.024
	OPDR	0.082	0.105	0.111	0.101	0.270(NS)	0.071(NS)	0.501(NS)	0.519(NS)	0.029	0.139(NS)	0.007	0.011
	SF	0.000	0.009	0.127	0.001	0.025	0.019	0.062(NS)	0.524(NS)	0.003	0.000	0.188(NS)	0.012
	DF	0.003	0.001	0.002	0.001	0.011	0.001	0.001	0.002	0.000	0.002	0.018	0.001
Katla	R	0.141	0.000	0.029	0.086	0.123(NS)	0.874(NS)	0.001	0.775(NS)	0.158(NS)	0.000	0.048	0.021
	B	0.017	0.002	0.022	0.008	0.033	0.003	0.084(NS)	0.589(NS)	0.014	0.065(NS)	0.005	0.022
	OPDR	0.013	0.120	0.004	0.477	0.238(NS)	0.414(NS)	0.082(NS)	0.030	0.002	0.018	0.089(NS)	0.006
	SF	0.073	0.008	0.071	0.037	0.108(NS)	0.031	0.001	0.030	0.002	0.051(NS)	0.042	0.099(NS)
	DF	0.022	0.006	0.014	0.005	0.335(NS)	0.014	0.005	0.001	0.009	0.000	0.046	0.002
Prawn	R	0.017	0.027	0.016	0.022	0.000	0.038	0.097(NS)	0.089(NS)	0.025	0.103(NS)	0.230(NS)	0.986(NS)
	B	0.000	0.000	0.001	0.010	0.008	0.000	0.001	0.028	0.000	0.000	0.001	0.002
	OPDR	0.008	0.000	0.004	0.054	0.003	0.001	0.130(NS)	0.007	0.002	0.004	0.003	0.002
	SF	0.001	0.002	0.003	0.141	0.002	0.000	0.060	0.049	0.003	0.019	0.002	0.002
	DF	0.000	0.001	0.013	0.405	0.053(NS)	0.000	0.012	0.004	0.000	0.011	0.002	0.004
Lobster	R	0.142	0.056	0.093	0.068	0.034	0.018	0.103(NS)	0.039	0.015	0.074(NS)	0.139(NS)	0.854(NS)
	B	0.002	0.015	0.003	0.009	0.005	0.046	0.010	0.026	0.005	0.022	0.005	0.012
	OPDR	0.028	0.000	0.102	0.001	0.005	0.005	0.004	0.019	0.016	0.001	0.004	0.001
	SF	0.000	0.000	0.009	0.105	0.010	0.002	0.021	0.001	0.000	0.009	0.009	0.000
	DF	0.000	0.000	0.000	0.038	0.000	0.001	0.000	0.006	0.000	0.002	0.015	0.000
Pomfret	R	0.076	0.054	0.076	0.145	0.010	0.306(NS)	0.100(NS)	0.012	0.038	0.056(NS)	0.144(NS)	0.006
	B	0.004	0.002	0.001	0.000	0.007	0.001	0.016	0.001	0.432(NS)	0.013	0.001	0.022
	OPDR	0.034	0.008	0.004	0.014	0.059(NS)	0.000	0.001	0.005	0.003	0.141(NS)	0.082(NS)	0.001
	SF	0.153	0.001	0.016	0.287	0.707(NS)	0.110(NS)	0.003	0.115(NS)	0.019	0.174(NS)	0.002	0.062(NS)
	DF	0.000	0.000	0.000	0.006	0.001	0.002	0.000	0.410(NS)	0.000	0.000	0.000	0.046
Hilsa	R	0.001	0.087	0.001	0.040	0.001	0.000	0.000	0.119(NS)	0.426(NS)	0.004	0.003	0.005
	B	0.001	0.010	0.000	0.005	0.018	0.005	0.004	0.001	0.001	0.102(NS)	0.001	0.000
	OPDR	0.007	0.001	0.121	0.008	0.826(NS)	0.000	0.002	0.001	0.016	0.000	0.169(NS)	0.009
	SF	0.000	0.004	0.001	0.003	0.000	0.037	0.006	0.010	0.000	0.018	0.771(NS)	0.003
	DF	0.000	0.008	0.000	0.431	0.000	0.012	0.011	0.007	0.016	0.000	0.090(NS)	0.000

NS= Non-Significant values that mean there is no significant difference present among the samples, preserved with the combination of salt and turmeric, potassium metabisulphite and without preservative in respect to the raw and cooked conditions. R= Raw, B= Boiling, DR= Dry roasting, SF= Shallow frying, DF= Deep frying.

This table shows the p values of the moisture content among the preserved samples with and without preservatives. Preservation without preservative and combination of salt and turmeric preservation show that all the values are significant in case of all the samples, which means significant differences present among the samples preserved without preservative and preserved with the combination of salt and turmeric. It indicates that the salt and turmeric preservation is effective to restore moisture content than preservation without preservative for all the samples.

Rohu shows non-significant p values for the raw state and open pan dry roasting in 24 hours and the raw state, boiling and open pan dry roasting in 48 hours, and the raw state, open pan dry roasting and shallow frying in 14 days, and the raw state, boiling, open pan dry roasting and shallow frying in 15 days control preservation without preservative and KMS preservation. In the case of the raw state and boiling in 24 hours, and the raw state, open pan dry roasting in 48 hours, and the raw state, boiling and shallow frying in 14 days, and the raw state in 15 days show non-significant p values by preservation with salt and turmeric and KMS. It indicates that there is no such significant difference present between the preservation without preservative and KMS preservation. But some significant differences present between the salt and turmeric preservation and KMS preservation. Thus the effect of salt and turmeric is prominent to restore moisture content in *rohu*.

Katla shows non-significant p values for the raw state, open pan dry roasting, shallow frying in 24 hours, and the raw state and open pan dry roasting in 48 hours, and boiling and open pan dry roasting in 14 days, and the raw state and boiling in 15 days control preservation without preservative and KMS preservation. In the case of the raw state in 24 hours, and boiling and shallow frying in 48 hours, and open pan dry roasting in 14 days, and shallow frying in 15 days show non-significant p values by preservation with salt and turmeric and KMS. It indicates that there is no such significant difference present between preservation without preservative and KMS preservation as well as some significant differences present between salt and turmeric preservation and KMS preservation. Thus here the effect of combination of salt and turmeric is prominent to restore moisture content in *katla.*

Prawn shows non-significant p values for deep frying in 24 hours, and the raw state, open pan dry roasting and shallow frying in 14 days, and the raw state in 15 days control preservation without preservative and KMS preservation. In the case of the raw state in 48 hours, 14 days, 15 days show non-significant p values by preservation with salt and turmeric and KMS. It indicates that there are some significant differences present between the preservation without preservative and KMS preservation as well as between the salt and turmeric preservation and KMS preservation. Thus the effects of both the preservatives are prominent to restore moisture content in prawn.

Lobster shows non-significant p value for the raw state in 48 hours preservation without preservative and KMS preservation. In the case of the raw state in 48 hours, 14 days and 15 days show non-significant p values by the preservation with salt and turmeric and KMS. It indicates that there is significant differences present between the preservation without preservative and KMS preservation as well as between the salt-turmeric preservation and KMS preservation. Thus the effects of both the preservative are prominent to restore moisture content in lobster.

Pomfret shows non-significant p values for open pan dry roasting, shallow frying in 24 hours, and the raw state and shallow frying in 48 hours, and the raw state in 14 days, and shallow frying and deep frying in 15 days control preservation without preservative and KMS preservation. In the case of boiling in 24 hours, and the raw state, open pan dry roasting and shallow frying in 48 hours, and the raw state, open pan dry roasting in 14 days, and shallow frying in 15 days show non-significant p value by preservation with salt and turmeric and KMS. It indicates that there are some significant differences present between the preservation without preservative and KMS preservation as well as between the salt and turmeric preservation and KMS preservation. Here also both the preservatives are effective to restore moisture content.

Hilsa shows non-significant p values for open pan dry roasting in 24 hours, and the raw state in 15 days preservation between without preservative and KMS preservation. In the case of the raw state in 24 hours, and boiling in 48 hours, and open pan dry roasting, shallow frying and deep frying in 14 days show non-significant p values by the preservation between the combination of salt-turmeric and KMS preservation. It indicates that there is significant differences present between the preservation without preservative and KMS preservation. But no such significant difference present between the salt and turmeric preservation and KMS preservation. Here KMS is more effective than salt and turmeric to restore moisture content.

Overall analysis reveals that the salt and turmeric preservation is effective to restore moisture content as compared to the preservation of samples without preservative, whereas it is also effective than KMS preservation for *rohu* and *katla.* KMS preservation is more effective than salt and turmeric for *hilsa.* Both the preservatives are similarly effective for prawn, lobster and pomfret preservation to restore moisture content.

Table no 5.11.5 Ash content (WOP= Without preservative, **ST**= Salt & Turmeric, **KMS**= Potassium metabisulphite)

		WOP vs. ST				WOP vs. KMS				ST vs. KMS			
		24Hr	48Hr	14D	15D	24Hr	48Hr	14D	15D	24Hr	48Hr	14D	15D
Rohu	R	0.000	0.000	0.000	0.010	0.000	0.000	0.011	0.001	0.000	0.000	0.000	0.000
	B	0.000	0.002	0.042	0.001	0.000	0.001	0.438(NS)	0.000	0.000	0.012	0.016	0.000
	OPDR	0.001	0.004	0.000	0.000	0.001	0.001	0.003	0.187(NS)	0.017	0.028	0.000	0.000
	SF	0.003	0.000	0.000	0.001	0.000	0.001	0.012	0.000	0.000	0.000	0.000	0.001
	DF	0.000	0.000	0.005	0.000	0.005	0.000	0.002	0.035	0.001	0.000	0.017	0.001
Katla	R	0.054	0.000	0.000	0.000	0.000	0.000	0.000	0.000	0.001	0.001	0.003	0.001
	B	0.006	0.001	0.000	0.000	0.000	0.002	0.000	0.000	0.000	0.001	0.001	0.000
	OPDR	0.001	0.000	0.000	0.001	0.000	0.000	0.000	0.000	0.000	0.001	0.001	0.001
	SF	0.000	0.021	0.000	0.000	0.000	0.000	0.000	0.000	0.461(NS)	0.041	0.000	0.000
	DF	0.002	0.000	0.000	0.000	0.000	0.000	0.000	0.000	0.000	0.001	0.000	0.001
Prawn	R	0.023	0.000	0.000	0.001	0.086(NS)	0.002	0.000	0.000	0.011	0.001	0.000	0.000
	B	0.000	0.000	0.000	0.001	0.000	0.001	0.001	0.002	0.001	0.000	0.003	0.001
	OPDR	0.000	0.000	0.001	0.000	0.001	0.001	0.001	0.000	0.184(NS)	0.000	0.009	0.000
	SF	0.000	0.000	0.000	0.001	0.000	0.000	0.000	0.004	0.000	0.000	0.000	0.000
	DF	0.157	0.000	0.001	0.000	0.001	0.032	0.000	0.000	0.005	0.206(NS)	0.000	0.000
Lobster	R	0.000	0.000	0.000	0.000	0.032	0.000	0.000	0.002	0.000	0.000	0.002	0.000
	B	0.019	0.383	0.001	0.000	0.223(NS)	0.002	0.002	0.005	0.014	0.004	0.000	0.000
	OPDR	0.101	0.000	0.000	0.000	0.499(NS)	0.000	0.000	0.015	0.010	0.002	0.012	0.000
	SF	0.001	0.000	0.000	0.000	0.000	0.000	0.001	0.000	0.000	0.002	0.000	0.000
	DF	0.000	0.001	0.008	0.000	0.000	0.000	0.006	0.000	0.000	0.000	0.005	0.000
Pomfret	R	0.003	0.000	0.000	0.001	0.000	0.423(NS)	0.001	0.100(NS)	0.001	0.000	0.000	0.004
	B	0.001	0.001	0.002	0.005	0.013	0.204(NS)	0.000	0.044	0.001	0.000	0.002	0.000
	OPDR	0.000	0.000	0.017	0.105	0.096(NS)	0.013	0.013	0.040	0.000	0.001	0.057(NS)	0.015
	SF	0.006	0.000	0.003	0.003	0.170(NS)	0.006	0.007	0.002	0.002	0.005	0.001	0.005
	DF	0.000	0.000	0.055	0.045	0.000	0.001	0.000	0.000	0.000	0.000	0.005	0.000
Hilsa	R	0.034	0.001	0.000	0.001	0.027	0.034	0.225(NS)	0.853(NS)	0.423(NS)	0.007	0.000	0.000
	B	0.005	0.006	0.000	0.001	0.000	0.009	0.034	0.063(NS)	0.020	0.199(NS)	0.000	0.001
	OPDR	0.001	0.003	0.000	0.001	0.009	0.079(NS)	0.001	0.001	0.007	0.000	0.000	0.005
	SF	0.000	0.010	0.000	0.000	0.001	0.003	0.009	0.000	0.001	0.000	0.000	0.000
	DF	0.000	0.015	0.000	0.000	0.001	0.711(NS)	0.000	0.004	0.002	0.001	0.000	0.000

NS= Non-Significant values that mean there is no significant difference present among the samples, preserved with the combination of salt and turmeric, potassium metabisulphite and without preservative in respect to the raw and cooked conditions. R= Raw, B= Boiling, DR= Dry roasting, SF= Shallow frying, DF= Deep frying.

This table shows the p values of the ash content among the preserved samples with and without preservatives. Preservation without preservative and combination of salt and turmeric preservation show that all the values are significant in case of all the samples, which means significant differences present among the samples preserved without preservative and preserved with the combination of salt and turmeric. It indicates that salt and turmeric preservation is effective to restore ash content as compared to the preservation without preservative for all the samples.

Rohu shows non-significant p values for boiling in 14 days, and open pan dry roasting in 15 days preservation without preservative and KMS preservation, whereas all the p values are significant by preservation with salt and turmeric and KMS. It indicates that there are some significant differences present between the preservation without preservative and with KMS preservation, but on the other hand, significant differences present between the salt and turmeric preservation and KMS preservation. Thus the effect of salt and turmeric is prominent to restore ash content in *rohu.*

Katla shows significant p values for all the cooking methods with respect to the preservation without preservative and KMS preservation. In the case of shallow frying in 24 hours shows non-significant p value by preservation with salt and turmeric and KMS. It indicates that there is overall significant difference present between the preservation without preservative and KMS preservation, and some significant difference present between the salt and turmeric preservation and KMS preservation. Thus here the effect of KMS is prominent to restore ash content in *katla.*

Prawn shows non-significant p value for the raw state in 24 hours preservation without preservative and KMS preservation. In the case of open pan dry roasting in 24 hours, and deep frying in 48 hours shows non-significant p value by preservation with salt-turmeric and KMS. It indicates that there is some significant differences present between the preservation without preservative and with KMS preservation as well as between the salt and turmeric preservation and KMS preservation. Thus the effects of both the preservatives are prominent to restore ash content in prawn.

Lobster shows non-significant p values for boiling and open pan dry roasting in 24 hours preservation without preservative and KMS preservation, whereas all the p values are significant by the preservation with salt and turmeric and KMS. It indicates that there are some significant differences present between the preservation without preservative and KMS preservation, and overall significant difference present between the salt and turmeric preservation and KMS preservation. Thus the effect of salt and turmeric is prominent to restore ash content in lobster.

Pomfret shows non-significant p values for open pan dry roasting and shallow frying in 24 hours, and the raw state and boiling in 48 hours, and the raw state in 15 days control preservation without preservative and KMS preservation. Open pan dry roasting in 14 days shows non-significant p value by preservation with salt-turmeric and KMS. It indicates that there is no such significant difference present between the preservation without preservative and with KMS preservation, and some significant differences present between the salt and turmeric preservation and KMS preservation. Here also the combination of salt and turmeric is effective to restore ash content.

Hilsa shows non-significant p values for open pan dry roasting and deep frying in 48 hours, and the raw state in 14 days, and the raw state, boiling in 15 days preservation without preservative and KMS preservation. In the case of the raw state in 24 hours, and boiling in 48 hours show non-significant p values by preservation between the combination of salt-turmeric and KMS preservation. It indicates that there is no such significant difference present between the preservation without preservative and KMS preservation. But some significant differences present between the salt and turmeric preservation and KMS preservation. Here salt and turmeric preservation is more effective than KMS preservation to restore ash content.

Overall analysis reveals that salt and turmeric preservation is effective to restore ash content as compared to the preservation of samples without preservative, whereas it is also effective than KMS preservation for *rohu,* lobster, pomfret and *hilsa.* KMS preservation is more effective than salt and turmeric for *katla.* Both the preservatives are similarly effective for prawn preservation to restore ash content.

Table no 5.11.6 Calcium content (**WOP**= Without preservative, **ST**= Salt & Turmeric, **KMS**= Potassium metabisulphite)

		WOP vs. ST				WOP vs. KMS				ST vs. KMS			
		24Hr	48Hr	14D	15D	24Hr	48Hr	14D	15D	24Hr	48Hr	14D	15D
Rohu	R	0.001	0.002	0.000	0.000	0.000	0.107(NS)	0.000	0.001	0.000	0.012	0.000	0.000
	B	0.001	0.011	0.355	0.000	0.000	0.001	0.208(NS)	0.000	0.000	0.001	0.042	0.012
	OPDR	0.000	0.001	0.000	0.000	0.001	0.001	0.000	0.000	0.000	0.003	0.003	0.000
	SF	0.001	0.000	0.000	0.000	0.000	0.000	0.000	0.000	0.000	0.000	0.000	0.000
	DF	0.002	0.000	0.001	0.000	0.000	0.000	0.000	0.001	0.000	0.000	0.000	0.000
Katla	R	0.000	0.000	0.000	0.000	0.000	0.000	0.000	0.000	0.001	0.000	0.003	0.000
	B	0.004	0.000	0.000	0.000	0.000	0.000	0.102(NS)	0.000	0.011	0.000	0.001	0.013
	OPDR	0.000	0.000	0.001	0.000	0.000	0.000	0.000	0.000	0.001	0.000	0.185(NS)	0.000
	SF	0.001	0.001	0.000	0.000	0.000	0.000	0.000	0.000	0.002	0.000	0.000	0.000
	DF	0.000	0.000	0.000	0.000	0.002	0.000	0.000	0.000	0.000	0.010	0.000	0.000
Prawn	R	0.000	0.000	0.001	0.004	0.002	0.002	0.001	0.001	0.000	0.000	0.034	0.187(NS)
	B	0.000	0.000	0.002	0.000	0.000	0.000	0.001	0.000	0.000	0.001	0.000	0.002
	OPDR	0.000	0.000	0.004	0.874	0.085(NS)	0.000	0.001	0.008	0.000	0.000	0.003	0.014
	SF	0.000	0.000	0.001	0.000	0.000	0.000	0.000	0.000	0.001	0.001	0.001	0.001
	DF	0.000	0.000	0.023	0.002	0.008	0.000	0.000	0.000	0.000	0.014	0.000	0.000
Lobster	R	0.347	0.000	0.000	0.000	0.000	0.000	0.000	0.000	0.000	0.000	0.000	0.000
	B	0.000	0.000	0.000	0.002	0.000	0.000	0.000	0.000	0.000	0.000	0.000	0.000
	OPDR	0.000	0.003	0.000	0.002	0.000	0.000	0.001	0.001	0.006	0.000	0.000	0.000
	SF	0.002	0.002	0.002	0.000	0.003	0.000	0.000	0.000	0.002	0.000	0.005	0.000
	DF	0.000	0.001	0.009	0.001	0.000	0.000	0.000	0.000	0.000	0.001	0.000	0.000
Pomfret	R	0.000	0.000	0.000	0.000	0.000	0.000	0.004	0.000	0.000	0.000	0.000	0.000
	B	0.001	0.000	0.000	0.000	0.000	0.000	0.000	0.000	0.000	0.000	0.000	0.000
	OPDR	0.001	0.000	0.000	0.000	0.000	0.000	0.000	0.000	0.000	0.000	0.000	0.000
	SF	0.000	0.000	0.000	0.000	0.000	0.003	0.000	0.000	0.001	0.001	0.001	0.000
	DF	0.000	0.001	0.001	0.000	0.001	0.001	0.000	0.000	0.000	0.000	0.000	0.000
Hilsa	R	0.000	0.000	0.000	0.000	0.000	0.000	0.003	0.000	0.000	0.000	0.000	0.000
	B	0.000	0.000	0.000	0.000	0.001	0.000	0.001	0.000	0.000	0.009	0.001	0.001
	OPDR	0.001	0.000	0.000	0.000	0.000	0.003	0.000	0.000	0.000	0.000	0.000	0.000
	SF	0.000	0.000	0.001	0.000	0.000	0.000	0.000	0.000	0.184((NS)	0.000	0.000	0.001
	DF	0.286	0.000	0.000	0.000	0.000	0.000	0.001	0.000	0.001	0.001	0.000	0.000

NS= Non-Significant values that mean there is no significant difference present among the samples, preserved with the combination of salt and turmeric, potassium metabisulphite and without preservative in respect to the raw and cooked conditions. R= Raw, B= Boiling, DR= Dry roasting, SF= Shallow frying, DF= Deep frying.

This table shows the p values of the calcium content among the preserved samples with and without preservatives. Preservation without preservative and the combination of salt and turmeric preservation show that all the values are significant in case of all the samples, which means significant differences present among the samples preserved without preservative and preserved with the combination of salt and turmeric. It indicates that salt and turmeric preservation is effective to restore calcium content than the preservation without preservative for all the samples.

Rohu shows non-significant p values for the raw state in 48 hours, and boiling in 14 days preservation without preservative and KMS preservation, whereas all the p values are significant by preservation with salt and turmeric and KMS. It indicates that there are some significant differences present between the preservation without preservative and KMS preservation, but on the other hand, overall significant difference present between the salt and turmeric preservation and KMS preservation. Thus the effect of the salt and turmeric is prominent to restore calcium content in *rohu.*

Katla shows non-significant p values for boiling in 14 days preservation without preservative and KMS preservation. Open pan dry roasting in 14 days preservation shows non-significant p value by the preservation with salt-turmeric and KMS. It indicates that there are some significant differences present between the preservation without preservative and KMS preservation as well as between the salt and turmeric preservation and KMS preservation. Thus here the effects of both the preservatives are prominent to restore calcium content in *katla.*

Prawn shows non-significant p values for open pan dry roasting in 24 hours control preservation without preservative and KMS preservation. In case of the raw state in 15 days shows non-significant p value by preservation with salt and turmeric and KMS. It indicates that there are some significant differences present between the preservation without preservative and KMS preservation as well as between the salt-turmeric preservation and KMS preservation. Thus the effects of both the preservatives are prominent to restore calcium content in prawn.

Lobster and pomfret show significant p values for all cooking methods with respect to the preservation without preservative and KMS preservation as well as preservation with salt-turmeric and KMS. It indicates that there is overall significant difference present between the preservation without preservative and KMS preservation as well as between the salt and turmeric preservation and KMS preservation. Thus the effects of both the preservatives are prominent to restore calcium content in lobster and pomfret.

Hilsa shows significant p values for all cooking methods with respect to the preservation without preservative and KMS preservation. Shallow frying in 24 hours shows non-significant p values by preservation between the combination of salt-turmeric and KMS preservation. It indicates that there is significant difference present between the preservation without preservative and KMS preservation. But some significant differences present between the salt and turmeric preservation and KMS preservation. Here KMS is more effective than salt and turmeric preservation to restore calcium content.

Overall analysis reveals that the salt and turmeric preservation is effective to restore calcium content as compared to the preservation of samples without preservative, whereas it is also effective than KMS preservation for *rohu.* KMS preservation is more effective than salt and turmeric for *hilsa.* Both the preservatives are similarly effective for *katla*, prawn, lobster and pomfret preservation to restore calcium content.

Table no 5.11.7 Iron content (WOP= Without preservative, **ST**= Salt & Turmeric, **KMS**= Potassium metabisulphite)

		WOP vs. ST				WOP vs. KMS				ST vs. KMS			
		24Hr	48Hr	14D	15D	24Hr	48Hr	14D	15D	24Hr	48Hr	14D	15D
Rohu	R	0.000	0.000	0.004	0.002	0.000	0.070(NS)	0.005	0.002	0.001	0.001	0.096(NS)	0.000
	B	0.000	0.000	0.150	0.000	0.000	0.016	0.001	0.005	0.000	0.001	0.000	0.000
	OPDR	0.000	0.000	0.028	0.469	0.001	0.010	0.000	0.003	0.000	0.000	0.003	0.006
	SF	0.001	0.004	0.000	0.003	0.937(NS)	0.000	0.000	0.011	0.000	0.000	0.000	0.001
	DF	0.004	0.000	0.002	0.002	0.002	0.000	0.011	0.058(NS)	0.002	0.003	0.000	0.000
Katla	R	0.006	0.013	0.011	0.001	0.003	0.002	0.011	0.058(NS)	0.001	0.000	0.011	0.002
	B	0.147	0.001	0.000	0.004	0.002	0.001	0.000	0.001	0.000	0.004	0.164(NS)	0.000
	OPDR	0.001	0.000	0.001	0.021	0.018	0.000	0.015	0.003	0.004	0.072(NS)	0.013	0.000
	SF	0.002	0.000	0.001	0.000	0.002	0.000	0.002	0.000	0.010	0.008	0.018	0.000
	DF	0.001	0.074	0.000	0.000	0.000	0.000	0.000	0.002	0.002	0.000	0.003	0.000
Prawn	R	0.000	0.009	0.000	0.000	0.000	0.002	0.000	0.001	0.003	0.001	0.002	0.000
	B	0.003	0.057	0.000	0.002	0.004	0.001	0.000	0.005	0.014	0.000	0.000	0.000
	OPDR	0.001	0.012	0.000	0.002	0.001	0.000	0.000	0.000	0.001	0.004	0.124(NS)	0.000
	SF	0.000	0.000	0.005	0.000	0.000	0.000	0.000	0.019	0.003	0.673(NS)	0.101(NS)	0.000
	DF	0.002	0.001	0.001	0.000	0.001	0.000	0.001	0.000	0.000	0.001	0.014	0.000
Lobster	R	0.003	0.002	0.250	0.003	0.109(NS)	0.034	0.110(NS)	0.007	0.001	0.000	0.012	0.038
	B	0.003	0.003	0.000	0.000	0.001	0.004	0.001	0.000	0.138(NS)	0.057(NS)	0.006	0.000
	OPDR	0.022	0.001	0.010	0.000	0.001	0.001	0.000	0.000	0.032	0.000	0.000	0.000
	SF	0.000	0.001	0.026	0.000	0.005	0.001	0.002	0.000	0.000	0.002	0.002	0.000
	DF	0.010	0.044	0.007	0.000	0.115(NS)	0.000	0.000	0.001	0.000	0.000	0.000	0.000
Pomfret	R	0.000	0.000	0.000	0.000	0.000	0.000	0.000	0.000	0.013	0.000	0.002	0.000
	B	0.000	0.000	0.000	0.000	0.000	0.001	0.000	0.001	0.004	0.866(NS)	0.000	0.000
	OPDR	0.000	0.000	0.000	0.000	0.000	0.000	0.000	0.840(NS)	0.002	0.007	0.012	0.002
	SF	0.000	0.000	0.000	0.002	0.000	0.000	0.000	0.000	0.011	0.000	0.000	0.000
	DF	0.000	0.000	0.001	0.000	0.000	0.000	0.001	0.000	0.002	0.002	0.002	0.009
Hilsa	R	0.001	0.031	0.005	0.000	0.000	0.002	0.009	0.002	0.000	0.004	0.001	0.000
	B	0.020	0.001	0.000	0.000	0.001	0.222(NS)	0.000	0.000	0.002	0.002	0.076(NS)	0.005
	OPDR	0.001	0.040	0.038	0.000	0.000	0.000	0.000	0.000	0.000	0.001	0.000	0.000
	SF	0.001	0.000	0.000	0.000	0.000	0.000	0.618(NS)	0.021	0.005	0.005	0.001	0.005
	DF	0.000	0.000	0.003	0.000	0.000	0.000	0.003	0.000	0.001	0.000	0.005	0.014

NS= Non-Significant values that mean there is no significant difference present among the samples, preserved with the combination of salt and turmeric, potassium metabisulphite and without preservative in respect to the raw and cooked conditions. R= Raw, B= Boiling, DR= Dry roasting, SF= Shallow frying, DF= Deep frying.

This table shows the p values of the iron content among the preserved samples with and without preservatives. Preservation without preservative and the combination of salt and turmeric preservation show that all the values are significant in case of all the samples, that means significant differences present among the samples preserved without preservative and preserved with the combination of salt and turmeric. It indicates that salt and turmeric preservation is effective to restore iron content as compared to the preservation without preservative for all the samples.

Rohu shows non-significant p values for shallow frying in 24 hours, and the raw state in 48 hours, and deep frying in 15 days control preservation without preservative and KMS preservation. In the case of the raw state shows non-significant p value in 14 days preservation with salt and turmeric and KMS. It indicates that there is some significant difference present between the preservation without preservative and KMS preservation as well as between the salt and turmeric preservation and KMS preservation. Thus the effects of both the preservatives are prominent to restore iron content in *rohu.*

Katla shows non-significant p value for the raw state in 15 days preservation without preservative and KMS preservation. In the case of open pan dry roasting in 48 hours, and boiling in 14 days preservation show non-significant p values by the preservation with salt and turmeric and KMS. It indicates that there are some significant differences present between the preservation without preservative and KMS preservation as well as between the salt and turmeric preservation and KMS preservation. Thus here the effects of both the preservatives are prominent to restore iron content in *katla.*

Prawn shows significant p values for all the cooking methods with respect to the preservation without preservative and KMS preservation. In the case of shallow frying in 48 hours and open pan dry roasting and shallow frying in 14 days show non-significant p value by the preservation with salt and turmeric and KMS. It indicates that there is significant difference present between the preservation without preservative and KMS preservation. But some significant differences present between the salt and turmeric preservation and KMS preservation. Thus the effect of KMS is more prominent as compared to the salt and turmeric preservation to restore iron content in prawn.

Lobster shows significant p values for the raw state and deep frying in 24 hours, and the raw state in 14 days control preservation without preservative and KMS preservation. In 24 hours and 48 hours boiling shows non-significant p values by preservation with salt-turmeric and KMS. It indicates that there are some significant differences present between the preservation without preservative and KMS preservation as well as between the salt and turmeric preservation and KMS preservation. Thus the effects of both the preservatives are prominent to restore iron content in lobster.

Pomfret shows significant p values for open pan dry roasting in 15 days preservation without preservative and KMS preservation. In the case of boiling in 48 hours shows non-significant p value by preservation with salt and turmeric and KMS. It indicates that there are some significant differences present between the preservation without preservative and KMS preservation as well as between the salt and turmeric preservation and KMS preservation. Thus the effects of both the preservatives are prominent to restore iron content in pomfret.

Hilsa shows non-significant p values for boiling in 48 hours, and shallow frying in 14 days preservation without preservative and KMS preservation. In the case of boiling in 48 hours shows non-significant p value by preservation between the combination of salt-turmeric and KMS preservation. It indicates that there are some significant differences present between the preservation without preservative and KMS preservation as well as between the salt and turmeric preservation and KMS preservation. Here salt and turmeric is more effective as compared to KMS preservation to restore iron content in *hilsa.*

Overall analysis reveals that the salt and turmeric preservation is effective to restore iron content as compared to the preservation of samples without preservative, whereas it is also effective than KMS preservation for *hilsa.* KMS preservation is more effective than salt and turmeric for prawn. Both the preservatives are similarly effective for *rohu*, *katla*, lobster and pomfret preservation to restore iron content.

Table no 5.11.8 Energy content (WOP= without preservative, ST= Salt & Turmeric, KMS= Potassium metabisulphite)

		WOP vs. ST				WOP vs. KMS				ST vs. KMS			
		24Hr	48Hr	14D	15D	24Hr	48Hr	14D	15D	24Hr	48Hr	14D	15D
Rohu	R	0.000	0.195	0.000	0.000	0.003	0.000	0.000	0.001	0.003	0.000	0.001	0.000
	B	0.002	0.000	0.013	0.001	0.000	0.002	0.002	0.027	0.014	0.000	0.000	0.001
	OPDR	0.000	0.001	0.001	0.000	0.009	0.001	0.010	0.001	0.000	0.000	0.000	0.008
	SF	0.000	0.000	0.000	0.003	0.002	0.002	0.044	0.005	0.000	0.001	0.000	0.001
	DF	0.001	0.000	0.001	0.004	0.001	0.020	0.007	0.003	0.000	0.001	0.219(NS)	0.020
Katla	R	0.000	0.000	0.009	0.001	0.386(NS)	0.000	0.005	0.001	0.000	0.003	0.060(NS)	0.001
	B	0.003	0.002	0.110	0.003	0.000	0.005	0.001	0.001	0.000	0.001	0.002	0.000
	OPDR	0.000	0.001	0.003	0.004	0.000	0.107(NS)	0.003	0.001	0.001	0.002	0.883(NS)	0.001
	SF	0.003	0.000	0.016	0.000	0.014	0.000	0.093(NS)	0.001	0.004	0.000	0.128(NS)	0.000
	DF	0.005	0.001	0.132	0.000	0.002	0.005	0.015	0.001	0.002	0.080(NS)	0.021	0.000
Prawn	R	0.099	0.000	0.001	0.047	0.004	0.010	0.031	0.002	0.002	0.000	0.014	0.403(NS)
	B	0.060	0.016	0.014	0.009	0.001	0.001	0.003	0.001	0.000	0.011	0.717(NS)	0.000
	OPDR	0.006	0.005	0.001	0.005	0.001	0.077(NS)	0.003	0.005	0.001	0.005	0.001	0.231(NS)
	SF	0.000	0.000	0.005	0.921	0.002	0.001	0.002	0.015	0.003	0.006	0.013	0.035
	DF	0.003	0.000	0.110	0.001	0.000	0.001	0.005	0.095(NS)	0.124(NS)	0.007	0.007	0.010
Lobster	R	0.016	0.001	0.005	0.012	0.200(NS)	0.008	0.050	0.000	0.011	0.004	0.145(NS)	0.072(NS)
	B	0.000	0.118	0.005	0.145	0.089(NS)	0.004	0.004	0.025	0.001	0.014	0.019	0.028
	OPDR	0.004	0.000	0.029	0.028	0.009	0.001	0.007	0.001	0.151(NS)	0.002	0.004	0.001
	SF	0.003	0.545	0.053	0.321	0.003	0.000	0.003	0.005	0.001	0.000	0.003	0.000
	DF	0.004	0.084	0.000	0.014	0.011	0.004	0.015	0.008	0.002	0.001	0.002	0.008
Pomfret	R	0.000	0.001	0.011	0.000	0.000	0.000	0.001	0.000	0.001	0.000	0.000	0.002
	B	0.000	0.000	0.001	0.348	0.000	0.001	0.001	0.003	0.001	0.002	0.008	0.012
	OPDR	0.000	0.000	0.001	0.050	0.000	0.002	0.007	0.002	0.001	0.007	0.023	0.016
	SF	0.000	0.496	0.000	0.001	0.000	0.000	0.001	0.002	0.000	0.001	0.008	0.019
	DF	0.000	0.000	0.004	0.091	0.000	0.000	0.000	0.002	0.003	0.008	0.004	0.002
Hilsa	R	0.001	0.000	0.002	0.001	0.001	0.001	0.004	0.014	0.005	0.000	0.003	0.000
	B	0.001	0.000	0.000	0.011	0.000	0.000	0.001	0.000	0.003	0.004	0.057(NS)	0.000
	OPDR	0.002	0.005	0.177	0.013	0.001	0.003	0.024	0.000	0.003	0.002	0.001	0.000
	SF	0.000	0.002	0.004	0.004	0.091(NS)	0.001	0.062(NS)	0.018	0.000	0.018	0.002	0.035
	DF	0.001	0.011	0.000	0.024	0.001	0.000	0.126(NS)	0.000	0.000	0.001	0.000	0.001

NS= Non-Significant values that mean there is no significant difference present among the samples, preserved with the combination of salt and turmeric, potassium metabisulphite and without preservative in respect to the raw and cooked conditions. R= Raw, B= Boiling, DR= Dry roasting, SF= Shallow frying, DF= Deep frying.

This table shows the p values of the energy content among the preserved samples with and without preservatives. Preservation without preservative and combination of the salt and turmeric preservation show that all the values are significant in case of all the samples, which means significant differences present among the samples preserved without preservative and preserved with the combination of salt and turmeric. It indicates that salt and turmeric preservation is effective to restore energy content as compared to the preservation without preservative for all the samples.

Rohu shows significant p values for all the cooking methods with respect to the preservation without preservative and KMS preservation. In the case of deep frying shows non-significant p value in 14 days preservation with salt and turmeric and KMS. It indicates that there are significant differences present between the preservation without preservative and KMS preservation, and some significant differences present between the salt and turmeric preservation and KMS preservation. Thus the effect of KMS is more prominent than salt and turmeric to restore energy content in *rohu.*

Katla shows non-significant p values for the raw state in 24 hours, open pan dry roasting in 48 hours and shallow frying in 14 days preservation without preservative and KMS preservation. In the case of deep frying in 48 hours, and open pan dry roasting and shallow frying in 14 days preservation show non-significant p values by preservation with salt and turmeric and KMS. It indicates that there are some significant differences present between the preservation without preservative and KMS preservation as well as between the salt and turmeric preservation and KMS preservation. Thus here the effects of both the preservatives are prominent to restore energy content in *katla.*

Prawn shows significant p values for open pan dry roasting in 48 hours, and deep frying in 15 days preservation without preservative and KMS preservation. In the case of deep frying in 24 hours, and boiling in 14 days, and the raw state and open pan dry roasting in 15 days show non-significant p values by the preservation with salt and turmeric and KMS. It indicates that there are some significant differences present between the preservation without preservative and KMS preservation as well as between the salt and turmeric preservation and KMS preservation. Thus the effects of both the preservatives are prominent to restore energy content in prawn.

Lobster shows significant p values for the raw state and boiling in 24 hours preservation without preservative and KMS preservation. Open pan dry roasting in 24 hours and the raw state in 14 days and 15 days show non-significant difference by preservation with salt-turmeric and KMS. It indicates that there are some significant differences present between the preservation without preservative and KMS preservation as well as salt and turmeric preservation and KMS preservation. Thus the effects of both the preservatives are prominent to restore energy content in lobster.

Pomfret shows significant p values for all cooking methods with respect to the preservation without preservative and KMS preservation as well as preservation with salt and turmeric and KMS. It indicates that there is significant difference present between the preservation without preservative and with KMS preservation as well as between the salt and turmeric preservation and KMS preservation. Thus the effects of both the preservatives are prominent to restore energy content in pomfret.

Hilsa shows non-significant p values for shallow frying in 24 hours, and shallow frying and deep frying in 14 days preservation without preservative and KMS preservation. In the case of boiling in 14 days shows non-significant p value by preservation between the combination of the salt-turmeric and KMS preservation. It indicates that there are some significant differences present between the preservation without preservative and KMS preservation as well as between the salt and turmeric preservation and KMS preservation. Here salt and turmeric is more effective than KMS preservation to restore energy content in *hilsa*.

Overall analysis reveals that the salt and turmeric preservation is effective to restore energy content as compared to the preservation of samples without preservative, whereas it is also effective than KMS preservation for *hilsa.* KMS preservation is more effective than salt and turmeric for *rohu.* Both the preservatives are similarly effective for *katla*, prawn, lobster and pomfret preservation to restore energy content.

5.12 Correlation matrix

This statistical analysis is carried out to estimate the correlation among the raw conditions and different cooking methods (boiling, open pan dry roasting, shallow frying and deep frying) with respect to the nutrient content (carbohydrate, protein, fat, moisture, ash, calcium, iron and energy) under different preservation conditions for the studied fish and edible aquatic species.

5.12.1 *Rohu* (*Labeo rohita*)

5.12.1.1 Carbohydrate

Table no 5.12.1.1.1 Correlation of cooking methods in fresh condition

Condition	RS	B	OPDR	SF	DF
Raw State(RS)	1	-.974(S)	.533	.983(S)	.330
Boiling (B)	-.974(S)	1	-.327	-.999*(S)	-.536
Open Pan Dry Roasting (OPDR)	.533	-.327	1	.366	-.623
Shallow Frying (SF)	.983(S)	-.999*(S)	.366	1	.500
Deep Frying (DF)	.330	-.536	-.623	.500	1

**. Correlation is highly significant at the 0.05 level (2-tailed)* ▢ Positive ▢ Negative *S= Significant*

This table shows the correlation of carbohydrate content of *rohu* with cooking methods. In fresh condition, there is significant negative correlation present between the raw state and boiling, and positive correlation between the raw state and shallow frying. Again boiling is negatively correlated with shallow frying. This table indicates that there is a strong correlation present among the **raw state, boiling and shallow frying** in fresh condition.

Table no 5.12.1.1.2 Correlation of cooking methods in 24 hours preservation without preservative

Condition	RS	B	OPDR	SF	DF
Raw State (RS)	1	1.000*(S)	.610	.980(S)	-.759
Boiling (B)	1.000*(S)	1	.612	.979(S)	-.757
Open Pan Dry Roasting (OPDR)	.610	.612	1	.439	.053
Shallow Frying (SF)	.980(S)	.979(S)	.439	1	-.874(S)
Deep Frying (DF)	-.759	-.757	.053	-.874(S)	1

**. Correlation is highly significant at the 0.05 level (2-tailed)* ▢ Positive ▢ Negative *S= Significant*

This table shows the correlation of carbohydrate content of *rohu* with cooking methods. In 24 hours control preservation condition, there is significant negative correlation present between the raw state and boiling, and positive correlation between the raw state and shallow frying. Again boiling is positively correlated with shallow frying. Moreover, shallow frying is negatively correlated with deep frying. This table indicates that there is a strong correlation present among the **raw state, boiling, shallow frying and deep frying** in 24 hours control preservation without preservative.

Table no 5.12.1.1.3 Correlation of cooking methods in 48 hours preservation without preservative

Condition	RS	B	OPDR	SF	DF
Raw State(RS)	1	.724	.042	.487	.130
Boiling (B)	.724	1	.719	.955(S)	.778
Open Pan Dry Roasting (OPDR)	.042	.719	1	.893(S)	.996(S)
Shallow Frying (SF)	.487	.955(S)	.893(S)	1	.929(S)
Deep Frying (DF)	.130	.778	.996(S)	.929(S)	1

**. Correlation is highly significant at the 0.05 level (2-tailed)* ▢ Positive *S= Significant*

This table shows the correlation of carbohydrate content of *rohu* with cooking methods. In 48 hours control preservation condition, there is significant positive correlation present between boiling and shallow frying, and also positive correlation between open pan dry roasting with shallow frying and deep frying. Again shallow frying is positively correlated with deep frying. This table indicates that there is a strong correlation present among **boiling, open pan dry roasting, shallow frying and deep frying** in 48 hours control preservation without preservative.

Table no 5.12.1.1.4 Correlation of cooking methods in 14 days preservation without preservative

Condition	RS	B	OPDR	SF	DF
Raw State (RS)	1	.950(S)	-.914(S)	.117	.834(S)
Boiling (B)	.950(S)	1	-.995(S)	-.198	.621
Open Pan Dry Roasting (OPDR)	-.914(S)	-.995(S)	1	.295	-.539
Shallow Frying (SF)	.117	-.198	.295	1	.646
Deep Frying (DF)	.834(S)	.621	-.539	.646	1

**. Correlation is highly significant at the 0.05 level (2-tailed)* ▢ Positive ▢ Negative *S= Significant*

This table shows the correlation of carbohydrate content of *rohu* with cooking methods. In 14 days control preservation, there is significant positive correlation present between the raw state with boiling and deep frying, and also negative correlation present between the raw state with open pan dry roasting. Again open pan dry roasting is negatively correlated with boiling. This table indicates that there is a strong correlation present among the **raw state, boiling, open pan dry roasting and deep frying** in 14 days control preservation without preservative.

Table no 5.12.1.1.5 Correlation of cooking methods in 15 days preservation without preservative

Condition	RS	B	OPDR	SF	DF
Raw State (RS)	1	.948(S)	-.808(S)	-.914(S)	-.967(S)
Boiling (B)	.948(S)	1	-.953(S)	-.738	-.998*(S)
Open Pan Dry Roasting (OPDR)	-.808(S)	-.953(S)	1	.500	.931(S)
Shallow Frying (SF)	-.914(S)	-.738	.500	1	.781
Deep Frying (DF)	-.967(S)	-.998*(S)	.931(S)	.781	1

**. Correlation is highly significant at the 0.05 level (2-tailed)* ▢ Positive ▢ Negative *S= Significant*

This table shows the correlation of carbohydrate content of *rohu* with cooking methods. In 15 days control preservation condition, there is significant positive correlation present between the raw state and boiling, and also negative correlation present with open pan dry roasting, shallow frying and deep frying. Again boiling is negatively correlated with open pan dry roasting and deep frying, whereas open pan dry roasting is positively correlated with deep frying. This table indicates that there is a strong correlation present among the **raw state, boiling, open pan dry roasting, shallow frying and deep frying** in 15 days control preservation without preservative.

Table no 5.12.1.1.6 Correlation of cooking methods in 24 hours preservation with salt and turmeric

Condition	RS	B	OPDR	SF	DF
Raw State (RS)	1	-.771	.962(S)	.905(S)	.969(S)
Boiling (B)	-.771	1	-.569	-.427	-.904(S)
Open Pan Dry Roasting (OPDR)	.962(S)	-.569	1	.986(S)	.866(S)
Shallow Frying (SF)	.905(S)	-.427	.986(S)	1	.772
Deep Frying (DF)	.969(S)	-.904(S)	.866(S)	.772	1

**. Correlation is highly significant at the 0.05 level (2-tailed)* ▢ Positive ▢ Negative *S= Significant*

This table shows the correlation of carbohydrate content of *rohu* with cooking methods. In 24 hours salt and turmeric preservation, there is significant positive correlation present between the raw state with open pan dry roasting, shallow frying and deep frying. Again boiling is negatively correlated with deep frying, whereas open pan dry roasting is positively correlated with shallow frying and deep frying. This data indicates that there is a strong correlation present among the **raw state, boiling, open pan dry roasting, shallow frying and deep frying** in 24 hours salt and turmeric preservation.

Table no 5.12.1.1.7 Correlation of cooking methods in 48 hours preservation with salt and turmeric

Condition	RS	B	OPDR	SF	DF
Raw State (RS)	1	-.756	-.029	-.954(S)	.133
Boiling (B)	-.756	1	.676	.524	.548
Open Pan Dry Roasting (OPDR)	-.029	.676	1	-.273	.987(S)
Shallow Frying (SF)	-.954(S)	.524	-.273	1	-.425
Deep Frying (DF)	.133	.548	.987(S)	-.425	1

**. Correlation is highly significant at the 0.05 level (2-tailed)* ▢ Positive ▢ Negative *S= Significant*

This table shows the correlation of carbohydrate content of *rohu* with cooking methods. In 48 hours salt and turmeric preservation, there is significant negative correlation present between the raw state and shallow frying. Again open pan dry roasting is positively correlated with deep frying. This table indicates that there is a strong correlation present among the **raw state, open pan dry roasting, shallow frying and deep frying** in 48 hours salt and turmeric preservation.

Table no 5.12.1.1.8 Correlation of cooking methods in 14 days preservation with salt and turmeric

Condition	RS	B	OPDR	SF	DF
Raw State (RS)	1	.975(S)	-.797	-.233	-.749
Boiling (B)	.975(S)	1	-.645	-.013	-.877(S)
Open Pan Dry Roasting (OPDR)	-.797	-.645	1	.772	.198
Shallow Frying (SF)	-.233	-.013	.772	1	-.470
Deep Frying (DF)	-.749	-.877(S)	.198	-.470	1

**. Correlation is highly significant at the 0.05 level (2-tailed)* ▢ Positive ▢ Negative *S= Significant*

This table shows the correlation of carbohydrate content of *rohu* with cooking methods. In 14 days salt and turmeric preservation, there is significant positive correlation present between the raw state and boiling. Again boiling is negatively correlated with deep frying. This table indicates that there is a strong correlation present among the **raw state, boiling and deep frying** in 14 days salt and turmeric preservation.

Table no 5.12.1.1.9 Correlation of cooking methods in 15 days preservation with salt and turmeric

Condition	RS	B	OPDR	SF	DF
Raw State (RS)	1	.135	-.997*(S)	.916(S)	.187
Boiling (B)	.135	1	-.212	-.273	.999*(S)
Open Pan Dry Roasting (OPDR)	-.997*(S)	-.212	1	-.882(S)	-.263
Shallow Frying (SF)	.916(S)	-.273	-.882(S)	1	-.222
Deep Frying (DF)	.187	.999*(S)	-.263	-.222	1

**. Correlation is highly significant at the 0.05 level (2-tailed)* ▢ Positive ▢ Negative *S= Significant*

This table shows the correlation of carbohydrate content of *rohu* with cooking methods. In 15 days salt and turmeric preservation, there is significant negative correlation present between the raw state and open pan dry roasting and positive correlation present with shallow frying. Again boiling is positively correlated with deep frying. Open pan dry roasting is positively correlated with shallow frying. This table indicates that there is a strong correlation present among the **raw state, boiling, open pan dry roasting, shallow frying and deep frying** in 15 days salt and turmeric preservation.

Table no 5.12.1.1.10 Correlation of cooking methods in 24 hours preservation with KMS

Condition	RS	B	OPDR	SF	DF
Raw State (RS)	1	.652	-.957(S)	-.992(S)	.980(S)
Boiling (B)	.652	1	-.844(S)	-.743	.790
Open Pan Dry Roasting (OPDR)	-.957(S)	-.844(S)	1	.986(S)	-.996(S)
Shallow Frying (SF)	-.992(S)	-.743	.986(S)	1	-.997*(S)
Deep Frying (DF)	.980(S)	.790	-.996(S)	-.997*(S)	1

**. Correlation is highly significant at the 0.05 level (2-tailed)* ▢ Positive ▢ Negative *S= Significant*

This table shows the correlation of carbohydrate content of *rohu* with cooking methods. In 24 hours KMS preservation, there is significant positive correlation present between the raw state and deep frying, and also negative correlation present with open pan dry roasting and shallow frying. Again boiling is negatively correlated with open pan dry roasting, whereas open pan dry roasting is positively correlated with both shallow frying and deep frying. Moreover, shallow frying is negatively correlated with deep frying. This table indicates that there is a strong correlation present among the **raw state, boiling, open pan dry roasting, shallow frying and deep frying** in 24 hours KMS preservation.

Table no 5.12.1.1.11 Correlation of cooking methods in 48 hours preservation with KMS

Condition	RS	B	OPDR	SF	DF
Raw State (RS)	1	.999*(S)	.996(S)	.747	.577
Boiling (B)	.999*(S)	1	.990(S)	.781	.619
Open Pan Dry Roasting (OPDR)	.996(S)	.990(S)	1	.683	.500
Shallow Frying (SF)	.747	.781	.683	1	.974(S)
Deep Frying (DF)	.577	.619	.500	.974(S)	1

**. Correlation is highly significant at the 0.05 level (2-tailed)* ▭ Positive *S= Significant*

This table shows the correlation of carbohydrate content of *rohu* with cooking methods. In 48 hours KMS preservation, there is significant positive correlation present between the raw state with boiling and open pan dry roasting. Again boiling is positively correlated with open pan dry roasting. Moreover, shallow frying is positively correlated with deep frying. This table indicates that there is a strong correlation present among the **raw state, boiling, open pan dry roasting, shallow frying and deep frying** in 48 hours KMS preservation.

Table no 5.12.1.1.12 Correlation of cooking methods in 14 days preservation with KMS

Condition	RS	B	OPDR	SF	DF
Raw State (RS)	1	.445	-.996(S)	.998*(S)	-.987(S)
Boiling (B)	.445	1	-.363	.391	-.294
Open Pan Dry Roasting (OPDR)	-.996(S)	-.363	1	-1.000*(S)	.997*(S)
Shallow Frying (SF)	.998*(S)	.391	-1.000*(S)	1	-.995(S)
Deep Frying (DF)	-.987(S)	-.294	.997*(S)	-.995(S)	1

**. Correlation is highly significant at the 0.05 level (2-tailed)* Positive Negative *S= Significant*

This table shows the correlation of carbohydrate content of *rohu* with cooking methods. In 14 days KMS preservation, there is significant positive correlation present between the raw state and shallow frying, and also negative correlation present with open pan dry roasting and deep frying. Again open pan dry roasting is negatively correlated with shallow frying and positively correlated with deep frying, whereas shallow frying is negatively correlated with deep frying. This table indicates that there is a strong correlation present among the **raw state, open pan dry roasting, shallow frying and deep frying** in 14 days KMS preservation.

Table no 5.12.1.1.13 Correlation of cooking methods in 15 days preservation with KMS

Condition	RS	B	OPDR	SF	DF
Raw State (RS)	1	-.462	-.715	.993(S)	-.355
Boiling (B)	-.462	1	-.291	-.563	-.665
Open Pan Dry Roasting (OPDR)	-.715	-.291	1	-.627	.908(S)
Shallow Frying (SF)	.993(S)	-.563	-.627	1	-.243
Deep Frying (DF)	-.355	-.665	.908(S)	-.243	1

**. Correlation is highly significant at the 0.05 level (2-tailed)* Positive *S= Significant*

This table shows the correlation of carbohydrate content of *rohu* with cooking methods. In 15 days KMS preservation, there is significant positive correlation present between the raw state and shallow frying. Again open pan dry roasting is positively correlated with deep frying. This table indicates that there is a strong correlation present among the **raw state, open pan dry roasting, shallow frying and deep frying** in 15 days KMS preservation.

Overall analysis reveals that the raw state is highly significant positively correlated with boiling in 24 hours preservation without preservative, whereas significant negatively correlated with open pan dry roasting in 15 days preservation with salt and turmeric, significant positively correlated with shallow frying in 14 days KMS preservation, and negatively correlated with deep frying in 14 days KMS preservation. Boiling is significant negatively correlated with open pan dry roasting in 14 days control preservation without preservative, whereas highly significant negatively correlated with shallow frying in fresh condition, and highly significant positively correlated with deep frying in 15 days salt and turmeric preservation. Open pan dry roasting is highly significant negatively correlated with shallow frying and highly significant positively correlated with deep frying in 14 days KMS preservation.

Shallow frying is highly significant negatively correlated with deep frying in 24 hours KMS preservation. Most of the correlation of the carbohydrate content of *rohu* is found in **14 days KMS preservation** with respect to different cooking conditions.

5.12.1.2 Protein

Table no 5.12.1.2.1 Correlation of cooking methods in fresh condition

Condition	RS	B	OPDR	SF	DF
Raw State (R)	1	.376	.638	.322	-.179
Boiling (B)	.376	1	.953(S)	.998*(S)	.844(S)
Open Pan Dry Roasting (OPDR)	.638	.953(S)	1	.934(S)	.643
Shallow Frying (SF)	.322	.998*(S)	.934(S)	1	.874(S)
Deep Frying (DF)	-.179	.844(S)	.643	.874(S)	1

**. Correlation is highly significant at the 0.05 level (2-tailed)* Positive *S= Significant*

This table shows the correlation of protein content of *rohu* with cooking methods. In fresh condition, there is significant positive correlation present between boiling with open pan dry roasting, shallow frying and deep frying. Again open pan dry roasting is positively correlated with shallow frying, whereas shallow frying is also positively correlated with deep frying. This table indicates that there is a strong correlation present among **boiling, open pan dry roasting, shallow frying and deep frying** in fresh condition.

Table no 5.12.1.2.2 Correlation of cooking methods in 24 hours preservation without preservative

Condition	RS	B	OPDR	SF	DF
Raw State (RS)	1	.003	-.334	.542	-.990(S)
Boiling (B)	.003	1	.942(S)	.842(S)	-.143
Open Pan Dry Roasting (OPDR)	-.334	.942(S)	1	.611	.199
Shallow Frying (SF)	.542	.842(S)	.611	1	-.655
Deep Frying (DF)	-.990(S)	-.143	.199	-.655	1

Positive Negative *S= Significant*

This table shows the correlation of protein content of *rohu* with cooking methods. In 24 hours control preservation without preservative, there is significant negative correlation present between the raw state and deep frying. Again boiling is positively correlated with open pan dry roasting and shallow frying. This table indicates that there is a strong correlation present among the **raw state**, **boiling, open pan dry roasting, shallow frying and deep frying** in 24 hours preservation.

Table no 5.12.1.2.3 Correlation of cooking methods in 48 hours preservation without preservative

Condition	RS	B	OPDR	SF	DF
Raw State (RS)	1	-.391	-.193	-.965(S)	.710
Boiling (B)	-.391	1	.979(S)	.619	.371
Open Pan Dry Roasting (OPDR)	-.193	.979(S)	1	.444	.554
Shallow Frying (SF)	-.965(S)	.619	.444	1	-.500
Deep Frying (DF)	.710	.371	.554	-.500	1

Positive Negative *S= Significant*

This table shows the correlation of protein content of *rohu* with cooking methods. In 48 hours control preservation without preservative, there is significant negative correlation present between the raw state and shallow frying. Again boiling is positively correlated with open pan dry roasting. This table indicates that there is a strong correlation present among the **raw state**, **boiling**, **open pan dry roasting and shallow frying** in 48 hours control preservation.

Table no 5.12.1.2.4 Correlation of cooking methods in 14 days preservation without preservative

Condition	RS	B	OPDR	SF	DF
Raw State (RS)	1	.989(S)	.026	.620	.752
Boiling (B)	.989(S)	1	.171	.500	.840(S)
Open Pan Dry Roasting (OPDR)	.026	.171	1	-.768	.678
Shallow Frying (SF)	.620	.500	-.768	1	-.050
Deep Frying (DF)	.752	.840(S)	.678	-.050	1

Positive *S= Significant*

This table shows the correlation of protein content of *rohu* with cooking methods. In 14 days control preservation without preservative, there is significantly positive correlation present between the raw state and boiling. Again boiling is positively correlated with deep frying. This table indicates that there is a strong correlation present among the **raw state**, **boiling and deep frying** in 14 days control preservation.

Table no 5.12.1.2.5 Correlation of cooking methods in 15 days preservation without preservative

Condition	RS	B	OPDR	SF	DF
Raw State (RS)	1	-.493	.763	.500	.758
Boiling (B)	-.493	1	-.938(S)	.507	.194
Open Pan Dry Roasting (OPDR)	.763	-.938(S)	1	-.178	.157
Shallow Frying (SF)	.500	.507	-.178	1	.944(S)
Deep Frying (DF)	.758	.194	.157	.944(S)	1

Positive Negative *S= Significant*

This table shows the correlation of protein content of *rohu* with cooking methods. In 15 days control preservation without preservative, there is significant negative correlation present between boiling and open pan dry roasting. Again shallow frying is positively correlated with deep frying. This table indicates that there is a strong correlation present among **boiling, open pan dry roasting, shallow frying and deep frying** in 15 days control preservation.

Table no 5.12.1.2.6 Correlation of cooking methods in 24 hours preservation with salt and turmeric

Condition	RS	B	OPDR	SF	DF
Raw State (RS)	1	.110	.524	.121	.080
Boiling (B)	.110	1	-.789	1.000**(S)	-.982(S)
Open Pan Dry Roasting (OPDR)	.524	-.789	1	-.782	.891(S)
Shallow Frying (SF)	.121	1.000**(S)	-.782	1	-.980(S)
Deep Frying (DF)	.080	-.982(S)	.891(S)	-.980(S)	1

***. Correlation is highly significant at the 0.01 level (2-tailed)* Positive Negative *S= Significant*

This table shows the correlation of protein content of *rohu* with cooking methods. In 24 hours salt and turmeric preservation, there is significant positive correlation present between boiling and shallow frying, and also negative correlation present with deep frying. Again open pan dry roasting is positively correlated with deep frying, whereas shallow frying is negatively correlated with deep frying. This table indicates that there is a strong correlation present among **boiling, open pan dry roasting, shallow frying and deep frying** in 24 hours salt and turmeric preservation.

Table no 5.12.1.2.7 Correlation of cooking methods in 48 hours preservation with salt and turmeric

Condition	RS	B	OPDR	SF	DF
Raw State (RS)	1	.038	-.366	1.000**(S)	.993(S)
Boiling (B)	.038	1	.916(S)	.038	.157
Open Pan Dry Roasting (OPDR)	-.366	.916(S)	1	-.366	-.253
Shallow Frying (SF)	1.000**(S)	.038	-.366	1	.993(S)
Deep Frying (DF)	.993(S)	.157	-.253	.993(S)	1

***. Correlation is highly significant at the 0.01 level (2-tailed)* ▭ Positive *S= Significant*

This table shows the correlation of protein content of *rohu* with cooking methods. In 48 hours salt and turmeric preservation, there is significant positive correlation present between the raw state with shallow frying and deep frying. Again open pan dry roasting is positively correlated with boiling, whereas shallow frying is positively correlated with deep frying. This table indicates that there is a strong correlation present among the **raw state**, **boiling, open pan dry roasting, shallow frying and deep frying** in 48 hours salt and turmeric preservation.

Table no 5.12.1.2.8 Correlation of cooking methods in 14 days preservation with salt and turmeric

Condition	RS	B	OPDR	SF	DF
Raw State (RS)	1	.099	.419	-.775	-.923(S)
Boiling (B)	.099	1	.945(S)	.552	-.475
Open Pan Dry Roasting (OPDR)	.419	.945(S)	1	.249	-.737
Shallow Frying (SF)	-.775	.552	.249	1	.471
Deep Frying (DF)	-.923(S)	-.475	-.737	.471	1

▭ Positive ▭ Negative *S= Significant*

This table shows the correlation of protein content of *rohu* with cooking methods. In 14 days salt and turmeric preservation, there is significant negative correlation present between the raw state and deep frying. Again boiling is positively correlated with open pan dry roasting. This table indicates that there is a strong correlation present among the **raw state**, **boiling, open pan dry roasting and deep frying** in 14 days salt and turmeric preservation.

Table no 5.12.1.2.9 Correlation of cooking methods in 15 days preservation with salt and turmeric

Condition	RS	B	OPDR	SF	DF
Raw State (RS)	1	.977(S)	.099	.000	-.812(S)
Boiling (B)	.977(S)	1	.311	-.215	-.668
Open Pan Dry Roasting (OPDR)	.099	.311	1	-.995(S)	.500
Shallow Frying (SF)	.000	-.215	-.995(S)	1	-.583
Deep Frying (DF)	-.812(S)	-.668	.500	-.583	1

▭ Positive ▭ Negative *S= Significant*

This table shows the correlation of protein content of *rohu* with cooking methods. In 15 days salt and turmeric preservation, there is significant negative correlation present between the raw state and deep frying and also positive correlation present with boiling. Again open pan dry roasting is negatively correlated with shallow frying. This table indicates that there is a strong correlation present among the **raw state**, **boiling, open pan dry roasting, shallow frying and deep frying** in 15 days salt and turmeric preservation.

Table no 5.12.1.2.10 Correlation of cooking methods in 24 hours preservation with KMS

Condition	RS	B	OPDR	SF	DF
Raw State (RS)	1	-.990(S)	.696	-.989(S)	-.884(S)
Boiling (B)	-.990(S)	1	-.585	.958(S)	.942(S)
Open Pan Dry Roasting (OPDR)	.696	-.585	1	-.794	-.279
Shallow Frying (SF)	-.989(S)	.958(S)	-.794	1	.806(S)
Deep Frying (DF)	-.884(S)	.942(S)	-.279	.806(S)	1

Positive Negative *S= Significant*

This table shows the correlation of protein content of *rohu* with cooking methods. In 24 hours KMS preservation, there is significant negative correlation present between the raw state with boiling, shallow frying and deep frying. Again boiling is positively correlated with both shallow frying and deep frying. Shallow frying is positively correlated with deep frying. This table indicates that there is a strong correlation present among the **raw state**, **boiling, shallow frying and deep frying** in 24 hours KMS preservation.

Table no 5.12.1.2.11 Correlation of cooking methods in 48 hours preservation with KMS

Condition	RS	B	OPDR	SF	DF
Raw State (RS)	1	.959(S)	.755	.998*(S)	.990(S)
Boiling (B)	.959(S)	1	.910(S)	.975(S)	.990(S)
Open Pan Dry Roasting (OPDR)	.755	.910(S)	1	.794	.841(S)
Shallow Frying (SF)	.998* (S)	.975(S)	.794	1	.997(S)
Deep Frying (DF)	.990(S)	.990(S)	.841(S)	.997(S)	1

**. Correlation is highly significant at the 0.05 level (2-tailed)* Positive *S= Significant*

This table shows the correlation of protein content of *rohu* with cooking methods. In 48 hours KMS preservation, there is significant positive correlation present between the raw state with shallow frying and deep frying. Again boiling is positively correlated with open pan dry roasting, shallow frying and deep frying, whereas open pan dry roasting is positively correlated with deep frying. Shallow frying is positively correlated with deep frying. This table indicates that there is a strong correlation present among the **raw state**, **boiling, open pan dry roasting, shallow frying and deep frying** in 48 hours KMS preservation.

Table no 5.12.1.2.12 Correlation of cooking methods in 14 days preservation with KMS

Condition	RS	B	OPDR	SF	DF
Raw State (RS)	1	.099	.419	-.775	-.923(S)
Boiling (B)	.099	1	.945(S)	.552	-.475
Open Pan Dry Roasting (OPDR)	.419	.945(S)	1	.249	-.737
Shallow Frying (SF)	-.775	.552	.249	1	.471
Deep Frying (DF)	-.923(S)	-.475	-.737	.471	1

Positive Negative *S= Significant*

This table shows the correlation of protein content of *rohu* with cooking methods. In 14 days KMS preservation, there is significant negative correlation present between the raw state and deep frying. Again boiling is positively correlated with open pan dry roasting. This table indicates that there is a strong correlation present among the **raw state**, **boiling, open pan dry roasting and deep frying** in 14 days KMS preservation.

Table no 5.12.1.2.13 Correlation of cooking methods in 15 days preservation with KMS

Condition	RS	B	OPDR	SF	DF
Raw State (RS)	1	.977(S)	.099	.000	-.812(S)
Boiling (B)	.977(S)	1	.311	-.215	-.668
Open Pan Dry Roasting (OPDR)	.099	.311	1	-.995(S)	.500
Shallow Frying (SF)	.000	-.215	-.995(S)	1	-.583
Deep Frying (DF)	-.812(S)	-.668	.500	-.583	1

Positive Negative *S= Significant*

This table shows the correlation of protein content of *rohu* with cooking methods. In 15 days KMS preservation, there is significant positive correlation present between the raw state and boiling, and also negative correlation with deep frying. Again open pan dry roasting is positively correlated with shallow frying. This table indicates that there is a strong correlation present among the **raw state**, **boiling, open pan dry roasting, shallow frying and deep frying** in 15 days KMS preservation.

Overall analysis reveals that the raw state is significant negatively correlated with boiling in 24 hours KMS preservation, whereas significant positively correlated with open pan dry roasting in 48 hours preservation with KMS, and positively correlated with shallow frying and deep frying in 48 hours salt and turmeric preservation. Boiling is significant positively correlated with open pan dry roasting in 48 hours control preservation without preservative, whereas highly significant positively correlated with shallow frying in 24 hours salt and turmeric preservation, and significant positively correlated with deep frying in 48 hours KMS preservation. Open pan dry roasting is significant negatively correlated with shallow frying in 15 days salt and turmeric preservation and 15 days KMS preservation, and positively correlated with deep frying in 24 hours salt and turmeric preservation. Shallow frying is positively correlated with deep frying in 48 hours KMS preservation. Most of the correlation of the protein content of *rohu* is found in **24 hours, 48 hours salt and turmeric preservation and 48 hours KMS preservation** with respect to different cooking conditions.

5.12.1.3 Fat

Table no 5.12.1.3.1 Correlation of cooking methods in fresh condition

Condition	RS	B	OPDR	SF	DF
Raw State (RS)	1	-.427	.541	-.807(S)	.221
Boiling (B)	-.427	1	.529	-.189	-.976(S)
Open Pan Dry Roasting (OPDR)	.541	.529	1	-.933(S)	-.700
Shallow Frying (SF)	-.807(S)	-.189	-.933(S)	1	.397
Deep Frying (DF)	.221	-.976(S)	-.700	.397	1

Negative *S= Significant*

This table shows the correlation of fat content of *rohu* with cooking methods. In fresh condition, there is significant negative correlation present between the raw state and shallow frying. Again boiling is negatively correlated with deep frying, whereas shallow frying is negatively correlated with open pan dry roasting. This table indicates that there is a strong correlation present among the **raw state**, **boiling, open pan dry roasting, shallow and deep frying** in fresh condition.

Table no 5.12.1.3.2 Correlation of cooking methods in 24 hours preservation without preservative

Condition	RS	B	OPDR	SF	DF
Raw State (RS)	1	-.974(S)	-.400	-.988(S)	.634
Boiling (B)	-.974(S)	1	.596	.927(S)	-.444
Open Pan Dry Roasting (OPDR)	-.400	.596	1	.252	.455
Shallow Frying (SF)	-.988(S)	.927(S)	.252	1	-.747
Deep Frying (DF)	.634	-.444	.455	-.747	1

Positive Negative *S= Significant*

This table shows the correlation of fat content of *rohu* with cooking methods. In 24 hours control preservation without preservative, there is significant negative correlation present between the raw state with boiling and shallow frying. Again boiling is positively correlated with shallow frying. This table indicates that there is a strong correlation present among the **raw state**, **boiling, shallow frying and deep frying** in 24 hours control preservation.

Table no 5.12.1.3.3 Correlation of cooking methods in 48 hours preservation without preservative

Condition	RS	B	OPDR	SF	DF
Raw State (RS)	1	-.993(S)	.997(S)	-.993(S)	-.990(S)
Boiling (B)	-.993(S)	1	-.999*(S)	1.000**(S)	.967(S)
Open Pan Dry Roasting (OPDR)	.997(S)	-.999*(S)	1	-.999*(S)	-.975(S)
Shallow Frying (SF)	-.993(S)	1.000**(S)	-.999*(S)	1	.967(S)
Deep Frying (DF)	-.990(S)	.967(S)	-.975(S)	.967(S)	1

**. Correlation is highly significant at the 0.05 level (2-tailed)* Positive Negative *S= Significant*

***.Correlation is highly significant at the 0.01 level (2-tailed)*

This table shows the correlation of fat content of *rohu* with cooking methods. In 48 hours control preservation without preservative, there is significant negative correlation present between the raw state with boiling, shallow frying and deep frying, and also positive correlation present with boiling. Again boiling is positively correlated with shallow frying and deep frying, and negative correlation present with open pan dry roasting, whereas open pan dry roasting is negatively correlated with shallow frying and deep frying. Shallow frying is positively correlated with deep frying. This table indicates that there is a strong correlation present among the **raw state**, **boiling, open pan dry roasting, shallow frying and deep frying** in 48 hours control preservation.

Table no 5.12.1.3.4 Correlation of cooking methods in 14 days preservation without preservative

Condition	RS	B	OPDR	SF	DF
Raw State (RS)	1	-.982(S)	-.500	-.976(S)	-.189
Boiling (B)	-.982(S)	1	.655	.918(S)	.000
Open Pan Dry Roasting (OPDR)	-.500	.655	1	.300	-.756
Shallow Frying (SF)	-.976(S)	.918(S)	.300	1	.397
Deep Frying (DF)	-.189	.000	-.756	.397	1

Positive Negative *S= Significant*

This table shows the correlation of fat content of *rohu* with cooking methods. In 14 days control preservation without preservative, there is significant negative correlation present between the raw state with boiling and shallow frying. Again boiling is positively correlated with shallow frying. This table indicates that there is a strong correlation present among the **raw state**, **boiling, and shallow frying** in 14 days control preservation.

Table no 5.12.1.3.5 Correlation of cooking methods in 15 days preservation without preservative

Condition	RS	B	OPDR	SF	DF
Raw State (RS)	1	.619	.052	-.500	-.749
Boiling (B)	.619	1	.817(S)	.371	.058
Open Pan Dry Roasting (OPDR)	.052	.817(S)	1	.839(S)	.623
Shallow Frying (SF)	-.500	.371	.839(S)	1	.948(S)
Deep Frying (DF)	-.749	.058	.623	.948(S)	1

Positive *S= Significant*

This table shows the correlation of fat content of *rohu* with cooking methods. In 15 days control preservation without preservative, there is significant positive correlation present between boiling and open pan dry roasting. Again open pan dry roasting is positively correlated with shallow frying, whereas shallow frying is correlated with deep frying. This table indicates that there is a strong correlation present among **boiling, open pan dry roasting, shallow frying and deep frying** in 15 days control preservation.

Table no 5.12.1.3.6 Correlation of cooking methods in 24 hours preservation with salt and turmeric

Condition	RS	B	OPDR	SF	DF
Raw State (RS)	1	.986(S)	-.434	.652	-.338
Boiling (B)	.986(S)	1	-.577	.518	-.178
Open Pan Dry Roasting (OPDR)	-.434	-.577	1	.401	-.702
Shallow Frying (SF)	.652	.518	.401	1	-.934(S)
Deep Frying (DF)	-.338	-.178	-.702	-.934(S)	1

Positive Negative *S= Significant*

This table shows the correlation of fat content of *rohu* with cooking methods. In 24 hours salt and turmeric preservation, there is significant positive correlation present between the raw state and boiling. Again shallow frying is positively correlated with deep frying. This table indicates that there is a strong correlation present among the **raw state, boiling, shallow frying and deep frying** in 24 hours salt and turmeric preservation.

Table no 5.12.1.3.7 Correlation of cooking methods in 48 hours preservation with salt and turmeric

Condition	RS	B	OPDR	SF	DF
Raw State (RS)	1	-.545	.091	-.307	.750
Boiling (B)	-.545	1	.786	.965(S)	-.963(S)
Open Pan Dry Roasting (OPDR)	.091	.786	1	.920(S)	-.590
Shallow Frying (SF)	-.307	.965(S)	.920(S)	1	-.859(S)
Deep Frying (DF)	.750	-.963(S)	-.590	-.859(S)	1

Positive Negative *S= Significant*

This table shows the correlation of fat content of *rohu* with cooking methods. In 48 hours salt and turmeric preservation, there is significant positive correlation present between boiling and shallow frying and negative correlation with deep frying. Again shallow frying is positively correlated with open pan dry roasting and negative with deep frying. This table indicates that there is a strong correlation present among **boiling, shallow frying and deep frying** in 48 hours salt and turmeric preservation.

Table no 5.12.1.3.8 Correlation of cooking methods in 14 days preservation with salt and turmeric

Condition	RS	B	OPDR	SF	DF
Raw State (RS)	1	-.974(S)	-.236	-.636	1.000**(S)
Boiling (B)	-.974(S)	1	.008	.795	-.974(S)
Open Pan Dry Roasting (OPDR)	-.236	.008	1	-.600	-.236
Shallow Frying (SF)	-.636	.795	-.600	1	-.636
Deep Frying (DF)	1.000**(S)	-.974(S)	-.236	-.636	1

***.Correlation is highly significant at the 0.01 level (2-tailed)* Positive Negative *S= Significant*

This table shows the correlation of fat content of *rohu* with cooking methods. In 14 days salt and turmeric preservation, there is significant positive correlation present between the raw state and deep frying and negative correlation present with boiling. Again boiling is negatively correlated with deep frying. This table indicates that there is a strong correlation present among the **raw state**, **boiling and deep frying** in 14 days salt and turmeric preservation.

Table no 5.12.1.3.9 Correlation of cooking methods in 15 days preservation with salt and turmeric

Condition	RS	B	OPDR	SF	DF
Raw State (RS)	1	-.974(S)	-.596	1.000**(S)	-.434
Boiling (B)	-.974(S)	1	.397	-.974(S)	.217
Open Pan Dry Roasting (OPDR)	-.596	.397	1	-.596	.982(S)
Shallow Frying (SF)	1.000**(S)	-.974(S)	-.596	1	-.434
Deep Frying (DF)	-.434	.217	.982(S)	-.434	1

***.Correlation is highly significant at the 0.01 level (2-tailed)* Positive Negative *S= Significant*

This table shows the correlation of fat content of *rohu* with cooking methods. In 15 days salt and turmeric preservation, there is significantly positive correlation present between the raw state and shallow frying and negative correlation present with boiling. Again boiling is negatively correlated with shallow frying. Open pan dry roasting is positively correlated with deep frying. This table indicates that there is a strong correlation present among the **raw state**, **boiling, open pan dry roasting, shallow and deep frying** in 15 days salt and turmeric preservation.

Table no 5.12.1.3.10 Correlation of cooking methods in 24 hours preservation with KMS

Condition	RS	B	OPDR	SF	DF
Raw State (RS)	1	.845(S)	.289	-.500	.974(S)
Boiling (B)	.845(S)	1	.756	.040	.945(S)
Open Pan Dry Roasting (OPDR)	.289	.756	1	.684	.500
Shallow Frying (SF)	-.500	.040	.684	1	-.289
Deep Frying (DF)	.974(S)	.945(S)	.500	-.289	1

Positive *S= Significant*

This table shows the correlation of fat content of *rohu* with cooking methods. In 24 hours KMS preservation, there is significantly positive correlation present between the raw state with boiling and deep frying. Again boiling is positively correlated with deep frying. This table indicates that there is a strong correlation present among the **raw state**, **boiling and deep frying** in 24 hours KMS preservation.

Table no 5.12.1.3.11 Correlation of cooking methods in 48 hours preservation with KMS

Condition	RS	B	OPDR	SF	DF
Raw State (RS)	1	.982(S)	.954(S)	-.997*(S)	-.500
Boiling (B)	.982(S)	1	.993(S)	-.993(S)	-.327
Open Pan Dry Roasting (OPDR)	.954(S)	.993(S)	1	-.974(S)	-.217
Shallow Frying (SF)	-.997*(S)	-.993(S)	-.974(S)	1	.434
Deep Frying (DF)	-.500	-.327	-.217	.434	1

**.Correlation is highly significant at the 0.05 level (2-tailed)* ■ Positive □ Negative *S= Significant*

This table shows the correlation of fat content of *rohu* with cooking methods. In 48 hours KMS preservation, there is significant positive correlation present between the raw state with boiling and open pan dry roasting and negative correlation present with shallow frying. Again boiling is positively correlated with open pan dry roasting and negative with shallow frying. Open pan dry roasting is negatively correlated with shallow frying. This table indicates that there is a strong correlation present among the **raw state**, **boiling, open pan dry roasting, shallow frying** in 48 hours KMS days preservation.

Table no 5.12.1.3.12 Correlation of cooking methods in 14 days preservation with KMS

Condition	RS	B	OPDR	SF	DF
Raw State (RS)	1	-.990(S)	.405	-.194	-.682
Boiling (B)	-.990(S)	1	-.269	.333	.781
Open Pan Dry Roasting (OPDR)	.405	-.269	1	.818(S)	.392
Shallow Frying (SF)	-.194	.333	.818(S)	1	.849(S)
Deep Frying (DF)	-.682	.781	.392	.849(S)	1

■ Positive □ Negative *S= Significant*

This table shows the correlation of fat content of *rohu* with cooking methods. In 14 days KMS preservation, there is significantly negative correlation present between the raw state and boiling. Again open pan dry roasting is positively correlated with shallow frying, whereas shallow frying is positively correlated with deep frying. This table indicates that there is a strong correlation present among the **raw state**, **boiling, open pan dry roasting, shallow frying and deep frying** in 14 days KMS preservation.

Table no 5.12.1.3.13 Correlation of cooking methods in 15 days preservation with KMS

Condition	RS	B	OPDR	SF	DF
Raw State (RS)	1	-.923(S)	.958(S)	.937(S)	.197
Boiling (B)	-.923(S)	1	-.774	-.729	-.560
Open Pan Dry Roasting (OPDR)	.958(S)	-.774	1	.998*(S)	-.092
Shallow Frying (SF)	.937(S)	-.729	.998*(S)	1	-.159
Deep Frying (DF)	.197	-.560	-.092	-.159	1

**.Correlation is highly significant at the 0.05 level (2-tailed)* ■ Positive □ Negative *S= Significant*

This table shows the correlation of fat content of *rohu* with cooking methods. In 15 days KMS preservation, there is significantly positive correlation present between the raw state with shallow frying and open pan dry roasting, and negative correlation with boiling. Again open pan dry roasting is positively correlated with shallow frying. This table indicates that there is a strong correlation present among the **raw state**, **boiling, open pan dry roasting, shallow frying** in 15 days KMS preservation.

Overall analysis reveals that the raw state is significant negatively correlated with boiling in 48 hours control preservation without preservative, whereas significant positively correlated with open pan dry roasting in 48 hours control preservation without preservative, perfect positively correlated with shallow frying and deep frying in 15 days and 14 days salt and turmeric preservation respectively. Boiling is highly significant negatively correlated with open pan dry roasting in 48 hours preservation without preservative, whereas significant positively correlated with shallow frying in 48 hours control preservation without preservative, and significant negatively correlated with deep frying in fresh condition. Open pan dry roasting is highly significant negatively correlated with shallow frying in 48 hours control preservation without preservative and significant positively correlated with deep frying in 15 days salt and turmeric preservation. Shallow frying is significant positively correlated with deep frying in 48 hours control preservation without preservation. Most of the correlation of the fat content of *rohu* is found in **48 hours control preservation without preservative** with respect to different cooking conditions.

5.12.1.4 Moisture

Table no 5.12.1.4.1 Correlation of cooking methods in fresh condition

Condition	RS	B	OPDR	SF	DF
Raw State (RS)	1	.029	.975(S)	.983(S)	-.561
Boiling (B)	.029	1	-.193	-.157	-.844(S)
Open Pan Dry Roasting (OPDR)	.975(S)	-.193	1	.999*(S)	-.364
Shallow Frying (SF)	.983(S)	-.157	.999*(S)	1	-.398
Deep Frying (DF)	-.561	-.844(S)	-.364	-.398	1

**.Correlation is highly significant at the 0.05 level (2-tailed)* ☐ Positive ☐ Negative *S= Significant*

This table shows the correlation of moisture content of *rohu* with cooking methods. In fresh condition, there is significant positive correlation present between the raw state with shallow frying and open pan dry roasting. Again boiling is negatively correlated with deep frying, whereas open pan dry roasting is positively correlated with shallow frying. This table indicates that there is a strong correlation present among the **raw state**, **boiling, open pan dry roasting, shallow frying and deep frying** in fresh condition.

Table no 5.12.1.4.2 Correlation of cooking methods in 24 hours preservation without preservative

Condition	RS	B	OPDR	SF	DF
Raw State (RS)	1	.939(S)	-.423	-.097	-.507
Boiling (B)	.939(S)	1	-.086	.251	-.773
Open Pan Dry Roasting (OPDR)	-.423	-.086	1	.943(S)	-.566
Shallow Frying (SF)	-.097	.251	.943(S)	1	-.808(S)
Deep Frying (DF)	-.507	-.773	-.566	-.808(S)	1

**.Correlation is highly significant at the 0.05 level (2-tailed)* ☐ Positive ☐ Negative *S= Significant*

This table shows the correlation of moisture content of *rohu* with cooking methods. In 24 hours preservation without preservative, there is significant positive correlation present between the raw state and boiling. Again open pan dry roasting is positively correlated with shallow frying, whereas shallow frying is negatively correlated with deep frying. This table indicates that there is a strong correlation present among the **raw state**, **boiling, open pan dry roasting, shallow frying** in 15 days KMS preservation.

Table no 5.12.1.4.3 Correlation of cooking methods in 48 hours preservation without preservative

Condition	RS	B	OPDR	SF	DF
Raw State (RS)	1	-.496	1.000** (S)	1.000* (S)	1.000** (S)
Boiling (B)	-.496	1	-.494	-.479	-.499
Open Pan Dry Roasting (OPDR)	1.000** (S)	-.494	1	1.000* (S)	1.000** (S)
Shallow Frying (SF)	1.000* (S)	-.479	1.000* (S)	1	1.000* (S)
Deep Frying (DF)	1.000** (S)	-.499	1.000** (S)	1.000* (S)	1

***.Correlation is highly significant at the 0.01 level (2-tailed)* Positive *S= Significant*

This table shows the correlation of moisture content of *rohu* with cooking methods. In 48 hours control preservation without preservative, there is highly significant positive correlation present between the raw state with shallow frying, deep frying and open pan dry roasting. Again open pan dry roasting is positively correlated with shallow frying and deep frying. Shallow frying is positively correlated with deep frying. This table indicates that there is a strong correlation present among the **raw state**, **open pan dry roasting, shallow frying** in 48 hours control preservation.

Table no 5.12.1.4.4 Correlation of cooking methods in 14 days preservation without preservative

Condition	RS	B	OPDR	SF	DF
Raw State (RS)	1	1.000** (S)	1.000** (S)	1.000** (S)	-.967(S)
Boiling (B)	1.000** (S)	1	1.000** (S)	1.000** (S)	-.969(S)
Open Pan Dry Roasting (OPDR)	1.000** (S)	1.000** (S)	1	1.000** (S)	-.970(S)
Shallow Frying (SF)	1.000** (S)	1.000** (S)	1.000** (S)	1	-.971(S)
Deep Frying (DF)	-.967(S)	-.969(S)	-.970(S)	-.971(S)	1

***.Correlation is highly significant at the 0.01 level (2-tailed)* Positive Negative *S= Significant*

This table shows the correlation of moisture content of *rohu* with cooking methods. In 14 days control preservation without preservative, there is highly significant positive correlation present between the raw state and shallow frying, boiling and open pan dry roasting, but negative correlation present with deep frying. Again boiling is positively correlated with open pan dry roasting, shallow frying and negatively correlated with deep frying. Open pan dry roasting is positively correlated with shallow frying and negatively correlated with deep frying. This table indicates that there is a highly strong correlation present among the **raw state**, **boiling, open pan dry roasting, shallow frying and deep frying** in 14 days control preservation.

Table no 5.12.1.4.5 Correlation of cooking methods in 15 days preservation without preservative

Condition	RS	B	OPDR	SF	DF
Raw State (RS)	1	1.000** (S)	-1.000** (S)	.446	.754
Boiling (B)	1.000** (S)	1	-1.000** (S)	.444	.756
Open Pan Dry Roasting (OPDR)	-1.000** (S)	-1.000** (S)	1	-.437	-.761
Shallow Frying (SF)	.446	.444	-.437	1	-.251
Deep Frying (DF)	.754	.756	-.761	-.251	1

***.Correlation is highly significant at the 0.01 level (2-tailed)* Positive Negative *S= Significant*

This table shows the correlation of moisture content of *rohu* with cooking methods. In 15 days control preservation without preservative, there is highly significant positive correlation present between the raw state and boiling, but negative correlation with open pan dry roasting. Again boiling is negatively correlated with open pan dry roasting. This table indicates that there is a strong correlation present among the **raw state, boiling, open pan dry roasting** in 15 days control preservation.

Table no 5.12.1.4.6 Correlation of cooking methods in 24 hours preservation with salt and turmeric

Condition	RS	B	OPDR	SF	DF
Raw State (RS)	1	-.999* (S)	.561	-.256	.472
Boiling (B)	-.999*(S)	1	-.597	.297	-.509
Open Pan Dry Roasting (OPDR)	.561	-.597	1	-.944(S)	.995(S)
Shallow Frying (SF)	-.256	.297	-.944(S)	1	-.973(S)
Deep Frying (DF)	.472	-.509	.995(S)	-.973(S)	1

**.Correlation is highly significant at the 0.05 level (2-tailed)* ▭ Positive ▭ Negative *S= Significant*

This table shows the correlation of moisture content of *rohu* with cooking methods. In 24 hours salt and turmeric preservation, there is significant negative correlation present between the raw state and boiling. Again open pan dry roasting is positively correlated with deep frying and negatively correlated with shallow frying. Shallow frying is negatively correlated with deep frying. This table indicates that there is a strong correlation present among the **raw state, boiling, open pan dry roasting, shallow frying and deep frying** in 24 hours salt and turmeric preservation.

Table no 5.12.1.4.7 Correlation of cooking methods in 48 hours preservation with salt and turmeric

Condition	RS	B	OPDR	SF	DF
Raw State (RS)	1	.992(S)	-.075	-.954(S)	.976(S)
Boiling (B)	.992(S)	1	.052	-.984(S)	.996(S)
Open Pan Dry Roasting (OPDR)	-.075	.052	1	-.228	.142
Shallow Frying (SF)	-.954(S)	-.984(S)	-.228	1	-.996(S)
Deep Frying (DF)	.976(S)	.996(S)	.142	-.996(S)	1

▭ Positive ▭ Negative *S= Significant*

This table shows the correlation of moisture content of *rohu* with cooking methods. In 48 hours salt and turmeric preservation, there is significant positive correlation present between the raw state with boiling and deep frying. Again boiling is positively correlated with deep frying and negatively correlated with shallow frying. Shallow frying is negatively correlated with deep frying. This table indicates that there is a strong correlation present among the **raw state, boiling, shallow frying and deep frying** in 48 hours salt and turmeric preservation.

Table no 5.12.1.4.8 Correlation of cooking methods in 14 days preservation with salt and turmeric

Condition	RS	B	OPDR	SF	DF
Raw State (RS)	1	.321	-.934(S)	-.493	.138
Boiling (B)	.321	1	-.638	.666	.982(S)
Open Pan Dry Roasting (OPDR)	-.934(S)	-.638	1	.149	-.483
Shallow Frying (SF)	-.493	.666	.149	1	.794
Deep Frying (DF)	.138	.982(S)	-.483	.794	1

▭ Positive ▭ Negative *S= Significant*

This table shows the correlation of moisture content of *rohu* with cooking methods. In 14 days salt and turmeric preservation, there is significant negative correlation present between the raw state and open pan dry roasting. Again boiling is positively correlated with deep frying. This table indicates that there is a strong correlation present among the **raw state**, **boiling, open and deep frying** in 14 days salt and turmeric preservation.

Table no 5.12.1.4.9 Correlation of cooking methods in 15 days preservation with salt and turmeric

Condition	RS	B	OPDR	SF	DF
Raw State (RS)	1	-.114	-.802(S)	.836(S)	.251
Boiling (B)	-.114	1	.685	-.640	.933(S)
Open Pan Dry Roasting (OPDR)	-.802(S)	.685	1	-.998* (S)	.377
Shallow Frying (SF)	.836(S)	-.640	-.998* (S)	1	-.321
Deep Frying (DF)	.251	.933(S)	.377	-.321	1

**.Correlation is highly significant at the 0.05 level (2-tailed)* Positive Negative *S= Significant*

This table shows the correlation of moisture content of *rohu* with cooking methods. In 15 days salt and turmeric preservation, there is significant negative correlation present between the raw state and open pan dry roasting, but positive correlation present with shallow frying. Boiling is positively correlated with deep frying. Again open pan dry roasting is negatively correlated with shallow frying. This table indicates that there is a strong correlation present among the **raw state**, **boiling, open pan dry roasting, shallow frying and deep frying** in 15 days salt and turmeric preservation.

Table no 5.12.1.4.10 Correlation of cooking methods in 24 hours preservation with KMS

Condition	RS	B	OPDR	SF	DF
Raw State (RS)	1	.821(S)	.427	-.744	-.964(S)
Boiling (B)	.821(S)	1	.867(S)	-.992(S)	-.944(S)
Open Pan Dry Roasting (OPDR)	.427	.867(S)	1	-.922(S)	-.653
Shallow Frying (SF)	-.744	-.992(S)	-.922(S)	1	.895(S)
Deep Frying (DF)	-.964(S)	-.944(S)	-.653	.895(S)	1

Positive Negative *S= Significant*

This table shows the correlation of moisture content of *rohu* with cooking methods. In 24 hours KMS preservation, there is significant negative correlation present between the raw state and deep frying and positive correlation present with boiling. Boiling is positively correlated with open pan dry roasting, but negatively correlated with shallow frying and deep frying. Again open pan dry roasting is negatively correlated with shallow frying, whereas shallow frying is positively correlated with deep frying. This table indicates that there is a strong correlation present among the **raw state**, **boiling, open pan dry roasting, shallow frying and deep frying** in 24 hours KMS s preservation.

Table no 5.12.1.4.11 Correlation of cooking methods in 48 hours preservation with KMS

Condition	RS	B	OPDR	SF	DF
Raw State (RS)	1	.925(S)	-.832(S)	.930(S)	-.736
Boiling (B)	.925(S)	1	-.980(S)	1.000** (S)	-.425
Open Pan Dry Roasting (OPDR)	-.832(S)	-.980(S)	1	-.978(S)	.236
Shallow Frying (SF)	.930(S)	1.000**(S)	-.978(S)	1	-.435
Deep Frying (DF)	-.736	-.425	.236	-.435	1

***.Correlation is highly significant at the 0.01 level (2-tailed)* Positive Negative *S= Significant*

This table shows the correlation of moisture content of *rohu* with cooking methods. In 48 hours KMS preservation, there is significant negative correlation present between the raw state and open pan dry roasting, but positive correlation present with boiling and shallow frying. Boiling is positively correlated with shallow frying and negatively correlated with open pan dry roasting. Again open pan dry roasting is negatively correlated with shallow frying. This table indicates that there is a strong correlation present among the **raw state**, **boiling, open pan dry roasting, shallow frying** in 48 hours KMS preservation.

Table no 5.12.1.4.12 Correlation of cooking methods in 14 days preservation with KMS

Condition	RS	B	OPDR	SF	DF
Raw State (RS)	1	.926(S)	.961(S)	.841(S)	-.066
Boiling (B)	.926(S)	1	.785	.983(S)	.317
Open Pan Dry Roasting (OPDR)	.961(S)	.785	1	.659	-.340
Shallow Frying (SF)	.841(S)	.983(S)	.659	1	.484
Deep Frying (DF)	-.066	.317	-.340	.484	1

***.Correlation is highly significant at the 0.01 level (2-tailed)* Positive *S= Significant*

This table shows the correlation of moisture content of *rohu* with cooking methods. In 14 days KMS preservation, there is significant positive correlation present between the raw state with open pan dry roasting, boiling and shallow frying. Boiling is positively correlated with shallow frying. This table indicates that there is a strong correlation present among the **raw state**, **boiling, open pan dry roasting and shallow frying** in 14 days KMS preservation.

Table no 5.12.1.4.13 Correlation of cooking methods in 15 days preservation with KMS

Condition	RS	B	OPDR	SF	DF
Raw State (RS)	1	.927(S)	.333	-.719	.658
Boiling (B)	.927(S)	1	.662	-.927(S)	.328
Open Pan Dry Roasting (OPDR)	.333	.662	1	-.895(S)	-.491
Shallow Frying (SF)	-.719	-.927(S)	-.895(S)	1	.050
Deep Frying (DF)	.658	.328	-.491	.050	1

Positive Negative *S= Significant*

This table shows the correlation of moisture content of *rohu* with cooking methods. In 15 days KMS preservation, there is significant positive correlation present between the raw state and boiling. Both boiling and open pan dry roasting is negatively correlated with shallow frying. This table indicates that there is a strong correlation present among the **raw state**, **boiling, open pan dry roasting and shallow frying** in 15 days KMS preservation.

Overall analysis reveals that the raw state is perfect positively correlated with boiling in 14 days and 15 days control preservation without preservative, whereas perfect positively correlated with open pan dry roasting in 48 hours, 14 days and 15 days control preservation without preservative, and perfect positively correlated with shallow frying and deep frying in 48 hours and 14 days control preservation without preservative. Boiling is perfect positively correlated with open pan dry roasting in 14 days and 15 days control preservation without preservative, whereas perfect positively correlated with shallow frying in 14 days control preservation without preservative and 48 hours KMS preservation, and significant positively correlated with deep frying in 14 days salt and turmeric preservation. Open pan dry roasting is perfect positively correlated with shallow frying in 48 hours and 14 days control preservation without preservative, and perfect positively correlated with deep frying in 48 hours control preservation without preservative. Shallow frying is positively correlated with deep frying in 48 hours control preservation without preservative. Most of the correlation of the moisture content of *rohu* is found in **48 hours and 14 days control preservation without preservative** with respect to different cooking conditions.

5.12.1.5 Ash

Table no 5.12.1.5.1 Correlation of cooking methods in fresh condition

Condition	RS	B	OPDR	SF	DF
Raw State (RS)	1	-.052	.997* (S)	.996(S)	-.693
Boiling (B)	-.052	1	.019	-.143	.756
Open Pan Dry Roasting (OPDR)	.997* (S)	.019	1	.987(S)	-.640
Shallow Frying (SF)	.996(S)	-.143	.987(S)	1	-.756
Deep Frying (DF)	-.693	.756	-.640	-.756	1

**.Correlation is highly significant at the 0.05 level (2-tailed)* ▢ Positive *S= Significant*

This table shows the correlation of ash content of *rohu* with cooking methods. In fresh condition, there is significant positive correlation present between the raw state with open pan dry roasting and shallow frying. Again open pan dry roasting is positively correlated with shallow frying. This table indicates that there is a strong correlation present among the **raw state**, **open pan dry roasting and shallow frying** in fresh condition.

Table no 5.12.1.5.2 Correlation of cooking methods in 24 hours preservation without preservative

Condition	RS	B	OPDR	SF	DF
Raw State (RS)	1	.630	-.846(S)	-.866(S)	-.165
Boiling (B)	.630	1	-.119	-.157	-.870(S)
Open Pan Dry Roasting (OPDR)	-.846(S)	-.119	1	.999* (S)	-.386
Shallow Frying (SF)	-.866(S)	-.157	.999* (S)	1	-.350
Deep Frying (DF)	-.165	-.870(S)	-.386	-.350	1

**.Correlation is highly significant at the 0.05 level (2-tailed)* ▢ Positive ▢ Negative *S= Significant*

This table shows the correlation of ash content of *rohu* with cooking methods. In 24 hours control preservation without preservative, there is significant negative correlation present between the raw state with open pan dry roasting and shallow frying. Boiling is negatively correlated with deep frying. Again open pan dry roasting positively correlated with shallow frying. This table indicates that there is a strong correlation present among the **raw state**, **boiling, open pan dry roasting, shallow frying and deep frying** in 24 hours control preservation.

Table no 5.12.1.5.3 Correlation of cooking methods in 48 hours preservation without preservative

Condition	RS	B	OPDR	SF	DF
Raw State (RS)	1	-.285	.980(S)	.697	1.000** (S)
Boiling (B)	-.285	1	-.470	-.886(S)	-.295
Open Pan Dry Roasting (OPDR)	.980(S)	-.470	1	.826(S)	.982(S)
Shallow Frying (SF)	.697	-.886(S)	.826(S)	1	.705
Deep Frying (DF)	1.000** (S)	-.295	.982(S)	.705	1

***.Correlation is highly significant at the 0.01 level (2-tailed)* ▢ Positive ▢ Negative *S= Significant*

This table shows the correlation of ash content of *rohu* with cooking methods. In 48 hours control preservation without preservative, there is significant positive correlation present between the raw state with open pan dry roasting and deep frying. Boiling is negatively correlated with shallow frying. Again open pan dry roasting positively correlated with shallow frying and deep frying. This table indicates that there is a strong correlation present among the **raw state**, **boiling, open pan dry roasting, shallow frying and deep frying** in 48 hours control preservation.

Table no 5.12.1.5.4 Correlation of cooking methods in 14 days preservation without preservative

Condition	RS	B	OPDR	SF	DF
Raw State (RS)	1	.655	-.997*(S)	.434	.419
Boiling (B)	.655	1	-.596	-.397	.961(S)
Open Pan Dry Roasting (OPDR)	-.997*(S)	-.596	1	-.500	-.350
Shallow Frying (SF)	.434	-.397	-.500	1	-.636
Deep Frying (DF)	.419	.961(S)	-.350	-.636	1

**.Correlation is highly significant at the 0.05 level (2-tailed)* Positive Negative *S= Significant*

This table shows the correlation of ash content of *rohu* with cooking methods. In 14 days control preservation without preservative, there is significant negative correlation present between the raw state and open pan dry roasting. Boiling is positively correlated with deep frying. This table indicates that there is a strong correlation present among the **raw state**, **boiling, open pan dry roasting and deep frying** in 14 days control preservation.

Table no 5.12.1.5.5 Correlation of cooking methods in 15 days preservation without preservative

Condition	RS	B	OPDR	SF	DF
Raw State (RS)	1	.945(S)	.540	-.812(S)	.903(S)
Boiling (B)	.945(S)	1	.786	-.577	.994(S)
Open Pan Dry Roasting (OPDR)	.540	.786	1	.052	.850(S)
Shallow Frying (SF)	-.812(S)	-.577	.052	1	-.482
Deep Frying (DF)	.903(S)	.994(S)	.850(S)	-.482	1

Positive Negative *S= Significant*

This table shows the correlation of ash content of *rohu* with cooking methods. In 15 days control preservation without preservative, there is significant negative correlation present between the raw state and shallow frying, but positive correlation present with boiling and deep frying. Boiling is positively correlated with deep frying. Open pan dry roasting is positively correlated with deep frying. This table indicates that there is a strong correlation present among the **raw state**, **boiling, open pan dry roasting, shallow and deep frying** in 15 days control preservation.

Table no 5.12.1.5.6 Correlation of cooking methods in 24 hours preservation with salt and turmeric

Condition	RS	B	OPDR	SF	DF
Raw State (RS)	1	-.569	-.756	1.000**(S)	.945(S)
Boiling (B)	-.569	1	-.108	-.569	-.269
Open Pan Dry Roasting (OPDR)	-.756	-.108	1	-.756	-.929(S)
Shallow Frying (SF)	1.000**(S)	-.569	-.756	1	.945(S)
Deep Frying (DF)	.945(S)	-.269	-.929(S)	.945(S)	1

***.Correlation is highly significant at the 0.01 level (2-tailed)* Positive Negative *S= Significant*

This table shows the correlation of ash content of *rohu* with cooking methods. In 24 hours salt and turmeric preservation, there is significant positive correlation present between the raw state with shallow frying and deep frying. Open pan dry roasting is negatively correlated with deep frying, whereas shallow frying is positively correlated with deep frying. This table indicates that there is a strong correlation present among the **raw state, open pan dry roasting, shallow frying and deep frying** in 24 hours salt and turmeric preservation.

Table no 5.12.1.5.7 Correlation of cooking methods in 48 hours preservation with salt and turmeric

Condition	RS	B	OPDR	SF	DF
Raw State (RS)	1	.945(S)	.817(S)	-.990(S)	-.397
Boiling (B)	.945(S)	1	.961(S)	-.888(S)	-.075
Open Pan Dry Roasting (OPDR)	.817(S)	.961(S)	1	-.726	.204
Shallow Frying (SF)	-.990(S)	-.888(S)	-.726	1	.524
Deep Frying (DF)	-.397	-.075	.204	.524	1

Positive Negative *S= Significant*

This table shows the correlation of ash content of *rohu* with cooking methods. In 48 hours salt and turmeric preservation, there is significant positive correlation present between the raw state with boiling and open pan dry roasting, and negative correlation present with shallow frying. Boiling is positively correlated with open pan dry roasting, but negatively correlated with shallow frying. This table indicates that there is a strong correlation present among the **raw state**, **boiling, open pan dry roasting and shallow frying** in 48 hours salt and turmeric preservation.

Table no 5.12.1.5.8 Correlation of cooking methods in 14 days preservation with salt and turmeric

Condition	RS	B	OPDR	SF	DF
Raw State (RS)	1	.359	.655	.000	.866(S)
Boiling (B)	.359	1	.941(S)	.933(S)	-.156
Open Pan Dry Roasting (OPDR)	.655	.941(S)	1	.756	.189
Shallow Frying (SF)	.000	.933(S)	.756	1	-.500
Deep Frying (DF)	.866(S)	-.156	.189	-.500	1

Positive *S= Significant*

This table shows the correlation of ash content of *rohu* with cooking methods. In 14 days salt and turmeric preservation, there is significantly positive correlation present between the raw state and deep frying. Boiling is positively correlated with open pan dry roasting and shallow frying. This table indicates that there is a strong correlation present among the **raw state**, **open pan dry roasting, shallow frying and deep frying** in 14 days salt and turmeric preservation.

Table no 5.12.1.5.9 Correlation of cooking methods in 15 days preservation with salt and turmeric

Condition	RS	B	OPDR	SF	DF
Raw State (RS)	1	.645	.999*(S)	.041	.968(S)
Boiling (B)	.645	1	.619	-.737	.434
Open Pan Dry Roasting (OPDR)	.999*(S)	.619	1	.075	.976(S)
Shallow Frying (SF)	.041	-.737	.075	1	.289
Deep Frying (DF)	.968(S)	.434	.976(S)	.289	1

**.Correlation is highly significant at the 0.05 level (2-tailed)* Positive *S= Significant*

This table shows the correlation of ash content of *rohu* with cooking methods. In 15 days salt and turmeric preservation, there is significant positive correlation present between the raw state with open pan dry roasting and deep frying. Open pan dry roasting is positively correlated with deep frying. This table indicates that there is a strong correlation present among the **raw state**, **open pan dry roasting and deep frying** in 15 days salt and turmeric preservation.

Table no 5.12.1.5.10 Correlation of cooking methods in 24 hours preservation with KMS

Condition	RS	B	OPDR	SF	DF
Raw State (RS)	1	1.000**(S)	-.327	.961(S)	.891(S)
Boiling (B)	1.000**(S)	1	-.327	.961(S)	.891(S)
Open Pan Dry Roasting (OPDR)	-.327	-.327	1	-.577	-.721
Shallow Frying (SF)	.961(S)	.961(S)	-.577	1	.982(S)
Deep Frying (DF)	.891(S)	.891(S)	-.721	.982(S)	1

***.Correlation is highly significant at the 0.01 level (2-tailed)* Positive *S= Significant*

This table shows the correlation of ash content of *rohu* with cooking methods. In 24 hours KMS preservation, there is significant positive correlation present between the raw state with boiling, shallow frying and deep frying. Boiling is positively correlated with shallow frying and deep frying. Shallow frying is positively correlated with deep frying. This table indicates that there is a strong correlation present among the **raw state**, **boiling, shallow frying and deep frying** in 24 hours KMS preservation.

Table no 5.12.1.5.11 Correlation of cooking methods in 48 hours preservation with KMS

Condition	RS	B	OPDR	SF	DF
Raw State (RS)	1	-.564	-.371	.737	.434
Boiling (B)	-.564	1	.976(S)	-.974(S)	.500
Open Pan Dry Roasting (OPDR)	-.371	.976(S)	1	-.901(S)	.676
Shallow Frying (SF)	.737	-.974(S)	-.901(S)	1	-.289
Deep Frying (DF)	.434	.500	.676	-.289	1

Positive Negative *S= Significant*

This table shows the correlation of ash content of *rohu* with cooking methods. In 48 hours KMS preservation, there is significant positive correlation present between boiling with open pan dry roasting, and negative correlation with shallow frying. Open pan dry roasting is positively correlated with shallow frying. This table indicates that there is a strong correlation present among **boiling, open pan dry roasting and shallow frying** in 48 hours KMS preservation.

Table no 5.12.1.5.12 Correlation of cooking methods in 14 days preservation with KMS

Condition	RS	B	OPDR	SF	DF
Raw State (RS)	1	.893(S)	.673	.712	.485
Boiling (B)	.893(S)	1	.269	.951(S)	.826(S)
Open Pan Dry Roasting (OPDR)	.673	.269	1	-.041	-.321
Shallow Frying (SF)	.712	.951(S)	-.041	1	.960(S)
Deep Frying (DF)	.485	.826(S)	-.321	.960(S)	1

Positive *S= Significant*

This table shows the correlation of ash content of *rohu* with cooking methods. In 14 days KMS preservation, there is significant positive correlation present between the raw state and boiling. Boiling is positively correlated with shallow frying and deep frying. Shallow frying is positively correlated with deep frying. This table indicates that there is a strong correlation present among the **raw state**, **boiling, shallow frying and deep frying** in 14 days KMS preservation.

Table no 5.12.1.5.13 Correlation of cooking methods in 15 days preservation with KMS

Condition	RS	B	OPDR	SF	DF
Raw State (RS)	1	.233	.890(S)	.996(S)	.998*(S)
Boiling (B)	.233	1	-.236	.321	.289
Open Pan Dry Roasting (OPDR)	.890(S)	-.236	1	.845(S)	.862(S)
Shallow Frying (SF)	.996(S)	.321	.845(S)	1	.999**(S)
Deep Frying (DF)	.998*(S)	.289	.862	.999*(S)	1

**.Correlation is highly significant at the 0.05 level (2-tailed)* Positive *S= Significant*

This table shows the correlation of ash content of *rohu* with cooking methods. In 15 days KMS preservation, there is significant positive correlation present between the raw state with open pan dry roasting, shallow frying and deep frying. Open pan dry roasting is positively correlated with shallow frying and deep frying, whereas shallow frying is positively correlated with deep frying. This indicates that there is a strong correlation present among the **raw state**, **open pan dry roasting, shallow frying and deep frying** in 15 days KMS preservation.

Overall analysis reveals that the raw state is perfect positively correlated with boiling in 24 hours KMS preservation, whereas highly significant positively correlated with open pan dry roasting in 15 days salt and turmeric preservation, highly significant positively correlated with shallow frying in 24 hours salt and turmeric preservation, and perfect positively correlated with deep frying in 48 hours control preservation without preservative. Boiling is significant positively correlated with open pan dry roasting in 48 hours KMS preservation, whereas significant negatively correlated with shallow frying in 48 hours KMS preservation, and significant positively correlated with deep frying in 15 days control preservation without preservative. Open pan dry roasting is highly significant positively correlated with shallow frying in 24 hours control preservation without preservative, and significant positively correlated with deep frying in 48 hours control preservation without preservative. Shallow frying is perfect positively correlated with deep frying in 15 days KMS preservation. Most of the correlation of the ash content of *rohu* is found in **48 hours control preservation without preservative and 48 hours KMS preservation** with respect to different cooking conditions.

5.12.1.6 Calcium

Table no 5.12.1.6.1 Correlation of cooking methods in fresh condition

Condition	RS	B	OPDR	SF	DF
Raw State (RS)	1	.397	.500	.189	.619
Boiling (B)	.397	1	.993(S)	.976(S)	.967(S)
Open Pan Dry Roasting (OPDR)	.500	.993(S)	1	.945(S)	.990(S)
Shallow Frying (SF)	.189	.976(S)	.945(S)	1	.888(S)
Deep Frying (DF)	.619	.967(S)	.990(S)	.888(S)	1

Positive *S= Significant*

This table shows the correlation of calcium content of *rohu* with cooking methods. In fresh condition, there is significant positive correlation present between boiling with open pan dry roasting, shallow frying and deep frying. Open pan dry roasting is positively correlated with shallow frying and deep frying, whereas shallow frying is positively correlated with deep frying. This table indicates that there is a strong correlation present among **boiling**, **open pan dry roasting, shallow frying and deep frying** in fresh condition.

Table no 5.12.1.6.2 Correlation of cooking methods in 24 hours preservation without preservative

Condition	RS	B	OPDR	SF	DF
Raw State (RS)	1	.655	-.954(S)	-.655	.371
Boiling (B)	.655	1	-.397	-1.000**(S)	.945(S)
Open Pan Dry Roasting (OPDR)	-.954(S)	-.397	1	.397	-.075
Shallow Frying (SF)	-.655	-1.000**(S)	.397	1	-.945(S)
Deep Frying (DF)	.371	.945(S)	-.075	-.945(S)	1

***.Correlation is highly significant at the 0.01 level (2-tailed)* ▭ Positive ▭ Negative *S= Significant*

This table shows the correlation of calcium content of *rohu* with cooking methods. In 24 hours control preservation without preservative, there is significant negative correlation present between the raw state and open pan dry roasting. Boiling is positively correlated with deep frying and negatively correlated with shallow frying, whereas shallow frying is negatively correlated with deep frying. This table indicates that there is a strong correlation present among the **raw state** , **boiling, open pan dry roasting, shallow frying and deep frying** in 24 hours control preservation.

Table no 5.12.1.6.3 Correlation of cooking methods in 48 hours preservation without preservative

Condition	RS	B	OPDR	SF	DF
Raw State (RS)	1	-.052	-.240	.091	-.500
Boiling (B)	-.052	1	.982(S)	.990(S)	.891(S)
Open Pan Dry Roasting (OPDR)	-.240	.982(S)	1	.945(S)	.961(S)
Shallow Frying (SF)	.091	.990(S)	.945(S)	1	.817(S)
Deep Frying (DF)	-.500	.891(S)	.961(S)	.817(S)	1

▭ Positive *S= Significant*

This table shows the correlation of calcium content of *rohu* with cooking methods. In 48 hours control preservation without preservative, there is significant positive correlation present between boiling with open pan dry roasting, shallow frying and deep frying. Open pan dry roasting is positively correlated with shallow frying and deep frying, whereas shallow frying is positively correlated with deep frying. This table indicates that there is a strong correlation present among **boiling, open pan dry roasting, shallow frying and deep frying** in 48 hours control preservation.

Table no 5.12.1.6.4 Correlation of cooking methods in 14 days preservation without preservative

Condition	RS	B	OPDR	SF	DF
Raw State (RS)	1	1.000** (S)	.982(S)	.982(S)	1.000** (S)
Boiling (B)	1.000** (S)	1	.982(S)	.982(S)	1.000**(S)
Open Pan Dry Roasting (OPDR)	.982(S)	.982(S)	1	1.000**(S)	.982(S)
Shallow Frying (SF)	.982(S)	.982(S)	1.000**(S)	1	.982(S)
Deep Frying (DF)	1.000**(S)	1.000**(S)	.982(S)	.982(S)	1

***.Correlation is highly significant at the 0.01 level (2-tailed)* ▭ Positive *S= Significant*

This table shows the correlation of calcium content of *rohu* with cooking methods. In 14 days control preservation without preservative, there is perfect significant positive correlation present between the raw state with boiling and deep frying, and also significant positive correlation present with open pan dry roasting and shallow frying. Boiling is perfect positively correlated with deep frying, and significant positively correlated with open pan dry roasting and shallow frying. Open pan dry roasting is perfect positively correlated with shallow frying and significant positively correlated with deep frying. Again shallow frying is significant positively correlated with deep frying. This table indicates that there is a strong correlation present among the **raw state**, **boiling, open pan dry roasting, shallow frying and deep frying** in 14 days control preservation.

Table no 5.12.1.6.5 Correlation of cooking methods in 15 days preservation without preservative

Condition	RS	B	OPDR	SF	DF
Raw State (RS)	1	-.500	.990(S)	.756	.866(S)
Boiling (B)	-.500	1	-.371	-.945(S)	.000
Open Pan Dry Roasting (OPDR)	.990(S)	-.371	1	.655	.929(S)
Shallow Frying (SF)	.756	-.945(S)	.655	1	.327
Deep Frying (DF)	.866(S)	.000	.929(S)	.327	1

Positive Negative *S= Significant*

This table indicates the correlation of calcium content of *rohu* with cooking methods. In 15 days control preservation without preservative, there is significant positive correlation present between the raw state with open pan dry roasting and deep frying. Boiling is negatively correlated with shallow frying, whereas open pan dry roasting is positively correlated with deep frying. This table indicates that there is a strong correlation present among the **raw state**, **boiling, open pan dry roasting, shallow frying and deep frying** in 15 days control preservation.

Table no 5.12.1.6.6 Correlation of cooking methods in 24 hours preservation with salt and turmeric

Condition	RS	B	OPDR	SF	DF
Raw State (RS)	1	.052	.923(S)	.923(S)	.923(S)
Boiling (B)	.052	1	.434	.434	.434
Open Pan Dry Roasting (OPDR)	.923(S)	.434	1	1.000** (S)	1.000** (S)
Shallow Frying (SF)	.923(S)	.434	1.000** (S)	1	1.000** (S)
Deep Frying (DF)	.923(S)	.434	1.000** (S)	1.000** (S)	1

***.Correlation is highly significant at the 0.01 level (2-tailed)* Positive *S= Significant*

This table shows the correlation of calcium content of *rohu* with cooking methods. In 24 hours salt and turmeric preservation, there is significant positive correlation present between the raw state with open pan dry roasting, shallow frying and deep frying. Open pan dry roasting is perfect positively correlated with shallow frying and deep frying, whereas shallow frying is perfect positively correlated with deep frying. This table indicates that there is a strong correlation present among the **raw state**, **open pan dry roasting, shallow frying and deep frying** in 24 hours salt and turmeric preservation.

Table no 5.12.1.6.7 Correlation of cooking methods in 48 hours preservation with salt and turmeric

Condition	RS	B	OPDR	SF	DF
Raw State (RS)	1	.901(S)	.993(S)	.993(S)	1.000**(S)
Boiling (B)	.901(S)	1	.945(S)	.945(S)	.901(S)
Open Pan Dry Roasting (OPDR)	.993(S)	.945	1	1.000**(S)	.993(S)
Shallow Frying (SF)	.993(S)	.945(S)	1.000**(S)	1	.993(S)
Deep Frying (DF)	1.000**(S)	.901(S)	.993(S)	.993(S)	1

***.Correlation is highly significant at the 0.01 level (2-tailed)* ▭ Positive *S= Significant*

This table shows the correlation of calcium content of *rohu* with cooking methods. In 48 hours salt and turmeric preservation, there is significant positive correlation present between the raw state with boiling, open pan dry roasting, shallow frying and perfect positive correlation with deep frying. Boiling is significant positively correlated with open pan dry roasting, shallow frying and deep frying. Open pan dry roasting is perfect positively correlated with shallow frying and significant positively correlated with deep frying, whereas shallow frying is significant positively correlated with deep frying. This table indicates that there is a strong correlation present among the **raw state**, **boiling, open pan dry roasting, shallow frying and deep frying** in 48 hours salt and turmeric preservation.

Table no 5.12.1.6.8 Correlation of cooking methods in 14 days preservation with salt and turmeric

Condition	RS	B	OPDR	SF	DF
Raw State (RS)	1	.986(S)	-.596	.993(S)	1.000**(S)
Boiling (B)	.986(S)	1	-.721	.961(S)	.986(S)
Open Pan Dry Roasting (OPDR)	-.596	-.721	1	-.500	-.596
Shallow Frying (SF)	.993(S)	.961(S)	-.500	1	.993(S)
Deep Frying (DF)	1.000**(S)	.986(S)	-.596	.993(S)	1

***.Correlation is highly significant at the 0.01 level (2-tailed)* ▭ Positive *S= Significant*

This table shows the correlation of calcium content of *rohu* with cooking methods. In 14 days salt and turmeric preservation, there is significant positive correlation present between the raw state with boiling and shallow frying, but perfect positive correlation present with deep frying. Boiling is significant positively correlated with shallow frying and deep frying, whereas shallow frying is significant positively correlated with deep frying. This table indicates that there is a strong correlation present among the **raw state**, **boiling, shallow frying and deep frying** in 14 days salt and turmeric preservation.

Table no 5.12.1.6.9 Correlation of cooking methods in 15 days preservation with salt and turmeric

Condition	RS	B	OPDR	SF	DF
Raw State (RS)	1	.976(S)	.976(S)	.974(S)	.993(S)
Boiling (B)	.976(S)	1	1.000**(S)	.901(S)	.945(S)
Open Pan Dry Roasting (OPDR)	.976(S)	1.000**(S)	1	.901(S)	.945(S)
Shallow Frying (SF)	.974(S)	.901(S)	.901(S)	1	.993(S)
Deep Frying (DF)	.993(S)	.945(S)	.945(S)	.993(S)	1

***.Correlation is highly significant at the 0.01 level (2-tailed)* ▭ Positive *S= Significant*

This table shows the correlation of calcium content of *rohu* with cooking methods. In 15 days salt and turmeric preservation, there is significant positive correlation present between the raw state with boiling, open pan dry roasting, shallow frying and deep frying. Boiling is perfect positively correlated with open pan dry roasting and significant positively correlated with shallow frying and deep frying, whereas open pan dry roasting is significant positively correlated with shallow frying and deep frying. Again shallow frying is significant positively correlated with deep frying. This table indicates that there is a strong correlation present among the **raw state**, **boiling, open pan dry roasting, shallow frying and deep frying** in 15 days salt and turmeric preservation.

Table no 5.12.1.6.10 Correlation of cooking methods in 24 hours preservation with KMS

Condition	RS	B	OPDR	SF	DF
Raw State (RS)	1	.240	-.240	1.000**(S)	-.619
Boiling (B)	.240	1	-1.000**(S)	.240	-.911(S)
Open Pan Dry Roasting (OPDR)	-.240	-1.000**(S)	1	-.240	.911(S)
Shallow Frying (SF)	1.000**(S)	.240	-.240	1	-.619
Deep Frying (DF)	-.619	-.911(S)	.911(S)	-.619	1

***.Correlation is highly significant at the 0.01 level (2-tailed)* Positive Negative *S= Significant*

This table shows the correlation of calcium content of *rohu* with cooking methods. In 24 hours KMS preservation, there is perfect positive correlation present between the raw state and shallow frying. Boiling is perfect negatively correlated with open pan dry roasting and significant negatively correlated with deep frying, whereas open pan dry roasting is significant positively correlated with deep frying. This table indicates that there is a strong correlation present among the **raw state**, **boiling, open pan dry roasting, shallow frying and deep frying** in 24 hours KMS preservation.

Table no 5.12.1.6.11 Correlation of cooking methods in 48 hours preservation with KMS

Condition	RS	B	OPDR	SF	DF
Raw State (RS)	1	.540	-.371	.371	-.459
Boiling (B)	.540	1	-.982(S)	.982(S)	.500
Open Pan Dry Roasting (OPDR)	-.371	-.982(S)	1	-1.000**(S)	-.655
Shallow Frying (SF)	.371	.982(S)	-1.000**(S)	1	.655
Deep Frying (DF)	-.459	.500	-.655	.655	1

***.Correlation is highly significant at the 0.01 level (2-tailed)* Positive Negative *S= Significant*

This table shows the correlation of calcium content of *rohu* with cooking methods. In 48 hours KMS preservation, there is significant positive correlation present between boiling with shallow frying and negative correlation with open pan dry roasting. Again open pan dry roasting is perfect negatively correlated with shallow frying. This table indicates that there is a strong correlation present among **boiling, open pan dry roasting and shallow frying** in 48 hours KMS preservation.

Table no 5.12.1.6.12 Correlation of cooking methods in 14 days preservation with KMS

Condition	RS	B	OPDR	SF	DF
Raw State (RS)	1	.974(S)	.636	1.000**(S)	.997*(S)
Boiling (B)	.974(S)	1	.795	.974(S)	.954(S)
Open Pan Dry Roasting (OPDR)	.636	.795	1	.636	.577
Shallow Frying (SF)	1.000**(S)	.974(S)	.636	1	.997*(S)
Deep Frying (DF)	.997*(S)	.954(S)	.577	.997*(S)	1

***.Correlation is highly significant at the 0.01 level (2-tailed)* Positive *S= Significant*
**.Correlation is highly significant at the 0.05 level (2-tailed)*

This table shows the correlation of calcium content of *rohu* with cooking methods. In 14 days KMS preservation, there is perfect positive correlation present between the raw state with shallow frying and significant positive correlation present with boiling and deep frying. Again boiling is significant positively correlated with shallow frying and deep frying. Shallow frying is significant positively correlated with deep frying. This table indicates that there is a strong correlation present among the **raw state, boiling, shallow frying and deep frying** in 14 days KMS preservation.

Table no 5.12.1.6.13 Correlation of cooking methods in 15 days preservation with KMS

Condition	RS	B	OPDR	SF	DF
Raw State (RS)	1	1.000**(S)	-.419	-.350	.127
Boiling (B)	1.000**(S)	1	-.419	-.350	.127
Open Pan Dry Roasting (OPDR)	-.419	-.419	1	.997*(S)	-.954(S)
Shallow Frying (SF)	-.350	-.350	.997*(S)	1	-.974(S)
Deep Frying (DF)	.127	.127	-.954(S)	-.974(S)	1

***.Correlation is highly significant at the 0.01 level (2-tailed)* ▭ Positive *S= Significant*
**.Correlation is highly significant at the 0.05 level (2-tailed)*

This table shows the correlation of calcium content of *rohu* with cooking methods. In 15 days KMS preservation, there is a perfect positive correlation present between the raw state and boiling. Again open pan dry roasting is significant positively correlated with shallow frying and deep frying. Shallow frying is significant positively correlated with deep frying. This table indicates that there is a strong correlation present among the **raw state, boiling, open pan dry roasting, shallow frying and deep frying** in 15 days KMS preservation.

Overall analysis reveals that the raw state is perfect positively correlated with boiling in 14 days control preservation without preservative and 15 days KMS preservation, whereas significant positively correlated with open pan dry roasting in 48 hours salt and turmeric preservation, and perfect positively correlated with shallow frying in 24 hours, 14 days KMS preservation, and perfect positively correlated with deep frying in 48 hours, 14 days control preservation without preservative and 14 days salt and turmeric preservation. Boiling is perfect positively correlated with open pan dry roasting in 15 days salt and turmeric preservation, whereas perfect negatively correlated with shallow frying in 24 hours KMS preservation and 24 hours control preservation without preservation, and perfect positively correlated with deep frying in 14 days control preservation without preservative. Open pan dry roasting is perfect positively correlated with shallow frying in 14 days control preservation without preservative, 24 hours, 48 hours salt and turmeric preservation, and perfect positively correlated with deep frying in 24 hours salt and turmeric preservation. Shallow frying is perfect positively correlated with deep frying in 24 hours salt and turmeric preservation. Most of the correlation of the calcium content of *rohu* is found in **14 days control preservation without preservative** with respect to different cooking conditions.

5.13.1.7 Iron

Table no 5.13.1.7.1 Correlation of cooking methods in fresh condition

Condition	RS	B	OPDR	SF	DF
Raw state (RS)	1	-1.000**(S)	-.319	.197	-.681
Boiling (B)	-1.000**(S)	1	.332	-.184	.691
Open Pan Dry Roasting (OPDR)	-.319	.332	1	.866 (S)	.911(S)
Shallow Frying (SF)	.197	-.184	.866(S)	1	.583
Deep Frying (DF)	-.681	.691	.911(S)	.583	1

***.Correlation is highly significant at the 0.01 level (2-tailed)* Positive Negative *S= Significant*

This table shows the correlation of iron content of *rohu* with cooking methods. In fresh condition, there is perfect negative correlation present between the raw state and boiling. Again open pan dry roasting is significant positively correlated with shallow frying and deep frying. This table indicates that there is a strong correlation present among the **raw state, boiling, open pan dry roasting, shallow frying and deep frying** in fresh condition.

Table no 5.13.1.7.2 Correlation of cooking methods in 24 hours preservation without preservative

Condition	RS	B	OPDR	SF	DF
Raw State (RS)	1	.993(S)	.999*(S)	-1.000**(S)	.993(S)
Boiling (B)	.993(S)	1	.997(S)	-.995(S)	1.000**(S)
Open Pan Dry Roasting (OPDR)	.999*(S)	.997(S)	1	-1.000*(S)	.997(S)
Shallow Frying (SF)	-1.000**(S)	-.995(S)	-1.000*(S)	1	-.995(S)
Deep Frying (DF)	.993(S)	1.000**(S)	.997(S)	-.995(S)	1

***.Correlation is highly significant at the 0.01 level (2-tailed)* Positive Negative *S= Significant*
**.Correlation is highly significant at the 0.05 level (2-tailed)*

This table shows the correlation of iron content of *rohu* with cooking methods. In 24 hours control preservation without preservative, there is significant positive correlation present between the raw state with boiling, open pan dry roasting and deep frying, but perfect negative correlation present with shallow frying. Again boiling is significant positively correlated with open pan dry roasting and perfect positive correlation present with deep frying, and significant positive correlation present with open pan dry roasting, but negative correlation present with shallow frying. Again open pan dry roasting is positive correlated with deep frying and perfectly negatively correlated with shallow frying. Shallow frying is significant negatively correlated with deep frying. This table indicates that there is a strong correlation present among the **raw state, boiling, open pan dry roasting, shallow frying and deep frying** in 24 hours control preservation.

Table no 5.13.1.7.3 Correlation of cooking methods in 48 hours preservation without preservative

Condition	RS	B	OPDR	SF	DF
Raw State (RS)	1	.717	.977(S)	-.273	-.663
Boiling (B)	.717	1	.849(S)	.475	.047
Open Pan Dry Roasting (OPDR)	.977(S)	.849(S)	1	-.062	-.489
Shallow Frying (SF)	-.273	.475	-.062	1	.901(S)
Deep Frying (DF)	-.663	.047	-.489	.901(S)	1

Positive *S= Significant*

This table shows the correlation of iron content of *rohu* with cooking methods. In 48 hours control preservation without preservative, there is significant positive correlation present between the raw state with open pan dry roasting, whereas boiling also significant positively correlated with open pan dry roasting. Shallow frying is significantly positively correlated with deep frying. This table indicates that there is a strong correlation present among the **raw state, boiling, open pan dry roasting, shallow frying and deep frying** in 48 hours control preservation.

Table no 5.13.1.7.4 Correlation of cooking methods in 14 days preservation without preservative

Condition	RS	B	OPDR	SF	DF
Raw State (RS)	1	.041	-.984(S)	.500	.992(S)
Boiling (B)	.041	1	-.217	.886(S)	.165
Open Pan Dry Roasting (OPDR)	-.984(S)	-.217	1	-.645	-.999*(S)
Shallow Frying (SF)	.500	.886(S)	-.645	1	.604
Deep Frying (DF)	.992(S)	.165	-.999*(S)	.604	1

*.*Correlation is highly significant at the 0.05 level (2-tailed)* Positive Negative *S= Significant*

This table shows the correlation of iron content of *rohu* with cooking methods. In 14 days control preservation without preservative, there is significant negative correlation present between the raw state and open pan dry roasting and positive correlation present with deep frying. Again boiling is positively correlated with shallow frying, whereas open pan dry roasting is significant negatively correlated with deep frying. This table indicates that there is a strong correlation present among the **raw state, boiling, open pan dry roasting, shallow frying and deep frying** in 14 days control preservation.

Table no 5.12.1.7.5 Correlation of cooking methods in 15 days preservation without preservative

Condition	RS	B	OPDR	SF	DF
Raw State (RS)	1	.970(S)	.962(S)	-.948(S)	-.273
Boiling (B)	.970(S)	1	1.000*(S)	-.997*(S)	-.500
Open Pan Dry Roasting (OPDR)	.962(S)	1.000*(S)	1	-.999*(S)	-.524
Shallow Frying (SF)	-.948(S)	-.997*(S)	-.999*(S)	1	.564
Deep Frying (DF)	-.273	-.500	-.524	.564	1

*.*Correlation is highly significant at the 0.05 level (2-tailed)* Positive Negative *S= Significant*

This table shows the correlation of iron content of *rohu* with cooking methods. In 15 days control preservation without preservative, there is significant positive correlation present between the raw state and boiling. Again open pan dry roasting is significant positively correlated with shallow frying and deep frying. This table indicates that there is a strong correlation present among the **raw state, boiling, open pan dry roasting, shallow frying and deep frying** in 15 days control preservation.

Table no 5.12.1.7.6 Correlation of cooking methods in 24 hours preservation with salt and turmeric

Condition	RS	B	OPDR	SF	DF
Raw State (RS)	1	.500	.684	.500	.500
Boiling (B)	.500	1	.974(S)	1.000**(S)	1.000**(S)
Open Pan Dry Roasting (OPDR)	.684	.974(S)	1	.974(S)	.974(S)
Shallow Frying (SF)	.500	1.000**(S)	.974(S)	1	1.000**(S)
Deep Frying (DF)	.500	1.000**(S)	.974(S)	1.000**(S)	1

*.*Correlation is highly significant at the 0.05 level (2-tailed)* Positive *S= Significant*

This table shows the correlation of iron content of *rohu* with cooking methods. In 24 hours salt and turmeric preservation, there is significant positive correlation present between boiling with open pan dry roasting, shallow frying and deep frying. Open pan dry roasting is positively correlated with shallow frying and deep frying, whereas shallow frying is also positively correlated with deep frying. This table indicates that there is a strong correlation present among **boiling, open pan dry roasting, shallow frying and deep frying** in 24 hours salt and turmeric preservation.

Table no 5.12.1.7.7 Correlation of cooking methods in 48 hours preservation with salt and turmeric

Condition	RS	B	OPDR	SF	DF
Raw State (RS)	1	.803(S)	-.705	-.500	-.705
Boiling (B)	.803(S)	1	-.143	-.918(S)	-.143
Open Pan Dry Roasting (OPDR)	-.705	-.143	1	-.262	1.000**(S)
Shallow Frying (SF)	-.500	-.918(S)	-.262	1	-.262
Deep Frying (DF)	-.705	-.143	1.000**(S)	-.262	1

**.Correlation is highly significant at the 0.05 level (2-tailed)* Positive Negative *S= Significant*

This table shows the correlation of iron content of *rohu* with cooking methods. In 48 hours salt and turmeric preservation, there is significant positive correlation present between the raw state and boiling. Again boiling is negatively correlated with shallow frying. Open pan dry roasting is perfect positively correlated with deep frying. This table indicates that there is a strong correlation present among the **raw state, boiling, open pan dry roasting, shallow frying and deep frying** in 48 hours salt and turmeric preservation.

Table no 5.12.1.7.8 Correlation of cooking methods in 14 days preservation with salt and turmeric

Condition	RS	B	OPDR	SF	DF
Raw State (RS)	1	.289	.475	.803(S)	.289
Boiling (B)	.289	1	-.705	.803(S)	1.000**(S)
Open Pan Dry Roasting (OPDR)	.475	-.705	1	-.143	-.705
Shallow Frying (SF)	.803(S)	.803(S)	-.143	1	.803(S)
Deep Frying (DF)	.289	1.000**(S)	-.705	.803(S)	1

***.Correlation is highly significant at the 0.01 level (2-tailed)* Positive *S= Significant*

This table shows the correlation of iron content of *rohu* with cooking methods. In 14 days salt and turmeric preservation, there is significant positive correlation present between the raw state and shallow frying. Boiling is positively correlated with shallow frying and highly significant positively correlated with deep frying. Shallow frying is positively correlated with deep frying. This table indicates that there is a strong correlation present among the **raw state, boiling, shallow frying and deep frying** in 14 days salt and turmeric preservation.

Table no 5.12.1.7.9 Correlation of cooking methods in 15 days preservation with salt and turmeric

Condition	RS	B	OPDR	SF	DF
Raw State (RS)	1	-.217	1.000**(S)	-.993(S)	-.993(S)
Boiling (B)	-.217	1	-.217	.327	.327
Open Pan Dry Roasting (OPDR)	1.000**(S)	-.217	1	-.993(S)	-.993(S)
Shallow Frying (SF)	-.993(S)	.327	-.993(S)	1	1.000**(S)
Deep Frying (DF)	-.993(S)	.327	-.993(S)	1.000**(S)	1

***.Correlation is highly significant at the 0.01 level (2-tailed)* Positive Negative *S= Significant*

This table shows the correlation of iron content of *rohu* with cooking methods. In 15 days salt and turmeric preservation, there is perfect positive correlation present between the raw state and open pan dry roasting, but negatively correlated with shallow frying and deep frying. Open pan dry roasting is negatively correlated with shallow frying and deep frying, whereas shallow frying is perfect positively correlated with deep frying. This table indicates that there is a strong correlation present among the **raw state, open pan dry roasting, shallow frying and deep frying** in 15 days salt and turmeric preservation.

Table no 5.12.1.7.10 Correlation of cooking methods in 24 hours preservation with KMS

Condition	RS	B	OPDR	SF	DF
Raw State (RS)	1	.500	.459	.986(S)	-.888(S)
Boiling (B)	.500	1	.999*(S)	.637	-.047
Open Pan Dry Roasting (OPDR)	.459	.999*(S)	1	.600	.000
Shallow Frying (SF)	.986(S)	.637	.600	1	-.800(S)
Deep Frying (DF)	-.888(S)	-.047	.000	-.800(S)	1

**.Correlation is highly significant at the 0.05 level (2-tailed)* Positive Negative *S= Significant*

This table shows the correlation of iron content of *rohu* with cooking methods. In 24 hours KMS preservation, there is positive correlation present between the raw state and shallow frying, but negatively correlated with deep frying. Open pan dry roasting is positively correlated with boiling, whereas shallow frying is negatively correlated with deep frying. This table indicates that there is a strong correlation present among the **raw state, boiling, open pan dry roasting, shallow frying and deep frying** in 24 hours KMS preservation.

Table no 5.12.1.7.11 Correlation of cooking methods in 48 hours preservation with KMS

Condition	RS	B	OPDR	SF	DF
Raw State (RS)	1	.304	-.998*(S)	1.000*(S)	-.245
Boiling (B)	.304	1	-.368	.321	-.998*(S)
Open Pan Dry Roasting (OPDR)	-.998*(S)	-.368	1	-.999*(S)	.311
Shallow Frying (SF)	1.000*(S)	.321	-.999*(S)	1	-.262
Deep Frying (DF)	*-.245*	*-.998*(S)*	*.311*	*-.262*	*1*

**.Correlation is highly significant at the 0.05 level (2-tailed)* Positive Negative *S= Significant*

This table shows the correlation of iron content of *rohu* with cooking methods. In 48 hours KMS preservation, there is positive correlation present between the raw state and shallow frying, but significant negative correlation present with open pan dry roasting. Boiling is significant negatively correlated with deep frying. Open pan dry roasting is significant negatively correlated with shallow frying. This table indicates that there is a strong correlation present among the **raw state, boiling, open pan dry roasting, shallow frying and deep frying** in 48 hours KMS preservation.

Table no 5.12.1.7.12 Correlation of cooking methods in 14 days preservation with KMS

Condition	RS	B	OPDR	SF	DF
Raw State (RS)	1	1.000*(S)	1.000**(S)	-.524	.859(S)
Boiling (B)	1.000*(S)	1	1.000*(S)	-.500	.844(S)
Open Pan Dry Roasting (OPDR)	1.000**(S)	1.000*(S)	1	-.524	.859(S)
Shallow Frying (SF)	-.524	-.500	-.524	1	-.886(S)
Deep Frying (DF)	.859(S)	.844	.859(S)	-.886(S)	1

**.Correlation is highly significant at the 0.05 level (2-tailed)* Positive Negative *S= Significant*
***.Correlation is highly significant at the 0.01 level (2-tailed)*

This table shows the correlation of iron content of *rohu* with cooking methods. In 14 days KMS preservation, there is perfect positive correlation present between the raw state with boiling and open pan dry roasting and significantly positive correlation with deep frying. Boiling is perfect positively correlated with open pan dry roasting and significant positively correlated with deep frying, but shallow frying is negatively correlated with deep frying. This table indicates that there is a strong correlation present among the **raw state, boiling, open pan dry roasting, shallow frying and deep frying** in 14 days KMS preservation.

Table no 5.12.1.7.13 Correlation of cooking methods in 15 days preservation with KMS

Condition	RS	B	OPDR	SF	DF
Raw State (RS)	1	-.959(S)	-.959(S)	-.812(S)	-.705
Boiling (B)	-.959(S)	1	1.000**(S)	.614	.475
Open Pan Dry Roasting (OPDR)	-.959(S)	1.000**(S)	1	.614	.475
Shallow Frying (SF)	-.812(S)	.614	.614	1	.986(S)
Deep Frying (DF)	-.705	.475	.475	.986(S)	1

***.Correlation is highly significant at the 0.01 level (2-tailed)* ▭ Positive ▭ Negative *S= Significant*

This table shows the correlation of iron content of *rohu* with cooking methods. In 15 days KMS preservation, there is negative correlation present between the raw state with boiling and open pan dry roasting and shallow frying. Boiling is perfect positively correlated with open pan dry roasting, whereas shallow frying is positively correlated with deep frying. This table indicates that there is a strong correlation present among the **raw state, boiling, open pan dry roasting, shallow frying and deep frying** in 15 days KMS preservation.

Overall analysis reveals that the raw state is perfect positively correlated with boiling in 14 days KMS preservation, whereas perfect positively correlated with open pan dry roasting in 15 days salt and turmeric preservation and 14 days KMS preservation, and perfect negatively correlated with shallow frying in 24 hours control preservation and 48 hours KMS preservation, and perfect positively correlated with deep frying in 24 hours control preservation without preservative and also perfect negatively correlated with deep frying in 15 days salt and turmeric preservation. Boiling is perfect positively correlated with open pan dry roasting in 15 days control preservation without preservative, 14 days and 15 days KMS preservation, whereas perfect positively correlated with shallow frying in 24 hours salt and turmeric preservation, and perfect positively correlated with deep frying in 24 hours control preservation without preservative, 24 hours and 14 days salt and turmeric preservation. Open pan dry roasting is perfect negatively correlated with shallow frying in 24 hours control preservation without preservative, and perfect positively correlated with deep frying in 48 hours salt and turmeric preservation. Shallow frying is perfect positively correlated with deep frying in 24 hours and 15 days salt and turmeric preservation. Most of the correlation of the iron content of *rohu* is found in **24 hours control preservation without preservative** with respect to different cooking conditions.

5.12.1.8 Energy

Table no 5.12.1.8.1 Correlation of cooking methods in fresh condition

Condition	RS	B	OPDR	SF	DF
Raw State (RS)	1	-.126	.315	.631	-.123
Boiling (B)	-.126	1	-.981(S)	-.849(S)	-.969(S)
Open Pan Dry Roasting (OPDR)	.315	-.981(S)	1	.935(S)	.903(S)
Shallow Frying (SF)	.631	-.849(S)	.935(S)	1	.693
Deep Frying (DF)	-.123	-.969(S)	.903(S)	.693	1

Positive Negative *S= Significant*

This table shows the correlation of energy content of *rohu* with cooking methods. In fresh condition, there is negative correlation present between the raw state with open pan dry roasting, shallow frying and deep frying. Open pan dry roasting is positively correlated with shallow frying and deep frying. This table indicates that there is a strong correlation present among **boiling, open pan dry roasting, shallow frying and deep frying** in fresh condition.

Table no 5.12.1.8.2 Correlation of cooking methods in 24 hours preservation without preservative

Condition	RS	B	OPDR	SF	DF
Raw State (RS)	1	-.494	.553	-.277	-.480
Boiling (B)	-.494	1	-.998*(S)	.972(S)	-.526
Open Pan Dry Roasting (OPDR)	.553	-.998*(S)	1	-.954(S)	.466
Shallow Frying (SF)	-.277	.972(S)	-.954(S)	1	-.710
Deep Frying (DF)	-.480	-.526	.466	-.710	1

**.Correlation is highly significant at the 0.05 level (2-tailed)* Positive Negative *S= Significant*

This table shows the correlation of energy content of *rohu* with cooking methods. In 24 hours control preservation without preservative, there is significant negative correlation present between boiling with open pan dry roasting and shallow frying. Open pan dry roasting is significant negatively correlated with shallow frying. This table indicates that there is a strong correlation present among **boiling, open pan dry roasting and shallow frying** in 24 hours control preservation.

Table no 5.12.1.8.3 Correlation of cooking methods in 48 hours preservation without preservative

Condition	RS	B	OPDR	SF	DF
Raw State (RS)	1	.750	-.905(S)	.517	.344
Boiling (B)	.750	1	-.960(S)	-.178	-.363
Open Pan Dry Roasting (OPDR)	-.905(S)	-.960(S)	1	-.104	.089
Shallow Frying (SF)	.517	-.178	-.104	1	.981(S)
Deep Frying (DF)	.344	-.363	.089	.981(S)	1

Positive Negative *S= Significant*

This table shows the correlation of energy content of *rohu* with cooking methods. In 48 hours control preservation without preservative, there is significant negative correlation present between the raw state with open pan dry roasting. Boiling is negatively correlated with open pan dry roasting. Shallow frying is positively correlated with deep frying. This table indicates that there is a strong correlation present among the **raw state, boiling, open pan dry roasting, shallow frying and deep frying** in 48 hours control preservation.

Table no 5.12.1.8.4 Correlation of cooking methods in 14 days preservation without preservative

Condition	RS	B	OPDR	SF	DF
Raw State (RS)	1	.970(S)	-.896(S)	-.107	.864(S)
Boiling (B)	.970(S)	1	-.760	.139	.961(S)
Open Pan Dry Roasting (OPDR)	-.896(S)	-.760	1	.538	-.550
Shallow Frying (SF)	-.107	.139	.538	1	.408
Deep Frying (DF)	.864(S)	.961(S)	-.550	.408	1

Positive Negative *S= Significant*

This table shows the correlation of energy content of *rohu* with cooking methods. In 14 days control preservation without preservative, there is significant negative correlation present between the raw state with open pan dry roasting and positive correlation with boiling and deep frying. Boiling is positively correlated with deep frying. This table indicates that there is a strong correlation present among the **raw state, boiling, open pan dry roasting and deep frying** in 14 days control preservation.

Table no 5.12.1.8.5 Correlation of cooking methods in 15 days preservation without preservative

Condition	RS	B	OPDR	SF	DF
Raw State (RS)	1	-.555	.900(S)	.966(S)	.886(S)
Boiling (B)	-.555	1	-.862(S)	-.323	-.106
Open Pan Dry Roasting (OPDR)	.900(S)	-.862(S)	1	.758	.596
Shallow Frying (SF)	.966(S)	-.323	.758	1	.975(S)
Deep Frying (DF)	.886(S)	-.106	.596	.975(S)	1

Positive Negative *S= Significant*

This table shows the correlation of energy content of *rohu* with cooking methods. In 15 days control preservation without preservative, there is significant positive correlation present between the raw state with open pan dry roasting, shallow frying and deep frying. Boiling is negatively correlated with open pan dry roasting. Shallow frying is positively correlated with deep frying. This table indicates that there is a strong correlation present among **the raw state, boiling, open pan dry roasting, shallow frying and deep frying** in 15 days control preservation.

Table no 5.12.1.8.6 Correlation of cooking methods in 24 hours preservation with salt and turmeric

Condition	RS	B	OPDR	SF	DF
Raw State (RS)	1	.409	-.093	-.153	.809(S)
Boiling (B)	.409	1	-.947(S)	.839(S)	-.205
Open Pan Dry Roasting (OPDR)	-.093	-.947(S)	1	-.970(S)	.509
Shallow Frying (SF)	-.153	.839(S)	-.970(S)	1	-.704
Deep Frying (DF)	.809(S)	-.205	.509	-.704	1

Positive Negative *S= Significant*

This table shows the correlation of energy content of *rohu* with cooking methods. In 24 hours salt and turmeric preservation, there is significant positive correlation present between the raw state and deep frying. Boiling is positively correlated with shallow frying and negatively correlated with open pan dry roasting. Again open pan dry roasting is negatively correlated with shallow frying. This table indicates that there is a strong correlation present among the **raw state, boiling, open pan dry roasting, shallow and deep frying** in 24 hours salt and turmeric preservation.

Table no 5.12.1.8.7 Correlation of cooking methods in 48 hours preservation with salt and turmeric

Condition	RS	B	OPDR	SF	DF
Raw State (RS)	1	-.888(S)	-.651	-.995(S)	.786
Boiling (B	-.888(S)	1	.928(S)	.836(S)	-.413
Open Pan Dry Roasting (OPDR)	-.651	.928(S)	1	.571	-.043
Shallow Frying (SF)	-.995(S)	.836(S)	.571	1	-.845(S)
Deep Frying (DF)	.786	-.413	-.043	-.845(S)	1

Positive Negative *S= Significant*

This table shows the correlation of energy content of *rohu* with cooking methods. In 48 hours salt and turmeric preservation, there is significant negative correlation present between the raw state with open pan dry roasting and boiling. Boiling is positively correlated with open pan dry roasting and shallow frying, whereas shallow frying is negatively correlated with deep frying. This table indicates that there is a strong correlation present among **the raw state, boiling, open pan dry roasting, shallow frying and deep frying** in 48 hours salt and turmeric preservation.

Table no 5.12.1.8.8 Correlation of cooking methods in 14 days preservation with salt and turmeric

Condition	RS	B	OPDR	SF	DF
Raw State (RS)	1	.243	.503	-.206	-.994(S)
Boiling (B)	.243	1	-.716	-.999* (S)	-.344
Open Pan Dry Roasting (OPDR)	.503	-.716	1	.742	-.409
Shallow Frying (SF)	-.206	-.999* (S)	.742	1	.308
Deep Frying (DF)	-.994(S)	-.344	-.409	.308	1

**.Correlation is highly significant at the 0.05 level (2-tailed)* Negative *S= Significant*

This table shows the correlation of energy content of *rohu* with cooking methods. In 14 days salt and turmeric preservation, there is significant negative correlation present between the raw state and deep frying. Boiling is highly negatively correlated with shallow frying. This table indicates that there is a strong correlation present among the **raw state, boiling, shallow frying and deep frying** in 14 days salt and turmeric preservation.

Table no 5.12.1.8.9 Correlation of cooking methods in 15 days preservation with salt and turmeric

Condition	RS	B	OPDR	SF	DF
Raw State (RS)	1	.210	-1.000*(S)	.877(S)	-.647
Boiling (B)	.210	1	-.191	-.285	.609
Open Pan Dry Roasting (OPDR)	-1.000*(S)	-.191	1	-.887(S)	.663
Shallow Frying (SF)	.877(S)	-.285	-.887(S)	1	-.934(S)
Deep Frying (DF)	-.647	.609	.663	-.934(S)	1

**.Correlation is highly significant at the 0.05 level (2-tailed)* Positive Negative *S= Significant*

This table shows the correlation of energy content of *rohu* with cooking methods. In 15 days salt and turmeric preservation, there is perfect negative correlation present between the raw state and open pan dry roasting, and significant positive correlation present between the raw state and shallow frying. Open pan dry roasting is negatively correlated with shallow frying. Again shallow frying is negatively correlated with deep frying. This table indicates that there is a strong correlation present among **the raw**

state, open pan dry roasting, shallow frying and deep frying in 15 days salt and turmeric preservation.

Table no 5.12.1.8.10 Correlation of cooking methods in 24 hours preservation with KMS

Condition	RS	B	OPDR	SF	DF
Raw State (RS)	1	.301	-.784	-.983(S)	.966(S)
Boiling (B)	.301	1	.357	-.469	.538
Open Pan Dry Roasting (OPDR)	-.784	.357	1	.658	-.596
Shallow Frying (SF)	-.983(S)	-.469	.658	1	-.997(S)
Deep Frying (DF)	.966(S)	.538	-.596	-.997(S)	1

Positive Negative *S= Significant*

This table shows the correlation of energy content of *rohu* with cooking methods. In 24 hours KMS preservation, there is significant negative correlation present between the raw state and shallow frying and positive correlation with deep frying. Shallow frying is negatively correlated with deep frying. This table indicates that there is a strong correlation present among the **raw state, shallow frying and deep frying** in 24 hours KMS preservation.

Table no 5.12.1.8.11 Correlation of cooking methods in 48 hours preservation with KMS

Condition	RS	B	OPDR	SF	DF
Raw State (RS)	1	.988(S)	-.341	-.564	-.461
Boiling (B)	.988(S)	1	-.481	-.683	-.320
Open Pan Dry Roasting (OPDR)	-.341	-.481	1	.969(S)	-.677
Shallow Frying (SF)	-.564	-.683	.969(S)	1	-.473
Deep Frying (DF)	-.461	-.320	-.677	-.473	1

Positive *S= Significant*

This table shows the correlation of energy content of *rohu* with cooking methods. In 48 hours KMS preservation, there is significant positive correlation present between the raw state and boiling. Again shallow frying is positively correlated with open pan dry roasting. This table indicates that there is a strong correlation present among the **raw state, boiling, open pan dry roasting and shallow frying** in 48 hours KMS preservation.

Table no 5.12.1.8.12 Correlation of cooking methods in 14 days preservation with KMS

Condition	RS	B	OPDR	SF	DF
Raw State (RS)	1	.713	.901(S)	-.955(S)	.860(S)
Boiling (B)	.713	1	.339	-.474	.971(S)
Open Pan Dry Roasting (OPDR)	.901(S)	.339	1	-.989(S)	.553
Shallow Frying (SF)	-.955(S)	-.474	-.989(S)	1	-.670
Deep Frying (DF)	.860(S)	.971(S)	.553	-.670	1

Positive Negative *S= Significant*

This table shows the correlation of energy content of *rohu* with cooking methods. In 14 days KMS preservation, there is significant negative correlation present between the raw state and shallow frying and positive correlation present with open pan dry roasting and deep frying. Boiling is positively correlated with deep frying. Shallow frying is negatively correlated with open pan dry roasting. This table indicates that there is a strong correlation present among the **raw state, boiling, open pan dry roasting, shallow frying and deep frying** in 14 days KMS preservation.

Table no 5.12.1.8.13 Correlation of cooking methods in 15 days preservation with KMS

Condition	RS	B	OPDR	SF	D
Raw State (RS)	1	-.402	.572	-.798	-.969(S)
Boiling (B)	-.402	1	.522	-.231	.163
Open Pan Dry Roasting (OPDR)	.572	.522	1	-.951(S)	-.757
Shallow Frying (SF)	-.798	-.231	-.951(S)	1	.922(S)
Deep Frying (DF)	-.969(S)	.163	-.757	.922(S)	1

Positive Negative *S= Significant*

This table shows the correlation of energy content of *rohu* with cooking methods. In 15 days KMS preservation, there is significant negative correlation present between the raw state and deep frying. Shallow frying is negatively correlated with open pan dry roasting and positively correlated with deep frying. This table indicates that there is a strong correlation present among the **raw state, open pan dry roasting, shallow frying and deep frying** in 15 days KMS preservation.

Overall analysis reveals that the raw state is significant negatively correlated with boiling in 48 hours KMS preservation, whereas perfect positively correlated with open pan dry roasting in 15 days salt and turmeric preservation, and significant negatively correlated with shallow frying and deep frying in 48 hours and 14 days salt and turmeric preservation. Boiling is significant negatively correlated with open pan dry roasting in 24 hours control preservation without preservative, whereas highly significant negatively correlated with shallow frying in 14 days salt and turmeric preservation, and significant positively correlated with deep frying in 14 days KMS preservation. Open pan dry roasting is significant negatively correlated with shallow frying in 14 days KMS preservation, and significant positively correlated with deep frying in fresh condition. Shallow frying is significant negatively correlated with deep frying in 24 hours KMS preservation. Most of the correlation of the energy content of *rohu* is found in **14 days salt and turmeric preservation and 14 days KMS preservation** with respect to different cooking conditions.

5.12.2 *Katla (Catla catla)*

5.12.2.1 Carbohydrate

Table no 5.12.2.1.1 Correlation of cooking methods in fresh condition

Condition	RS	B	OPDR	SF	DF
Raw State (RS)	1	.232	-.993(S)	-.701	-.843(S)
Boiling (B)	.232	1	-.343	.531	.327
Open Pan Dry Roasting (OPDR)	-.993(S)	-.343	1	.614	.776
Shallow Frying (SF)	-.701	.531	.614	1	.975(S)
Deep Frying (DF)	-.843(S)	.327	.776	.975(S)	1

Positive Negative *S= Significant*

This table shows the correlation of carbohydrate content of *katla* with cooking methods. In fresh condition, there is significant negative correlation present between the raw state with open pan dry roasting and deep frying. Shallow frying is positively correlated with deep frying. This table indicates that there is a strong correlation present among **the raw state, open pan dry roasting, shallow frying and deep frying** in fresh condition.

Table no 5.12.2.1.2 Correlation of cooking methods in 24 hours preservation without preservative

Condition	RS	B	OPDR	SF	DF
Raw State (RS)	1	.961(S)	.971(S)	.596	.514
Boiling (B)	.961(S)	1	.866(S)	.350	.732
Open Pan Dry Roasting (OPDR)	.971(S)	.866(S)	1	.771	.293
Shallow Frying (SF)	.596	.350	.771	1	-.382
Deep Frying (DF)	.514	.732	.293	-.382	1

Positive *S= Significant*

This table shows the correlation of carbohydrate content of *katla* with cooking methods. In 24 hours control preservation without preservative, there is significant positive correlation present between the raw state with boiling and open pan dry roasting. Again boiling is positively correlated with open pan dry roasting. This table indicates that there is a strong correlation present among the **raw state, boiling and open pan dry roasting** in 24 hours preservation without preservative.

Table no 5.12.2.1.3 Correlation of cooking methods in 48 hours preservation without preservative

Condition	RS	B	OPDR	SF	DF
Raw State (RS)	1	-.430	.295	.573	.380
Boiling (B)	-.430	1	.736	.494	-.999*
Open Pan Dry Roasting (OPDR)	.295	.736	1	.952	-.772
Shallow Frying (SF)	.573	.494	.952	1	-.541
Deep Frying (DF)	.380	-.999*	-.772	-.541	1

**.Correlation is highly significant at the 0.05 level (2-tailed)* Negative *S= Significant*

This table shows the correlation of carbohydrate content of *katla* with cooking methods. In 48 hours control preservation without preservative, there is highly significant negative correlation present between boiling and deep frying. This table indicates that there is a strong correlation present between **boiling and deep frying only** in 48 hours control preservation without preservative.

Table no 5.12.2.1.4 Correlation of cooking methods in 14 days preservation without preservative

Condition	RS	B	OPDR	SF	DF
Raw State (RS)	1	-.721	.596	.667	.286
Boiling (B)	-.721	1	-.986(S)	.036	.458
Open Pan Dry Roasting (OPDR)	.596	-.986(S)	1	-.200	-.599
Shallow Frying (SF)	.667	.036	-.200	1	.905(S)
Deep Frying (DF)	.286	.458	-.599	.905(S)	1

Positive Negative *S= Significant*

This table shows the correlation of carbohydrate content of *katla* with cooking methods. In 14 days control preservation without preservative, there is highly significant negative correlation present between boiling and open pan dry roasting. Again shallow frying is significant positively correlated with deep frying. This table indicates that there is a strong correlation present between **boiling and open pan dry roasting and also between shallow frying and deep frying** in 14 days control preservation without preservative.

Table no 5.12.2.1.5 Correlation of cooking methods in 15 days preservation without preservative

Condition	RS	B	OPDR	SF	DF
Raw State (RS)	1	-.089	-.419	-.587	-.677
Boiling (B)	-.089	1	-.867(S)	.858(S)	.793
Open Pan Dry Roasting (OPDR)	-.419	-.867(S)	1	-.488	-.384
Shallow Frying (SF)	-.587	.858(S)	-.488	1	.993(S)
Deep Frying (DF)	-.677	.793	-.384	.993(S)	1

Positive Negative *S= Significant*

This table shows the correlation of carbohydrate content of *katla* with cooking methods. In 15 days control preservation without preservative, there is highly significant negative correlation present between boiling and open pan dry roasting, and also positive correlation between boiling and shallow frying. Again shallow frying is significant positively correlated with deep frying. This table indicates that there is a strong correlation present among **boiling, open pan dry roasting, shallow frying and deep frying** in 15 days control preservation without preservative.

Table no 5.12.2.1.6 Correlation of cooking methods in 24 hours preservation with salt and turmeric

Condition	RS	B	OPDR	SF	DF
Raw State(RS)	1	.120	.977(S)	.860(S)	.868(S)
Boiling (B)	.120	1	.327	-.403	-.389
Open Pan Dry Roasting (OPDR)	.977(S)	.327	1	.733	.743
Shallow Frying (SF)	.860(S)	-.403	.733	1	1.000**(S)
Deep Frying (DF)	.868(S)	-.389	.743	1.000**(S)	1

***.Correlation is highly significant at the 0.01 level (2-tailed)* Positive *S= Significant*

This table shows the correlation of carbohydrate content of *katla* with cooking methods. In 24 hours salt and turmeric preservation, there is highly significant positive correlation present between the raw state with open pan dry roasting, shallow frying and deep frying. Again shallow frying is perfect positively correlated with deep frying. This table indicates that there is a strong correlation present among **the raw state, open pan dry roasting, shallow frying and deep frying** in 24 hours salt and turmeric preservation.

Table no 5.12.2.1.7 Correlation of cooking methods in 48 hours preservation with salt and turmeric

Condition	RS	B	OPDR	SF	DF
Raw State (RS)	1	-.074	-.933(S)	.947(S)	.924(S)
Boiling (B)	-.074	1	-.289	.250	.311
Open Pan Dry Roasting (OPDR)	-.933(S)	-.289	1	-.999*(S)	-1.000*(S)
Shallow Frying (SF)	.947(S)	.250	-.999*(S)	1	.998*(S)
Deep Frying (DF)	.924(S)	.311	-1.000*(S)	.998*(S)	1

**.Correlation is highly significant at the 0.05 level (2-tailed)* Positive Negative *S= Significant*

This table shows the correlation of carbohydrate content of *katla* with cooking methods. In 48 hours salt and turmeric preservation, there is highly significant negative correlation present between the raw state and open pan dry roasting, and positive correlation present between the raw state with shallow frying and deep frying. Open pan dry roasting is significant negatively correlated with shallow frying, and perfect negative correlation present between open pan dry roasting and deep frying, whereas shallow frying is significant positively correlated with deep frying. This table indicates that there is a strong correlation present among **the raw state, open pan dry roasting, shallow frying and deep frying** in 48 hours salt and turmeric preservation.

Table no 5.12.2.1.8 Correlation of cooking methods in 14 days preservation with salt and turmeric

Condition	RS	B	OPDR	SF	DF
Raw State(RS)	1	.931(S)	.775	.860(S)	.983(S)
Boiling (B)	.931(S)	1	.953(S)	.614	.847(S)
Open Pan Dry Roasting (OPDR)	.775	.953(S)	1	.344	.646
Shallow Frying (SF)	.860(S)	.614	.344	1	.939(S)
Deep Frying (DF)	.983(S)	.847(S)	.646	.939(S)	1

Positive *S= Significant*

This table shows the correlation of carbohydrate content of *katla* with cooking methods. In 14 days salt and turmeric preservation, there is highly significant positive correlation present between the raw state with boiling, shallow frying and deep frying. Again boiling is positively correlated with open pan dry roasting and deep frying, whereas shallow frying is significant positively correlated with deep frying. This table indicates that there is a strong correlation present among **the raw state, boiling, open pan dry roasting, shallow frying and deep frying** in 14 days salt and turmeric preservation.

Table no 5.12.2.1.9 Correlation of cooking methods in 15 days preservation with salt and turmeric

Condition	RS	B	OPDR	SF	DF
Raw State (RS)	1	-.934(S)	.999*(S)	.938(S)	.966(S)
Boiling (B)	-.934(S)	1	-.950(S)	-1.000**(S)	-.995(S)
Open Pan Dry Roasting (OPDR)	.999*(S)	-.950(S)	1	.954(S)	.977(S)
Shallow Frying (SF)	.938(S)	-1.000**(S)	.954(S)	1	.996(S)
Deep Frying (DF)	.966(S)	-.995(S)	.977(S)	.996(S)	1

**.Correlation is highly significant at the 0.05 level (2-tailed)* Positive Negative *S= Significant*
***.Correlation is highly significant at the 0.01 level (2-tailed)*

This table shows the correlation of carbohydrate content of *katla* with cooking methods. In 15 days salt and turmeric preservation, there is significant negative correlation present between the raw state and boiling, and positive correlation present between the raw state with open pan dry roasting, shallow frying and deep frying. Boiling is significant negatively correlated with open pan dry roasting and deep frying and perfect negatively correlated with shallow frying. Open pan dry roasting is significant positively correlated with shallow frying and deep frying, whereas shallow frying is significant positively correlated with deep frying. This table indicates that there is a strong correlation present among **the raw state, boiling, open pan dry roasting, shallow frying and deep frying** in 15 days salt and turmeric preservation.

Table no 5.12.2.1.10 Correlation of cooking methods in 24 hours preservation with KMS

Condition	RS	B	OPDR	SF	DF
Raw State (RS)	1	.987(S)	.902(S)	.933(S)	.996(S)
Boiling (B)	.987(S)	1	.960(S)	.862(S)	.970(S)
Open Pan Dry Roasting (OPDR)	.902(S)	.960(S)	1	.685	.861(S)
Shallow Frying (SF)	.933(S)	.862(S)	.685	1	.960(S)
Deep Frying (DF)	.996(S)	.970(S)	.861(S)	.960(S)	1

Positive *S= Significant*

This table shows the correlation of carbohydrate content of *katla* with cooking methods. In 24 hours KMS preservation, there is highly significant positive correlation present between the raw state with boiling, open pan dry roasting, shallow frying and deep frying. Boiling is also significant positively correlated with open pan dry roasting, shallow frying and deep frying. Open pan dry roasting is significant positively correlated with deep frying, whereas shallow frying is significant positively correlated with deep frying. This table indicates that there is a strong correlation present among the **raw state, boiling, open pan dry roasting, shallow frying and deep frying** in 24 hours KMS preservation.

Table no 5.12.2.1.11 Correlation of cooking methods in 48 hours preservation with KMS

Condition	RS	B	OPDR	SF	DF
Raw State (RS)	1	1.000**(S)	.795	1.000**(S)	.661
Boiling (B)	1.000**(S)	1	.795	1.000**(S)	.661
Open Pan Dry Roasting (OPDR)	.795	.795	1	.795	.981(S)
Shallow Frying (SF)	1.000**(S)	1.000**(S)	.795	1	.661
Deep Frying (DF)	.661	.661	.981(S)	.661	1

***.Correlation is highly significant at the 0.01 level (2-tailed)* ▭ Positive *S= Significant*

This table shows the correlation of carbohydrate content of *katla* with cooking methods. In 48 hours KMS preservation, there is perfect positive correlation present between the raw state with boiling and shallow frying. Boiling is also perfect positively correlated with shallow frying. Open pan dry roasting is significant positively correlated with deep frying. This table indicates that there is a strong correlation present among **the raw state, boiling, open pan dry roasting, shallow frying and deep frying** in 48 hours KMS preservation.

Table no 5.12.2.1.12 Correlation of cooking methods in 14 days preservation with KMS

Condition	RS	B	OPDR	SF	DF
Raw State (RS)	1	.954(S)	.959(S)	.972(S)	.998*(S)
Boiling (B)	.954(S)	1	.831(S)	.998*(S)	.935(S)
Open Pan Dry Roasting (OPDR)	.959(S)	.831(S)	1	.866(S)	.974(S)
Shallow Frying (SF)	.972(S)	.998*(S)	.866(S)	1	.957(S)
Deep Frying (DF)	.998*(S)	.935(S)	.974(S)	.957(S)	1

***.Correlation is highly significant at the 0.01 level (2-tailed)* ▭ Positive *S= Significant*

This table shows the correlation of carbohydrate content of *katla* with cooking methods. In 14 days KMS preservation, there is highly significant positive correlation present between the raw state with boiling, open pan dry roasting and shallow frying and highly significant positive correlation with deep frying. Boiling is also significant positively correlated with open pan dry roasting and deep frying and highly significant positively correlated with shallow frying. Open pan dry roasting is significant positively correlated with shallow frying and deep frying, whereas shallow frying is significant positively correlated with deep frying. This table indicates that there is a very strong correlation present among **the raw state, boiling, open pan dry roasting, shallow frying and deep frying** in 14 days KMS preservation.

Table no 5.12.2.1.13 Correlation of cooking methods in 15 days preservation with KMS

Condition	RS	B	OPDR	SF	DF
Raw State (RS)	1	.619	.929(S)	-.106	.986(S)
Boiling (B)	.619	1	.866(S)	-.847(S)	.741
Open Pan Dry Roasting (OPDR)	.929(S)	.866(S)	1	-.468	.977(S)
Shallow Frying (SF)	-.106	-.847(S)	-.468	1	-.270
Deep Frying (DF)	.986(S)	.741	.977(S)	-.270	1

Positive Negative *S= Significant*

This table shows the correlation of carbohydrate content of *katla* with cooking methods. In 15 days KMS preservation, there is highly significant positive correlation present between the raw state with open pan dry roasting and deep frying. Boiling is also significant positively correlated with open pan dry roasting and negatively correlated with deep frying. Open pan dry roasting is significant positively correlated with deep frying. This table indicates that there is a strong correlation present among **the raw state, boiling, open pan dry roasting, shallow frying and deep frying** in 15 days KMS preservation.

Overall analysis reveals that the raw state is positively correlated with boiling in 48 hours KMS preservation, whereas highly significant positively correlated with open pan dry roasting in 15 days salt and turmeric preservation, and perfect positively correlated with shallow frying in 48 hours KMS preservation, and highly significant positively correlated with 14 days KMS preservation. Boiling is significant negatively correlated with open pan dry roasting in 14 days control preservation without preservative, whereas perfect positively correlated with shallow frying in 48 hours KMS preservation and perfect negatively correlated with 15 days salt and turmeric preservation, and highly significant negatively correlated with deep frying in 48 hours preservation without preservative. Open pan dry roasting is significant negatively correlated with shallow frying and deep frying in 48 hours salt and turmeric preservation. Shallow frying is perfect positively correlated with deep frying in 24 hours salt and turmeric preservation. Most of the correlation of the carbohydrate content of *katla* is found in **48 hours KMS preservation** with respect to different cooking conditions.

5.12.2.2 Protein

Table no 5.12.2.2.1 Correlation of cooking methods in fresh condition

Condition	RS	B	OPDR	SF	DF
Raw State (RS)	1	-.786	-.824(S)	.851(S)	-.705
Boiling (B)	-.786	1	.998*(S)	-.993(S)	.115
Open Pan Dry Roasting (OPDR)	-.824(S)	.998*(S)	1	-.999*(S)	.178
Shallow Frying (SF)	.851(S)	-.993(S)	-.999*(S)	1	-.228
Deep Frying (DF)	-.705	.115	.178	-.228	1

**.Correlation is highly significant at the 0.05 level (2-tailed)* Positive Negative *S= Significant*

This table shows the correlation of protein content of *katla* with cooking methods. In fresh condition, there is significant negative correlation present between the raw state and open pan dry roasting. Boiling is also highly significant positively correlated with open pan dry roasting and negatively correlated with shallow frying. Open pan dry roasting is highly significant negatively correlated with shallow frying.

This table indicates that there is a strong correlation present among the **raw state, boiling, open pan dry roasting and shallow frying** in fresh condition.

Table no 5.12.2.2.2 Correlation of cooking methods in 24 hours preservation without preservative

Condition	RS	B	OPDR	SF	DF
Raw State (RS)	1	-.977(S)	-.262	.792	.985(S)
Boiling (B)	-.977(S)	1	.052	-.646	-.999*(S)
Open Pan Dry Roasting (OPDR)	-.262	.052	1	-.796	-.091
Shallow Frying (SF)	.792	-.646	-.796	1	.675
Deep Frying (DF)	.985(S)	-.999*(S)	-.091	.675	1

**.Correlation is highly significant at the 0.05 level (2-tailed)* Positive Negative *S= Significant*

This table shows the correlation of protein content of *katla* with cooking methods. In 24 hours control preservation without preservative, there is significant negative correlation present between the raw state and boiling, and positive correlation present with deep frying. Boiling is also highly significant negatively correlated with deep frying. This table indicates that there is a strong correlation present among the **raw state, boiling and deep frying** in 24 hours control preservation.

Table no 5.12.2.2.3 Correlation of cooking methods in 48 hours preservation without preservative

Condition	RS	B	OPDR	SF	DF
Raw State (RS)	1	.081	-.198	.659	.881(S)
Boiling (B)	.081	1	-.993(S)	.803(S)	.543
Open Pan Dry Roasting (OPDR)	-.198	-.993(S)	1	-.868(S)	-.639
Shallow Frying (SF)	.659	.803(S)	-.868(S)	1	.937(S)
Deep Frying (DF)	.881(S)	.543	-.639	.937(S)	1

Positive Negative *S= Significant*

This table shows the correlation of protein content of *katla* with cooking methods. In 48 hours control preservation without preservative, there is significant positive correlation present between the raw state and deep frying. Boiling is also significant positively correlated with shallow frying and negatively correlated with open pan dry roasting. Open pan dry roasting is significant negatively correlated with shallow frying, whereas shallow frying is positively correlated with deep frying. This table indicates that there is a strong correlation present among the **raw state, boiling, open pan dry roasting, shallow frying and deep frying** in 48 hours control preservation.

Table no 5.12.2.2.4 Correlation of cooking methods in 14 days preservation without preservative

Condition	RS	B	OPDR	SF	DF
Raw State (RS)	1	-.974(S)	-.963(S)	.985(S)	-.906(S)
Boiling (B)	-.974(S)	1	.999*(S)	-.920(S)	.978(S)
Open Pan Dry Roasting (OPDR)	-.963(S)	.999*(S)	1	-.902(S)	.986(S)
Shallow Frying (SF)	.985(S)	-.920(S)	-.902(S)	1	-.818(S)
Deep Frying (DF)	-.906(S)	.978(S)	.986(S)	-.818(S)	1

**.Correlation is highly significant at the 0.05 level (2-tailed)* Positive Negative *S= Significant*

This table shows the correlation of protein content of *katla* with cooking methods. In 14 days control preservation without preservative, there is significant negative correlation present between the raw state with boiling, open pan dry roasting and deep frying, and positive correlation with shallow frying. Boiling is also highly significant positively correlated with open pan dry roasting and deep frying, and negatively correlated with shallow frying. Open pan dry roasting is significant negatively correlated with shallow frying and positively correlated with deep frying, whereas shallow frying is negatively correlated with deep frying. This table indicates that there is a strong correlation present among the **raw state, boiling, open pan dry roasting, shallow frying and deep frying** in 14 days control preservation.

Table no 5.12.2.2.5 Correlation of cooking methods in 15 days preservation without preservative

Condition	RS	B	OPDR	SF	DF
Raw State (RS)	1	.040	-.640	-.682	.702
Boiling (B)	.040	1	-.793	-.758	.740
Open Pan Dry Roasting (OPDR)	-.640	-.793	1	.998*(S)	-.997(S)
Shallow Frying (SF)	-.682	-.758	.998*(S)	1	-1.000*(S)
Deep Frying (DF)	.702	.740	-.997(S)	-1.000*(S)	1

**.Correlation is highly significant at the 0.05 level (2-tailed)* Positive Negative *S= Significant*

This table shows the correlation of protein content of *katla* with cooking methods. In 15 days control preservation without preservative, there is significant negative correlation present between open pan dry roasting and deep frying and positive correlation present with shallow frying, whereas shallow frying is negatively correlated with deep frying. This table indicates that there is a strong correlation present among **open pan dry roasting, shallow frying and deep frying** in 15 days control preservation.

Table no 5.12.2.2.6 Correlation of cooking methods in 24 hours preservation with salt and turmeric

Condition	RS	B	OPDR	SF	DF
Raw State (RS)	1	.895(S)	.573	.922(S)	.680
Boiling (B)	.895(S)	1	.878(S)	.998*(S)	.935(S)
Open Pan Dry Roasting (OPDR)	.573	.878(S)	1	.846(S)	.991(S)
Shallow Frying (SF)	.922(S)	.998*(S)	.846(S)	1	.911(S)
Deep Frying (DF)	.680	.935(S)	.991(S)	.911(S)	1

**.Correlation is highly significant at the 0.05 level (2-tailed)* Positive *S= Significant*

This table shows the correlation of protein content of *katla* with cooking methods. In 24 hours salt and turmeric preservation, there is significant positive correlation present between the raw state with boiling, shallow frying and deep frying. Boiling is also highly significant positively correlated with shallow frying along with open pan dry roasting and deep frying. Open pan dry roasting is significant positively correlated with shallow frying and deep frying, whereas shallow frying is positively correlated with deep frying. This table shows that there is a strong correlation present among the **raw state, boiling, open pan dry roasting, shallow frying and deep frying** in 24 hours salt and turmeric preservation.

Table no 5.12.2.2.7 Correlation of cooking methods in 48 hours preservation with salt and turmeric

Condition	RS	B	OPDR	SF	DF
Raw state (RS)	1	-.898(S)	-.618	-.798	-.618
Boiling (B)	-.898(S)	1	.901(S)	.450	.901(S)
Open Pan Dry Roasting (OPDR)	-.618	.901(S)	1	.019	1.000**(S)
Shallow Frying (SF)	-.798	.450	.019	1	.019
Deep Frying (DF)	-.618	.901(S)	1.000**(S)	.019	1

***.Correlation is highly significant at the 0.01 level (2-tailed)* Positive Negative *S= Significant*

This table shows the correlation of protein content of *katla* with cooking methods. In 48 hours salt and turmeric preservation, there is significant negative correlation present between the raw state and boiling. Boiling is significant positively correlated with open pan dry roasting and deep frying. Open pan dry roasting is perfect positively correlated with deep frying. This table indicates that there is a strong correlation present among the **raw state, boiling, open pan dry roasting and deep frying** in 48 hours salt and turmeric preservation.

Table no 5.12.2.2.8 Correlation of cooking methods in 14 days preservation with salt and turmeric

Condition	RS	B	OPDR	SF	DF
Raw State (RS)	1	-.277	.860(S)	.048	-.649
Boiling (B)	-.277	1	-.729	-.973(S)	.911(S)
Open Pan Dry Roasting (OPDR)	.860(S)	-.729	1	.551	-.947(S)
Shallow Frying (SF)	.048	-.973(S)	.551	1	-.790
Deep Frying (DF)	-.649	.911(S)	-.947(S)	-.790	1

Positive Negative *S= Significant*

This table shows the correlation of protein content of *katla* with cooking methods. In 14 days salt and turmeric preservation, there is significant positive correlation present between the raw state and open pan dry roasting. Boiling is significant positively correlated with deep frying and negatively correlated with shallow frying. Open pan dry roasting is negatively correlated with deep frying. This table indicates that there is a strong correlation present among the **raw state, boiling, open pan dry roasting, shallow frying and deep frying** in 14 days salt and turmeric preservation.

Table no 5.12.2.2.9 Correlation of cooking methods in 15 days preservation with salt and turmeric

Condition	RS	B	OPDR	SF	DF
Raw State (RS)	1	.843(S)	.102	-.828(S)	-.938(S)
Boiling (B)	.843(S)	1	.621	-1.000*(S)	-.977(S)
Open Pan Dry Roasting (OPDR)	.102	.621	1	-.642	-.439
Shallow Frying (SF)	-.828(S)	-1.000*(S)	-.642	1	.971(S)
Deep Frying (DF)	-.938(S)	-.977(S)	-.439	.971(S)	1

**.Correlation is highly significant at the 0.05 level (2-tailed)* Positive Negative *S= Significant*

This table shows the correlation of protein content of *katla* with cooking methods. In 15 days salt and turmeric preservation, there is significant negative correlation present between the raw state with shallow frying and deep frying and positive correlation present with boiling. Boiling is perfect negatively correlated with shallow frying and significant negatively correlated with deep frying. Shallow frying is significant positively correlated with deep frying. This table indicates that there is a strong correlation present among the **raw state, boiling, shallow frying and deep frying** in 15 days salt and turmeric preservation.

Table no 5.12.2.2.10 Correlation of cooking methods in 24 hours preservation with KMS

Condition	RS	B	OPDR	SF	DF
Raw State (RS)	1	.954(S)	.997*(S)	-.878(S)	.926(S)
Boiling (B)	.954(S)	1	.929(S)	-.981(S)	.771
Open Pan Dry Roasting (OPDR)	.997*(S)	.929(S)	1	-.839(S)	.952(S)
Shallow Frying (SF)	-.878(S)	-.981(S)	-.839(S)	1	-.633
Deep Frying (DF)	.926(S)	.771	.952(S)	-.633	1

**.Correlation is highly significant at the 0.05 level (2-tailed)* Positive Negative *S= Significant*

This table shows the correlation of protein content of *katla* with cooking methods. In 24 hours KMS preservation, there is significant negative correlation present between the raw state and shallow frying, and significant positive correlation present with boiling and deep frying, and highly significant positive correlation present with open pan dry roasting. Boiling is significant negatively correlated with shallow frying and positively correlated with open pan dry roasting. Again open pan dry roasting is positively correlated with deep frying and negatively correlated with shallow frying. This table indicates that there is a strong correlation present among the **raw state, boiling, open pan dry roasting, shallow frying and deep frying** in 24 hours KMS preservation.

Table no 5.12.2.2.11 Correlation of cooking methods in 48 hours preservation with KMS

Condition	RS	B	OPDR	SF	DF\
Raw State (RS)	1	.993(S)	.126	.986(S)	-.325
Boiling (B)	.993(S)	1	.239	.998*(S)	-.215
Open Pan Dry Roasting (OPDR)	.126	.239	1	.292	.897(S)
Shallow Frying (SF)	.986(S)	.998*(S)	.292	1	-.160
Deep Frying (DF)	-.325	-.215	.897(S)	-.160	1

**.Correlation is highly significant at the 0.05 level (2-tailed)* ▭ Positive *S= Significant*

This table shows the correlation of protein content of *katla* with cooking methods. In 48 hours KMS preservation, there is significant negative correlation present between the raw state with boiling and shallow frying. Boiling is highly significant positively correlated with shallow frying. Again open pan dry roasting is positively correlated with deep frying. This table indicates that there is a strong correlation present among the **raw state, boiling, open pan dry roasting, shallow frying and deep frying** in 48 hours KMS preservation.

Table no 5.12.2.2.12 Correlation of cooking methods in 14 days preservation with KMS

Condition	RS	B	OPDR	SF	DF
Raw State (RS)	1	.639	1.000**(S)	-.862(S)	.391
Boiling (B)	.639	1	.639	-.940(S)	.958(S)
Open Pan Dry Roasting (OPDR)	1.000**(S)	.639	1	-.862(S)	.391
Shallow Frying (SF)	-.862(S)	-.940(S)	-.862(S)	1	-.803(S)
Deep Frying (DF)	.391	.958(S)	.391	-.803(S)	1

***.Correlation is highly significant at the 0.01 level (2-tailed)* ▭ Positive ▭ Negative *S= Significant*

This table shows the correlation of protein content of *katla* with cooking methods. In 14 days KMS preservation, there is significant negative correlation present between the raw state and shallow frying and perfect positive correlation present with open pan dry roasting. Boiling is significant negatively correlated with shallow frying and positively correlated with deep frying. Again open pan dry roasting is negatively correlated with shallow frying, whereas shallow frying is also negatively correlated with deep frying. This table indicates that there is a strong correlation present among the **raw state, boiling, open pan dry roasting, shallow frying and deep frying** in 14 days KMS preservation.

Table no 5.12.2.2.13 Correlation of cooking methods in 15 days preservation with KMS

Condition	RS	B	OPDR	SF	DF
Raw State (RS)	1	-.648	-.334	.909(S)	.844(S)
Boiling (B)	-.648	1	-.502	-.906(S)	-.139
Open Pan Dry Roasting (OPDR)	-.334	-.502	1	.089	-.787
Shallow Frying (SF)	.909(S)	-.906(S)	.089	1	.545
Deep Frying (DF)	.844(S)	-.139	-.787	.545	1

**.Correlation is highly significant at the 0.05 level (2-tailed)* ▭ Positive ▭ Negative *S= Significant*

This table shows the correlation of protein content of *katla* with cooking methods. In 15 days KMS preservation, there is significant positive correlation present between the raw state with shallow frying and deep frying. Boiling is significant negatively correlated with shallow frying. This table indicates that there is a strong correlation present among the **raw state, boiling, shallow frying and deep frying** in 15 days KMS preservation.

Overall analysis reveals that the raw state is significant positively correlated with boiling in 48 hours KMS preservation, whereas perfect positively correlated with open pan dry roasting in 14 days KMS preservation, significant positively correlated with shallow frying and deep frying in 15 days KMS preservation and 24 hours control preservation without preservative respectively. Boiling is highly significant positively correlated with open pan dry roasting in 14 days control preservation without preservative, whereas highly significant negatively correlated with shallow frying in 15 days salt and turmeric preservation, and highly significant negatively correlated with deep frying in 24 hours control preservation without preservative. Open pan dry roasting is highly significant negatively correlated with shallow frying in fresh condition, and significant negatively correlated with deep frying in 15 days control preservation without preservative. Shallow frying is perfect negatively correlated with deep frying in 15 days control preservation without preservative. Most of the correlation of the protein content of *katla* is found in **15 days control preservation without preservative** with respect to different cooking conditions.

5.12.2.3 Fat

Table no 5.12.2.3.1 Correlation of cooking methods in fresh condition

Condition	RS	B	OPDR	SF	DF
Raw State (RS)	1	-.818(S)	.485	-.895(S)	.951(S)
Boiling (B)	-.818(S)	1	.107	.475	-.956(S)
Open Pan Dry Roasting (OPDR)	.485	.107	1	-.824(S)	.190
Shallow Frying (SF)	-.895(S)	.475	-.824(S)	1	-.713
Deep Frying (DF)	.951(S)	-.956(S)	.190	-.713	1

▭ Positive ▭ Negative *S= Significant*

This table shows the correlation of fat content of *katla* with cooking methods. In fresh condition, there is significant positive correlation present between the raw state and deep frying, and negative correlation present between the raw state with boiling and shallow frying. Boiling is significant negatively correlated with deep frying. Open pan dry roasting is negatively correlated with shallow frying. This table indicates that there is a strong correlation present among the **raw state, boiling, open pan dry roasting, shallow frying and deep frying** in fresh condition.

Table no 5.12.2.3.2 Correlation of cooking methods in 24 hours preservation without preservative

Condition	RS	B	OPDR	SF	DF
Raw State (RS)	1	.991(S)	-.668	-.412	-.524
Boiling (B)	.991(S)	1	-.763	-.533	-.636
Open Pan Dry Roasting (OPDR)	-.668	-.763	1	.953(S)	.984(S)
Shallow Frying (SF)	-.412	-.533	.953(S)	1	.992(S)
Deep Frying (DF)	-.524	-.636	.984(S)	.992(S)	1

Positive *S= Significant*

This table shows the correlation of fat content of *katla* with cooking methods. In 24 hours control preservation without preservative, there is significant positive correlation present between the raw state and boiling. Open pan dry roasting is significant positively correlated with shallow frying and deep frying, whereas shallow frying is significant positively correlated with deep frying. This table indicates that there is a strong correlation present among the **raw state, boiling, open pan dry roasting, shallow frying and deep frying** in 24 hours control preservation.

Table no 5.12.2.3.3 Correlation of cooking methods in 48 hours preservation without preservative

Condition	RS	B	OPDR	SF	DF
Raw state (RS)	1	-.569	-.500	-.980(S)	.989(S)
Boiling (B)	-.569	1	-.427	.721	-.444
Open Pan Dry Roasting (OPDR)	-.500	-.427	1	.319	-.621
Shallow Frying (SF)	-.980(S)	.721	.319	1	-.941(S)
Deep Frying (DF)	.989(S)	-.444	-.621	-.941(S)	1

Positive Negative *S= Significant*

This table shows the correlation of protein content of *katla* with cooking methods. In 48 hours control preservation, there is significant positive correlation present between the raw state and deep frying, and negative correlation present between the raw state and shallow frying. Shallow frying is significant negatively correlated with deep frying. This table indicates that there is a strong correlation present among the **raw state, shallow frying and deep frying** in 48 hours control preservation.

Table no 5.12.2.3.4 Correlation of cooking methods in 14 days preservation without preservative

Condition	RS	B	OPDR	SF	DF
Raw State (RS)	1	-.028	.272	-.500	.880(S)
Boiling (B)	-.028	1	-.970(S)	-.851(S)	-.500
Open Pan Dry Roasting (OPDR)	.272	-.970(S)	1	.697	.697
Shallow Frying (SF)	-.500	-.851(S)	.697	1	-.028
Deep Frying (DF)	.880(S)	-.500	.697	-.028	1

Positive Negative *S= Significant*

This table shows the correlation of fat content of *katla* with cooking methods. In 14 days control preservation without preservative, there is significant positive correlation present between the raw state and deep frying. Boiling is significant negatively correlated with open pan dry roasting and shallow frying. This table indicates that there is a strong correlation present among the **raw state, boiling, open pan dry roasting, shallow frying and deep frying** in 14 days control preservation.

Table no 5.12.2.3.5 Correlation of cooking methods in 15 days preservation without preservative

Condition	RS	B	OPDR	SF	DF
Raw State (RS)	1	.986(S)	-.733	.990(S)	-.099
Boiling (B)	.986(S)	1	-.836(S)	.952(S)	.068
Open Pan Dry Roasting (OPDR)	-.733	-.836(S)	1	-.629	-.604
Shallow Frying (SF)	.990(S)	.952(S)	-.629	1	-.240
Deep Frying (DF)	-.099	.068	-.604	-.240	1

Positive Negative *S= Significant*

This table shows the correlation of fat content of *katla* with cooking methods. In 15 days control preservation, there is significant positive correlation present between the raw state with boiling and shallow frying. Boiling is significant negatively correlated with open pan dry roasting and positively correlated with shallow frying. This table indicates that there is a strong correlation present among the **raw state, boiling, open pan dry roasting and shallow frying** in 15 days control preservation.

Table no 5.12.2.3.6 Correlation of cooking methods in 24 hours preservation with salt and turmeric

Condition	RS	B	OPDR	SF	DF
Raw State (RS)	1	-.226	-.471	.901(S)	.975(S)
Boiling (B)	-.226	1	-.752	-.627	-.438
Open Pan Dry Roasting (OPDR)	-.471	-.752	1	-.041	-.262
Shallow Frying (SF)	.901(S)	-.627	-.041	1	.975(S)
Deep Frying (DF)	.975(S)	-.438	-.262	.975(S)	1

Positive *S= Significant*

This table shows the correlation of fat content of *katla* with cooking methods. In 24 hours salt and turmeric preservation, there is significant positive correlation present between the raw state with shallow frying and deep frying. Shallow frying is significant positively correlated with deep frying. This table indicates that there is a strong correlation present among the **raw state, shallow frying and deep frying** in 24 hours salt and turmeric preservation.

Table no 5.12.2.3.7 Correlation of cooking methods in 48 hours preservation with salt and turmeric

Condition	RS	B	OPDR	SF	DF
Raw State (RS)	1	-.318	.452	-.873(S)	.979(S)
Boiling (B)	-.318	1	-.989(S)	-.185	-.503
Open Pan Dry Roasting (OPDR)	.452	-.989(S)	1	.041	.623
Shallow Frying (SF)	-.873(S)	-.185	.041	1	-.756
Deep Frying (DF)	.979(S)	-.503	.623	-.756	1

Positive Negative *S= Significant*

This table shows the correlation of fat content of *katla* with cooking methods. In 48 hours salt and turmeric preservation, there is significant positive correlation present between the raw state and deep frying, and negative correlation present between the raw state and shallow frying. Boiling is significant negatively correlated with open pan dry roasting. This table indicates that there is a strong correlation present among the **raw state, boiling, open pan dry roasting and deep frying** in 48 hours salt and turmeric preservation.

Table no 5.12.2.3.8 Correlation of cooking methods in 14 days preservation with salt and turmeric

Condition	RS	B	OPDR	SF	DF
Raw State (RS)	1	.993(S)	.610	-.581	.982(S)
Boiling (B)	.993(S)	1	.697	-.483	.954(S)
Open Pan Dry Roasting (OPDR)	.610	.697	1	.291	.449
Shallow Frying (SF)	-.581	-.483	.291	1	-.724
Deep Frying (DF)	.982(S)	.954(S)	.449	-.724	1

Positive *S= Significant*

This table shows the correlation of fat content of *katla* with cooking methods. In 14 days salt and turmeric preservation, there is significant positive correlation present between the raw state with boiling and deep frying. Boiling is significant positively correlated with deep frying. This table indicates that there is a strong correlation present among the **raw state, boiling and deep frying** in 14 days salt and turmeric preservation.

Table no 5.12.2.3.9 Correlation of cooking methods in 15 days preservation with salt and turmeric

Condition	RS	B	OPDR	SF	DF
Raw State (RS)	1	-.500	-.933(S)	-.721	-.466
Boiling (B)	-.500	1	.778	.961(S)	.999*(S)
Open Pan Dry Roasting (OPDR)	-.933(S)	.778	1	.922(S)	.753
Shallow Frying (SF)	-.721	.961(S)	.922(S)	1	.949(S)
Deep Frying (DF)	-.466	.999*(S)	.753	.949(S)	1

**.Correlation is highly significant at the 0.05 level (2-tailed)* Positive Negative *S= Significant*

This table shows the correlation of fat content of *katla* with cooking methods. In 15 days salt and turmeric preservation, there is significant negative correlation present between the raw state and open pan dry roasting. Boiling is significant positively correlated with shallow frying and highly significant positively correlated with deep frying. Open pan dry roasting is significant positively correlated with shallow frying, whereas shallow frying is positively correlated with deep frying. This table indicates that there is a strong correlation present among the **raw state, boiling, open pan dry roasting, shallow frying and deep frying** in 15 days salt and turmeric preservation.

Table no 5.12.2.3.10 Correlation of cooking methods in 24 hours preservation with KMS

Condition	RS	B	OPDR	SF	DF
Raw State (RS)	1	-.024	.906(S)	.000	.681
Boiling (B)	-.024	1	.401	1.000*(S)	-.749
Open Pan Dry Roasting (OPDR)	.906(S)	.401	1	.423	.307
Shallow Frying (SF)	.000	1.000*(S)	.423	1	-.732
Deep Frying (DF)	.681	-.749	.307	-.732	1

Positive *S= Significant*

This table shows the correlation of fat content of *katla* with cooking methods. In 24 hours KMS preservation, there is significant positive correlation present between the raw state with open pan dry roasting. Boiling is perfect positively correlated with shallow frying. This table indicates that there is a strong correlation present among the **raw state, boiling, open pan dry roasting and shallow frying** in 24 hours KMS preservation.

Table no 5.12.2.3.11 Correlation of cooking methods in 48 hours preservation with KMS

Condition	RS	B	OPDR	SF	DF
Raw State (RS)	1	.442	.975(S)	.947(S)	.941(S)
Boiling (B)	.442	1	.630	.130	.111
Open Pan Dry Roasting (OPDR)	.975(S)	.630	1	.852(S)	.842
Shallow Frying (SF)	.947(S)	.130	.852(S)	1	1.000*(S)
Deep Frying (DF)	.941(S)	.111	.842(S)	1.000*(S)	1

**.Correlation is highly significant at the 0.05 level (2-tailed)* Positive *S= Significant*

This table shows the correlation of fat content of *katla* with cooking methods. In 48 hours KMS preservation, there is significant positive correlation present between the raw state with open pan dry roasting, shallow frying and deep frying. Open pan dry roasting is positively correlated with shallow frying. Shallow frying is perfect positively correlated with deep frying. This table indicates that there is a strong correlation present between the **raw state, open pan dry roasting, shallow frying and deep frying** in 48 hours KMS preservation.

Table no 5.12.2.3.12 Correlation of cooking methods in 14 days preservation with KMS

Condition	RS	B	OPDR	SF	DF
Raw State (RS)	1	.676	.990(S)	.676	.686
Boiling (B)	.676	1	.564	1.000**(S)	1.000**(S)
Open Pan Dry Roasting (OPDR)	.990(S)	.564	1	.564	.575
Shallow Frying (SF)	.676	1.000**(S)	.564	1	1.000**(S)
Deep Frying (DF)	.686	1.000**(S)	.575	1.000**(S)	1

***.Correlation is highly significant at the 0.01 level (2-tailed)* Positive *S= Significant*

This table shows the correlation of fat content of *katla* with cooking methods. In 14 days KMS preservation, there is significant positive correlation present between the raw state and open pan dry roasting. Boiling is perfect positively correlated with both shallow frying and deep frying. Shallow frying is perfect positively correlated with deep frying. This table indicates that there is a strong correlation present among the **raw state, boiling, open pan dry roasting, shallow frying and deep frying** in 14 days KMS preservation.

Table no 5.12.2.3.13 Correlation of cooking methods in 15 days preservation with KMS

Condition	RS	B	OPDR	SF	DF
Raw State (RS)	1	.906(S)	-.388	.454	-.454
Boiling (B)	.906(S)	1	-.742	.034	-.034
Open Pan Dry Roasting (OPDR)	-.388	-.742	1	.645	-.645
Shallow Frying (SF)	.454	.034	.645	1	-1.000**(S)
Deep Frying (DF)	-.454	-.034	-.645	-1.000**(S)	1

***.Correlation is highly significant at the 0.01 level (2-tailed)* Positive Negative *S= Significant*

This table shows the correlation of fat content of *katla* with cooking methods. In 15 days KMS preservation, there is significant positive correlation present between the raw state and boiling. Shallow frying is perfect negatively correlated with deep frying. This table indicates that there is a strong correlation present between the **raw state and boiling and also between shallow frying and deep frying** in 15 days KMS preservation.

Overall analysis reveals that the raw state is significant positively correlated with boiling, open pan dry roasting, shallow frying and deep frying in 14 days salt-turmeric preservation and 48 hours KMS preservation, 15 days salt-turmeric preservation and 48 hours salt-turmeric preservation respectively. Boiling is significant negatively correlated with open pan dry roasting in 48 hours salt-turmeric preservation, whereas perfect positively correlated with shallow frying in 24 hours and 14 days KMS preservation, and again perfect positively correlated with deep frying in 14 days KMS preservation. Open pan dry roasting is significant positively correlated with shallow frying and deep frying in 24 hours control preservation without preservative. Shallow frying is perfect positively correlated with deep frying in 48 hours and 14 days KMS preservation, and perfect negatively correlated with deep frying in 15 days KMS preservation. Most of the correlation of the fat content of *katla* is found in **14 days KMS preservation** with respect to different cooking conditions.

5.12.2.4 Moisture

Table no 5.12.2.4.1 Correlation of cooking methods in fresh condition

Condition	RS	B	OPDR	SF	DF
Raw State (RS)	1	-.656	-.437	-.704	-.973(S)
Boiling (B)	-.656	1	-.392	-.073	.814(S)
Open Pan Dry Roasting (OPDR)	-.437	-.392	1	.946(S)	.216
Shallow Frying (SF)	-.704	-.073	.946(S)	1	.520
Deep Frying (DF)	-.973(S)	.814(S)	.216	.520	1

Positive Negative *S= Significant*

This table shows the correlation of moisture content of *katla* with cooking methods. In fresh condition, there is significant negative correlation present between the raw state and deep frying. Boiling is significant positively correlated with deep frying, whereas shallow frying is positively correlated with open pan dry roasting. This table indicates that there is a strong correlation present among the **raw state, boiling, open pan dry roasting, shallow frying and deep frying** in fresh condition.

Table no 5.12.2.4.2 Correlation of cooking methods in 24 hours preservation without preservative

Condition	RS	B	OPDR	SF	DF
Raw State (RS)	1	.955(S)	.329	-.241	-.313
Boiling (B)	.955(S)	1	.595	.058	-.017
Open Pan Dry Roasting (OPDR)	.329	.595	1	.837(S)	.794
Shallow Frying (SF)	-.241	.058	.837(S)	1	.997*(S)
Deep Frying (DF)	-.313	-.017	.794	.997*(S)	1

**.Correlation is highly significant at the 0.05 level (2-tailed)* Positive Negative *S= Significant*

This table shows the correlation of moisture content of *katla* with cooking methods. In 24 hours control preservation without preservative, there is significant positive correlation present between the raw state and boiling. Open pan dry roasting is significant positively correlated with shallow frying, whereas shallow frying is highly significant positively correlated with deep frying. This table indicates that there is a strong correlation present among the **raw state, boiling, open pan dry roasting, shallow frying and deep frying** in 24 hours control preservation.

Table no 5.12.2.4.3 Correlation of cooking methods in 48 hours preservation without preservative

Condition	RS	B	OPDR	SF	DF
Raw State (RS)	1	.890(S)	.807(S)	-.972(S)	.993(S)
Boiling (B)	.890(S)	1	.449	-.973(S)	.831(S)
Open Pan Dry Roasting (OPDR)	.807(S)	.449	1	-.644	.871(S)
Shallow Frying (SF)	-.972(S)	-.973(S)	-.644	1	-.937(S)
Deep Frying (DF)	.993(S)	.831(S)	.871(S)	-.937(S)	1

Positive Negative *S= Significant*

This table shows the correlation of moisture content of *katla* with cooking methods. In 48 hours control preservation without preservative, there is significant negative correlation present between the raw state and shallow frying, and positive correlation present between the raw state with boiling, open pan dry roasting and deep frying. Boiling is significant positively correlated with deep frying, but negatively correlated with shallow frying. Open pan dry roasting is positively correlated with deep frying, whereas shallow frying is negatively correlated with deep frying. This table indicates that there is a strong correlation present among the **raw state, boiling, open pan dry roasting, shallow frying and deep frying** in 48 hours control preservation.

Table no 5.12.2.4.4 Correlation of cooking methods in 14 days preservation without preservative

Condition	RS	B	OPDR	SF	DF
Raw State (RS)	1	.958(S)	-.653	-.713	.176
Boiling (B)	.958(S)	1	-.843(S)	-.884(S)	.450
Open Pan Dry Roasting (OPDR)	-.653	-.843(S)	1	.997(S)	-.860(S)
Shallow Frying (SF)	-.713	-.884(S)	.997(S)	1	-.815(S)
Deep Frying (DF)	.176	.450	-.860(S)	-.815(S)	1

Positive Negative *S= Significant*

This table shows the correlation of moisture content of *katla* with cooking methods. In 14 days control preservation without preservative, there is significant positive correlation present between the raw state and boiling. Boiling is negatively correlated with open pan dry roasting and shallow frying. Open pan dry roasting is positively correlated with shallow frying and negatively correlated with deep frying, whereas shallow frying is negatively correlated with deep frying. This table indicates that there is a strong correlation present among the **raw state, boiling, open pan dry roasting, shallow frying and deep frying** in 14 days control preservation.

Table no 5.12.2.4.5 Correlation of cooking methods in 15 days preservation without preservative

Condition	RS	B	OPDR	SF	DF
Raw State (RS)	1	.122	-.967(S)	-.444	.517
Boiling (B)	.122	1	-.371	.835(S)	-.787
Open Pan Dry Roasting (OPDR)	-.967(S)	-.371	1	.200	-.281
Shallow Frying (SF)	-.444	.835(S)	.200	1	-.997(S)
Deep Frying (DF)	.517	-.787	-.281	-.997(S)	1

Positive Negative *S= Significant*

This table shows the correlation of moisture content of *katla* with cooking methods. In 15 days control preservation without preservative, there is significant negative correlation present between the raw state and open pan dry roasting Boiling is significant positively correlated with shallow frying, whereas shallow frying is negatively correlated with deep frying. This table indicates that there is a strong correlation present among the **raw state, boiling, open pan dry roasting, shallow frying and deep frying** in 15 days control preservation.

Table no 5.12.2.4.6 Correlation of cooking methods in 24 hours preservation with salt and turmeric

Condition	RS	B	OPDR	SF	DF
Raw State (RS)	1	.072	.072	.115	-.718
Boiling (B)	.072	1	1.000**(S)	-.983(S)	-.746
Open Pan Dry Roasting (OPDR)	.072	1.000**(S)	1	-.983(S)	-.746
Shallow Frying (SF)	.115	-.983(S)	-.983(S)	1	.610
Deep Frying (DF)	-.718	-.746	-.746	.610	1

**.Correlation is highly significant at the 0.05 level (2-tailed)* ▭ Negative *S= Significant*

This table shows the correlation of moisture content of *katla* with cooking methods. In 24 hours salt and turmeric preservation, there is perfect negative correlation present between boiling and open pan dry roasting and significant positive correlation between the raw state and shallow frying. Open pan dry roasting is negatively correlated with shallow frying. This table indicates that there is a strong correlation present among **boiling, open pan dry roasting and shallow frying** in 24 hours salt and turmeric preservation.

Table no 5.12.2.4.7 Correlation of cooking methods in 48 hours preservation with salt and turmeric

Condition	RS	B	OPDR	SF	DF
Raw State (RS)	1	-.937(S)	.973(S)	.694	.989(S)
Boiling (B)	-.937(S)	1	-.831(S)	-.399	-.874(S)
Open Pan Dry Roasting (OPDR)	.973(S)	-.831(S)	1	.842(S)	.997(S)
Shallow Frying (SF)	.694	-.399	.842(S)	1	.794
Deep Frying (DF)	.989	-.874(S)	.997(S)	.794	1

▭ Positive ▭ Negative *S= Significant*

This table shows the correlation of moisture content of *katla* with cooking methods. In 48 hours salt and turmeric preservation, there is significant negative correlation present between the raw state and boiling, and positive correlation present between the raw state with open pan dry roasting and deep frying. Boiling is significant negatively correlated with open pan dry roasting and shallow frying. Open pan dry roasting is positively correlated with shallow frying and deep frying. This table indicates that there is a strong correlation present among the **raw state, boiling, open pan dry roasting, shallow frying and deep frying** in 48 hours salt and turmeric preservation.

Table no 5.12.2.4.8 Correlation of cooking methods in 14 days preservation with salt and turmeric

Condition	RS	B	OPDR	SF	DF
Raw State (RS)	1	.539	-.613	-1.000**(S)	.967(S)
Boiling (B)	.539	1	.335	-.526	.737
Open Pan Dry Roasting (OPDR)	-.613	.335	1	.625	-.391
Shallow Frying (SF)	-1.000**(S)	-.526	.625	1	-.963(S)
Deep Frying (DF)	.967(S)	.737	-.391	-.963(S)	1

***.Correlation is highly significant at the 0.01 level (2-tailed)* ▭ Positive ▭ Negative *S= Significant*

This table shows the correlation of moisture content of *katla* with cooking methods. In 14 days salt and turmeric preservation, there is perfect negative correlation present between the raw state and shallow frying, and significant positive correlation present between the raw state and deep frying. Shallow frying is negatively correlated with deep frying. This table indicates that there is a strong correlation present among the **raw state, shallow frying and deep frying** in 14 days salt and turmeric preservation.

Table no 5.12.2.4.9 Correlation of cooking methods in 15 days preservation with salt and turmeric

Condition	RS	B	OPDR	SF	DF
Raw State (RS)	1	-.624	-1.000**(S)	.996(S)	.174
Boiling (B)	-.624	1	.621	-.554	.661
Open Pan Dry Roasting (OPDR)	-1.000**(S)	.621	1	-.997(S)	-.178
Shallow Frying (SF)	.996(S)	-.554	-.997(S)	1	.259
Deep Frying (DF)	.174	.661	-.178	.259	1

***.Correlation is highly significant at the 0.01 level (2-tailed)* Positive Negative *S= Significant*

This table shows the correlation of moisture content of *katla* with cooking methods. In 15 days salt and turmeric preservation, there is perfect negative correlation present between the raw state and open pan dry roasting, and significant positive correlation present between the raw state and shallow frying. Open pan dry roasting is negatively correlated with shallow frying. This table indicates that there is a strong correlation present among the **raw state, open dry roasting and shallow frying** in 15 days salt and turmeric preservation.

Table no 5.12.2.4.10 Correlation of cooking methods in 24 hours preservation with KMS

Condition	RS	B	OPDR	SF	DF
Raw State (RS)	1	.742	-.927(S)	-.669	.887(S)
Boiling (B)	.742	1	-.437	-.995(S)	.348
Open Pan Dry Roasting (OPDR)	-.927(S)	-.437	1	.342	-.995(S)
Shallow Frying (SF)	-.669	-.995(S)	.342	1	-.250
Deep Frying (DF)	.887(S)	.348	-.995(S)	-.250	1

Positive Negative *S= Significant*

This table shows the correlation of moisture content of *katla* with cooking methods. In 24 hours KMS preservation, there is significant negative correlation present between the raw state and open pan dry roasting, and significant positive correlation present between the raw state and deep frying. Boiling is significant negatively correlated with shallow frying. Open pan dry roasting is negatively correlated with deep frying. This table indicates that there is a strong correlation present among the **raw state, boiling, open pan dry roasting, shallow frying and deep frying** in 24 hours KMS preservation.

Table no 5.12.2.4.11 Correlation of cooking methods in 48 hours preservation with KMS

Condition	RS	B	OPDR	SF	DF
Raw State (RS)	1	-.550	.815(S)	-.741	.536
Boiling (B)	-.550	1	-.932(S)	-.154	.411
Open Pan Dry Roasting (OPDR)	.815(S)	-.932(S)	1	-.215	-.052
Shallow Frying (SF)	-.741	-.154	-.215	1	-.964(S)
Deep Frying (DF)	.536	.411	-.052	-.964(S)	1

Positive Negative *S= Significant*

This table shows the correlation of moisture content of *katla* with cooking methods. In 48 hours KMS preservation, there is significant positive correlation present between the raw state and open pan dry roasting. Boiling is significant negatively correlated with open pan dry roasting. Shallow frying is negatively correlated with deep frying. This table indicates that there is a strong correlation present among the **raw state, boiling, open dry roasting, shallow frying and deep frying** in 48 hours KMS preservation.

Table no 5.12.2.4.12 Correlation of cooking methods in 14 days preservation with KMS

Condition	RS	B	OPDR	SF	DF
Raw State (RS)	1	.473	-.365	.978(S)	-.945(S)
Boiling (B)	.473	1	-.993(S)	.648	-.734
Open Pan Dry Roasting (OPDR)	-.365	-.993(S)	1	-.553	.648
Shallow Frying (SF)	.978(S)	.648	-.553	1	-.993(S)
Deep Frying (DF)	-.945(S)	-.734	.648	-.993(S)	1

Positive Negative *S= Significant*

This table shows the correlation of moisture content of *katla* with cooking methods. In 14 days KMS preservation, there is significant negative correlation present between the raw state and deep frying and significant positive correlation present between the raw state and shallow frying. Boiling is significant negatively correlated with open pan dry roasting. Shallow frying is significant negatively correlated with deep frying. This table indicates that there is a strong correlation present among the **raw state, boiling, open dry roasting, shallow frying and deep frying** in 14 days KMS preservation.

Table no 5.12.2.4.13 Correlation of cooking methods in 15 days preservation with KMS

Condition	RS	B	OPDR	SF	DF
Raw State (RS)	1	-.985(S)	-.997(S)	.388	.500
Boiling (B)	-.985(S)	1	.968(S)	-.539	-.344
Open Pan Dry Roasting (OPDR)	-.997(S)	.968(S)	1	-.311	-.568
Shallow Frying (SF)	.388	-.539	-.311	1	-.605
Deep Frying (DF)	.500	-.344	-.568	-.605	1

Positive Negative *S= Significant*

This table shows the correlation of moisture content of *katla* with cooking methods. In 15 days KMS preservation, there is significant negative correlation present between the raw state with open pan dry roasting and boiling. Boiling is significant positively correlated with open pan dry roasting. This table indicates that there is a strong correlation present among the **raw state, boiling, and open dry roasting** in 15 days KMS preservation.

Overall analysis reveals that the raw state is significant negatively correlated with boiling in 15 days KMS preservation, whereas perfect negatively correlated with open pan dry roasting and shallow frying in 15 days and 14 days salt-turmeric preservation respectively, and significant positively correlated with deep frying in 48 hours control preservation without preservative. Boiling is perfect positively correlated with open pan dry roasting in 24 hours salt-turmeric preservation, whereas significant negatively correlated with both shallow frying and deep frying in 24 hours KMS preservation and 48 hours salt-turmeric preservation respectively. Open pan dry roasting is highly significant negatively correlated with shallow frying in 15 days salt and turmeric and significant positively correlated with 14 days control preservation without preservative, and significant positively correlated with deep frying in 48 hours salt and turmeric preservation. Shallow frying is highly significant positively correlated with deep frying in 24 hours control preservation without preservative and significant negatively correlated with deep frying in 15 days control preservation without preservative. Most of the correlation of the moisture content of *katla* is found in **48 hours and 15 days salt and turmeric preservation** with respect to different cooking conditions.

5.12.2.5 Ash

Table no 5.12.2.5.1 Correlation of cooking methods in fresh condition

Condition	RS	B	OPDR	SF	DF
Raw State (RS)	1	.670	.909(S)	.275	.368
Boiling (B)	.670	1	.300	.898(S)	.937(S)
Open Pan Dry Roasting (OPDR)	.909(S)	.300	1	-.150	-.052
Shallow Frying (SF)	.275	.898(S)	-.150	1	.995(S)
Deep Frying (DF)	.368	.937(S)	-.052	.995(S)	1

Positive *S= Significant*

This table shows the correlation of ash content of *katla* with cooking methods. In fresh condition, there is significant positive correlation present between the raw state and open pan dry roasting. Boiling is significant positively correlated with shallow frying and deep frying, whereas shallow frying is significant positively correlated with deep frying. This table indicates that there is a strong correlation present among the **raw state, boiling, open dry roasting, shallow frying and deep frying** in fresh condition.

Table no 5.12.2.5.2 Correlation of cooking methods in 24 hours preservation without preservative

Condition	RS	B	OPDR	SF	DF
Raw State (RS)	1	-.992(S)	.978(S)	.110	.103
Boiling (B)	-.992(S)	1	-.943(S)	.017	.025
Open Pan Dry Roasting (OPDR)	.978(S)	-.943(S)	1	.316	.310
Shallow Frying (SF)	.110	.017	.316	1	1.000** (S)
Deep Frying (DF)	.103	.025	.310	1.000** (S)	1

***.Correlation is highly significant at the 0.01 level (2-tailed)* Positive Negative *S= Significant*

This table shows the correlation of ash content of *katla* with cooking methods. In 24 hours control preservation without preservative, there is significant negative correlation present between the raw state and boiling, and positive correlation present between the raw state and open pan dry roasting. Boiling is significant negatively correlated with open pan dry roasting. Shallow frying is perfect positively correlated with deep frying. This table indicates that there is a strong correlation present among the **raw state, boiling, open dry roasting, shallow frying and deep frying** in 24 hours control preservation.

Table no 5.12.2.5.3 Correlation of cooking methods in 48 hours preservation without preservative

Condition	RS	B	OPDR	SF	DF
Raw State (RS)	1	.989(S)	.974(S)	1.000**(S)	.991(S)
Boiling (B)	.989(S)	1	.930(S)	.991(S)	.961(S)
Open Pan Dry Roasting (OPDR)	.974(S)	.930(S)	1	.972(S)	.995(S)
Shallow Frying (SF)	1.000**(S)	.991(S)	.972(S)	1	.990(S)
Deep Frying (DF)	.991(S)	.961(S)	.995(S)	.990(S)	1

***.Correlation is highly significant at the 0.01 level (2-tailed)* ▭ Positive *S= Significant*

This table shows the correlation of ash content of *katla* with cooking methods. In 48 hours control preservation without preservative, there is significant positive correlation present between the raw state with boiling, open pan dry roasting and deep frying, and perfect positive correlation present between the raw state and shallow frying. Boiling is significant positively correlated with open pan dry roasting, shallow frying and deep frying, whereas shallow frying is also significant positively correlated with deep frying. This table indicates that there is a strong correlation present among the **raw state, boiling, open dry roasting, shallow frying and deep frying** in 48 hours control preservation.

Table no 5.12.2.5.4 Correlation of cooking methods in 14 days preservation without preservative

Condition	RS	B	OPDR	SF	DF
Raw State (RS)	1	.954(S)	-.189	.817(S)	.954(S)
Boiling (B)	.954(S)	1	-.475	.606	1.000**(S)
Open Pan Dry Roasting (OPDR)	-.189	-.475	1	.412	-.475
Shallow Frying (SF)	.817(S)	.606	.412	1	.606
Deep Frying (DF)	.954(S)	1.000**(S)	-.475	.606	1

***.Correlation is highly significant at the 0.01 level (2-tailed)* ▭ Positive *S= Significant*

This table shows the correlation of ash content of *katla* with cooking methods. In 14 days control preservation without preservative, there is significant positive correlation present between the raw state with boiling, shallow frying and deep frying. Boiling is perfect positively correlated with deep frying. This table indicates that there is a strong correlation present among the **raw state, boiling, shallow frying and deep frying** in 14 days control preservation.

Table no 5.12.2.5.5 Correlation of cooking methods in 15 days preservation without preservative

Condition	RS	B	OPDR	SF	DF
Raw State (RS)	1	-.934(S)	.961(S)	-.795	.332
Boiling (B)	-.934(S)	1	-.798	.960(S)	.027
Open Pan Dry Roasting (OPDR)	.961(S)	-.798	1	-.596	.581
Shallow Frying (SF)	-.795	.960(S)	-.596	1	.308
Deep Frying (DF)	.332	.027	.581	.308	1

▭ Positive ▭ Negative *S= Significant*

This table shows the correlation of ash content of *katla* with cooking methods. In 15 days control preservation without preservative, there is significant negative correlation present between the raw state and boiling, and positive correlation present between the raw state and open pan dry roasting. Boiling is significant positively correlated with shallow frying. This table indicates that there is a strong correlation present among the **raw state, boiling, open dry roasting and shallow frying** in 15 days control preservation.

Table no 5.12.2.5.6 Correlation of cooking methods in 24 hours preservation with salt and turmeric

Condition	RS	B	OPDR	SF	DF
Raw States (RS)	1	-.797	-.999*(S)	-.797	-.680
Boiling (B)	-.797	1	.771	1.000**(S)	.099
Open Pan Dry Roasting (OPDR)	-.999*(S)	.771	1	.771	.710
Shallow Frying (SF)	-.797	1.000**(S)	.771	1	.099
Deep Frying (DF)	-.680	.099	.710	.099	1

***.Correlation is highly significant at the 0.01 level (2-tailed)* Positive Negative *S= Significant*

This table shows the correlation of ash content of *katla* with cooking methods. In 24 hours salt and turmeric preservation, there is significant negative correlation present between the raw state and boiling. Boiling is perfect positively correlated with shallow frying. This table indicates that there is a strong correlation present between the **raw state and open dry roasting and also between boiling and shallow frying** in 24 hours salt and turmeric preservation.

Table no 5.12.2.5.7 Correlation of cooking methods in 48 hours preservation with salt and turmeric

Condition	RS	B	OPDR	SF	DF
Raw state (RS)	1	.737	-.997*(S)	.282	-.037
Boiling (B)	.737	1	-.684	.856(S)	.648
Open Pan Dry Roasting (OPDR)	-.997*(S)	-.684	1	-.209	.112
Shallow Frying (SF)	.282	.856(S)	-.209	1	.948(S)
Deep Frying (DF)	-.037	.648	.112	.948(S)	1

**.Correlation is highly significant at the 0.05 level (2-tailed)* Positive Negative *S= Significant*

This table shows the correlation of ash content of *katla* with cooking methods. In 48 hours salt and turmeric preservation, there is significant negative correlation present between the raw state and open pan dry roasting. Boiling is positively correlated with shallow frying. Again shallow frying is positively correlated with deep frying. This table indicates that there is a strong correlation present among the **raw state, boiling, open pan dry roasting, shallow frying and deep frying** in 48 hours salt and turmeric preservation.

Table no 5.12.2.5.8 Correlation of cooking methods in 14 days preservation with salt and turmeric

Condition	RS	B	OPDR	SF	DF
Raw State (RS)	1	.988(S)	.679	.894(S)	.666
Boiling (B)	.988(S)	1	.786	.812(S)	.540
Open Pan Dry Roasting (OPDR)	.679	.786	1	.277	-.096
Shallow Frying (SF)	.894(S)	.812(S)	.277	1	.930(S)
Deep Frying (DF)	.666	.540	-.096	.930(S)	1

Positive *S= Significant*

This table shows the correlation of ash content of *katla* with cooking methods. In 14 days salt and turmeric preservation, there is significant positive correlation present between the raw state with boiling and shallow frying. Boiling is positively correlated with shallow frying. Again shallow frying is positively correlated with deep frying. This table indicates that there is a strong correlation present among the **raw state, boiling, shallow frying and deep frying** in 14 days salt and turmeric preservation.

Table no 5.12.2.5.9 Correlation of cooking methods in 15 days preservation with salt and turmeric

Condition	RS	B	OPDR	SF	DF
Raw State (RS)	1	.882(S)	.749	.786	.786
Boiling (B)	.882(S)	1	.973(S)	.984(S)	.984(S)
Open Pan Dry Roasting (OPDR)	.749	.973(S)	1	.998*(S)	.998*(S)
Shallow Frying (SF)	.786	.984(S)	.998*(S)	1	1.000**(S)
Deep Frying (DF)	.786	.984(S)	.998*(S)	1.000**(S)	1

**.Correlation is highly significant at the 0.05 level (2-tailed)* Positive *S= Significant*
***.Correlation is highly significant at the 0.01 level (2-tailed)*

This table shows the correlation of ash content of *katla* with cooking methods. In 15 days salt and turmeric preservation, there is significant positive correlation present between the raw state and boiling. Boiling is positively correlated with open pan dry roasting, shallow frying and deep frying. Again open pan dry roasting is highly significant positively correlated with shallow frying and deep frying, whereas shallow frying is perfect positively correlated with deep frying. This table indicates that there is a strong correlation present among the **raw state, boiling, open dry roasting, shallow frying and deep frying** in 15 days salt and turmeric preservation.

Table no 5.12.2.5.10 Correlation of cooking methods in 24 hours preservation with KMS

Condition	RS	B	OPDR	SF	DF
Raw state (RS)	1	.893(S)	.893(S)	.948(S)	-.717
Boiling (B)	.893(S)	1	1.000**(S)	.990(S)	-.327
Open Pan Dry Roasting (OPDR)	.893(S)	1.000**(S)	1	.990(S)	-.327
Shallow Frying (SF)	.948(S)	.990(S)	.990(S)	1	-.459
Deep Frying (DF)	-.717	-.327	-.327	-.459	1

***.Correlation is highly significant at the 0.01 level (2-tailed)* Positive *S= Significant*

This table shows the correlation of ash content of *katla* with cooking methods. In 24 hours KMS preservation, there is significant positive correlation present between the raw state with boiling, open pan dry roasting and shallow frying. Boiling is significant positively correlated with shallow frying and perfect positively correlated with open pan dry roasting. Again open pan dry roasting is significant positively correlated with shallow frying. This table indicates that there is a strong correlation present among the **raw state, boiling, open dry roasting and shallow frying** in 24 hours KMS preservation.

Table no 5.12.2.5.11 Correlation of cooking methods in 48 hours preservation with KMS

Condition	RS	B	OPDR	SF	DF
Raw State (RS)	1	.999*(S)	-.404	-.404	-.999*(S)
Boiling (B)	.999*(S)	1	-.446	-.446	-.996(S)
Open Pan Dry Roasting (OPDR)	-.404	-.446	1	1.000**(S)	.364
Shallow Frying (SF)	-.404	-.446	1.000**(S)	1	.364
Deep Frying (DF)	-.999*(S)	-.996(S)	.364	.364	1

***.Correlation is highly significant at the 0.01 level (2-tailed)* Positive Negative *S= Significant*
**.Correlation is highly significant at the 0.05 level (2-tailed)*

This table shows the correlation of ash content of *katla* with cooking methods. In 48 hours KMS preservation, there is highly significant positive correlation present between the raw state and boiling, and highly negative correlation present between the raw state and deep frying. Boiling is also highly significant negatively correlated with deep frying, whereas open pan dry roasting is perfect positively correlated with shallow frying. This table indicates that there is a strong correlation present among the **raw state, boiling, open dry roasting, shallow frying and deep frying** in 48 hours KMS preservation.

Table no 5.12.2.5.12 Correlation of cooking methods in 14 days preservation with KMS

Condition	RS	B	OPDR	SF	DF
Raw State (RS)	1	.459	.327	.217	.839(S)
Boiling (B)	.459	1	.990(S)	.967(S)	-.099
Open Pan Dry Roasting (OPDR)	.327	.990(S)	1	.993(S)	-.240
Shallow Frying (SF)	.217	.967(S)	.993(S)	1	-.350
Deep Frying (DF)	.839(S)	-.099	-.240	-.350	1

Positive *S= Significant*

This table shows the correlation of ash content of *katla* with cooking methods. In 14 days KMS preservation, there is significant positive correlation present between the raw state and deep frying. Boiling is significant positively correlated with shallow frying and open pan dry roasting. Again open pan dry roasting is significant positively correlated with shallow frying. This table indicates that there is a strong correlation present among the **raw state, boiling, open dry roasting, shallow frying and deep frying** in 14 days KMS preservation.

Table no 5.12.2.5.13 Correlation of cooking methods in 15 days preservation with KMS

Condition	RS	B	OPDR	SF	DF
Raw State (RS)	1	.915(S)	-.569	.981(S)	.041
Boiling (B)	.915(S)	1	-.189	.976(S)	.441
Open Pan Dry Roasting (OPDR)	-.569	-.189	1	-.397	.798
Shallow Frying (SF)	.981(S)	.976(S)	-.397	1	.236
Deep Frying (DF)	.041	.441	.798	.236	1

Positive *S= Significant*

This table shows the correlation of ash content of *katla* with cooking methods. In 15 days KMS preservation, there is significant positive correlation present between the raw state with boiling and shallow frying. Boiling is significant positively correlated with shallow frying. This table indicates that there is a strong correlation present among the **raw state, boiling and shallow frying** in 15 days KMS preservation.

Overall analysis reveals that the raw state is highly significant positively correlated with boiling in 48 hours KMS preservation, whereas highly significant negatively correlated with open pan dry roasting and deep frying in 24 hours salt-turmeric preservation and 48 hours KMS preservation respectively, and perfect positively correlated with shallow frying in 48 hours control preservation without preservative. Boiling is perfect positively correlated with open pan dry roasting, shallow frying and deep frying in 24 hours KMS preservation, 24 hours salt-turmeric preservation and in 14 days control preservation without preservative respectively. Open pan dry roasting is significant positively correlated with shallow frying and deep frying in 14 days KMS preservation and 48 hours control preservation without preservative respectively. Shallow frying is perfect positively correlated with deep frying in 15 days salt-turmeric preservation and 24 hours control preservation without preservative. Most of the correlation of the ash content of *katla* is found in **24 hours salt-turmeric preservation, 48 hours KMS preservation and 48 hours control preservation without preservative** with respect to different cooking conditions.

5.12.2.6 Calcium

Table no 5.12.2.6.1 Correlation of cooking methods in fresh condition

Condition	RS	B	OPDR	SF	DF
Raw State (RS)	1	1.000**(S)	.976(S)	.803(S)	.993(S)
Boiling (B)	1.000**(S)	1	.976(S)	.803(S)	.993(S)
Open Pan Dry Roasting (OPDR)	.976(S)	.976(S)	1	.655	.945(S)
Shallow Frying (SF)	.803(S)	.803(S)	.655	1	.866(S)
Deep Frying (DF)	.993(S)	.993(S)	.945(S)	.866(S)	1

***.Correlation is highly significant at the 0.01 level (2-tailed)* Positive *S= Significant*

This table shows the correlation of calcium content of *katla* with cooking methods. In fresh condition, there is perfect positive correlation present between the raw state and boiling, and significant positive correlation present between the raw state with open pan dry roasting, shallow frying and deep frying. Boiling is significant positively correlated with shallow frying, deep frying and open pan dry roasting. Again open pan dry roasting is significant positively correlated with shallow frying, whereas shallow frying is significant positively correlated with deep frying. This table indicates that there is a strong correlation present among the **raw state, boiling, open dry roasting, shallow frying and deep frying** in fresh condition.

Table no 5.12.2.6.2 Correlation of cooking methods in 24 hours preservation without preservative

Condition	RS	B	OPDR	SF	DF
Raw State (RS)	1	.996(S)	.954(S)	.954(S)	.929(S)
Boiling (B)	.996(S)	1	.923(S)	.923(S)	.891(S)
Open Pan Dry Roasting (OPDR)	.954(S)	.923(S)	1	1.000**(S)	.997*(S)
Shallow Frying (SF)	.954(S)	.923(S)	1.000**(S)	1	.997*(S)
Deep Frying (DF)	.929(S)	.891(S)	.997*(S)	.997*(S)	1

***.Correlation is highly significant at the 0.01 level (2-tailed)* Positive *S= Significant*

**.Correlation is highly significant at the 0.05 level (2-tailed)*

This table shows the correlation of calcium content of *katla* with cooking methods. In 24 hours control preservation without preservative, there is significant positive correlation present between the raw state and boiling, open pan dry roasting, shallow frying and deep frying. Boiling is significant positively correlated with shallow frying, deep frying and open pan dry roasting. Again open pan dry roasting is perfect positively correlated with shallow frying and highly significant positively correlated with deep frying, whereas shallow frying is highly significant positively correlated with deep frying. This table indicates that there is a strong correlation present among the **raw state, boiling, open dry roasting, shallow frying and deep frying** in 24 hours control preservation.

Table no 5.12.2.6.3 Correlation of cooking methods in 48 hours preservation without preservative

Condition	RS	B	OPDR	SF	DF
Raw State (RS)	1	.901(S)	.901(S)	1.000**(S)	1.000**(S)
Boiling (B)	.901(S)	1	1.000**(S)	.901(S)	.901(S)
Open Pan Dry Roasting (OPDR)	.901(S)	1.000**(S)	1	.901(S)	.901(S)
Shallow Frying (SF)	1.000**(S)	.901(S)	.901(S)	1	1.000**(S)
Deep Frying (DF)	1.000**(S)	.901(S)	.901(S)	1.000**(S)	1

***.Correlation is highly significant at the 0.01 level (2-tailed)* Positive *S= Significant*

This table shows the correlation of calcium content of *katla* with cooking methods. In 48 hours control preservation without preservative, there is significant positive correlation present between the raw state with boiling and open pan dry roasting, and perfect positive correlation present between the raw state with shallow frying and deep frying. Boiling is significant positively correlated with shallow frying, deep frying and perfect positively correlated with open pan dry roasting. Again open pan dry roasting is significant positively correlated with shallow frying and deep frying, whereas shallow frying is perfect significant positively correlated with deep frying. This table indicates that there is a strong correlation present among the **raw state, boiling, open dry roasting, shallow frying and deep frying** in 48 hours control preservation.

Table no 5.12.2.6.4 Correlation of cooking methods in 14 days preservation without preservative

Condition	RS	B	OPDR	SF	DF
Raw State (RS)	1	.993(S)	.997*(S)	.886(S)	.993(S)
Boiling (B)	.993(S)	1	.982(S)	.933(S)	1.000**(S)
Open Pan Dry Roasting (OPDR)	.997*(S)	.982(S)	1	.849(S)	.982(S)
Shallow Frying (SF)	.886(S)	.933(S)	.849(S)	1	.933(S)
Deep Frying (DF)	.993(S)	1.000**(S)	.982(S)	.933(S)	1

***.Correlation is highly significant at the 0.01 level (2-tailed)* ▭ Positive *S= Significant*

**.Correlation is highly significant at the 0.05 level (2-tailed)*

This table shows the correlation of calcium content of *katla* with cooking methods. In 14 days control preservation without preservative, there is significant positive correlation present between the raw state with boiling, shallow frying and deep frying and highly significant positive correlation present with open pan dry roasting. Boiling is significant positively correlated with shallow frying, open pan dry roasting and perfect positively correlated with deep frying. Again open pan dry roasting is significant positively correlated with shallow frying and deep frying, whereas shallow frying is significant positively correlated with deep frying. This table indicates that there is a strong correlation present among the **raw state, boiling, open dry roasting, shallow frying and deep frying** in 14 days control preservation.

Table no 5.12.2.6.5 Correlation of cooking methods in 15 days preservation without preservative

Condition	RS	B	OPDR	SF	DF
Raw state (RS)	1	.327	.778	.993(S)	.189
Boiling (B)	.327	1	.849(S)	.434	.990(S)
Open Pan Dry Roasting (OPDR)	.778	.849(S)	1	.845(S)	.764
Shallow Frying (SF)	.993(S)	.434	.845(S)	1	.300
Deep Frying (DF)	.189	.990(S)	.764	.300	1

▭ Positive *S= Significant*

This table shows the correlation of calcium content of *katla* with cooking methods. In 15 days control preservation without preservative, there is significant positive correlation present between the raw state and shallow frying. Boiling is significant positively correlated with deep frying and open pan dry roasting. Again open pan dry roasting is significant positively correlated with shallow frying. This table indicates that there is a strong correlation present among the **raw state, boiling, open dry roasting, shallow frying and deep frying** in 15 days control preservation.

Table no 5.12.2.6.6 Correlation of cooking methods in 24 hours preservation with salt and turmeric

Condition	RS	B	OPDR	SF	DF
Raw State (RS)	1	-.596	1.000**(S)	-.997*	.993(S)
Boiling (B)	-.596	1	-.596	.655	-.500
Open Pan Dry Roasting (OPDR)	1.000**(S)	-.596	1	-.997*(S)	.993(S)
Shallow Frying (SF)	-.997*(S)	.655	-.997*(S)	1	-.982(S)
Deep Frying (DF)	.993(S)	-.500	.993(S)	-.982(S)	1

***.Correlation is highly significant at the 0.01 level (2-tailed)* Positive Negative *S= Significant*
**.Correlation is highly significant at the 0.05 level (2-tailed)*

This table shows the correlation of calcium content of *katla* with cooking methods. In 24 hours salt and turmeric preservation, there is significant positive correlation present between the raw state and deep frying and perfect positive correlation present with open pan dry roasting, and highly significant negative correlation present between the raw state and shallow frying. Again open pan dry roasting is significant positively correlated with deep frying and highly significant negative correlation present with shallow frying, whereas shallow frying is significant negatively correlated with deep frying. This table indicates that there is a strong correlation present among the **raw state, open dry roasting, shallow frying and deep frying** in 24 hours salt and turmeric preservation.

Table no 5.12.2.6.7 Correlation of cooking methods in 48 hours preservation with salt and turmeric

Condition	RS	B	OPDR	SF	DF
Raw state (RS)	1	-.371	.705	.459	-.524
Boiling (B)	-.371	1	.397	.655	-.596
Open Pan Dry Roasting (OPDR)	.705	.397	1	.954(S)	-.974(S)
Shallow Frying (SF)	.459	.655	.954(S)	1	-.997*(S)
Deep Frying (DF)	-.524	-.596	-.974(S)	-.997*(S)	1

**.Correlation is highly significant at the 0.05 level (2-tailed)* Positive Negative *S= Significant*

This table shows the correlation of calcium content of *katla* with cooking methods. In 48 hours salt and turmeric preservation, there is significant positive correlation present between open pan dry roasting and shallow frying, and negative correlation present between boiling and deep frying. Again shallow frying is highly significant negatively correlated with deep frying. This table indicates that there is a strong correlation present among **open dry roasting, shallow frying and deep frying** in 48 hours salt and turmeric preservation.

Table no 5.12.2.6.8 Correlation of cooking methods in 14 days preservation with salt and turmeric

Condition	RS	B	OPDR	SF	DF
Raw State (RS)	1	-.500	.684	-.997*(S)	-.397
Boiling (B)	-.500	1	.289	.434	.993(S)
Open Pan Dry Roasting (OPDR)	.684	.289	1	-.737	.397
Shallow Frying (SF)	-.997*(S)	.434	-.737	1	.327
Deep Frying (DF)	-.397	.993(S)	.397	.327	1

**.Correlation is highly significant at the 0.05 level (2-tailed)* Positive Negative *S= Significant*

This table shows the correlation of calcium content of *katla* with cooking methods. In 14 days salt and turmeric preservation, there is highly significant negative correlation present between the raw state and shallow frying. Again boiling is significant positively correlated with deep frying. This table indicates that there is a strong correlation present among the **raw state, boiling, shallow frying and deep frying** in 14 days salt and turmeric preservation.

Table no 5.12.2.6.9 Correlation of cooking methods in 15 days preservation with salt and turmeric

Condition	R	B	OPDR	SF	DF
Raw State (RS)	1	.993(S)	.993(S)	1.000**(S)	.986(S)
Boiling (B)	.993(S)	1	1.000**(S)	.993(S)	.961(S)
Open Pan Dry Roasting (OPDR)	.993(S)	1.000**(S)	1	.993(S)	.961(S)
Shallow Frying (SF)	1.000**(S)	.993(S)	.993(S)	1	.986(S)
Deep Frying (DF)	.986(S)	.961(S)	.961(S)	.986(S)	1

***.Correlation is highly significant at the 0.01 level (2-tailed)* ▭ Positive *S= Significant*

This table shows the correlation of calcium content of *katla* with cooking methods. In 15 days salt and turmeric preservation, there is significant positive correlation present between the raw state with open pan dry roasting, boiling, deep frying, and perfect positive correlation present between the raw state and shallow frying. Again boiling is significant positively correlated with shallow frying and deep frying and perfect positively correlated with open pan dry roasting. Open pan dry roasting is significant positively correlated with shallow frying and deep frying, whereas shallow frying is significant positively correlated with deep frying. This table indicates that there is a strong correlation present among the **raw state, boiling, open pan dry roasting, shallow frying and deep frying** in 15 days salt and turmeric preservation.

Table no 5.12.2.6.10 Correlation of cooking methods in 24 hours preservation with KMS

Condition	RS	B	OPDR	SF	DF
Raw State (RS)	1	.993(S)	.993(S)	1.000**(S)	1.000**(S)
Boiling (B)	.993(S)	1	1.000**(S)	.993(S)	.993(S)
Open Pan Dry Roasting (OPDR)	.993(S)	1.000**(S)	1	.993(S)	.993(S)
Shallow Frying (SF)	1.000**(S)	.993(S)	.993(S)	1	1.000**(S)
Deep Frying (DF)	1.000**(S)	.993(S)	.993(S)	1.000**(S)	1

***.Correlation is highly significant at the 0.01 level (2-tailed)* ▭ Positive *S= Significant*

This table shows the correlation of calcium content of *katla* with cooking methods. In 24 hours KMS preservation, there is significant positive correlation present between the raw state with open pan dry roasting, boiling and perfect positive correlation present between the raw state with shallow frying and deep frying. Again boiling is significant positively correlated with shallow frying and deep frying and perfect positively correlated with open pan dry roasting. Open pan dry roasting is significant positively correlated with shallow frying rand deep frying, whereas shallow frying is perfect positively correlated with deep frying. This table indicates that there is a strong correlation present among the **raw state, boiling, open pan dry roasting, shallow frying and deep frying** in 24 hours KMS preservation.

Table no 5.12.2.6.11 Correlation of cooking methods in 48 hours preservation with KMS

Condition	RS	B	OPDR	SF	DF
Raw state (RS)	1	.397	.993(S)	.993(S)	.993(S)
Boiling (B)	.397	1	.500	.500	.500
Open Pan Dry Roasting (OPDR)	.993(S)	.500	1	1.000**(S)	1.000**(S)
Shallow Frying (SF)	.993(S)	.500	1.000**(S)	1	1.000**(S)
Deep Frying (DF)	.993(S)	.500	1.000**(S)	1.000**(S)	1

***.Correlation is highly significant at the 0.01 level (2-tailed)* ▭ Positive *S= Significant*

This table shows the correlation of calcium content of *katla* with cooking methods. In 48 hours KMS preservation, there is significant positive correlation present between the raw state with open pan dry roasting, shallow frying and deep frying. Open pan dry roasting is perfect positively correlated with shallow frying and deep frying, whereas shallow frying is perfect positively correlated with deep frying. This table indicates that there is a strong correlation present among the **raw state, open pan dry roasting, shallow frying and deep frying** in 48 hours KMS preservation.

Table no 5.12.2.6.12 Correlation of cooking methods in 14 days preservation with KMS

Condition	RS	B	OPDR	SF	DF
Raw State (RS)	1	-.500	.961(S)	.327	1.000**(S)
Boiling (B)	-.500	1	-.240	.655	-.500
Open Pan Dry Roasting (OPDR)	.961(S)	-.240	1	.577	.961(S)
Shallow Frying (SF)	.327	.655	.577	1	.327
Deep Frying (DF)	1.000**(S)	-.500	.961(S)	.327	1

***.Correlation is highly significant at the 0.01 level (2-tailed)* ▭ Positive *S= Significant*

This table shows the correlation of calcium content of *katla* with cooking methods. In 14 days KMS preservation, there is significant positive correlation present between the raw state and open pan dry roasting, and perfect positive correlation present between the raw state with deep frying. Open pan dry roasting is significant positively correlated with deep frying. This table indicates that there is a strong correlation present among the **raw state, open pan dry roasting and deep frying** in 14 days KMS preservation.

Table no 5.12.2.6.13 Correlation of cooking methods in 15 days preservation with KMS

Condition	RS	B	OPDR	SF	DF
Raw State (RS)	1	.982(S)	.929(S)	1.000**(S)	.945(S)
Boiling (B)	.982(S)	1	.982(S)	.982(S)	.866(S)
Open Pan Dry Roasting (OPDR)	.929(S)	.982(S)	1	.929(S)	.756
Shallow Frying (SF)	1.000**(S)	.982(S)	.929(S)	1	.945(S)
Deep Frying (DF)	.945(S)	.866(S)	.756	.945(S)	1

***.Correlation is highly significant at the 0.01 level (2-tailed)* ▭ Positive *S= Significant*

This table shows the correlation of calcium content of *katla* with cooking methods. In 14 days KMS preservation, there is significant positive correlation present between the raw state with boiling, open pan dry roasting and deep frying, and perfect positive correlation present between the raw state with shallow frying. Again boiling is significant positively correlated with open pan dry roasting, shallow frying and deep frying. Open pan dry roasting is significant positively correlated with shallow frying, whereas shallow frying is significant positively correlated with deep frying. This table indicates that there is a strong correlation present among the **raw state, boiling, open pan dry roasting, shallow and deep frying** in 15 days KMS preservation.

Overall analysis reveals that the raw state is perfect positively correlated with boiling and open pan dry roasting in fresh condition and 24 hours salt-turmeric respectively, whereas perfect positively correlated with shallow frying in 48 hours control preservation without preservative, 24 hours and 15 days salt-turmeric preservation and 24 hours KMS preservation, and also perfect positively correlated with deep frying in 48 hours control preservation without preservative, 24 hours and 14 days KMS preservation. Boiling is perfect positively correlated with open pan dry roasting in 48 hours control preservation without preservative, 15 days salt-turmeric preservation and 24 hours KMS preservation, whereas significant positively correlated with shallow frying in 15 days salt and turmeric preservation and 24 hours KMS preservation, and perfect positively correlated with deep frying in 48 hours control preservation without preservative. Open pan dry roasting is perfect positively correlated with shallow frying in 24 hours control preservation without preservative and 48 hours KMS preservation, and again perfect positively correlated with deep frying in 48 hours KMS preservation. Shallow frying is perfect positively correlated with deep frying in 48 hours control preservation without preservative, 24 hours and 48 hours KMS preservation. Most of the correlation of the calcium content of *katla* is found in **24 hours KMS preservation** with respect to different cooking conditions.

5.12.2.7 Iron

Table no 5.12.2.7.1 Correlation of cooking methods in fresh condition

Condition	RS	B	OPDR	SF	DF
Raw State (RS)	1	-.581	-.778	-.311	.991(S)
Boiling (B)	-.581	1	.963(S)	.954(S)	-.683
Open Pan Dry Roasting (OPDR)	-.778	.963(S)	1	.840(S)	-.854(S)
Shallow Frying (SF)	-.311	.954(S)	.840(S)	1	-.434
Deep Frying (DF)	.991(S)	-.683	-.854(S)	-.434	1

Positive Negative *S= Significant*

This table shows the correlation of iron content of *katla* with cooking methods. In fresh condition, there is significant positive correlation present between the raw state and deep frying. Boiling is significant positively correlated with open pan dry roasting and shallow frying. Open pan dry roasting is significant positively correlated with shallow frying and negatively correlated with deep frying. This table indicates that there is a strong correlation present among the **raw state, boiling, open pan dry roasting, shallow frying and deep frying** in fresh condition.

Table no 5.12.2.7.2 Correlation of cooking methods in 24 hours preservation with preservative

Condition	RS	B	OPDR	SF	DF
Raw State (RS)	1	-.441	-.704	.572	-.798
Boiling (B)	-.441	1	-.327	.484	-.189
Open Pan Dry Roasting (OPDR)	-.704	-.327	1	-.985(S)	.990(S)
Shallow Frying (SF)	.572	.484	-.985(S)	1	-.951(S)
Deep Frying (DF)	-.798	-.189	.990(S)	-.951(S)	1

Positive Negative *S= Significant*

This table shows the correlation of iron content of *katla* with cooking methods. In 24 hours control preservation without preservative, there is significant positive correlation present between open pan dry roasting and deep frying, and significant negative correlation present between open pan dry roasting and shallow frying. Shallow frying is significant negatively correlated with deep frying. This table indicates that there is a strong correlation present among **open pan dry roasting, shallow frying and deep frying** in 24 hours control preservation.

Table no 5.12.2.7.3 Correlation of cooking methods in 48 hours preservation with preservative

Condition	RS	B	OPDR	SF	DF
Raw State (RS)	1	.113	-.890(S)	1.000**(S)	.327
Boiling (B)	.113	1	.353	.126	.976(S)
Open Pan Dry Roasting (OPDR)	-.890(S)	.353	1	-.884(S)	.140
Shallow Frying (SF)	1.000**(S)	.126	-.884(S)	1	.339
Deep Frying (DF)	.327	.976(S)	.140	.339	1

***.Correlation is highly significant at the 0.01 level (2-tailed)* Positive Negative *S= Significant*

This table shows the correlation of iron content of *katla* with cooking methods. In 48 hours control preservation without preservative, there is perfect positive correlation present between the raw state and shallow frying and significant negative correlation present with open pan dry roasting. Boiling is significant positively correlated with deep frying. Open pan dry roasting is significant negatively correlated with shallow frying. This table shows that there is a strong correlation present among the **raw state, boiling, open pan dry roasting, shallow frying and deep frying** in 48 hours control preservation.

Table no 5.12.2.7.4 Correlation of cooking methods in 14 days preservation with preservative

Condition	RS	B	OPDR	SF	DF
Raw State (R)	1	-.863(S)	-.458	-.516	.308
Boiling (B)	-.863(S)	1	.844(S)	.013	.215
Open Pan Dry Roasting (OPDR)	-.458	.844(S)	1	-.524	.705
Shallow Frying (SF)	-.516	.013	-.524	1	-.974(S)
Deep Frying (DF)	.308	.215	.705	-.974(S)	1

Positive Negative *S= Significant*

This table shows the correlation of iron content of *katla* with cooking methods. In 14 days control preservation without preservative, there is significant negative correlation present between the raw state and boiling. Boiling is significant positively correlated with open pan dry roasting. Shallow frying is significant negatively correlated with deep frying. This table indicates that there is a strong correlation present among the **raw state, boiling, open pan dry roasting, shallow frying and deep frying** in 14 days control preservation.

Table no 5.12.2.7.5 Correlation of cooking methods in 15 days preservation with preservative

Condition	RS	B	OPDR	SF	DF
Raw State (RS)	1	1.000**(S)	.286	.500	.500
Boiling (B)	1.000**(S)	1	.286	.500	.500
Open Pan Dry Roasting (OPDR)	.286	.286	1	.973(S)	.973(S)
Shallow Frying (SF)	.500	.500	.973(S)	1	1.000**(S)
Deep Frying (DF)	.500	.500	.973(S)	1.000**(S)	1

***.Correlation is highly significant at the 0.01 level (2-tailed)* Positive *S= Significant*

This table shows the correlation of iron content of *katla* with cooking methods. In 15 days control preservation without preservative, there is perfect positive correlation present between the raw state and boiling. Open pan dry roasting is significant positively correlated with shallow frying and deep frying. Shallow frying is perfect positively correlated with deep frying. This table indicates that there is a strong correlation present among the **raw state, boiling, open pan dry roasting, shallow frying and deep frying** in 15 days control preservation.

Table no 5.12.2.7.6 Correlation of cooking methods in 24 hours preservation with salt and turmeric

Condition	RS	B	OPDR	SF	DF
Raw State (RS)	1	.996(S)	.655	-.249	-.327
Boiling (B)	.996(S)	1	.721	-.160	.996(S)
Open Pan Dry Roasting (OPDR)	.655	.721	1	.569	.500
Shallow Frying (SF)	-.249	-.160	.569	1	.997(S)
Deep Frying (DF)	-.327	-.240	.500	.997(S)	1

Positive *S= Significant*

This table shows the correlation of iron content of *katla* with cooking methods. In 24 hours salt and turmeric preservation, there is positive correlation present between the raw state and boiling. Boiling is significant positively correlated with deep frying. Shallow frying is perfect positively correlated with deep frying. This table indicates that there is a strong correlation present among the **raw state, boiling, shallow frying and deep frying** in 24 hours salt and turmeric preservation.

Table no 5.12.2.7.7 Correlation of cooking methods in 48 hours preservation with salt and turmeric

Condition	RS	B	OPDR	SF	DF
Raw state (RS)	1	1.000**(S)	-.397	-.397	.596
Boiling (B)	1.000**(S)	1	-.397	-.397	.596
Open Pan Dry Roasting (OPDR)	-.397	-.397	1	1.000**(S)	.500
Shallow Frying (SF)	-.397	-.397	1.000**(S)	1	.500
Deep Frying (DF)	.596	.596	.500	.500	1

***.Correlation is highly significant at the 0.01 level (2-tailed)* Positive *S= Significant*

This table shows the correlation of iron content of *katla* with cooking methods. In 48 hours salt and turmeric preservation, there is perfect positive correlation present between the raw state and boiling. Open pan dry roasting is perfect positively correlated with shallow frying. This table indicates that there is a strong correlation present between the **raw state and boiling and also between shallow frying and deep frying** in 48 hours salt and turmeric preservation.

Table no 5.12.2.7.8 Correlation of cooking methods in 14 days preservation with salt and turmeric

Condition	RS	B	OPDR	SF	DF
Raw State (RS)	1	.967(S)	.967(S)	.786	-1.000*(S)
Boiling (B)	.967(S)	1	1.000**(S)	.918(S)	-.974(S)
Open Pan Dry Roasting (OPDR)	.967(S)	1.000**(S)	1	.918(S)	-.974(S)
Shallow Frying (SF)	.786	.918(S)	.918(S)	1	-.803(S)
Deep Frying (DF)	-1.000*(S)	-.974(S)	-.974(S)	-.803(S)	1

***.Correlation is highly significant at the 0.01 level (2-tailed)* ▭ Positive *S= Significant*
**.Correlation is highly significant at the 0.05 level (2-tailed)*

This table shows the correlation of iron content of *katla* with cooking methods. In 14 days salt and turmeric preservation, there is significant positive correlation present between the raw state with boiling, open pan dry roasting and perfect negative correlation present with deep frying. Boiling is perfect positively correlated with open pan dry roasting and significant positively correlated with shallow frying and significant negatively correlated with deep frying. Open pan dry roasting is significant positively correlated with shallow frying and significant negatively correlated with deep frying, whereas shallow frying is significant negatively correlated with deep frying. This table indicates that there is a strong correlation present among the **raw state, boiling, open pan dry roasting, shallow frying and deep frying** in 14 days salt and turmeric preservation.

Table no 5.12.2.7.9 Correlation of cooking methods in 15 days preservation with salt and turmeric

Condition	RS	B	OPDR	SF	DF
Raw State (RS)	1	-.705	1.000**(S)	-.524	-.262
Boiling (B)	-.705	1	-.705	.974(S)	-.500
Open Pan Dry Roasting (OPDR)	1.000**(S)	-.705	1	-.524	-.262
Shallow Frying (SF)	-.524	.974(S)	-.524	1	-.684
Deep Frying (DF)	-.262	-.500	-.262	-.684	1

***.Correlation is highly significant at the 0.01 level (2-tailed)* ▭ Positive *S= Significant*

This table shows the correlation of iron content of *katla* with cooking methods. In 15 days salt and turmeric preservation, there is perfect positive correlation present between the raw state and open pan dry roasting. Boiling is significant positively correlated with shallow frying. This table indicates that there is a strong correlation present between the **raw state and open pan dry roasting and also between boiling and shallow frying** in 15 days salt and turmeric preservation.

Table no 5.12.2.7.10 Correlation of cooking methods in 24 hours preservation with KMS

Condition	RS	B	OPDR	SF	DF
Raw State (RS)	1	.986(S)	-.812(S)	.923(S)	.986(S)
Boiling (B)	.986(S)	1	-.705	.974(S)	1.000**(S)
Open Pan Dry Roasting (OPDR)	-.812(S)	-.705	1	-.524	-.705
Shallow Frying (SF)	.923(S)	.974(S)	-.524	1	.974(S)
Deep Frying (DF)	.986(S)	1.000**(S)	-.705	.974(S)	1

***.Correlation is highly significant at the 0.01 level (2-tailed)* ▭ Positive ▭ Negative *S= Significant*

This table shows the correlation of iron content of *katla* with cooking methods. In 24 hours KMS preservation, there is significant positive correlation present between the raw state with boiling, shallow frying and deep frying, and significant negative correlation present between the raw state and open pan dry roasting. Boiling is perfect positively correlated with deep frying, whereas shallow frying is significant positively correlated with deep frying. This table indicates that there is a strong correlation present among the **raw state, boiling, open pan dry roasting, shallow frying and deep frying** in 24 hours KMS preservation.

Table no 5.12.2.7.11Correlation of cooking methods in 48 hours preservation with KMS

Condition	RS	B	OPDR	SF	DF
Raw state (RS)	1	.941(S)	.795	1.000**(S)	.986(S)
Boiling (B)	.941(S)	1	.543	.941(S)	.984(S)
Open Pan Dry Roasting (OPDR)	.795	.543	1	.795	.684
Shallow Frying (SF)	1.000**(S)	.941(S)	.795	1	.986(S)
Deep Frying (DF)	.986(S)	.984(S)	.684	.986(S)	1

***.Correlation is highly significant at the 0.01 level (2-tailed)* ▭ Positive *S= Significant*

This table shows the correlation of iron content of *katla* with cooking methods. In 48 hours KMS preservation, there is significant positive correlation present between the raw state with boiling and deep frying and perfect positive correlation present between the raw state and open pan dry roasting. Boiling is significant positively correlated with shallow frying and deep frying, whereas shallow frying is significant positively correlated with deep frying. This table indicates that there is a strong correlation present among the **raw state, boiling, shallow frying and deep frying** in 48 hours KMS preservation.

Table no 5.12.2.7.12 Correlation of cooking methods in 14 days preservation with KMS

Condition	RS	B	OPDR	SF	DF
Raw State (RS)	1	.997(S)	.475	.997(S)	1.000**(S)
Boiling (B)	.997(S)	1	.543	1.000**(S)	.997(S)
Open Pan Dry Roasting (OPDR)	.475	.543	1	.543	.475
Shallow Frying (SF)	.997(S)	1.000**(S)	.543	1	.997(S)
Deep Frying (DF)	1.000**(S)	.997(S)	.475	.997(S)	1

***.Correlation is highly significant at the 0.01 level (2-tailed)* ▭ Positive *S= Significant*

This table shows the correlation of iron content of *katla* with cooking methods. In 14 days KMS preservation, there is significant positive correlation present between the raw state with boiling, shallow frying, and perfect positive correlation present between the raw state and deep frying. Boiling is perfect positively correlated with shallow frying and significant positively correlated with deep frying, whereas shallow frying is significant positively correlated with deep frying. This table indicates that there is a strong correlation present among the **raw state, boiling, shallow frying and deep frying** in 14 days KMS preservation.

Table no 5.12.2.7.13 Correlation of cooking methods in 15 days preservation with KMS

Condition	RS	B	OPDR	SF	DF
Raw State (RS)	1	-.262	-.619	-.262	-.262
Boiling (B)	-.262	1	-.596	1.000**(S)	1.000**(S)
Open Pan Dry Roasting (OPDR)	-.619	-.596	1	-.596	-.596
Shallow Frying (SF)	-.262	1.000**(S)	-.596	1	1.000**(S)
Deep Frying (DF)	-.262	1.000**(S)	-.596	1.000**(S)	1

***.Correlation is highly significant at the 0.01 level (2-tailed)* ▭ Positive *S= Significant*

This table shows the correlation of iron content of *katla* with cooking methods. In 15 days KMS preservation, there is perfect positive correlation present between boiling with shallow frying and deep frying. Shallow frying is significant positively correlated with deep frying. This table indicates that there is a strong correlation present among **boiling, shallow frying and deep frying** in 15 days KMS preservation.

Overall analysis reveals that the raw state is perfect positively correlated with boiling in 15 days control preservation and 48 hours salt-turmeric preservation, whereas perfect positively correlated with open pan dry roasting in 15 days salt-turmeric preservation, perfect positively correlated with shallow frying in 48 hours salt and turmeric preservation and 48 hours KMS preservation, and again perfect positively correlated with deep frying in 14 days salt-turmeric and 14 days KMS preservation. Boiling is perfect positively correlated with open pan dry roasting in 14 days and 15 days salt-turmeric preservation, whereas perfect positively correlated with shallow frying in 14 days and 15 days KMS preservation, and perfect positively correlated with deep frying in 24 hours and 15 days KMS preservation. Open pan dry roasting is perfect positively correlated with shallow frying in 48 hours salt-turmeric preservation, and significant positively correlated with deep frying in 24 hours control preservation without preservative. Shallow frying is perfect positively correlated with deep frying in 15 days control preservation without preservative and 15 days KMS preservation. Most of the correlation of the iron content of *katla* is found in **15 days KMS preservation** with respect to different cooking conditions.

5.12.2.8 Energy

Table no 5.12.2.8.1 Correlation of cooking methods in fresh condition

Condition	RS	B	OPDR	SF	DF
Raw State (RS)	1	.498	.033	.028	.986(S)
Boiling (B)	.498	1	.883(S)	.881(S)	.344
Open Pan Dry Roasting (OPDR)	.033	.883(S)	1	1.000**(S)	-.137
Shallow Frying (SF)	.028	.881(S)	1.000**(S)	1	-.142
Deep Frying (DF)	.986(S)	.344	-.137	-.142	1

***.Correlation is highly significant at the 0.01 level (2-tailed)* ▭ Positive *S= Significant*

This table shows the correlation of energy content of *katla* with cooking methods. In fresh condition, there is significant positive correlation present between the raw state and deep frying. Boiling is significant positively correlated with open pan dry roasting and shallow frying, whereas shallow frying is perfect positively correlated with open pan dry roasting. This table indicates that there is a strong correlation present among the **raw state, boiling, open pan dry roasting, shallow frying** in fresh condition.

Table no 5.12.2.8.2 Correlation of cooking methods in 24 hours preservation without preservative

Condition	RS	B	OPDR	SF	DF
Raw State (RS)	1	.854(S)	.856(S)	.947(S)	.096
Boiling (B)	.854(S)	1	1.000**(S)	.642	-.437
Open Pan Dry Roasting (OPDR)	.856	1.000**(S)	1	.645	-.432
Shallow Frying (SF)	.947(S)	.642	.645	1	.410
Deep Frying (DF)	.096	-.437	-.432	.410	1

***.Correlation is highly significant at the 0.01 level (2-tailed)* ▭ Positive *S= Significant*

This table shows the correlation of energy content of *katla* with cooking methods. In 24 hours control preservation without preservative, there is significant positive correlation present between the raw state with boiling, shallow frying and open pan dry roasting. Boiling is perfect positively correlated with open pan dry roasting. This table indicates that there is a strong correlation present among the **raw state, boiling, open pan dry roasting and shallow frying** in 24 hours control preservation.

Table no 5.12.2.8.3 Correlation of cooking methods in 48 hours preservation without preservative

Condition	RS	B	OPDR	SF	DF
Raw State (RS)	1	-.875(S)	-.723	.895(S)	-.215
Boiling (B)	-.875(S)	1	.967(S)	-.999*(S)	-.285
Open Pan Dry Roasting (OPDR)	-.723	.967(S)	1	-.955(S)	-.519
Shallow Frying (SF)	.895(S)	-.999*(S)	-.955(S)	1	.243
Deep Frying (DF)	-.215	-.285	-.519	.243	1

**.Correlation is highly significant at the 0.05 level (2-tailed)* Positive Negative *S= Significant*

This table shows the correlation of energy content of *katla* with cooking methods. In 48 hours control preservation without preservative, there is significant positive correlation present between the raw state and shallow frying, and significant negative correlation present between the raw state and boiling. Boiling is significant positively correlated with open pan dry roasting and highly negatively correlated with shallow frying, whereas open pan dry roasting is negatively correlated with shallow frying. This table indicates that there is a strong correlation present among the **raw state, boiling, open pan dry roasting and shallow frying** in 48 hours control preservation.

Table no 5.12.2.8.4 Correlation of cooking methods in 14 days preservation without preservative

Condition	RS	B	OPDR	SF	DF
Raw State (RS)	1	-.966(S)	-1.000**(S)	.498	-.977(S)
Boiling (B)	-.966(S)	1	.962(S)	-.258	.889(S)
Open Pan Dry Roasting (OPDR)	-1.000**(S)	.962(S)	1	-.511	.980(S)
Shallow Frying (SF)	.498	-.258	-.511	1	-.672
Deep Frying (DF)	-.977(S)	.889(S)	.980(S)	-.672	1

***.Correlation is highly significant at the 0.01 level (2-tailed)* Positive Negative *S= Significant*

This table shows the correlation of energy content of *katla* with cooking methods. In 14 days control preservation without preservative, there is significant negative correlation present between the raw state with boiling and deep frying, and perfect negative correlation present between the raw state and open pan dry roasting. Boiling is significant positively correlated with open pan dry roasting and deep frying. This table indicates that there is a strong correlation present among the **raw state, boiling, open pan dry roasting and deep frying** in 14 days control preservation.

Table no 5.12.2.8.5 Correlation of cooking methods in 15 days preservation without preservative

Condition	RS	B	OPDR	SF	DF
Raw State (RS)	1	-.560	-.055	-.276	.586
Boiling (B)	-.560	1	-.796	.951(S)	-1.000*(S)
Open Pan Dry Roasting (OPDR)	-.055	-.796	1	-.944(S)	.777
Shallow Frying (SF)	-.276	.951(S)	-.944(S)	1	-.941(S)
Deep Frying (DF)	.586	-1.000*(S)	.777	-.941(S)	1

**.Correlation is highly significant at the 0.05 level (2-tailed)* Positive Negative *S= Significant*

This table shows the correlation of energy content of *katla* with cooking methods. In 15 days control preservation without preservative, there is significant negative correlation present between the raw state and shallow frying, and perfect negative correlation present between the raw state and deep frying. Open pan dry roasting is significant negatively correlated with shallow frying, whereas shallow frying is significant negatively correlated with deep frying. This table indicates that there is a strong correlation present among **boiling, open pan dry roasting, shallow frying and deep frying** in 15 days control preservation.

Table no 5.12.2.8.6 Correlation of cooking methods in 24 hours preservation with salt and turmeric

Condition	RS	B	OPDR	SF	DF
Raw State (RS)	1	.289	.999*(S)	.914	.904(S)
Boiling (B)	.289	1	.328	-.123	-.147
Open Pan Dry Roasting (OPDR)	.999*(S)	.328	1	.897(S)	.886(S)
Shallow Frying (SF)	.914(S)	-.123	.897(S)	1	1.000*(S)
Deep Frying (DF)	.904(S)	-.147	.886(S)	1.000*(S)	1

**.Correlation is highly significant at the 0.05 level (2-tailed)* Positive *S= Significant*

This table shows the correlation of energy content of *katla* with cooking methods. In 24 hours salt and turmeric preservation, there is highly significant positive correlation present between the raw state and open pan dry roasting, and significant positive correlation present between the raw state and deep frying. Open pan dry roasting is significant positively correlated with shallow frying and deep frying. This table indicates that there is a strong correlation present among the **raw state, open pan dry roasting, shallow frying and deep frying** in 24 hours salt and turmeric preservation.

Table no 5.12.2.8.7 Correlation of cooking methods in 48 hours preservation with salt and turmeric

Condition	RS	B	OPDR	SF	DF
Raw State (RS)	1	-.454	.395	-.558	.464
Boiling (B)	-.454	1	-.998*(S)	-.486	-1.000**(S)
Open Pan Dry Roasting (OPDR)	.395	-.998*(S)	1	.543	.997*(S)
Shallow Frying (SF)	-.558	-.486	.543	1	.476
Deep Frying (DF)	.464	-1.000**(S)	.997*(S)	.476	1

**.Correlation is highly significant at the 0.05 level (2-tailed)* Positive Negative *S= Significant*
***.Correlation is highly significant at the 0.01 level (2-tailed)*

This table shows the correlation of energy content of *katla* with cooking methods. In 48 hours salt and turmeric preservation, there is highly significant negative correlation present between the raw state and open pan dry roasting, and perfect negative correlation present between the raw state and deep frying. Open pan dry roasting is significant positively correlated with deep frying. This table indicates that there is a strong correlation present among **boiling, open pan dry roasting and deep frying** in 48 hours salt and turmeric preservation.

Table no 5.12.2.8.8 Correlation of cooking methods in 14 days preservation with salt and turmeric

Condition	RS	B	OPDR	SF	DF
Raw State (RS)	1	.995(S)	.996(S)	.273	.819(S)
Boiling (B)	.995(S)	1	1.000**(S)	.367	.872(S)
Open Pan Dry Roasting (OPDR)	.996(S)	1.000**(S)	1	.359	.868(S)
Shallow Frying (SF)	.273	.367	.359	1	.775
Deep Frying (DF)	.819(S)	.872(S)	.868(S)	.775	1

***.Correlation is highly significant at the 0.01 level (2-tailed)* Positive *S= Significant*

This table shows the correlation of energy content of *katla* with cooking methods. In 14 days salt and turmeric preservation, there is highly significant positive correlation present between the raw state with boiling, open pan dry roasting and deep frying. Boiling is perfect positively correlated open pan dry roasting and significant positively correlated with deep frying. Open pan dry roasting is significant positively correlated with deep frying. This table indicates that there is a strong correlation present among the **raw state, boiling, shallow frying and deep frying** in 14 days salt and turmeric preservation.

Table no 5.12.2.8.9 Correlation of cooking methods in 15 days preservation with salt and turmeric

Condition	RS	B	OPDR	SF	DF
Raw State (RS)	1	-.997* (S)	-.576	-.116	.554
Boiling (B)	-.997*(S)	1	.633	.186	-.494
Open Pan Dry Roasting (OPDR)	-.576	.633	1	.879(S)	.361
Shallow Frying (SF)	-.116	.186	.879(S)	1	.762
Deep Frying (DF)	.554	-.494	.361	.762	1

**.Correlation is highly significant at the 0.05 level (2-tailed)* Positive Negative *S= Significant*

This table shows the correlation of energy content of *katla* with cooking methods. In 15 days salt and turmeric preservation, there is highly significant negative correlation present between the raw state and boiling. Open pan dry roasting is significant positively correlated with shallow frying. This table indicates that there is a strong correlation present between the **raw state and boiling and also between open pan dry roasting and shallow frying** in 15 days salt and turmeric preservation.

Table no 5.12.2.8.10 Correlation of cooking methods in 24 hours preservation with KMS

Condition	RS	B	OPDR	SF	DF
Raw State (RS)	1	.992(S)	.820(S)	-.222	.148
Boiling (B)	.992(S)	1	.740	-.095	.019
Open Pan Dry Roasting (OPDR)	.820(S)	.740	1	-.740	.687
Shallow Frying (SF)	-.222	-.095	-.740	1	-.997*(S)
Deep Frying (DF)	.148	.019	.687	-.997*(S)	1

**.Correlation is highly significant at the 0.05 level (2-tailed)* Positive Negative *S= Significant*

This table shows the correlation of energy content of *katla* with cooking methods. In 24 hours salt and turmeric preservation, there is significant positive correlation present between the raw state with boiling and open pan dry roasting. Shallow frying is significant negatively correlated with deep frying. This table indicates that there is a strong correlation present among the **raw state, boiling, open pan dry roasting, shallow frying and deep frying** in 24 hours KMS preservation.

Table no 5.12.2.8.11 Correlation of cooking methods in 48 hours preservation with KMS

Condition	RS	B	OPDR	SF	DF
Raw State (RS)	1	.869(S)	.989(S)	.884(S)	.854(S)
Boiling (B)	.869(S)	1	.787	.537	.485
Open Pan Dry Roasting (OPDR)	.989(S)	.787	1	.943(S)	.921(S)
Shallow Frying (SF)	.884(S)	.537	.943(S)	1	.998*(S)
Deep Frying (DF)	.854(S)	.485(S)	.921(S)	.998*(S)	1

**.Correlation is highly significant at the 0.05 level (2-tailed)* ▭ Positive *S= Significant*

This table shows the correlation of energy content of *katla* with cooking methods. In 48 KMS preservation, there is significant positive correlation present between the raw state with boiling, open pan dry roasting, shallow frying and deep frying. Open pan dry roasting is positively correlated with shallow frying and deep frying. Shallow frying is highly significant positively correlated with deep frying. This table indicates that there is a strong correlation present among the **raw state, boiling, open pan dry roasting, shallow frying and deep frying** in 48 hours KMS preservation.

Table no 5.12.2.8.12 Correlation of cooking methods in 14 days preservation with KMS

Condition	RS	B	OPDR	SF	DF
Raw State (RS)	1	1.000**(S)	.962(S)	-.608	.977(S)
Boiling (B)	1.000**(S)	1	.959(S)	-.600	.979(S)
Open Pan Dry Roasting (OPDR)	.962(S)	.959(S)	1	-.802(S)	.882(S)
Shallow Frying (SF)	-.608	-.600	-.802(S)	1	-.426
Deep Frying (DF)	.977(S)	.979(S)	.882(S)	-.426	1

***.Correlation is highly significant at the 0.01 level (2-tailed)* ▭ Positive ▭ Negative *S= Significant*

This table shows the correlation of energy content of *katla* with cooking methods. In 14 days KMS preservation, there is significant positive correlation present between the raw state with open pan dry roasting and deep frying, and perfect positive correlation present between the raw state and boiling. Boiling is significant positively correlated with open pan dry roasting and deep frying. Open pan dry roasting is positively correlated with deep frying and negatively correlated with shallow frying. This table indicates that there is a strong correlation present among the **raw state, boiling, open pan dry roasting, shallow frying and deep frying** in 14 days KMS preservation.

Table no 5.12.2.8.13 Correlation of cooking methods in 15 days preservation with KMS

Condition	RS	B	OPDR	SF	DF
Raw State (RS)	1	-.314	-.147	.696	.770
Boiling (B)	-.314	1	-.893(S)	-.900(S)	.365
Open Pan Dry Roasting (OPDR)	-.147	-.893(S)	1	.608	-.745
Shallow Frying (SF)	.696	-.900(S)	.608	1	.077
Deep Frying (DF)	.770	.365	-.745	.077	1

▭ Negative *S= Significant*

This table shows the correlation of energy content of *katla* with cooking methods. In 15 days KMS preservation, there is significant negative correlation present between boiling with open pan dry roasting and shallow frying. This table indicates that there is a strong correlation present among **boiling, open pan dry roasting and shallow frying** in 15 days KMS preservation.

Overall analysis reveals that the raw state is perfect positively correlated with boiling and open pan dry roasting in 14 days KMS preservation and 14 days control preservation without preservative respectively, whereas significant positively correlated with shallow frying and deep frying in 24 hours control preservation without preservative and in fresh condition respectively. Boiling is perfect positively correlated with open pan dry roasting in 24 hours control preservation without preservative, whereas highly significant negatively correlated with shallow frying in 48 hours control preservation without preservative, and perfect negatively correlated with deep frying in 48 hours salt-turmeric preservation and 15 days control preservation without preservative. Open pan dry roasting is perfect positively correlated with shallow frying in fresh condition, and highly significant positively correlated with deep frying in 48 hours salt and turmeric preservation. Shallow frying is positively correlated with deep frying in 24 hours salt-turmeric preservation. Most of the correlation of the energy content of *katla* is found in **24 hours control preservation without preservative and 48 hours salt and turmeric preservation** with respect to different cooking conditions.

5.12.3 Prawn *(Fenneropenaeus indicus)*

5.12.3.1 Carbohydrate

Table no 5.12.3.1.1 Correlation of cooking methods in fresh condition

Condition	RS	B	OPDR	SF	DF
Raw State (RS)	1	.655	1.000*(S)	-.281	.979(S)
Boiling (B)	.655	1	.676	-.909(S)	.796
Open Pan Dry Roasting (OPDR)	1.000*(S)	.676	1	-.308	.984(S)
Shallow Frying (SF)	-.281	-.909(S)	-.308	1	-.472
Deep Frying (DF)	.979(S)	.796	.984(S)	-.472	1

**.Correlation is highly significant at the 0.05 level (2-tailed)* Positive Negative *S= Significant*

This table shows the correlation of carbohydrate content of prawn with cooking methods. In fresh condition, there is perfect positive correlation present between the raw state and open pan dry roasting, and significant positive correlation present between the raw state and deep frying. Boiling is significant negatively correlated with shallow frying. Open pan dry roasting is significant positively correlated with deep frying. This table indicates that there is a strong correlation present among the **raw state, boiling, open pan dry roasting, shallow frying and deep frying** in fresh condition.

Table no 5.12.3.1.2 Correlation of cooking methods in 24 hours preservation without preservative

Condition	RS	B	OPDR	SF	DF
Raw State (RS)	1	.573	.545	.885(S)	.775
Boiling (B)	.573	1	.999*(S)	.125	-.074
Open Pan Dry Roasting (OPDR)	.545	.999*(S)	1	.091	-.108
Shallow Frying (SF)	.885(S)	.125	.091	1	.980(S)
Deep Frying (DF)	.775	-.074	-.108	.980(S)	1

**.Correlation is highly significant at the 0.05 level (2-tailed)* Positive *S= Significant*

This table shows the correlation of carbohydrate content of prawn with cooking methods. In 24 hours preservation without preservative, there is significant positive correlation present between the raw state and shallow frying. Boiling is highly significant positively correlated with open pan dry roasting.

Shallow frying is significant positively correlated with deep frying. This table indicates that there is a strong correlation present among the **raw state, boiling, open pan dry roasting, shallow frying and deep frying** in 24 hours preservation without preservative.

Table no 5.12.3.1.3 Correlation of cooking methods in 48 hours preservation without preservative

Condition	RS	B	OPDR	SF	DF
Raw State (RS)	1	.923(S)	.395	-.982(S)	-.099
Boiling (B)	.923(S)	1	.719	-.833(S)	-.475
Open Pan Dry Roasting (OPDR)	.395	.719	1	-.214	-.953(S)
Shallow Frying (SF)	-.982(S)	-.833(S)	-.214	1	-.091
Deep Frying (DF)	-.099	-.475	-.953(S)	-.091	1

Positive Negative *S= Significant*

This table shows the correlation of carbohydrate content of prawn with cooking methods. In 48 hours preservation without preservative, there is significant positive correlation present between the raw state and boiling, and significant negative correlation present between the raw state and shallow frying. Boiling is significant negatively correlated with shallow frying. Open pan dry roasting is significant negatively correlated with deep frying. This table indicates that there is a strong correlation present among the **raw state, boiling, open pan dry roasting, shallow frying and deep frying** in 48 hours preservation without preservative.

Table no 5.12.3.1.4 Correlation of cooking methods in 14 days preservation without preservative

Condition	RS	B	OPDR	SF	DF
Raw State (RS)	1	.999*(S)	.220	.994(S)	.304
Boiling (B)	.999*(S)	1	.180	.998*(S)	.342
Open Pan Dry Roasting (OPDR)	.220	.180	1	.115	-.862(S)
Shallow Frying (SF)	.994(S)	.998*(S)	.115	1	.404
Deep Frying (DF)	.304	.342	-.862(S)	.404	1

**.Correlation is highly significant at the 0.05 level (2-tailed)* Positive Negative *S= Significant*

This table shows the correlation of carbohydrate content of prawn with cooking methods. In 14 days preservation without preservative, there is highly significant positive correlation present between the raw state with boiling and shallow frying. Boiling is highly significant positively correlated with shallow frying. Open pan dry roasting is significant negatively correlated with deep frying. This table indicates that there is a strong correlation present among the **raw state, boiling, open pan dry roasting, shallow frying and deep frying** in 14 days preservation without preservative.

Table no 5.12.3.1.5 Correlation of cooking methods in 15 days preservation without preservative

Condition	RS	B	OPDR	SF	DF
Raw State (RS)	1	.655	.955(S)	.997(S)	.051
Boiling (B)	.655	1	.850(S)	.715	-.722
Open Pan Dry Roasting (OPDR)	.955(S)	.850(S)	1	.976(S)	-.248
Shallow Frying (SF)	.997(S)	.715	.976(S)	1	-.031
Deep Frying (DF)	.051	-.722	-.248	-.031	1

Positive *S= Significant*

This table shows the correlation of carbohydrate content of prawn with cooking methods. In 15 days preservation without preservative, there is significant positive correlation present between the raw state with open pan dry roasting and shallow frying. Boiling is significant positively correlated with open pan dry roasting. Open pan dry roasting is significant positively correlated with shallow frying. This table indicates that there is a strong correlation present among the **raw state, boiling, open pan dry roasting and shallow frying** in 15 days preservation without preservative.

Table no 5.12.3.1.6 Correlation of cooking methods in 24 hours preservation with salt and turmeric

Condition	RS	B	OPDR	SF	DF
Raw State (RS)	1	.610	.778	-.397	-.973(S)
Boiling (B)	.610	1	.973(S)	.485	-.410
Open Pan Dry Roasting (OPDR)	.778	.973(S)	1	.268	-.611
Shallow Frying (SF)	-.397	.485	.268	1	.599
Deep Frying (DF)	-.973(S)	-.410	-.611	.599	1

Positive Negative *S= Significant*

This table shows the correlation of carbohydrate content of prawn with cooking methods. In 24 hours salt and turmeric preservation, there is highly significant negative correlation present between the raw state and deep frying. Boiling is highly significant positively correlated with open pan dry roasting. This table indicates that there is a strong correlation present between the **raw state and deep frying and also between boiling and open pan dry roasting** in 24 hours salt and turmeric preservation without preservative.

Table no 5.12.3.1.7 Correlation of cooking methods in 48 hours preservation with salt and turmeric

Condition	RS	B	OPDR	SF	DF
Raw State (RS)	1	.127	-.977(S)	.944(S)	.986(S)
Boiling (B)	.127	1	-.337	.448	-.038
Open Pan Dry Roasting (OPDR)	-.977(S)	-.337	1	-.993(S)	-.928(S)
Shallow Frying (SF)	.944(S)	.448	-.993(S)	1	.876(S)
Deep Frying (DF)	.986(S)	-.038	-.928(S)	.876(S)	1

Positive Negative *S= Significant*

This table shows the correlation of carbohydrate content of prawn with cooking methods. In 48 hours salt and turmeric preservation, there is significant negative correlation present between the raw state and open pan dry roasting, and significant positive correlation present between the raw state with shallow frying and deep frying. Open pan dry roasting is significant negatively correlated with shallow frying and deep frying. Shallow frying is significant positively correlated with deep frying. This table indicates that there is a strong correlation present among the **raw state, open pan dry roasting, shallow frying and deep frying** in 48 hours salt and turmeric preservation without preservative.

Table no 5.12.3.1.8 Correlation of cooking methods in 14 days preservation with salt and turmeric

Condition	RS	B	OPDR	SF	DF
Raw State (RS)	1	.979(S)	.965(S)	-.365	.019
Boiling (B)	.979(S)	1	.891(S)	-.167	.223
Open Pan Dry Roasting (OPDR)	.965(S)	.891(S)	1	-.596	-.243
Shallow Frying (SF)	-.365	-.167	-.596	1	.924(S)
Deep Frying (DF)	.019	.223	-.243	.924(S)	1

Positive *S= Significant*

This table shows the correlation of carbohydrate content of prawn with cooking methods. In 14 days salt and turmeric preservation, there is significant positive correlation present between the raw state with boiling and open pan dry roasting. Boiling is significant positively correlated with open pan dry roasting. Shallow frying is significant positively correlated with deep frying. This table indicates that there is a strong correlation present among the **raw state, boiling, open pan dry roasting, shallow frying and deep frying** in 14 days salt and turmeric preservation without preservative.

Table no 5.12.3.1.9 Correlation of cooking methods in 15 days preservation with salt and turmeric

Condition	RS	B	OPDR	SF	DF
Raw State (RS)	1	-.339	.261	.462	.998*(S)
Boiling (B)	-.339	1	-.997(S)	-.991(S)	-.274
Open Pan Dry Roasting (OPDR)	.261	-.997(S)	1	.977(S)	.195
Shallow Frying (SF)	.462	-.991(S)	.977(S)	1	.401
Deep Frying (DF)	.998*(S)	-.274	.195	.401	1

**.Correlation is highly significant at the 0.05 level (2-tailed)* ▭ Positive ▭ Negative *S= Significant*

This table shows the correlation of carbohydrate content of prawn with cooking methods. In 15 days salt and turmeric preservation, there is highly significant positive correlation present between the raw state and deep frying. Boiling is significant negatively correlated with open pan dry roasting and shallow frying. Open pan dry roasting is significant positively correlated with shallow frying. This table indicates that there is a strong correlation present among the **raw state, boiling, open pan dry roasting, shallow frying and deep frying** in 15days salt and turmeric preservation without preservative.

Table no 5.12.3.1.10 Correlation of cooking methods in 24 hours preservation with KMS

Condition	RS	B	OPDR	SF	DF
Raw State (RS)	1	.045	.843(S)	.769	.557
Boiling (B)	.045	1	-.500	-.604	-.805(S)
Open Pan Dry Roasting (OPDR)	.843(S)	-.500	1	.992(S)	.917(S)
Shallow Frying (SF)	.769	-.604	.992(S)	1	.959(S)
Deep Frying (DF)	.557	-.805(S)	.917	.959(S)	1

▭ Positive ▭ Negative *S= Significant*

This table shows the correlation of carbohydrate content of prawn with cooking methods. In 24 hours KMS preservation, there is highly significant positive correlation present between the raw state and open pan dry roasting. Boiling is significant negatively correlated with deep frying. Open pan dry roasting is significant positively correlated with shallow frying and deep frying. Shallow frying is significant positively correlated with deep frying. This table indicates that there is a strong correlation present among the **raw state, boiling, open pan dry roasting, shallow frying and deep frying** in 24 hours KMS preservation without preservative.

Table no 5.12.3.1.11 Correlation of cooking methods in 48 hours preservation with KMS

Condition	RS	B	OPDR	SF	DF
Raw State (RS)	1	.564	.954(S)	.362	.978(S)
Boiling (B)	.564	1	.786	.974(S)	.724
Open Pan Dry Roasting (OPDR)	.954(S)	.786	1	.625	.996(S)
Shallow Frying (SF)	.362	.974(S)	.625	1	.549
Deep Frying (DF)	.978(S)	.724	.996(S)	.549	1

▭ Positive *S= Significant*

This table shows the correlation of carbohydrate content of prawn with cooking methods. In 48 hours KMS preservation, there is highly significant positive correlation present between the raw state with open pan dry roasting and deep frying. Boiling is significant positively correlated with shallow frying. Open pan dry roasting is significant positively correlated with deep frying. This table indicates that there is a strong correlation present among the **raw state, boiling, open pan dry roasting, shallow frying and deep frying** in 48 hours KMS preservation without preservative.

Table no 5.12.3.1.12 Correlation of cooking methods in 14 days preservation with KMS

Condition	Rs	B	OPDR	SF	DF
Raw State (RS)	1	-.929(S)	.472	.500	.655
Boiling (B)	-.929(S)	1	-.111	-.143	-.327
Open Pan Dry Roasting (OPDR)	.472	-.111	1	.999*(S)	.975(S)
Shallow Frying (SF)	.500	-.143	.999*(S)	1	.982(S)
Deep Frying (DF)	.655	-.327	.975(S)	.982(S)	1

**.Correlation is highly significant at the 0.05 level (2-tailed)* ▭ Positive ▭ Negative *S= Significant*

This table shows the correlation of carbohydrate content of prawn with cooking methods. In 14 days KMS preservation, there is highly significant negative correlation present between the raw state and boiling. Boiling is highly significant positively correlated with shallow frying and deep frying. Open pan dry roasting is significant positively correlated with shallow frying and deep frying. Shallow frying is significant positively correlated with deep frying. This table indicates that there is a strong correlation present among the **raw state, boiling, open pan dry roasting, shallow frying and deep frying** in 14 days KMS preservation without preservative.

Table no 5.12.3.1.13 Correlation of cooking methods in 15 days preservation with KMS

Condition	RS	B	OPDR	SF	DF
Raw State (RS)	1	.817(S)	.005	.923(S)	.143
Boiling (B)	.817(S)	1	.581	.533	-.454
Open Pan Dry Roasting (OPDR)	.005	.581	1	-.379	-.989(S)
Shallow Frying (SF)	.923(S)	.533	-.379	1	.512
Deep Frying (DF)	.143	-.454	-.989(S)	.512	1

▭ Positive ▭ Negative *S= Significant*

This table shows the correlation of carbohydrate content of prawn with cooking methods. In 15 days KMS preservation, there is highly significant positive correlation present between the raw state with boiling and shallow frying. Open pan dry roasting is significant negatively correlated with deep frying. This table indicates that there is a strong correlation present among the **raw state, boiling, open pan dry roasting, shallow frying and deep frying** in 15 days KMS preservation without preservative.

Overall analysis reveals that the raw state is highly significant positively correlated with boiling and deep frying in 14 days control preservation without preservative and 15 days salt-turmeric preservation respectively, whereas perfect positively correlated with open pan dry roasting in fresh condition, and highly significant positively correlated with shallow frying in 15 days control preservation without preservative. Boiling is highly significant positively correlated with open pan dry roasting and shallow frying in 24 hours and 14 days control preservation without preservative respectively, whereas significant positively correlated with deep frying in fresh condition. Open pan dry roasting is perfect positively correlated with shallow frying in 14 days KMS preservation, and significant positively correlated with deep frying in 48 hours KMS preservation. Shallow frying is significant positively correlated with deep frying in 14 days KMS preservation. Most of the correlation of the carbohydrate content of prawn is found in **fresh condition, 14 days control preservation without preservative and 14 days KMS preservation** with respect to different cooking conditions.

5.12.3.2 Protein

Table no 5.12.3.2.1 Correlation of cooking methods in fresh condition

Condition	RS	B	OPDR	SF	DF
Raw State (RS)	1	.592	.038	.971(S)	.780
Boiling (B)	.592	1	.828(S)	.769	-.043
Open Pan Dry Roasting (OPDR)	.038	.828(S)	1	.277	-.596
Shallow Frying (SF)	.971(S)	.769	.277	1	.606
Deep Frying (DF)	.780	-.043	-.596	.606	1

Positive *S= Significant*

This table shows the correlation of protein content of prawn with cooking methods. In fresh condition, there is highly significant positive correlation present between the raw state and shallow frying. Boiling is significant positively correlated with open pan dry roasting. This table indicates that there is a strong correlation present between the **raw state and shallow frying and also between boiling and open pan dry roasting** in fresh condition.

Table no 5.12.3.2.2 Correlation of cooking methods in 24 hours preservation without preservative

Condition	RS	B	OPDR	SF	DF
Raw State (RS)	1	.143	.745	.689	.842(S)
Boiling (B)	.143	1	-.554	-.619	.655
Open Pan Dry Roasting (OPDR)	.745	-.554	1	.997(S)	.266
Shallow Frying (SF)	.689	-.619	.997(S)	1	.189
Deep Frying (DF)	.842(S)	.655	.266	.189	1

Positive *S= Significant*

This table shows the correlation of protein content of prawn with cooking methods. In 24 hours control preservation without preservative, there is highly significant positive correlation present between the raw state and deep frying. Boiling is significant positively correlated with open pan dry roasting. This table indicates that there is a strong correlation present between the **raw state and deep frying and also between boiling and open pan dry roasting** in 24 hours control preservation.

Table no 5.12.3.2.3 Correlation of cooking methods in 48 hours preservation without preservative

Condition	RS	B	OPDR	SF	DF
Raw State (RS)	1	.333	-.943(S)	-.983(S)	-.898(S)
Boiling (B)	.333	1	.000	-.500	.115
Open Pan Dry Roasting (OPDR)	-.943(S)	.000	1	.866(S)	.993(S)
Shallow Frying (SF)	-.983(S)	-.500	.866(S)	1	.803(S)
Deep Frying (DF)	-.898(S)	.115	.993(S)	.803(S)	1

Positive Negative *S= Significant*

This table shows the correlation of protein content of prawn with cooking methods. In 48 hours preservation without preservative, there is significant negative correlation present between the raw state with open pan dry roasting, shallow frying and deep frying. Open pan dry roasting is significant positively correlated with shallow frying and deep frying. Shallow frying is significant positively correlated with deep frying. This table indicates that there is a strong correlation present among the **raw state, open pan dry roasting, shallow frying and deep frying** in 48 hours preservation without preservative.

Table no 5.12.3.2.4 Correlation of cooking methods in 14 days preservation without preservative

Condition	RS	B	OPDR	SF	DF
Raw State (RS)	1	-.962(S)	-.680	.488	.962(S)
Boiling (B)	-.962(S)	1	.855(S)	-.708	-.850(S)
Open Pan Dry Roasting (OPDR)	-.680	.855	1	-.972(S)	-.454
Shallow Frying (SF)	.488	-.708	-.972(S)	1	.231
Deep Frying (DF)	.962(S)	-.850(S)	-.454	.231	1

Positive Negative *S= Significant*

This table shows the correlation of protein content of prawn with cooking methods. In 14 days preservation without preservative, there is significant negative correlation present between the raw state and boiling, and positive correlation present between the raw state and deep frying. Boiling is significant positively correlated with open pan dry roasting and significant negatively correlated with deep frying. Open pan dry roasting is significant positively correlated with shallow frying. This table indicates that there is a strong correlation present among the **raw state, open pan dry roasting, shallow frying and deep frying** in 14 days preservation without preservative.

Table no 5.12.3.2.5 Correlation of cooking methods in 15 days preservation without preservative

Condition	RS	B	OPDR	SF	DF
Raw State (RS)	1	1.000** (S)	.702	1.000**(S)	-.220
Boiling (B)	1.000**(S)	1	.696	1.000**(S)	-.228
Open Pan Dry Roasting (OPDR)	.702	.696	1	.692	.540
Shallow Frying (SF)	1.000**(S)	1.000**(S)	.692	1	-.234
Deep Frying (DF)	-.220	-.228	.540	-.234	1

***.Correlation is highly significant at the 0.01 level (2-tailed)* Positive *S= Significant*

This table shows the correlation of protein content of prawn with cooking methods. In 15 days preservation without preservative, there is perfect positive correlation present between the raw state with boiling and shallow frying. Boiling is perfect positively correlated with shallow frying. This table indicates that there is a strong correlation present among the **raw state, boiling and shallow frying** in 15 days preservation without preservative.

Table no 5.12.3.2.6 Correlation of cooking methods in 24 hours preservation with salt and turmeric

Condition	RS	B	OPDR	SF	DF
Raw State (RS)	1	.493	-.494	-.061	.500
Boiling (B)	.493	1	-1.000**(S)	.838(S)	1.000**(S)
Open Pan Dry Roasting (OPDR)	-.494	-1.000**(S)	1	-.838(S)	-1.000**(S)
Shallow Frying (SF)	-.061	.838(S)	-.838(S)	1	.834(S)
Deep Frying (DF)	.500	1.000**(S)	-1.000**(S)	.834(S)	1

***.Correlation is highly significant at the 0.01 level (2-tailed)* Positive Negative *S= Significant*

This table shows the correlation of protein content of prawn with cooking methods. In 24 hours salt and turmeric preservation, there is perfect positive correlation present between boiling and deep frying, and perfect negative correlation present between boiling and open pan dry roasting, and significant positive correlation present between boiling and shallow frying. Open pan dry roasting is perfect negatively correlated with deep frying and significant negatively correlated with shallow frying. Shallow frying is significant positively correlated with deep frying. This table indicates that there is a strong correlation present among **boiling, open pan dry roasting, shallow frying and deep frying** in 24 hours salt and turmeric preservation.

Table no 5.12.3.2.7 Correlation of cooking methods in 48 hours preservation with salt and turmeric

Condition	RS	B	OPDR	SF	DF
Raw State (RS)	1	.723	.494	.725	.895(S)
Boiling (B)	.723	1	-.243	1.000** (S)	.338
Open Pan Dry Roasting (OPDR)	.494	-.243	1	-.240	.830(S)
Shallow Frying (SF)	.725	1.000** (S)	-.240	1	.341
Deep Frying (DF)	.895(S)	.338	.830(S)	.341	1

***.Correlation is highly significant at the 0.01 level (2-tailed)* ▭ Positive *S= Significant*

This table shows the correlation of protein content of prawn with cooking methods. In 48 hours salt and turmeric preservation, there is perfect positive correlation present between boiling and shallow frying, whereas significant positive correlation present between the raw state and deep frying. Open pan dry roasting is significant positively correlated with deep frying. This table indicates that there is a strong correlation present among the **raw state, boiling, open pan dry roasting, shallow frying and deep frying** in 48 hours salt and turmeric preservation.

Table no 5.12.3.2.8 Correlation of cooking methods in 14 days preservation with salt and turmeric

Condition	RS	B	OPDR	SF	DF
Raw State (RS)	1	-.974(S)	-.998* (S)	.646	-.572
Boiling (B)	-.974(S)	1	.987(S)	-.457	.742
Open Pan Dry Roasting (OPDR)	-.998* (S)	.987(S)	1	-.595	.624
Shallow Frying (SF)	.646	-.457	-.595	1	.257
Deep Frying (DF)	-.572	.742	.624	.257	1

**.Correlation is highly significant at the 0.05 level (2-tailed)* ▭ Positive ▭ Negative *S= Significant*

This table shows the correlation of protein content of prawn with cooking methods. In 14 days salt and turmeric preservation, there is significant negative correlation present between the raw state and boiling, and highly significant negative correlation present between the raw state and open pan dry roasting, whereas significant positive correlation present between boiling and open pan dry roasting. This table indicates that there is a strong correlation present among the **raw state, boiling and open pan dry roasting** in 14 days salt and turmeric preservation.

Table no 5.12.3.2.9 Correlation of cooking methods in 15 days preservation with salt and turmeric

Condition	RS	B	OPDR	SF	DF
Raw State (RS)	1	-.506	-1.000**(S)	.659	.899(S)
Boiling (B)	-.506	1	.501	.315	-.078
Open Pan Dry Roasting (OPDR)	-1.000**(S)	.501	1	-.664	-.902(S)
Shallow Frying (SF)	.659	.315	-.664	1	.922(S)
Deep Frying (DF)	.899(S)	-.078	-.902(S)	.922(S)	1

***.Correlation is highly significant at the 0.01 level (2-tailed)* ▭ Positive ▭ Negative *S= Significant*

This table shows the correlation of protein content of prawn with cooking methods. In 15 days salt and turmeric preservation, there is perfect negative correlation present between the raw state and open pan dry roasting, and significant positive correlation present between the raw state and deep frying. Open pan dry roasting is significant negatively correlated with deep frying. Shallow frying is significant positively correlated with deep frying. This table indicates that there is a strong correlation present among the **raw state, open pan dry roasting, shallow frying and deep frying** in 15 days salt and turmeric preservation.

Table no 5.12.3.2.10 Correlation of cooking methods in 24 hours preservation with KMS

Condition	RS	B	OPDR	SF	DF
Raw State (RS)	1	1.000**(S)	-.657	.494	.928(S)
Boiling (B)	1.000**(S)	1	-.662	.500	.931(S)
Open Pan Dry Roasting (OPDR)	-.657	-.662	1	-.980(S)	-.890(S)
Shallow Frying (SF)	.494	.500	-.980(S)	1	.782
Deep Frying (DF)	.928(S)	.931	-.890(S)	.782	1

***.Correlation is highly significant at the 0.01 level (2-tailed)* ▭ Positive ▭ Negative *S= Significant*

This table shows the correlation of protein content of prawn with cooking methods. In 24 hours KMS preservation, there is perfect positive correlation present between the raw state and boiling, and significant positive correlation present between the raw state and deep frying. Boiling is positively correlated with deep frying. Open pan dry roasting is significant negatively correlated with shallow frying and deep frying. This table indicates that there is a strong correlation present among the **raw state, boiling, open pan dry roasting, shallow frying and deep frying** in 24 hours KMS preservation.

Table no 5.12.3.2.11 Correlation of cooking methods in 48 hours preservation with KMS

Condition	RS	B	OPDR	SF	DF
Raw State (RS)	1	.657	-.494	-.500	.825(S)
Boiling (B)	.657	1	-.980(S)	-.981(S)	.117
Open Pan Dry Roasting (OPDR)	-.494	-.980(S)	1	1.000**(S)	.083
Shallow Frying (SF)	-.500	-.981(S)	1.000**(S)	1	.076
Deep Frying (DF)	.825(S)	.117	.083	.076	1

***.Correlation is highly significant at the 0.01 level (2-tailed)* ▭ Positive ▭ Negative *S= Significant*

This table shows the correlation of protein content of prawn with cooking methods. In 48 hours KMS preservation, there is significant positive correlation present between the raw state and deep frying, whereas significant negative correlation present between the raw state with open pan dry roasting and shallow frying. Open pan dry roasting is perfect positively correlated with shallow frying. This table indicates that there is a strong correlation present among the **raw state, boiling, open pan dry roasting, shallow frying and deep frying** in 48 hours KMS preservation.

Table no 5.12.3.2.12 Correlation of cooking methods in 14 days preservation with KMS

Condition	RS	B	OPDR	SF	DF
Raw State (RS)	1	-.194	.981(S)	.746	.774
Boiling (B)	-.194	1	-.002	-.798	-.771
Open Pan Dry Roasting (OPDR)	.981(S)	-.002	1	.605	.638
Shallow Frying (SF)	.746	-.798	.605	1	.999*(S)
Deep Frying (DF)	.774	-.771	.638	.999*(S)	1

**.Correlation is highly significant at the 0.05 level (2-tailed)* ▭ Positive *S= Significant*

This table shows the correlation of protein content of prawn with cooking methods. In 14 days KMS preservation, there is significant positive correlation present between the raw state and open pan dry roasting, whereas shallow frying is highly significant positively correlated with deep frying. This table indicates that there is a strong correlation present between the **raw state and open pan dry roasting and also between shallow frying and deep frying** in 14 days KMS preservation.

Table no 5.12.3.2.13 Correlation of cooking methods in 15 days preservation with KMS

Condition	RS	B	OPDR	SF	DF
Raw State (RS)	1	.947(S)	-.943(S)	-.709	.189
Boiling (B)	.947(S)	1	-1.000**(S)	-.446	.493
Open Pan Dry Roasting (OPDR)	-.943(S)	-1.000**(S)	1	.433	-.506
Shallow Frying (SF)	-.709	-.446	.433	1	.559
Deep Frying (DF)	.189	.493	-.506	.559	1

***.Correlation is highly significant at the 0.01 level (2-tailed)* ▭ Positive ▭ Negative *S= Significant*

This table shows the correlation of protein content of prawn with cooking methods. In 15 days KMS preservation, there is significant positive correlation present between the raw state and boiling, and significant negative correlation present between the raw state and open pan dry roasting. Boiling is perfect negatively correlated with open pan dry roasting. This table indicates that there is a strong correlation present among the **raw state, boiling and open pan dry roasting** in 15 days KMS preservation.

Overall analysis reveals that the raw state is perfect positively correlated with boiling in 24 hours KMS preservation and 15 days control preservation without preservative, whereas perfect negatively correlated with open pan dry roasting in 15 days salt-turmeric preservation, perfect positively correlated with shallow frying in 15 days control preservation without preservative, and significant positively correlated with deep frying in 14 days control preservation without preservative. Boiling is perfect negatively correlated with open pan dry roasting and shallow frying in 24 hours salt-turmeric preservation and 15 days KMS preservation respectively, whereas perfect positively correlated with shallow frying in 15 days control preservation without preservative and 48 hours salt-turmeric preservation, and perfect positively correlated with deep frying in 24 hours salt-turmeric preservation. Open pan dry roasting is perfect positively correlated with shallow frying in 48 hours KMS preservation, and perfect negatively correlated with deep frying in 24 hours salt and turmeric preservation. Shallow frying is highly significant positively correlated with deep frying in 14 days KMS preservation. Most of the correlation of the protein content of prawn is found in **15 days control preservation without preservative and 24 hours salt and turmeric preservation** with respect to different cooking conditions.

5.12.3.3 Fat

Table no 5.12.3.3.1 Correlation of cooking methods in fresh condition

Condition	RS	B	OPDR	SF	DF
Raw State (RS)	1	-.681	-.886(S)	.861(S)	-.412
Boiling (B)	-.681	1	.943(S)	-.213	-.387
Open Pan Dry Roasting (OPDR)	-.886(S)	.943(S)	1	-.527	-.057
Shallow Frying (SF)	.861(S)	-.213	-.527	1	-.819(S)
Deep Frying (DF)	-.412	-.387	-.057	-.819(S)	1

Positive Negative *S= Significant*

This table shows the correlation of fat content of prawn with cooking methods. In fresh condition, there is significant positive correlation present between the raw state and shallow frying, and significant negative correlation present between the raw state and open pan dry roasting. Boiling is positively correlated with open pan dry roasting. Shallow frying is significant negatively correlated with deep frying. This table indicates that there is a strong correlation present among the **raw state, boiling, open pan dry roasting, shallow frying and deep frying** in fresh condition.

Table no 5.12.3.3.2 Correlation of cooking methods in 24 hours preservation without preservative

Condition	RS	B	OPDR	SF	DF
Raw State (RS)	1	.982(S)	.756	-.596	.500
Boiling (B)	.982(S)	1	.619	-.434	.327
Open Pan Dry Roasting (OPDR)	.756	.619	1	-.976(S)	.945(S)
Shallow Frying (SF)	-.596	-.434	-.976(S)	1	-.993(S)
Deep Frying (DF)	.500	.327	.945(S)	-.993(S)	1

Positive Negative *S= Significant*

This table shows the correlation of fat content of prawn with cooking methods. In 24 hours preservation without preservative, there is significant positive correlation present between the raw state and boiling, whereas open pan dry roasting is significant negatively correlated with shallow frying and significant positively correlated with deep frying. Shallow frying is significant negatively correlated with deep frying. This table indicates that there is a strong correlation present among the **raw state, boiling, open pan dry roasting, shallow frying and deep frying** in 24 hours preservation without preservative.

Table no 5.12.3.3.3 Correlation of cooking methods in 48 hours preservation without preservative

Condition	RS	B	OPDR	SF	DF
Raw State (RS)	1	1.000**(S)	.958(S)	.614	-.524
Boiling (B)	1.000**(S)	1	.958(S)	.614	-.524
Open Pan Dry Roasting (OPDR)	.958(S)	.958(S)	1	.363	-.746
Shallow Frying (SF)	.614	.614	.363	1	.350
Deep Frying (DF)	-.524	-.524	-.746	.350	1

***.Correlation is highly significant at the 0.01 level (2-tailed)* Positive Negative *S= Significant*

This table shows the correlation of fat content of prawn with cooking methods. In 48 hours preservation without preservative, there is significant positive correlation present between the raw state and open pan dry roasting and perfect positively correlated with boiling. Boiling is significant positively correlated with open pan dry roasting. This table indicates that there is a strong correlation present among the **raw state, boiling and open pan dry roasting** in 48 hours preservation without preservative.

Table no 5.12.3.3.4 Correlation of cooking methods in 14 days preservation without preservative

Condition	RS	B	OPDR	SF	DF
Raw State (RS)	1	-.500	.500	.596	.619
Boiling (B)	-.500	1	.500	-.993(S)	.371
Open Pan Dry Roasting (OPDR)	.500	.500	1	-.397	.990(S)
Shallow Frying (SF)	.596	-.993(S)	-.397	1	-.262
Deep Frying (DF)	.619	.371	.990(S)	-.262	1

Positive Negative *S= Significant*

This table shows the correlation of fat content of prawn with cooking methods. In 14 days preservation without preservative, there is significant negative correlation present between the raw state and shallow frying, whereas open pan dry roasting is significant positively correlated with deep frying. This table indicates that there is a strong correlation present between **boiling and shallow frying and also between open pan dry roasting and deep frying** in 14 days preservation without preservative.

Table no 5.12.3.3.5 Correlation of cooking methods in 15 days preservation without preservative

Condition	RS	B	OPDR	SF	DF
Raw State (RS)	1	-.034	-.952(S)	-.933(S)	-.860(S)
Boiling (B)	-.034	1	.339	-.327	.540
Open Pan Dry Roasting (OPDR)	-.952(S)	.339	1	.778	.975(S)
Shallow Frying (SF)	-.933(S)	-.327	.778	1	.619
Deep Frying (DF)	-.860(S)	.540	.975(S)	.619	1

Positive Negative *S= Significant*

This table shows the correlation of fat content of prawn with cooking methods. In 15 days preservation without preservative, there is significant negative correlation present between the raw state with open pan dry roasting, shallow frying and deep frying, whereas open pan dry roasting is significant positively correlated with deep frying. This table indicates that there is a strong correlation present among the **raw state, open pan dry roasting, shallow frying and deep frying** in 15 days preservation without preservative.

Table no 5.12.3.3.6 Correlation of cooking methods in 24 hours preservation with salt and turmeric

Condition	RS	B	OPDR	SF	DF
Raw State (RS)	1	-1.000**(S)	.434	.564	-.993(S)
Boiling (B)	-1.000**(S)	1	-.434	-.564	.993(S)
Open Pan Dry Roasting (OPDR)	.434	-.434	1	-.500	-.327
Shallow Frying (SF)	.564	-.564	-.500	1	-.655
Deep Frying (DF)	-.993(S)	.993(S)	-.327	-.655	1

***.Correlation is highly significant at the 0.01 level (2-tailed)* Positive Negative *S= Significant*

This table shows the correlation of fat content of prawn with cooking methods. In 24 hours salt and turmeric preservation, there is significant negative correlation present between the raw state and deep frying, and perfect negative correlation present between the raw state and boiling, whereas boiling is significant positively correlated with deep frying. This table indicates that there is a strong correlation present among the **raw state, boiling and deep frying** in 24 hours salt and turmeric preservation.

Table no 3.12.3.3.7 Correlation of cooking methods in 48 hours preservation with salt and turmeric

Condition	RS	B	OPDR	SF	DF
Raw State (RS)	1	-.908(S)	.945(S)	.908(S)	.982(S)
Boiling (B)	-.908(S)	1	-.721	-1.000**(S)	-.812(S)
Open Pan Dry Roasting (OPDR)	.945(S)	-.721	1	.721	.990(S)
Shallow Frying (SF)	.908(S)	-1.000**(S)	.721	1	.812(S)
Deep Frying (DF)	.982(S)	-.812(S)	.990(S)	.812(S)	1

***.Correlation is highly significant at the 0.01 level (2-tailed)* ▭ Positive ▭ Negative *S= Significant*

This table shows the correlation of fat content of prawn with cooking methods. In 48 hours salt and turmeric preservation, there is significant negative correlation present between the raw state and boiling, and significant negative correlation present between the raw state with open pan dry roasting, shallow frying and deep frying, whereas boiling is significant negatively correlated with deep frying and perfect negatively correlated with shallow frying. Open pan dry roasting is significant positively correlated with deep frying. Shallow frying is significant positively correlated with deep frying. This table indicates that there is a strong correlation present among the **raw state, boiling, open pan dry roasting, shallow frying and deep frying** in 48 hours salt and turmeric preservation.

Table no 3.12.3.3.8 Correlation of cooking methods in 14 days preservation with salt and turmeric

Condition	RS	B	OPDR	SF	DF
Raw State (RS)	1	.836(S)	.655	.000	-.327
Boiling (B)	.836(S)	1	.132	-.549	-.792
Open Pan Dry Roasting (OPDR)	.655	.132	1	.756	.500
Shallow Frying (SF)	.000	-.549	.756	1	.945(S)
Deep Frying (DF)	-.327	-.792	.500	.945(S)	1

▭ Positive *S= Significant*

This table shows the correlation of fat content of prawn with cooking methods. In 14 days salt and turmeric preservation, there is significant positive correlation present between the raw state and boiling, whereas shallow frying is significant positively correlated with deep frying. This table indicates that there is a strong correlation present between the **raw state and boiling and also between shallow frying and deep frying** in 14 days salt and turmeric preservation.

Table no 5.12.3.3.9 Correlation of cooking methods in 15 days preservation with salt and turmeric

Condition	RS	B	OPDR	SF	DF
Raw State (RS)	1	.999*(S)	-.971(S)	.277	-.992(S)
Boiling (B)	.999*(S)	1	-.982	.327	-.997*(S)
Open Pan Dry Roasting (OPDR)	-.971(S)	-.982(S)	1	-.500	.993(S)
Shallow Frying (SF)	.277	.327	-.500	1	-.397
Deep Frying (DF)	-.992(S)	-.997*(S)	.993(S)	-.397	1

**.Correlation is highly significant at the 0.05 level (2-tailed)* ▭ Positive ▭ Negative *S= Significant*

This table shows the correlation of fat content of prawn with cooking methods. In 15 days salt and turmeric preservation, there is significant negative correlation present between the raw state with open pan dry roasting and deep frying, and highly significant positive correlation present between the raw state and boiling, whereas boiling is significant negatively correlated with deep frying. Open pan dry roasting is significant positively correlated with deep frying. This table indicates that there is a strong correlation present among the **raw state, boiling, open pan dry roasting and deep frying** in 15 days salt and turmeric preservation.

Table no 5.12.3.3.10 Correlation of cooking methods in 24 hours preservation with KMS

Condition	RS	B	OPDR	SF	DF
Raw State (RS)	1	.125	-.901(S)	.156	-.013
Boiling (B)	.125	1	.319	-.961(S)	.991(S)
Open Pan Dry Roasting (OPDR)	-.901(S)	.319	1	-.569	.446
Shallow Frying (SF)	.156	-.961(S)	-.569	1	-.990(S)
Deep Frying (DF)	-.013	.991(S)	.446	-.990(S)	1

Positive Negative *S= Significant*

This table shows the correlation of fat content of prawn with cooking methods. In 24 hours KMS preservation, there is significant negative correlation present between the raw state and open pan dry roasting, and significant negative correlation present between boiling and shallow frying. Again boiling is significant positively correlated with deep frying. Shallow frying is significant negatively correlated with deep frying. This table indicates that there is a strong correlation present among the **raw state, boiling, open pan dry roasting, shallow frying and deep frying** in 24 hours KMS preservation.

Table no 5.12.3.3.11 Correlation of cooking methods in 48 hours preservation with KMS

Condition	RS	B	OPDR	SF	DF
Raw State (RS)	1	-.891(S)	.897(S)	-.189	.454
Boiling (B)	-.891(S)	1	-1.000**(S)	-.277	.000
Open Pan Dry Roasting (OPDR)	.897(S)	-1.000**(S)	1	.264	.014
Shallow Frying (SF)	-.189	-.277	.264	1	-.961(S)
Deep Frying (DF)	.454	.000	.014	-.961(S)	1

***.Correlation is highly significant at the 0.01 level (2-tailed)* Positive Negative *S= Significant*

This table shows the correlation of fat content of prawn with cooking methods. In 48 hours salt and turmeric preservation, there is significant negative correlation present between the raw state and boiling, and significant negative correlation present between the raw state with open pan dry roasting, shallow frying and deep frying, whereas boiling is significant negatively correlated with deep frying and perfect negatively correlated with shallow frying. Open pan dry roasting is significant positively correlated with deep frying. Shallow frying is significant positively correlated with deep frying. This table indicates that there is a strong correlation present among the **raw state, boiling, open pan dry roasting, shallow frying and deep frying** in 24 hours KMS preservation.

Table no 5.12.3.3.12 Correlation of cooking methods in 14 days preservation with KMS

Condition	RS	B	OPDR	SF	DF
Raw State (RS)	1	-.331	.397	.995(S)	-.268
Boiling (B)	-.331	1	.735	-.427	.998*(S)
Open Pan Dry Roasting (OPDR)	.397	.735	1	.300	.778
Shallow Frying (SF)	.995(S)	-.427	.300	1	-.366
Deep Frying (DF)	-.268	.998*(S)	.778	-.366	1

**.Correlation is highly significant at the 0.05 level (2-tailed)* Positive *S= Significant*

This table shows the correlation of fat content of prawn with cooking methods. In 48 hours KMS preservation, there is significant positive correlation present between the raw state and shallow frying, and highly significant positive correlation present between boiling and deep frying. This table indicates that there is a strong correlation present between the **raw state and shallow frying and also between boiling and deep frying** in 48 hours KMS preservation.

Table no 5.12.3.3.13 Correlation of cooking methods in 15 days preservation with KMS

Condition	RS	B	OPDR	SF	DF
Raw State (RS)	1	.472	.989(S)	-.816(S)	.997(S)
Boiling (B)	.472	1	.339	-.895(S)	.540
Open Pan Dry Roasting (OPDR)	.989(S)	.339	1	-.723	.975(S)
Shallow Frying (SF)	-.816(S)	-.895(S)	-.723	1	-.860(S)
Deep Frying (DF)	.997(S)	.540	.975(S)	-.860(S)	1

Positive Negative *S= Significant*

This table shows the correlation of fat content of prawn with cooking methods. In 14 days KMS preservation, there is significant negative correlation present between the raw state and shallow frying, and significant positive correlation present between the raw state with open pan dry roasting and deep frying, whereas boiling is significant negatively correlated with shallow frying. Open pan dry roasting is significant positively correlated with deep frying. Shallow frying is significant negatively correlated with deep frying. This table indicates that there is a strong correlation present among the **raw state, boiling, open pan dry roasting, shallow frying and deep frying** in 14 days KMS preservation.

Overall analysis reveals that the raw state is perfect positively correlated with boiling in 48 hours control preservation without preservative, whereas significant positively correlated with open pan dry roasting and deep frying in 15 days KMS preservation, and significant positively correlated with shallow frying in 14 days KMS preservation. Boiling is perfect negatively correlated with open pan dry roasting and shallow frying in 48 hours KMS preservation and 48 hours salt-turmeric preservation respectively, whereas highly significant positively correlated with deep frying in 14 days KMS preservation. Open pan dry roasting is significant negatively correlated with shallow frying in 24 hours control preservation without preservative, and significant positively correlated with deep frying in 15 days salt and turmeric preservation. Shallow frying is significant negatively correlated with deep frying in 24 hours control preservation without preservative. Most of the correlation of the fat content of prawn is found in **24 hours control preservation without preservative, 15 days salt and turmeric preservation, and 14 days and 15 days KMS preservation** with respect to different cooking conditions.

5.12.3.4 Moisture

Table no 5.12.3.4.1 Correlation of cooking methods in fresh condition

Condition	RS	B	OPDR	SF	DF
Raw State (RS)	1	.997(S)	-.838(S)	-.335	.993(S)
Boiling (B)	.997(S)	1	-.879(S)	-.408	.981(S)
Open Pan Dry Roasting (OPDR)	-.838(S)	-.879(S)	1	.794	-.769
Shallow Frying (SF)	-.335	-.408	.794	1	-.222
Deep Frying (DF)	.993(S)	.981(S)	-.769	-.222	1

Positive Negative *S= Significant*

This table shows the correlation of moisture content of prawn with cooking methods. In fresh condition, there is significant negative correlation present between the raw state and open pan dry roasting, and significant positive correlation present between the raw state with boiling and deep frying, whereas boiling is significant negatively correlated with open pan dry roasting and negatively correlated with deep frying. This table indicates that there is a strong correlation present among the **raw state, boiling, open pan dry roasting and deep frying** in fresh condition.

Table no 5.12.3.4.2 Correlation of cooking methods in 24 hours preservation without preservatives

Condition	RS	B	OPDR	SF	DF
Raw state (RS)	1	.328	-.546	.672	.705
Boiling (B)	.328	1	-.971(S)	.920(S)	.902(S)
Open Pan Dry Roasting (OPDR)	-.546	-.971(S)	1	-.987(S)	-.979(S)
Shallow Frying (SF)	.672	.920(S)	-.987(S)	1	.999*(S)
Deep Frying (DF)	.705	.902(S)	-.979(S)	.999*(S)	1

**.Correlation is highly significant at the 0.05 level (2-tailed)* Positive Negative *S= Significant*

This table shows the correlation of moisture content of prawn with cooking methods. In 24 hours preservation without preservative, there is significant negative correlation present between boiling and open pan dry roasting, and significant positive correlation present between boiling with shallow frying and deep frying, whereas open pan dry roasting is significant negatively correlated with shallow frying and deep frying. Shallow frying is highly significant positively correlated with deep frying. This table indicates that there is a strong correlation present among **boiling, open pan dry roasting and deep frying** in 24 hours preservation without preservative.

Table no 5.12.3.4.3 Correlation of cooking methods in 48 hours preservation without preservatives

Condition	RS	B	OPDR	SF	DF
Raw State (RS)	1	.729	-.357	-.946(S)	.611
Boiling (B)	.729	1	.379	-.911(S)	-.096
Open Pan Dry Roasting (OPDR)	-.357	.379	1	.035	-.957(S)
Shallow Frying (SF)	-.946(S)	-.911(S)	.035	1	-.323
Deep Frying (DF)	.611	-.096	-.957(S)	-.323	1

Negative *S= Significant*

This table shows the correlation of moisture content of prawn with cooking methods. In 48 hours preservation without preservative, there is significant negative correlation present between the raw state and shallow frying, whereas significant negative correlation present between boiling and shallow frying. Open pan dry roasting is significant negatively correlated with deep frying. This table indicates that there is a strong correlation present among the **raw state, boiling, open pan dry roasting, shallow frying and deep frying** in 48 hours preservation without preservative.

Table no 5.12.3.4.4 Correlation of cooking methods in 14 days preservation without preservatives

Condition	RS	B	OPDR	SF	DF
Raw State (RS)	1	.945(S)	-.500	-.156	-1.000*(S)
Boiling (B)	.945(S)	1	-.189	.176	-.953(S)
Open Pan Dry Roasting (OPDR)	-.500	-.189	1	.933(S)	.478
Shallow Frying (SF)	-.156	.176	.933(S)	1	.131
Deep Frying (DF)	-1.000*(S)	-.953(S)	.478	.131	1

**.Correlation is highly significant at the 0.05 level (2-tailed)* Positive Negative *S= Significant*

This table shows the correlation of moisture content of prawn with cooking methods. In 14 days preservation without preservative, there is significant positive correlation present between the raw state and boiling, and perfect positive correlation present between the raw state and deep frying, whereas open pan dry roasting is significant positively correlated with shallow frying. This table indicates that there is a strong correlation present among the **raw state, boiling, open pan dry roasting, shallow frying and deep frying** in 14 days preservation without preservative.

Table no 5.12.3.4.5 Correlation of cooking methods in 15 days preservation without preservatives

Condition	RS	B	OPDR	SF	DF
Raw State (RS)	1	-.589	-.143	.972(S)	.998*(S)
Boiling (B)	-.589	1	.884(S)	-.383	-.537
Open Pan Dry Roasting (OPDR)	-.143	.884(S)	1	.094	-.080
Shallow Frying (SF)	.972(S)	-.383	.094	1	.985(S)
Deep Frying (DF)	.998*(S)	-.537	-.080	.985(S)	1

**.Correlation is highly significant at the 0.05 level (2-tailed)* ▭ Positive *S= Significant*

This table shows the correlation of moisture content of prawn with cooking methods. In 15 days preservation without preservative, there is significant positive correlation present between the raw state and shallow frying, and highly significant positive correlation present between the raw state and deep frying, whereas open pan dry roasting is significant positively correlated with boiling. Shallow frying is highly significant positively correlated with deep frying. This table indicates that there is a strong correlation present among the **raw state, boiling, open pan dry roasting and deep frying** in 15 days preservation without preservative.

Table no 5.12.3.4.6 Correlation of cooking methods in 24 hours preservation with salt and turmeric

Condition	RS	B	OPDR	SF	DF
Raw State (RS)	1	.597	1.000**(S)	-.483	-.038
Boiling (B)	.597	1	.586	-.991(S)	.779
Open Pan Dry Roasting (OPDR)	1.000**(S)	.586	1	-.470	-.052
Shallow Frying (SF)	-.483	-.991(S)	-.470	1	-.857(S)
Deep Frying (DF)	-.038	.779	-.052	-.857(S)	1

**.Correlation is highly significant at the 0.05 level (2-tailed)* ▭ Positive ▭ Negative *S= Significant*

This table shows the correlation of moisture content of prawn with cooking methods. In 24 hours salt and turmeric preservation, there is perfect positive correlation present between the raw state and open pan dry roasting, whereas significant negative correlation present between boiling and shallow frying. Shallow frying is significant negatively correlated with deep frying. This table indicates that there is a strong correlation present among the **raw state, boiling, open pan dry roasting and deep frying** in 24 hours salt and turmeric preservation.

Table no 5.12.3.4.7 Correlation of cooking methods in 48 hours preservation with salt and turmeric

Condition	RS	B	OPDR	SF	DF
Raw State (RS)	1	-.603	-.464	-.462	-.998*(S)
Boiling (B)	-.603	1	.986(S)	-.429	.653
Open Pan Dry Roasting (OPDR)	-.464	.986(S)	1	-.572	.519
Shallow Frying (SF)	-.462	-.429	-.572	1	.404
Deep Frying (DF)	-.998*(S)	.653	.519	.404	1

**.Correlation is highly significant at the 0.05 level (2-tailed)* Positive Negative *S= Significant*

This table shows the correlation of moisture content of prawn with cooking methods. In 48 hours salt and turmeric preservation, there is highly significant negative correlation present between the raw state and deep frying, whereas significant positive correlation present between boiling and open pan dry roasting. This table indicates that there is a strong correlation present between the **raw state and deep frying and also between boiling and open pan dry roasting** in 48 hours salt and turmeric preservation.

Table no 5.12.3.4.8 Correlation of cooking methods in 14 days preservation with salt and turmeric

Condition	RS	B	OPDR	SF	DF
Raw State (RS)	1	-.265	.126	.738	-.689
Boiling (B)	-.265	1	.923(S)	.456	.881(S)
Open Pan Dry Roasting (OPDR)	.126	.923(S)	1	.763	.632
Shallow Frying (SF)	.738	.456	.763	1	-.019
Deep Frying (DF)	-.689	.881(S)	.632	-.019	1

Positive *S= Significant*

This table shows the correlation of moisture content of prawn with cooking methods. In 14 days salt and turmeric preservation, there is significant positive correlation present between boiling with open pan dry roasting and deep frying. This table indicates that there is a strong correlation present among **boiling, open pan dry roasting and deep frying** in 14 days salt and turmeric preservation.

Table no 5.12.3.4.9 Correlation of cooking methods in 15 days preservation with salt and turmeric

Condition	RS	B	OPDR	SF	DF
Raw State (RS)	1	-.623	-.610	.958(S)	-.077
Boiling (B)	-.623	1	1.000*(S)	-.822(S)	-.731
Open Pan Dry Roasting (OPDR)	-.610	1.000*(S)	1	-.812(S)	-.743
Shallow Frying (SF)	.958(S)	-.822(S)	-.812(S)	1	.213
Deep Frying (DF)	-.077	-.731	-.743	.213	1

**.Correlation is highly significant at the 0.05 level (2-tailed)* Positive Negative *S= Significant*

This table shows the correlation of moisture content of prawn with cooking methods. In 15 days salt and turmeric preservation, there is positive correlation present between the raw state and shallow frying, whereas significant negative correlation present between boiling and shallow frying, and perfect positive correlation present between boiling and open pan dry roasting. Shallow frying is significant negatively correlated with open pan dry roasting. This table indicates that there is a strong correlation present among the **raw state, boiling, open pan dry roasting and shallow frying** in 15 days salt and turmeric preservation.

Table no 5.12.3.4.10 Correlation of cooking methods in 24 hours preservation with KMS

Condition	RS	B	OPDR	SF	DF
Raw State (RS)	1	.890(S)	.235	-.994(S)	-.509
Boiling (B)	.890(S)	1	-.235	-.935(S)	-.060
Open Pan Dry Roasting (OPDR)	.235	-.235	1	-.126	-.956(S)
Shallow Frying (SF)	-.994(S)	-.935(S)	-.126	1	.410
Deep Frying (DF)	-.509	-.060	-.956(S)	.410	1

Positive Negative *S= Significant*

This table shows the correlation of moisture content of prawn with cooking methods. In 24 hours KMS preservation, there is significant positive correlation present between the raw state and boiling, and significant negative correlation present between the raw state and shallow frying, whereas significant negative correlation present between boiling and shallow frying. Deep frying is significant negatively correlated with open pan dry roasting. This table indicates that there is a strong correlation present among the **raw state, boiling, open pan dry roasting, shallow frying and deep frying** in 24 hours KMS preservation.

Table no 5.12.3.4.11 Correlation of cooking methods in 48 hours preservation with KMS

Condition	RS	B	OPDR	SF	DF
Raw State (RS)	1	.982(S)	-.821(S)	-.904(S)	-.204
Boiling (B)	.982(S)	1	-.914(S)	-.806(S)	-.016
Open Pan Dry Roasting (OPDR)	-.821(S)	-.914(S)	1	.498	-.390
Shallow Frying (SF)	-.904(S)	-.806(S)	.498	1	.604
Deep Frying (DF)	-.204	-.016	-.390	.604	1

Positive Negative *S= Significant*

This table shows the correlation of moisture content of prawn with cooking methods. In 48 hours KMS preservation, there is significant positive correlation present between the raw state and boiling, and significant negative correlation present between the raw state with open pan dry roasting and shallow frying, whereas significant negative correlation present between boiling with open pan dry roasting and shallow frying. This table indicates that there is a strong correlation present among the **raw state, boiling, open pan dry roasting and shallow frying** in 48 hours KMS preservation.

Table no 5.12.3.4.12 Correlation of cooking methods in 14 days preservation with KMS

Condition	RS	B	OPDR	SF	DF
Raw State (RS)	1	.387	.970(S)	.943(S)	.854(S)
Boiling (B)	.387	1	.151	.672	-.149
Open Pan Dry Roasting (OPDR)	.970(S)	.151	1	.834(S)	.955(S)
Shallow Frying (SF)	.943(S)	.672	.834(S)	1	.632
Deep Frying (DF)	.854(S)	-.149	.955(S)	.632	1

Positive *S= Significant*

This table shows the correlation of moisture content of prawn with cooking methods. In 14 days KMS preservation, there is significant positive correlation present between the raw state with open pan dry roasting, shallow frying and deep frying, whereas significant positive correlation present between boiling with shallow frying and deep frying. This table indicates that there is a strong correlation present among the **raw state, open pan dry roasting, shallow frying and deep frying** in 14 days KMS preservation.

Table no 5.12.3.4.13 Correlation of cooking methods in 15 days preservation with KMS

Condition	RS	B	OPDR	SF	DF\
Raw State (RS)	1	.755	-.097	-.555	.999*(S)
Boiling (B)	.755	1	-.727	-.965(S)	.725
Open Pan Dry Roasting (OPDR)	-.097	-.727	1	.882(S)	-.053
Shallow Frying (SF)	-.555	-.965(S)	.882(S)	1	-.518
Deep Frying (DF)	.999*(S)	.725	-.053	-.518	1

Positive Negative *S= Significant*

This table shows the correlation of moisture content of prawn with cooking methods. In 15 days KMS preservation, there is significant positive correlation present between the raw state and deep frying, and significant negative correlation present between boiling and shallow frying. Open pan dry roasting significant positively correlated with shallow frying. This table indicates that there is a strong correlation present among the **raw state, boiling, open pan dry roasting, shallow frying and deep frying** in 15 days KMS preservation.

Overall analysis reveals that the raw state is significant positively correlated with boiling in fresh condition, whereas perfect positively correlated with open pan dry roasting in 24 hours preservation with salt and turmeric, significant negatively correlated with shallow frying in 24 hours KMS preservation, and perfect negatively correlated with deep frying in 14 days control preservation without preservative. Boiling is perfect positively correlated with open pan dry roasting in 15 days salt-turmeric preservation, whereas significant negatively correlated with shallow frying in 24 hours salt and turmeric preservation, and significant positively correlated with deep frying in fresh condition. Open pan dry roasting is negatively correlated with shallow frying and deep frying in 24 hours control preservation without preservative. Shallow frying is highly significant positively correlated with deep frying in 24 hours control preservation without preservative. Most of the correlation of the moisture content of prawn is found in **24 hours control preservation without preservative** with respect to different cooking conditions.

5.12.3.5 Ash

Table no 5.12.3.5.1 Correlation of cooking methods in fresh condition

Condition	RS	B	OPDR	SF	DF
Raw State (RS)	1	.974(S)	.981(S)	.839(S)	.564
Boiling (B)	.974(S)	1	.911(S)	.941(S)	.737
Open Pan Dry Roasting (OPDR)	.981(S)	.911(S)	1	.718	.392
Shallow Frying (SF)	.839	.941(S)	.718	1	.922(S)
Deep Frying (DF)	.564	.737	.392	.922(S)	1

Positive *S= Significant*

This table shows the correlation of ash content of prawn with cooking methods. In fresh condition, there is significant positive correlation present between the raw state with boiling, open pan dry roasting, deep frying. Boiling is significant positively correlated with open pan dry roasting and shallow frying.

Shallow frying significant positively correlated with deep frying. This table indicates that there is a strong correlation present among the **raw state, boiling, open pan dry roasting, shallow frying and deep frying** in fresh condition.

Table no 5.12.3.5.2 Correlation of cooking methods in 24 hours preservation without preservative

Condition	RS	B	OPDR	SF	DF
Raw State (RS)	1	-.693	.246	.062	.030
Boiling (B)	-.693	1	.528	.676	.700
Open Pan Dry Roasting (OPDR)	.246	.528	1	.983(S)	.976(S)
Shallow Frying (SF)	.062	.676	.983(S)	1	.999*(S)
Deep Frying (DF)	.030	.700	.976(S)	.999*(S)	1

**.Correlation is highly significant at the 0.05 level (2-tailed)* ▭ Positive *S= Significant*

This table shows the correlation of ash content of prawn with cooking methods. In 24 hours control preservation without preservative, there is significant positive correlation present between open pan dry roasting with shallow frying and deep frying, whereas highly significant positive correlation present between shallow frying and deep frying. This table indicates that there is a strong correlation present among **open pan dry roasting, shallow frying and deep frying** in 24 hours preservation without preservative.

Table no 5.12.3.5.3 Correlation of cooking methods in 48 hours preservation without preservative

Condition	RS	B	OPDR	SF	DF
Raw State (RS)	1	.991(S)	.979(S)	.178	.916(S)
Boiling (B)	.991(S)	1	.998*(S)	.311	.962(S)
Open Pan Dry Roasting (OPDR)	.979(S)	.998*(S)	1	.375	.979(S)
Shallow Frying (SF)	.178	.311	.375	1	.558
Deep Frying (DF)	.916(S)	.962(S)	.979(S)	.558	1

**.Correlation is highly significant at the 0.05 level (2-tailed)* ▭ Positive *S= Significant*

This table shows the correlation of ash content of prawn with cooking methods. In 48 hours control preservation without preservative, there is significant positive correlation present between the raw state with open pan dry roasting, boiling and deep frying, whereas boiling is highly significant positively correlated with open pan dry roasting and significant positively correlated with deep frying. This table indicates that there is a strong correlation present among the **raw state, boiling, open pan dry roasting and deep frying** in 48 hours control preservation without preservative.

Table no 5.12.3.5.4 Correlation of cooking methods in 14 days preservation without preservative

Condition	RS	B	OPDR	SF	DF
Raw state (RS)	1	.991(S)	.721	.933(S)	.961(S)
Boiling (B)	.991(S)	1	.806(S)	.973(S)	.989(S)
Open Pan Dry Roasting (OPDR)	.721	.806(S)	1	.922(S)	.885(S)
Shallow Frying (SF)	.933(S)	.973(S)	.922(S)	1	.996(S)
Deep Frying (DF)	.961(S)	.989(S)	.885(S)	.996(S)	1

▭ Positive *S= Significant*

This table shows the correlation of ash content of prawn with cooking methods. In 14 days control preservation without preservative, there is significant positive correlation present between the raw state with boiling, shallow frying and deep frying, whereas boiling is significant positively correlated with open pan dry roasting, shallow frying and deep frying. Open pan dry roasting is significant positively correlated with shallow frying and deep frying. Again shallow frying is significant positively correlated with deep frying. This table indicates that there is a strong correlation present among the **raw state, boiling, open pan dry roasting, shallow frying and deep frying** in 14 days preservation without preservative.

Table no 5.12.3.5.5 Correlation of cooking methods in 15 days preservation without preservative

Condition	RS	B	OPDR	SF	DF
Raw State (RS)	1	-.486	.999*(S)	-.373	-.999*(S)
Boiling (B)	-.486	1	-.532	.992(S)	.532
Open Pan Dry Roasting (OPDR)	.999*(S)	-.532	1	-.421	-1.000**(S)
Shallow Frying (SF)	-.373	.992(S)	-.421	1	.421
Deep Frying (DF)	-.999*(S)	.532	-1.000**(S)	.421	1

**.Correlation is highly significant at the 0.05 level (2-tailed)* Positive Negative *S= Significant*
***.Correlation is highly significant at the 0.01 level (2-tailed)*

This table shows the correlation of ash content of prawn with cooking methods. In 15 days control preservation without preservative, there is highly significant positive correlation present between the raw state and open pan dry roasting, whereas highly significant negative correlation present between the raw state and deep frying. Again boiling is significant positively correlated with shallow frying. Open pan dry roasting is perfect negatively correlated with deep frying. This table indicates that there is a strong correlation present among the **raw state, boiling, open pan dry roasting, shallow frying and deep frying** in 15 days preservation without preservative.

Table no 5.12.3.5.6 Correlation of cooking methods in 24 hours preservation with salt and turmeric

Condition	RS	B	OPDR	SF	DF
Raw State (RS)	1	.991(S)	.980(S)	.623	-.110
Boiling (B)	.991(S)	1	.945(S)	.721	-.240
Open Pan Dry Roasting (OPDR)	.980(S)	.945(S)	1	.454	.091
Shallow Frying (SF)	.623	.721	.454	1	-.846(S)
Deep Frying (DF)	-.110	-.240	.091	-.846(S)	1

Positive Negative *S= Significant*

This table shows the correlation of ash content of prawn with cooking methods. In 24 hours salt and turmeric preservation, there is highly significant positive correlation present between the raw state with boiling and open pan dry roasting, whereas significant positive correlation present between boiling and open pan dry roasting. Again shallow frying is significant negatively correlated with deep frying. This table indicates that there is a strong correlation present among the **raw state, boiling, open pan dry roasting, shallow frying and deep frying** in 24 hours salt and turmeric preservation.

Table no 5.12.3.5.7 Correlation of cooking methods in 48 hours preservation with salt and turmeric

Condition	RS	B	OPDR	SF	DF
Raw state (RS)	1	-.971(S)	-.908(S)	-.971(S)	-.992(S)
Boiling (B)	-.971(S)	1	.982(S)	1.000**(S)	.993(S)
Open Pan Dry Roasting (OPDR)	-.908(S)	.982(S)	1	.982(S)	.954(S)
Shallow Frying (SF)	-.971(S)	1.000**(S)	.982(S)	1	.993(S)
Deep Frying (DF)	-.992(S)	.993(S)	.954(S)	.993(S)	1

***.Correlation is highly significant at the 0.01 level (2-tailed)* Positive Negative *S= Significant*

This table shows the correlation of ash content of prawn with cooking methods. In 48 hours salt and turmeric preservation, there is significant negative correlation present between the raw state with boiling, open pan dry roasting, shallow frying and deep frying, whereas significant positive correlation present between boiling with open pan dry roasting and deep frying, and perfect positive correlation present between boiling and shallow frying. Again open pan dry roasting is significant positively correlated with shallow frying and deep frying. Shallow frying is significant positively correlated with deep frying. This table indicates that there is a strong correlation present among the **raw state, boiling, open pan dry roasting, shallow frying and deep frying** in 48 hours salt and turmeric preservation.

Table no 5.12.3.5.8 Correlation of cooking methods in 14 hours preservation with salt and turmeric

Condition	RS	B	OPDR	SF	DF
Raw State (RS)	1	1.000**(S)	.945(S)	.990(S)	.235
Boiling (B)	1.000**(S)	1	.945(S)	.990(S)	.235
Open Pan Dry Roasting (OPDR)	.945(S)	.945(S)	1	.888(S)	-.096
Shallow Frying (SF)	.990(S)	.990(S)	.888(S)	1	.371
Deep Frying (DF)	.235	.235	-.096	.371	1

***.Correlation is highly significant at the 0.01 level (2-tailed)* Positive *S= Significant*

This table shows the correlation of ash content of prawn with cooking methods. In 14 days salt and turmeric preservation, there is significant positive correlation present between the raw state with open pan dry roasting and shallow frying and perfect positive correlation present between the raw state and boiling, whereas significant positive correlation present between boiling with open pan dry roasting and shallow frying. Again open pan dry roasting is significant positively correlated with shallow frying. This table indicates that there is a strong correlation present among the **raw state, boiling, open pan dry roasting and shallow frying** in 14 days salt and turmeric preservation.

Table no 5.12.3.5.9 Correlation of cooking methods in 15 days preservation with salt and turmeric

Condition	RS	B	OPDR	SF	DF
Raw State (RS)	1	-.500	-.419	.000	.189
Boiling (B)	-.500	1	.996(S)	.866(S)	.756
Open Pan Dry Roasting (OPDR)	-.419	.996(S)	1	.908(S)	.812(S)
Shallow Frying (SF)	.000	.866(S)	.908(S)	1	.982(S)
Deep Frying (DF)	.189	.756	.812(S)	.982(S)	1

Positive *S= Significant*

This table shows the correlation of ash content of Prawn with cooking methods. In 15 days salt and turmeric preservation, there is significant positive correlation present between boiling with open pan dry roasting and shallow frying, whereas significant positive correlation present between open pan dry roasting with shallow frying and deep frying Again shallow frying is significant positively correlated with shallow frying and deep frying. Shallow frying is significant positively correlated with deep frying. This table indicates that there is a strong correlation present among **boiling, open pan dry roasting, shallow frying and deep frying** in 15 days salt and turmeric preservation.

Table no 5.12.3.5.10 Correlation of cooking methods in 24 hours preservation with KMS

Condition	RS	B	OPDR	SF	DF
Raw State (Rs)	1	.540	.332	.540	-.483
Boiling (B)	.540	1	-.614	1.000**(S)	.475
Open Pan Dry Roasting (OPDR)	.332	-.614	1	-.614	-.986(S)
Shallow Frying (SF)	.540	1.000**(S)	-.614	1	.475
Deep Frying (DF)	-.483	.475	-.986(S)	.475	1

***.Correlation is highly significant at the 0.01 level (2-tailed)* Positive Negative *S= Significant*

This table shows the correlation of ash content of Prawn with cooking methods. In 24 hours KMS preservation, there is perfect positive correlation present between boiling and shallow frying, whereas significant negative correlation present between open pan dry roasting and deep frying. This table indicates that there is a strong correlation present between **boiling and shallow frying and also between open pan dry roasting and deep frying** in 24 hours KMS preservation.

Table no 5.12.3.5.11 Correlation of cooking methods in 48 hours preservation with KMS

Condition	RS	B	OPDR	SF	DF
Raw State (RS)	1	.161	.967(S)	.800(S)	.989(S)
Boiling (B)	.161	1	.407	.721	.013
Open Pan Dry Roasting (OPDR)	.967(S)	.407	1	.926(S)	.919(S)
Shallow Frying (SF)	.800(S)	.721	.926(S)	1	.703
Deep Frying (DF)	.989(S)	.013	.919(S)	.703	1

Positive *S= Significant*

This table shows the correlation of ash content of prawn with cooking methods. In 48 hours KMS preservation, there is perfect positive correlation present between the raw state with open pan roasting, shallow frying and deep frying, whereas significant positive correlation present between open pan dry roasting with shallow frying and deep frying. This table indicates that there is a strong correlation present among the **raw state, open pan dry roasting, shallow frying and deep frying in** 48 hours KMS preservation.

Table no 5.12.3.5.12 Correlation of cooking methods in 14 days preservation with KMS

Condition	RS	B	OPDR	SF	DF
Raw State (RS)	1	-.606	.995(S)	-.545	-.632
Boiling (B)	-.606	1	-.524	.997*(S)	.999*(S)
Open Pan Dry Roasting (OPDR)	.995(S)	-.524	1	-.459	-.552
Shallow Frying (SF)	-.545	.997*(S)	-.459	1	.994(S)
Deep Frying (DF)	-.632	.999*(S)	-.552	.994(S)	1

**.Correlation is highly significant at the 0.05 level (2-tailed)* Positive *S= Significant*

This table shows the correlation of ash content of prawn with cooking methods. In 14 days KMS preservation, there is significant positive correlation present between the raw state and open pan dry roasting, whereas highly significant positive correlation present between boiling with shallow frying and deep frying. Shallow frying is significant positively correlated with deep frying. This table indicates that there is a strong correlation present among the **raw state, boiling, open pan dry roasting, shallow frying and deep frying** in 14 days KMS preservation.

Table no 5.12.3.5.13 Correlation of cooking methods in 15 days preservation with KMS

Condition	RS	B	OPDR	SF	DF
Raw State (RS)	1	.999*(S)	-.815(S)	-.470	-.897(S)
Boiling (B)	.999*(S)	1	-.796	-.442	-.883(S)
Open Pan Dry Roasting (OPDR)	-.815(S)	-.796	1	.895(S)	.987(S)
Shallow Frying (SF)	-.470	-.442	.895(S)	1	.812(S)
Deep Frying (DF)	-.897(S)	-.883(S)	.987(S)	.812(S)	1

**.Correlation is highly significant at the 0.05 level (2-tailed)* Positive Negative *S= Significant*

This table shows the correlation of ash content of prawn with cooking methods. In 15 days KMS preservation, there is highly significant positive correlation present between the raw state and boiling, and significant negative correlation present between the raw state with open pan dry roasting and deep frying, whereas significant negative correlation present between boiling and deep frying. Open pan dry roasting is significant positively correlated with shallow frying and deep frying. Shallow frying is significant positively correlated with deep frying. This table indicates that there is a strong correlation present among the **raw state, boiling, open pan dry roasting, shallow frying and deep frying** in 15 days KMS preservation.

Overall analysis reveals that the raw state is perfect positively correlated with boiling in 14 days salt-turmeric preservation, whereas highly significant positively correlated with open pan dry roasting in 15 days control preservation without preservative, significant positively correlated with shallow frying in 14 days salt and turmeric preservation, and highly significant negatively correlated with deep frying in 15 days control preservation without preservative. Boiling is highly significant positively correlated with open pan dry roasting in 48 hours control preservation without preservative, whereas perfect positively correlated with shallow frying in 48 hours salt and turmeric preservation and 24 hours KMS preservation, and significant positively correlated with deep frying in 14 days control preservation without preservative. Open pan dry roasting is significant positively correlated with shallow frying in 48 hours salt and turmeric preservation, and perfect positively correlated with deep frying in 15 days control preservation without preservative. Shallow frying is highly significant positively correlated with deep frying in 24 hours control preservation without preservative. Most of the correlation of the ash content of prawn is found in **15 days control preservation without preservative** with respect to different cooking conditions.

5.12.3.6 Calcium

Table no 5.12.3.6.1 Correlation of cooking methods in fresh condition

Condition	RS	B	OPDR	SF	DF
Raw State (RS)	1	.961(S)	.961(S)	.961(S)	.891(S)
Boiling (B)	.961(S)	1	1.000**(S)	1.000**(S)	.982(S)
Open Pan Dry Roasting (OPDR)	.961(S)	1.000**(S)	1	1.000**(S)	.982(S)
Shallow Frying (SF)	.961(S)	1.000**(S)	1.000**(S)	1	.982(S)
Deep Frying (DF)	.891(S)	.982(S)	.982(S)	.982(S)	1

***.Correlation is highly significant at the 0.01 level (2-tailed)* Positive *S= Significant*

This table shows the correlation of calcium content of prawn with cooking methods. In fresh condition, there is significant positive correlation present between the raw state with boiling, open pan dry roasting, shallow frying and deep frying. Again boiling is perfect positively correlated with open pan dry roasting and shallow frying and significant positively correlated with deep frying. Open pan dry roasting is significant positively correlated with deep frying and perfect positively correlated with shallow frying. Shallow frying is significant positively correlated with deep frying. This table indicates that there is a strong correlation present among the **raw state, boiling, open pan dry roasting, shallow frying and deep frying** in fresh condition.

Table no 5.12.3.6.2 Correlation of cooking methods in 24 hours preservation without preservative

Condition	RS	B	OPDR	SF	DF
Raw State (RS)	1	.619	.327	.052	.500
Boiling (B)	.619	1	.945(S)	.817(S)	.990(S)
Open Pan Dry Roasting (OPDR)	.327	.945(S)	1	.961(S)	.982(S)
Shallow Frying (SF)	.052	.817(S)	.961(S)	1	.891(S)
Deep Frying (DF)	.500	.990(S)	.982(S)	.891(S)	1

Positive *S= Significant*

This table shows the correlation of calcium content of prawn with cooking methods. In 24 hours control preservation without preservative, there is significant positive correlation present between boiling with open pan dry roasting, shallow frying and deep frying. Open pan dry roasting is significant positively correlated with shallow frying and deep frying. Shallow frying is significant positively correlated with deep frying. This table indicates that there is a strong correlation present among **boiling, open pan dry roasting, shallow frying and deep frying** 24 hours control preservation without preservative.

Table no 5.12.3.6.3 Correlation of cooking methods in 48 hours preservation without preservative

Condition	RS	B	OPDR	SF	DF
Raw state (RS)	1	.929(S)	.982(S)	.891(S)	.929(S)
Boiling (B)	.929(S)	1	.982(S)	.996(S)	1.000**(S)
Open Pan Dry Roasting (OPDR)	.982(S)	.982(S)	1	.961(S)	.982(S)
Shallow Frying (SF)	.891(S)	.996(S)	.961(S)	1	.996(S)
Deep Frying (DF)	.929(S)	1.000**(S)	.982(S)	.996(S)	1

***.Correlation is highly significant at the 0.01 level (2-tailed)* Positive *S= Significant*

This table shows the correlation of calcium content of prawn with cooking methods. In 48 hours control preservation without preservative, there is significant positive correlation present between the raw state with boiling, open pan dry roasting, shallow frying and deep frying, whereas significant positive correlation present between boiling with open pan dry roasting and shallow frying and perfect positive correlation present between boiling and deep frying. Open pan dry roasting is significant positively correlated with shallow frying and deep frying. Shallow frying is significant positively correlated with deep frying. This table indicates that there is a strong correlation present among the **raw state, boiling, open pan dry roasting, shallow frying and deep frying** in 48 hours preservation without preservative.

Table no 5.12.3.6.4 Correlation of cooking methods in 14 days preservation without preservative

Condition	RS	B	OPDR	SF	DF
Raw State (RS)	1	.961(S)	.961(S)	.721	.961(S)
Boiling (B)	.961(S)	1	1.000**(S)	.500	1.000**(S)
Open Pan Dry Roasting (OPDR)	.961(S)	1.000**(S)	1	.500	1.000**(S)
Shallow Frying (SF)	.721	.500	.500	1	.500
Deep Frying (DF)	.961(S)	1.000**(S)	1.000**(S)	.500	1

***.Correlation is highly significant at the 0.01 level (2-tailed)* ▭ Positive *S= Significant*

This table shows the correlation of calcium content of prawn with cooking methods. In 14 days control preservation without preservative, there is significant positive correlation present between the raw state with boiling, open pan dry roasting and deep frying. Boiling is perfect positively correlated with open pan dry roasting and deep frying, whereas open pan dry roasting is perfect positively correlated with deep frying. This table indicates that there is a strong correlation present among the **raw state, boiling, open pan dry roasting and deep frying** in 14 days preservation without preservative.

Table no 5.12.3.6.5 Correlation of cooking methods in 15 days preservation without preservative

Condition	RS	B	OPDR	SF	DF
Raw State (RS)	1	.655	.982(S)	1.000**(S)	.982(S)
Boiling (B)	.655	1	.500	.655	.500
Open Pan Dry Roasting (OPDR)	.982(S)	.500	1	.982(S)	1.000**(S)
Shallow Frying (SF)	1.000**(S)	.655	.982(S)	1	.982(S)
Deep Frying (DF)	.982(S)	.500	1.000**(S)	.982(S)	1

***.Correlation is highly significant at the 0.01 level (2-tailed)* ▭ Positive *S= Significant*

This table shows the correlation of calcium content of prawn with cooking methods. In 15 days control preservation without preservative, there is significant positive correlation present between the raw state with open pan dry roasting and deep frying, and perfect positive correlation present between the raw state and shallow frying. Open pan dry roasting is perfect positively correlated with deep frying and significant positively correlated with shallow frying, whereas shallow frying is significant positively correlated with deep frying. This table indicates that there is a strong correlation present among the **raw state, open pan dry roasting, shallow frying and deep frying** in 15 days control preservation without preservative.

Table no 5.12.3.6.6 Correlation of cooking methods in 24 hours preservation with salt and turmeric

Condition	RS	B	OPDR	SF	DF
Raw State (RS)	1	1.000**(S)	.993(S)	1.000**(S)	-.397
Boiling (B)	1.000**(S)	1	.993(S)	1.000**(S)	-.397
Open Pan Dry Roasting (OPDR)	.993(S)	.993(S)	1	.993(S)	-.500
Shallow Frying (SF)	1.000**(S)	1.000**(S)	.993(S)	1	-.397
Deep Frying (DF)	-.397	-.397	-.500	-.397	1

***.Correlation is highly significant at the 0.01 level (2-tailed)* ▭ Positive *S= Significant*

This table shows the correlation of calcium content of prawn with cooking methods. In 24 hours salt and turmeric preservation, there is significant positive correlation present between the raw state with open pan dry roasting, and perfect positive correlation present between the raw state with boiling and shallow frying. Open pan dry roasting is significant positively correlated with boiling and shallow frying.

Boiling is perfect positively correlated with shallow frying. This table indicates that there is a strong correlation present among the **raw state, boiling, open pan dry roasting and shallow frying** in 24 hours salt and turmeric preservation.

Table no 5.12.3.6.7 Correlation of cooking methods in 48 hours preservation with salt and turmeric

Condition	RS	B	OPDR	SF	DF
Raw State (RS)	1	1.000**(S)	1.000**(S)	1.000**(S)	.993(S)
Boiling (B)	1.000**(S)	1	1.000**(S)	1.000**(S)	.993(S)
Open Pan Dry Roasting (OPDR)	1.000**(S)	1.000**(S)	1	1.000**(S)	.993(S)
Shallow Frying (SF)	1.000**(S)	1.000**(S)	1.000**(S)	1	.993(S)
Deep Frying (DF)	.993(S)	.993(S)	.993(S)	.993(S)	1

***.Correlation is highly significant at the 0.01 level (2-tailed)* Positive *S= Significant*

This table shows the correlation of calcium content of prawn with cooking methods. In 48 hours salt and turmeric preservation, there is significant positive correlation present between the raw state and deep frying, and perfect positive correlation present between the raw state with boiling, open pan dry roasting and shallow frying. Boiling is perfect positively correlated with open pan dry roasting and shallow frying and significant positive correlation present between boiling and deep frying. Open pan dry roasting is significant positively correlated with deep frying and perfect positively correlated with shallow frying, whereas shallow frying is significant positively correlated with deep frying. This table indicates that there is a strong correlation present among the **raw state, boiling, open pan dry roasting, shallow frying and deep frying** in 48 hours salt and turmeric preservation.

Table no 5.12.3.6.8 Correlation of cooking methods in 14 days preservation with salt and turmeric

Condition	RS	B	OPDR	SF	DF
Raw State (RS)	1	1.000**(S)	.434	.000	.327
Boiling (B)	1.000**(S)	1	.434	.000	.327
Open Pan Dry Roasting (OPDR)	.434	.434	1	.901(S)	.993(S)
Shallow Frying (SF)	.000	.000	.901(S)	1	.945(S)
Deep Frying (DF)	.327	.327	.993(S)	.945(S)	1

***.Correlation is highly significant at the 0.01 level (2-tailed)* Positive *S= Significant*

This table shows the correlation of calcium content of prawn with cooking methods. In 14 days salt and turmeric preservation, there is perfect positive correlation present between the raw state and boiling, whereas open pan dry roasting is significant positively correlated with shallow frying and deep frying. Again shallow frying is significant positively correlated with deep frying. This table indicates that there is a strong correlation present among the **raw state, boiling, open pan dry roasting, shallow frying and deep frying** in 14 days salt and turmeric preservation.

Table no 5.12.3.6.9 Correlation of cooking methods in 15 days preservation with salt and turmeric

Condition	RS	B	OPDR	SF	DF
Raw State (RS)	1	1.000** (S)	-.397	.397	-.721
Boiling (B)	1.000**(S)	1	-.397	.397	-.721
Open Pan Dry Roasting (OPDR)	-.397	-.397	1	.684	-.350
Shallow Frying (SF)	.397	.397	.684	1	-.923(S)
Deep Frying (DF)	-.721	-.721	-.350	-.923(S)	1

***.Correlation is highly significant at the 0.01 level (2-tailed)* Positive Negative *S= Significant*

This table shows the correlation of calcium content of prawn with cooking methods. In 15 days salt and turmeric preservation, there is perfect positive correlation present between the raw state and boiling, whereas shallow frying is significant positively correlated with shallow frying and deep frying. Again shallow frying is significant negatively correlated with deep frying. This table indicates that there is a strong correlation present between the **raw state and boiling and also between shallow frying and deep frying** in 15 days salt and turmeric preservation.

Table no 5.12.3.6.10 Correlation of cooking methods in 24 hours preservation with KMS

Condition	RS	B	OPDR	SF	DF
Raw State (RS)	1	.982(S)	.961(S)	.655	-.993(S)
Boiling (B)	.982(S)	1	.891(S)	.500	-.954(S)
Open Pan Dry Roasting (OPDR)	.961(S)	.891(S)	1	.839(S)	-.986(S)
Shallow Frying (SF)	.655	.500	.839(S)	1	-.737
Deep Frying (DF)	-.993(S)	-.954(S)	-.986(S)	-.737	1

Positive Negative *S= Significant*

This table shows the correlation of calcium content of prawn with cooking methods. In 24 hours KMS preservation, there is significant positive correlation present between the raw state with boiling and open pan dry roasting, and significant negative correlation present between the raw state and deep frying, whereas open pan dry roasting is significant positively correlated with boiling and shallow frying and significant negatively correlated with deep frying. Boiling is significant negatively correlated with deep frying. This table indicates that there is a strong correlation present among the **raw state, boiling, open pan dry roasting, shallow frying and deep frying** in 24 hours KMS preservation.

Table no 5.12.3.6.11 Correlation of cooking methods in 48 hours preservation with KMS

Condition	RS	B	OPDR	SF	DF
Raw State (RS)	1	.143	-.327	-.786	.982(S)
Boiling (B)	.143	1	-.982(S)	.500	.327
Open Pan Dry Roasting (OPDR)	-.327	-.982(S)	1	-.327	-.500
Shallow Frying (SF)	-.786	.500	-.327	1	-.655
Deep Frying (DF)	.982(S)	.327	-.500	-.655	1

Positive Negative *S= Significant*

This table shows the correlation of calcium content of prawn with cooking methods. In 48 hours KMS preservation, there is significant positive correlation present between the raw state with boiling and open pan dry roasting, and significant negative correlation present between the raw state and deep frying, whereas open pan dry roasting is significant positively correlated with boiling and shallow frying and significant negatively correlated with deep frying. Boiling is significant negatively correlated with deep frying. This table indicates that there is a strong correlation present between the **raw state and deep frying and also between boiling and open pan dry roasting** in 24 hours KMS preservation.

Table no 5.12.3.6.12 Correlation of cooking methods in 14 days preservation with KMS

Condition	RS	B	OPDR	SF	DF
Raw State (RS)	1	-.655	-.500	-.655	-.655
Boiling (B)	-.655	1	.982	1.000** (S)	1.000** (S)
Open Pan Dry Roasting (OPDR)	-.500	.982(S)	1	.982(S)	.982(S)
Shallow Frying (SF)	-.655	1.000** (S)	.982(S)	1	1.000** (S)
Deep Frying (DF)	-.655	1.000** (S)	.982(S)	1.000** (S)	1

***.Correlation is highly significant at the 0.01 level (2-tailed)* ▭ Positive *S= Significant*

This table shows the correlation of calcium content of prawn with cooking methods. In 14 days KMS preservation, there is perfect positive correlation present between boiling with shallow frying and deep frying. Open pan dry roasting is significant positively correlated with boiling, shallow frying and deep frying. Shallow frying is perfect positively correlated with deep frying. This table indicates that there is a strong correlation present among **boiling, open pan dry roasting, shallow frying and deep frying** in 14 days KMS preservation.

Table no 5.12.3.6.13 Correlation of cooking methods in 15 days preservation with KMS

Condition	RS	B	OPDR	SF	DF
Raw State (RS)	1	.961(S)	-.500	.982(S)	1.000** (S)
Boiling (B)	.961(S)	1	-.240	.891(S)	.961(S)
Open Pan Dry Roasting (OPDR)	-.500	-.240	1	-.655	-.500
Shallow Frying (SF)	.982(S)	.891(S)	-.655	1	.982(S)
Deep Frying (DF)	1.000** (S)	.961(S)	-.500	.982(S)	1

***.Correlation is highly significant at the 0.01 level (2-tailed)* ▭ Positive *S= Significant*

This table shows the correlation of calcium content of prawn with cooking methods. In 15 days KMS preservation, there is perfect positive correlation present between the raw state with deep frying and significant positive correlation present between the raw state with boiling and shallow frying. Boiling is significant positively correlated with shallow frying and deep frying. Shallow frying is significant positively correlated with deep frying. This table indicates that there is a strong correlation present among the **raw state, boiling, shallow frying and deep frying in** 15 days KMS preservation.

Overall analysis reveals that the raw state is perfect positively correlated with boiling in 24 hours, 48 hours, 14 days and 15 days salt and turmeric preservation, whereas perfect positively correlated with open pan dry roasting and shallow frying in 48 hours preservation with salt-turmeric, highly significant positively correlated with deep frying in 15 days KMS preservation. Boiling is perfect positively correlated with open pan dry roasting and shallow frying in 48 hours salt and turmeric preservation and in fresh condition respectively, and perfect positively correlated with deep frying in 48 hours and 14 days control preservation without preservative. Open pan dry roasting is perfect positively correlated with shallow frying in 48 hours salt and turmeric preservation and in fresh condition, and perfect positively correlated with deep frying in 14 days and 15 days control preservation without preservative. Shallow frying is perfect positively correlated with deep frying in 14 days KMS preservation. Most of the correlation of the calcium content of prawn is found in **48 hours salt and turmeric preservation** with respect to different cooking conditions.

5.12.3.7 Iron

Table no 5.12.3.7.1 Correlation of cooking methods in fresh condition

Condition	RS	B	OPDR	SF	DF
Raw State (RS)	1	.954(S)	-.327	1.000**(S)	.857(S)
Boiling (B)	.954(S)	1	-.596	.954(S)	.972(S)
Open Pan Dry Roasting (OPDR)	-.327	-.596	1	-.327	-.768
Shallow Frying (SF)	1.000**(S)	.954(S)	-.327	1	.857(S)
Deep Frying (DF)	.857(S)	.972(S)	-.768	.857(S)	1

***.Correlation is highly significant at the 0.01 level (2-tailed)* ▭ Positive *S= Significant*

This table shows the correlation of iron content of prawn with cooking methods. In fresh condition, there is perfect positive correlation present between the raw state and shallow frying, and significant positive correlation present between the raw state with boiling and deep frying. Boiling is significant positively correlated with shallow frying and deep frying. Shallow frying is significant positively correlated with deep frying. This table indicates that there is a strong correlation present among the **raw state, boiling, shallow frying and deep frying** in fresh condition.

Table no 5.12.3.7.2 Correlation of cooking methods in 24 hours preservation without preservative

Condition	RS	B	OPDR	SF	DF
Raw State (RS)	1	-.756	.929(S)	.756	.756
Boiling (B)	-.756	1	-.945(S)	-1.000**(S)	-1.000**(S)
Open Pan Dry Roasting (OPDR)	.929(S)	-.945(S)	1	.945(S)	.945
Shallow Frying (SF)	.756	-1.000**(S)	.945(S)	1	1.000**(S)
Deep Frying (DF)	.756	-1.000**(S)	.945(S)	1.000**(S)	1

***.Correlation is highly significant at the 0.01 level (2-tailed)* ▭ Positive ▭ Negative *S= Significant*

This table shows the correlation of iron content of prawn with cooking methods. In 24 hours control preservation without preservative, there is significant positive correlation present between the raw state and open pan dry roasting. Boiling is significant negatively correlated with open pan dry roasting and perfect negatively correlated with shallow frying and deep frying. Shallow frying is perfect positively correlated with deep frying. This table indicates that there is a strong correlation present among the **raw state, boiling, open pan dry roasting, shallow frying and deep frying** in 24 hours control preservation.

Table no 5.12.3.7.3 Correlation of cooking methods in 48 hours preservation without preservative

Condition	RS	B	OPDR	SF	DF
Raw State (RS)	1	-.976(S)	.737	-.075	.817(S)
Boiling (B)	-.976S)	1	-.866(S)	.289	-.923(S)
Open Pan Dry Roasting (OPDR)	.737	-.866(S)	1	-.729	.992(S)
Shallow Frying (SF)	-.075	.289	-.729	1	-.636
Deep Frying (DF)	.817(S)	-.923(S)	.992(S)	-.636	1

▭ Positive ▭ Negative *S= Significant*

This table shows the correlation of iron content of prawn with cooking methods. In 48 hours control preservation without preservative, there is significant positive correlation present between the raw state and deep frying, and significant negative correlation present between the raw state and boiling. Boiling is significant negatively correlated with open pan dry roasting and deep frying. Open pan dry roasting is significant positively correlated with deep frying. This table indicates that there is a strong correlation present among the **raw state, boiling, open pan dry roasting and deep frying** in 48 hours control preservation.

Table no 5.12.3.7.4 Correlation of cooking methods in 14 days preservation without preservative

Condition	RS	B	OPDR	SF	DF
Raw State (RS)	1	-.797	-.636	-.038	-.636
Boiling (B)	-.797	1	.041	-.573	.041
Open Pan Dry Roasting (OPDR)	-.636	.041	1	.795	1.000** (S)
Shallow Frying (SF)	-.038	-.573	.795	1	.795
Deep Frying (DF)	-.636	.041	1.000** (S)	.795	1

***.Correlation is highly significant at the 0.01 level (2-tailed)* ▭ Positive *S= Significant*

This table shows the correlation of iron content of prawn with cooking methods. In 14 days control preservation without preservative, there is perfect positive correlation present between open pan dry roasting and deep frying. This table indicates that there is a strong correlation present between **open pan dry roasting and deep frying in** 14 days control preservation.

Table no 5.12.3.7.5 Correlation of cooking methods in 15 days preservation without preservative

Condition	RS	B	OPDR	SF	DF
Raw State (RS)	1	-.075	.434	.596	-.262
Boiling (B)	-.075	1	.866(S)	.756	.982(S)
Open Pan Dry Roasting (OPDR)	.434	.866(S)	1	.982(S)	.756
Shallow Frying (SF)	.596	.756	.982(S)	1	.619
Deep Frying (DF)	-.262	.982	.756	.619	1

▭ Positive *S= Significant*

This table shows the correlation of iron content of prawn with cooking methods. In 15 days control preservation without preservative, there is significant positive correlation present between boiling with open pan dry roasting and deep frying. Open pan dry roasting is significant positively correlated with shallow frying. Shallow frying is perfect positively correlated with deep frying. This table indicates that there is a strong correlation present among **boiling, open pan dry roasting, shallow frying and deep frying** in 15 days control preservation.

Table no 5.12.3.7.6 Correlation of cooking methods in 24 hours preservation with salt and turmeric

Condition	RS	B	OPDR	SF	DF
Raw State (RS)	1	-.500	1.000** (S)	-.705	-.705
Boiling (B)	-.500	1	-.500	-.262	-.262
Open Pan Dry Roasting (OPDR)	1.000** (S)	-.500	1	-.705	-.705
Shallow Frying (SF)	-.705	-.262	-.705	1	1.000** (S)
Deep Frying (DF)	-.705	-.262	-.705	1.000** (S)	1

***.Correlation is highly significant at the 0.01 level (2-tailed)* ▭ Positive *S= Significant*

This table shows the correlation of iron content of prawn with cooking methods. In 24 hours salt and turmeric preservation, there is perfect positive correlation present between the raw state and open pan dry roasting. Shallow frying is perfect positively correlated with deep frying. This table indicates that there is a strong correlation present between the **raw state and open pan dry roasting and also between shallow frying and deep frying** in 24 hours salt and turmeric preservation.

Table no 5.12.3.7. Correlation of cooking methods in 48 hours preservation with salt and turmeric

Condition	RS	B	OPDR	SF	DF
Raw State (RS)	1	.564	.596	.475	.564
Boiling (B)	.564	1	-.327	-.459	1.000**(S)
Open Pan Dry Roasting (OPDR)	.596	-.327	1	.990(S)	-.327
Shallow Frying (SF)	.475	-.459	.990(S)	1	-.459
Deep Frying (DF)	.564	1.000**(S)	-.327	-.459	1

***.Correlation is highly significant at the 0.01 level (2-tailed)* ▭ Positive *S= Significant*

This table shows the correlation of iron content of prawn with cooking methods. In 48 hours salt and turmeric preservation, there is perfect positive correlation present between the raw state and boiling, whereas open pan dry roasting is significant positively correlated with shallow frying. This table indicates that there is a strong correlation present between **boiling and deep frying and also between open pan dry roasting and shallow frying** in 48 hours salt and turmeric preservation.

Table no 5.12.3.7.8 Correlation of cooking methods in 14 days preservation with salt and turmeric

Condition	RS	B	OPDR	SF	DF
Raw State (Rs)	1	.954(S)	.596	-.500	.803(S)
Boiling (B)	.954(S)	1	.327	-.737	.945(S)
Open Pan Dry Roasting (OPDR)	.596	.327	1	.397	.000
Shallow Frying (SF)	-.500	-.737	.397	1	-.918(S)
Deep Frying (DF)	.803(S)	.945(S)	.000	-.918(S)	1

▭ Positive ▭ Negative *S= Significant*

This table shows the correlation of iron content of prawn with cooking methods. In 14 days salt and turmeric preservation, there is significant positive correlation present between the raw state with boiling, deep frying. Boiling is significant positively correlated with deep frying. Shallow frying is significant negatively correlated with deep frying. This table indicates that there is a strong correlation present among the **raw state, boiling, shallow frying and deep frying** in 14 days salt and turmeric preservation.

Table no 5.12.3.7.9 Correlation of cooking methods in 15 days preservation with salt and turmeric

Condition	RS	B	OPDR	SF	DF
Raw State (RS)	1	-1.000**(S)	-.961(S)	.655	.500
Boiling (B)	-1.000**(S)	1	.961(S)	-.655	-.500
Open Pan Dry Roasting (OPDR)	-.961(S)	.961(S)	1	-.419	-.721
Shallow Frying (SF)	.655	-.655	-.419	1	-.327
Deep Frying (DF)	.500	-.500	-.721	-.327	1

***.Correlation is highly significant at the 0.01 level (2-tailed)* ▭ Positive ▭ Negative *S= Significant*

This table shows the correlation of iron content of prawn with cooking methods. In 15 days salt and turmeric preservation, there is perfect positive correlation present between the raw state and open pan dry roasting. Shallow frying is perfect positively correlated with deep frying. This table indicates that there is a strong correlation present among the **raw state, open pan dry roasting, shallow frying and deep frying** in 15 days salt and turmeric preservation.

Table no 5.12.3.7.10 Correlation of cooking methods in 24 hours preservation with KMS

Condition	RS	B	OPDR	SF	DF
Raw State (RS)	1	.945(S)	-.826(S)	.047	-.327
Boiling (B)	.945(S)	1	-.596	.371	-.619
Open Pan Dry Roasting (OPDR)	-.826(S)	-.596	1	.524	-.262
Shallow Frying (SF)	.047	.371	.524	1	-.959(S)
Deep Frying (DF)	-.327	-.619	-.262	-.959(S)	1

***.Correlation is highly significant at the 0.01 level (2-tailed)* Positive Negative *S= Significant*

This table shows the correlation of iron content of prawn with cooking methods. In 24 hours KMS preservation, there is significant positive correlation present between the raw state and boiling, and significant negative correlation present between the raw state and open pan dry roasting. Shallow frying is significant negatively correlated with deep frying. This table indicates that there is a strong correlation present among **the raw state, boiling, open pan dry roasting, shallow frying and deep frying** in 24 hours KMS preservation.

Table no 5.12.3.7.11 Correlation of cooking methods in 48 hours preservation with KMS

Condition	RS	B	OPDR	SF	DF
Raw State (RS)	1	.289	.981(S)	.676	.962(S)
Boiling (B)	.289	1	.098	.901(S)	.017
Open Pan Dry Roasting (OPDR)	.981(S)	.098	1	.520	.997(S)
Shallow Frying (SF)	.676	.901(S)	.520	1	.449
Deep Frying (DF)	.962(S)	.017	.997(S)	.449	1

Positive *S= Significant*

This table shows the correlation of iron content of prawn with cooking methods. In 48 hours KMS preservation, there is significant positive correlation present between the raw state with open pan dry roasting and deep frying. Boiling is significant positively correlated with shallow frying. Shallow frying is perfect positively correlated with open pan dry roasting. This table indicates that there is a strong correlation present among the **raw state, boiling, open pan dry roasting, shallow frying and deep frying** in 48 hours KMS preservation.

Table no 5.12.3.7.12 Correlation of cooking methods in 14 days preservation with KMS

Condition	RS	B	OPDR	SF	DF
Raw State (RS)	1	1.000**(S)	.993(S)	.923(S)	.999*(S)
Boiling (B)	1.000**(S)	1	.993(S)	.923(S)	.999*(S)
Open Pan Dry Roasting (OPDR)	.993(S)	.993(S)	1	.961(S)	.998*(S)
Shallow Frying (SF)	.923(S)	.923(S)	.961(S)	1	.941(S)
Deep Frying (DF)	.999*(S)	.999*(S)	.998*(S)	.941(S)	1

***.Correlation is highly significant at the 0.01 level (2-tailed)* Positive *S= Significant*
**.Correlation is highly significant at the 0.05 level (2-tailed)*

This table shows the correlation of iron content of prawn with cooking methods. In 14 days KMS preservation, there is perfect positive correlation present between the raw state and boiling, and significant correlation present between the raw state with open pan dry roasting, shallow frying, deep frying. Boiling is highly significant positively correlated with deep frying and significant positively correlated with boiling and open pan dry roasting. Open pan dry roasting is highly significant positively correlated with deep frying, whereas shallow frying is significant positively correlated with open pan dry roasting and deep frying. This table indicates that there is a strong correlation present among the **raw state, boiling, open pan dry roasting, shallow frying and deep frying** in 14 days KMS preservation.

Table no 5.12.3.7.13 Correlation of cooking methods in 15 days preservation with KMS

Condition	RS	B	OPDR	SF	DF
Raw State (RS)	1	-.596	.974(S)	-.997*(S)	1.000**(S)
Boiling (B)	-.596	1	-.397	.655	-.596
Open Pan Dry Roasting (OPDR)	.974(S)	-.397	1	-.954(S)	.974(S)
Shallow Frying (SF)	-.997*(S)	.655	-.954(S)	1	-.997*(S)
Deep Frying (DF)	1.000**(S)	-.596	.974(S)	-.997*(S)	1

***.Correlation is highly significant at the 0.01 level (2-tailed)* ▢ Positive ▢ Negative *S= Significant*
**.Correlation is highly significant at the 0.05 level (2-tailed)*

This table shows the correlation of iron content of prawn with cooking methods. In 15 days KMS preservation, there is perfect positive correlation present between the raw state and deep frying, and significant positive correlation present between the raw state and open pan dry roasting, and highly significant negative correlation present between the raw state and shallow frying. Open pan dry roasting is significant positively correlated with deep frying and significant negatively correlated with shallow frying. Shallow frying is highly significant negatively correlated with deep frying. This table indicates that there is a strong correlation present among the **raw state, open pan dry roasting, shallow frying and deep frying** in 15 days KMS preservation.

Overall analysis reveals that the raw state is perfect negatively correlated with boiling in 15 days salt-turmeric preservation and 14 days KMS preservation, whereas perfect positively correlated with open pan dry roasting in 24 hours preservation with salt-turmeric, and perfect positively correlated with shallow frying and deep frying in fresh condition and 15 days KMS preservation. Boiling is significant positively correlated with open pan dry roasting in 14 days KMS preservation, whereas perfect negatively correlated with shallow frying in 24 hours control preservation without preservative, and perfect negatively correlated with deep frying in 24 hours control preservation without preservative and perfect positively correlated with 48 hours salt-turmeric preservation. Open pan dry roasting is significant positively correlated with shallow frying in 48 hours salt and turmeric preservation, and perfect positively correlated with deep frying in 14 days control preservation without preservative. Shallow frying is perfect positively correlated with deep frying in 24 hours control preservation without preservative and 24 hours salt-turmeric preservation. Most of the correlation of the iron content of prawn is found in **24 hours control preservation without preservative** with respect to different cooking conditions.

5.12.3.8 Energy

Table no 5.12.3.8.1 Correlation of cooking methods in fresh condition

Condition	RS	B	OPDR	SF	DF
Raw State (RS)	1	.996(S)	-.253	.820(S)	.091
Boiling (B)	.996(S)	1	-.335	.866(S)	.005
Open Pan Dry Roasting (OPDR)	-.253	-.335	1	-.761	.941(S)
Shallow Frying (SF)	.820(S)	.866(S)	-.761	1	-.495
Deep Frying (DF)	.091	.005	.941(S)	-.495	1

Positive *S= Significant*

This table shows the correlation of energy content of prawn with cooking methods. In fresh condition, there is significant positive correlation present between the raw state with boiling and shallow frying, whereas boiling is significant positively correlated with shallow frying. Open pan dry roasting is significant positively correlated with deep frying This table indicates that there is a strong correlation present among the **raw state, boiling, open pan dry roasting, shallow frying and deep frying** in fresh condition.

Table no 5.12.3.8.2 Correlation of cooking methods in 24 hours preservation without preservative

Condition	RS	B	OPDR	SF	DF
Raw State (RS)	1	.997*(S)	.732	-.940(S)	.284
Boiling (B)	.997*(S)	1	.680	-.912(S)	.353
Open Pan Dry Roasting (OPDR)	.732	.680	1	-.921(S)	-.445
Shallow Frying (SF)	-.940(S)	-.912(S)	-.921(S)	1	.061
Deep Frying (DF)	.284	.353	-.445	.061	1

**.Correlation is highly significant at the 0.05 level (2-tailed)* Positive Negative *S= Significant*

This table shows the correlation of energy content of prawn with cooking methods. In 24 hours control preservation without preservative, there is highly significant positive correlation present between the raw state and boiling, and significant negative correlation present between the raw state and shallow frying. Boiling is significant negatively correlated with shallow frying. Open pan dry roasting is significant negatively correlated with shallow frying. This table indicates that there is a strong correlation present among the **raw state, boiling, open pan dry roasting and shallow frying** in 24 hours control preservation.

Table no 5.12.3.8.3 Correlation of cooking methods in 48 hours preservation without preservative

Condition	RS	B	OPDR	SF	DF
Raw State (RS)	1	.951(S)	.503	-.342	.353
Boiling (B)	.951(S)	1	.745	-.035	.625
Open Pan Dry Roasting (OPDR)	.503	.745	1	.640	.986(S)
Shallow Frying (SF)	-.342	-.035	.640	1	.758
Deep Frying (DF)	.353	.625	.986(S)	.758	1

Positive *S= Significant*

This table shows the correlation of energy content of prawn with cooking methods. In 48 hours control preservation without preservative, there is significant positive correlation present between the raw state and boiling, whereas open pan dry roasting is significant positively correlated with deep frying. This table indicates that there is a strong correlation present **between the raw state and boiling and also between open pan dry roasting and deep frying** in 48 hours control preservation.

Table no 5.12.3.8.4 Correlation of cooking methods in 14 days preservation without preservative

Condition	RS	B	OPDR	SF	DF
Raw State (RS)	1	.308	.196	.589	.895(S)
Boiling (B)	.308	1	.993(S)	-.588	.700
Open Pan Dry Roasting (OPDR)	.196	.993(S)	1	-.678	.613
Shallow Frying (SF)	.589	-.588	-.678	1	.166
Deep Frying (DF)	.895(S)	.700	.613	.166	1

Positive *S= Significant*

This table shows the correlation of energy content of prawn with cooking methods. In 14 days control preservation without preservative, there is significant positive correlation present between the raw state and deep frying, whereas open pan dry roasting is significant positively correlated with boiling. This table indicates that there is a strong correlation present **between the raw state and deep frying and also between open pan dry roasting and boiling** in 14 days control preservation.

Table no 5.12.3.8.5 Correlation of cooking methods in 15 days preservation without preservative

Condition	RS	B	OPDR	SF	DF
Raw State (RS)	1	.971(S)	.742	.968(S)	.651
Boiling (B)	.971(S)	1	.561	1.000^{**}(S)	.452
Open Pan Dry Roasting (OPDR)	.742	.561	1	.550	.992(S)
Shallow Frying (SF)	.968(S)	1.000^{**}(S)	.550	1	.440
Deep Frying (DF)	.651	.452	.992(S)	.440	1

***.Correlation is highly significant at the 0.01 level (2-tailed)* Positive *S= Significant*

This table shows the correlation of energy content of prawn with cooking methods. In 15 days control preservation without preservative, there is significant positive correlation present between the raw state with boiling and shallow frying. Boiling is perfect positively correlated with shallow frying. Open pan dry roasting is significant positively correlated with deep frying. This table indicates that there is a strong correlation present among the **raw state, boiling, open pan dry roasting, shallow frying and deep frying** in 15 days control preservation.

Table no 5.12.3.8.6 Correlation of cooking methods in 24 hours preservation with salt and turmeric

Condition	RS	B	OPDR	SF	DF
Raw State (RS)	1	-.729	.695	-.965(S)	-.577
Boiling (B)	-.729	1	$-.999^{*}$(S)	.883(S)	.980(S)
Open Pan Dry Roasting (OPDR)	.695	$-.999^{*}$(S)	1	-.858(S)	-.988(S)
Shallow Frying (SF)	-.965(S)	.883(S)	-.858(S)	1	.770
Deep Frying (DF)	-.577	.980(S)	-.988(S)	.770	1

***.Correlation is highly significant at the 0.01 level (2-tailed)* Positive Negative *S= Significant*

This table shows the correlation of energy content of prawn with cooking methods. In 24 hours salt and turmeric preservation, there is significant negative correlation present between the raw state and shallow frying. Boiling is significant positively correlated with shallow frying and deep frying and highly significant negatively correlated with open pan dry roasting. Open pan dry roasting is significant negatively correlated with shallow frying and deep frying. This table indicates that there is a strong correlation present among the **raw state, boiling, open pan dry roasting, shallow frying and deep frying** in 24 hours salt and turmeric preservation.

Table no 5.12.3.8.7 Correlation of cooking methods in 48 hours preservation with salt and turmeric

Condition	RS	B	OPDR	SF	DF
Raw State (RS)	1	.747	.474	-.043	.458
Boiling (B)	.747	1	-.230	.632	-.248
Open Pan Dry Roasting (OPDR)	.474	-.230	1	-.900(S)	1.000*(S)
Shallow Frying (SF)	-.043	.632	-.900(S)	1	-.908(S)
Deep Frying (DF)	.458	-.248	1.000*(S)	-.908(S)	1

*.Correlation is highly significant at the 0.05 level (2-tailed) Positive Negative S= Significant

This table shows the correlation of energy content of prawn with cooking methods. In 48 hours salt and turmeric preservation, there is significant negative correlation present between open pan dry roasting and shallow frying, and perfect positive correlation present between open pan dry roasting and deep frying. Shallow frying is significant negatively correlated with deep frying. This table indicates that there is a strong correlation present among **open pan dry roasting, shallow frying and deep frying** in 48 hours salt and turmeric preservation.

Table no 5.12.3.8.8 Correlation of cooking methods in 14 days preservation with salt and turmeric

Condition	RS	B	OPDR	SF	DF
Raw State (RS)	1	-.993(S)	-.149	.875(S)	-.910(S)
Boiling (B)	-.993(S)	1	.262	-.925(S)	.857(S)
Open Pan Dry Roasting (OPDR)	-.149	.262	1	-.609	-.273
Shallow Frying (SF)	.875(S)	-.925(S)	-.609	1	-.596
Deep Frying (DF)	-.910(S)	.857(S)	-.273	-.596	1

Positive Negative S= Significant

This table shows the correlation of energy content of prawn with cooking methods. In 14 days salt and turmeric preservation, there is significant negative correlation present between the raw state with boiling and deep frying, whereas boiling is significant positively correlated with deep frying and significant negatively correlated with shallow frying. This table indicates that there is a strong correlation present among the **raw state, boiling, shallow frying and deep frying** in 14 days salt and turmeric preservation.

Table no 5.12.3.8.9 Correlation of cooking methods in 15 days preservation with salt and turmeric

Condition	RS	B	OPDR	SF	DF
Raw State (RS)	1	-.333	-.991(S)	.570	.946(S)
Boiling (B)	-.333	1	.456	.585	-.011
Open Pan Dry Roasting (OPDR)	-.991(S)	.456	1	-.456	-.895(S)
Shallow Frying (SF)	.570	.585(S)	-.456	1	.805(S)
Deep Frying (DF)	.946(S)	-.011	-.895(S)	.805(S)	1

Positive Negative S= Significant

This table shows the correlation of energy content of prawn with cooking methods. In 15 days salt and turmeric preservation, there is significant negative correlation present between the raw state and open pan dry roasting, and significant positive correlation present between the raw state and deep frying, whereas open pan dry roasting is significant negatively correlated with deep frying. Shallow frying is significant positively correlated with deep frying. This table indicates that there is a strong correlation present among the **raw state, open pan dry roasting, shallow frying and deep frying** in 15 days salt and turmeric preservation.

Table no 5.12.3.8.10 Correlation of cooking methods in 24 hours preservation with KMS

Condition	RS	B	OPDR	SF	DF
Raw State (RS)	1	.953(S)	-.931(S)	.564	.924(S)
Boiling (B)	.953(S)	1	-.777	.287	.765
Open Pan Dry Roasting (OPDR)	-.931(S)	-.777	1	-.826(S)	-1.000*(S)
Shallow Frying (SF)	.564	.287	-.826(S)	1	.836(S)
Deep Frying (DF)	.924(S)	.765	-1.000*(S)	.836(S)	1

**.Correlation is highly significant at the 0.05 level (2-tailed)* ▭ Positive ▭ Negative *S= Significant*

This table shows the correlation of energy content of prawn with cooking methods. In 24 hours KMS preservation, there is significant negative correlation present between the raw state and open pan dry roasting, and significant positive correlation present between the raw state with boiling and deep frying, whereas open pan dry roasting is significant negatively correlated with shallow frying and perfect negatively correlated with deep frying. Shallow frying is significant positively correlated with deep frying. This table indicates that there is a strong correlation present among the **raw state, boiling, open pan dry roasting, shallow frying and deep frying** in 24 hours KMS preservation.

Table no 5.12.3.8.11 Correlation of cooking methods in 48 hours preservation with KMS

Condition	RS	B	OPDR	SF	DF
Raw State (RS)	1	.948(S)	-.085	-.657	.087
Boiling (B)	.948(S)	1	.237	-.383	-.234
Open Pan Dry Roasting (OPDR)	-.085	.237	1	.807(S)	-1.000**(S)
Shallow Frying (SF)	-.657	-.383	.807(S)	1	-.808(S)
Deep Frying (DF)	.087	-.234	-1.000**(S)	-.808(S)	1

***.Correlation is highly significant at the 0.05 level (2-tailed)* ▭ Positive ▭ Negative *S= Significant*

This table shows the correlation of energy content of prawn with cooking methods. In 48 hours KMS preservation, there is significant positive correlation present between the raw state and boiling, whereas open pan dry roasting is significant positively correlated with shallow frying and perfect negatively correlated with deep frying. Shallow frying is significant negatively correlated with deep frying. This table indicates that there is a strong correlation present among the **raw state, boiling, open pan dry roasting, shallow frying and deep frying** in 48 hours KMS preservation.

Table no 5.12.3.8.12 Correlation of cooking methods in 14 days preservation with KMS

Condition	RS	B	OPDR	SF	DF
Raw State (RS)	1	.175	.954(S)	.734	.159
Boiling (B)	.175	1	-.128	-.540	-.944(S)
Open Pan Dry Roasting (OPDR)	.954(S)	-.128	1	.904(S)	.447
Shallow Frying (SF)	.734	-.540	.904(S)	1	.787
Deep Frying (DF)	.159	-.944(S)	.447	.787	1

▭ Positive ▭ Negative *S= Significant*

This table shows the correlation of energy content of prawn with cooking methods. In 14 days KMS preservation, there is significant positive correlation present between the raw state and open pan dry roasting, whereas boiling is significant negatively correlated with deep frying. Shallow frying is significant positively correlated with open pan dry roasting. This table indicates that there is a strong correlation present among the **raw state, boiling, open pan dry roasting, shallow frying and deep frying** in 14 days KMS preservation.

Table no 5.12.3.8.13 Correlation of cooking methods in 15 days preservation with KMS

Condition	RS	B	OPDR	SF	DF
Raw State (RS)	1	-.999*(S)	.936(S)	-.184	-.752
Boiling (B)	-.999*(S)	1	-.950(S)	.142	.724
Open Pan Dry Roasting (OPDR)	.936(S)	-.950(S)	1	.175	-.471
Shallow Frying (SF)	-.184	.142	.175	1	.786
Deep Frying (DF)	-.752	.724	-.471	.786	1

** Correlation is highly significant at the 0.05 level (2-tailed)* ▢ Positive ▢ Negative *S= Significant*

This table shows the correlation of energy content of prawn with cooking methods. In 15 days KMS preservation, there is significant positive correlation present between the raw state and open pan dry roasting, and highly significant negative correlation present between the raw state and boiling, whereas boiling is significant negatively correlated with open pan dry roasting. This table indicates that there is a strong correlation present among the **raw state, boiling and open pan dry roasting** in 15 days KMS preservation.

Overall analysis reveals that the raw state is highly negatively correlated with boiling in 15 days KMS preservation and 15 days control preservation without preservative, whereas significant negatively correlated with open pan dry roasting and shallow frying in 15 days and 24 hours preservation with salt-turmeric respectively, and significant positively correlated with deep frying in 15 days salt-turmeric preservation. Boiling is highly significant negatively correlated with open pan dry roasting in 24 hours salt-turmeric preservation, whereas perfect positively correlated with shallow frying in 15 days control preservation without preservative, and significant positively correlated with deep frying in 24 hours salt-turmeric preservation. Open pan dry roasting is significant negatively correlated with shallow frying in 24 hours control preservation without preservative, and perfect positively correlated with deep frying in 48 hours salt and turmeric preservation, and again perfect negatively correlated with deep frying in 24 hours and 48 hours KMS preservation. Shallow frying is significant negatively correlated with deep frying in 24 hours KMS preservation. Most of the correlation of the energy content of prawn is found in **24 hours salt and turmeric preservation** with respect to different cooking conditions.

5.12.4 Lobster (*Macrobrachium rosenbergii)*

5.12.4.1 Carbohydrate

Table no 512.4.1.1 Correlation of cooking methods in fresh condition

Condition	RS	B	OPDR	SF	DF
Raw State (RS)	1	.997(S)	.504	.256	.223
Boiling (B)	.997(S)	1	.571	.332	.300
Open Pan Dry Roasting (OPDR)	.504	.571	1	.964(S)	.954(S)
Shallow Frying (SF)	.256	.332	.964(S)	1	.999*(S)
Deep Frying (DF)	.223	.300	.954(S)	.999*(S)	1

**.Correlation is highly significant at the 0.05 level (2-tailed)* ▭ Positive *S= Significant*

This table shows the correlation of carbohydrate content of lobster with cooking methods. In fresh condition, there is significant positive correlation present between the raw state and boiling, whereas significant positive correlation present between open pan dry roasting with shallow frying and deep frying. Shallow frying is highly significant positively correlated with deep frying. This table indicates that there is a strong correlation present among the **raw state, boiling, open pan dry roasting, shallow frying and deep frying** in fresh condition.

Table no 5.12.4.1.2 Correlation of cooking methods in 24 hours preservation without preservative

Condition	RS	B	OPDR	SF	DF
Raw State (RS)	1	-.854(S)	.891(S)	.857(S)	.449
Boiling (B)	-.854(S)	1	-.997*(S)	-1.000**(S)	-.849(S)
Open Pan Dry Roasting (OPDR)	.891(S)	-.997*(S)	1	.997*(S)	.806(S)
Shallow Frying (SF)	.857(S)	-1.000**(S)	.997*(S)	1	.846(S)
Deep Frying (DF)	.449	-.849(S)	.806(S)	.846(S)	1

**.Correlation is highly significant at the 0.05 level (2-tailed)* ▭ Positive ▭ Negative *S= Significant*
***.Correlation is highly significant at the 0.01 level (2-tailed)*

This table shows the correlation of carbohydrate content of lobster with cooking methods. In 24 hours preservation without preservative, there is significant positive correlation present between the raw state with open pan dry roasting and shallow frying, and significant negative correlation present between the raw state and boiling, whereas significant negative correlation present between boiling with open pan dry roasting and deep frying, and perfect negative correlation present between boiling and shallow frying. Shallow frying is significant positively correlated with shallow frying and deep frying and perfect negatively correlated with open pan dry roasting. This table indicates that there is a strong correlation present among the **raw state, boiling, open pan dry roasting, shallow frying and deep frying** in 24 hours preservation without preservative.

Table no 5.12.4.1.3 Correlation of cooking methods in 48 hours preservation without preservative

Condition	RS	B	OPDR	SF	DF
Raw State (RS)	1	.997(S)	.998*(S)	.686	.405
Boiling (B)	.997(S)	1	1.000*(S)	.625	.477
Open Pan Dry Roasting (OPDR)	.998*(S)	1.000*(S)	1	.638	.463
Shallow Frying (SF)	.686	.625	.638	1	-.388
Deep Frying (DF)	.405	.477	.463	-.388	1

**.Correlation is highly significant at the 0.05 level (2-tailed)* ▭ Positive *S= Significant*

This table shows the correlation of carbohydrate content of lobster with cooking methods. In 48 hours preservation without preservative, there is highly significant positive correlation present between the raw state with boiling and open pan dry roasting, whereas boiling is perfect positively correlated with open pan dry roasting. This table indicates that there is a strong correlation present among the **raw state, boiling and open pan dry roasting** in 48 hours control preservation without preservative.

Table no 5.12.4.1.4 Correlation of cooking methods in 14 days preservation without preservative

Condition	RS	B	OPDR	SF	DF
Raw State (RS)	1	-.349	-.682	-.761	-.291
Boiling (B)	-.349	1	-.448	-.343	-.795
Open Pan Dry Roasting (OPDR)	-.682	-.448	1	.993(S)	.898(S)
Shallow Frying (SF)	-.761	-.343	.993(S)	1	.842(S)
Deep Frying (DF)	-.291	-.795	.898(S)	.842(S)	1

**.Correlation is highly significant at the 0.05 level (2-tailed)* Positive *S= Significant*

This table shows the correlation of carbohydrate content of lobster with cooking methods. In 14 days preservation without preservative, there is significant positive correlation present between open pan dry roasting with shallow frying and deep frying, whereas shallow frying is perfect positively correlated with deep frying. This table indicates that there is a strong correlation present among **open pan dry roasting, shallow frying and deep frying** in 14 days control preservation without preservative.

Table no 5.12.4.1.5 Correlation of cooking methods in 15 days preservation without preservative

Condition	RS	B	OPDR	SF	DF
Raw State (RS)	1	.364	.525	.838(S)	.856(S)
Boiling (B)	.364	1	-.602	-.203	-.171
Open Pan Dry Roasting (OPDR)	.525	-.602	1	.904(S)	.890(S)
Shallow Frying (SF)	.838(S)	-.203	.904(S)	1	.999*(S)
Deep Frying (DF)	.856(S)	-.171	.890(S)	.999*(S)	1

**.Correlation is highly significant at the 0.05 level (2-tailed)* Positive *S= Significant*

This table shows the correlation of carbohydrate content of lobster with cooking methods. In 15 days preservation without preservative, there is significant positive correlation present between the raw state with shallow frying and deep frying, whereas open pan dry roasting is significant positively correlated with shallow frying and deep frying. Shallow frying is highly significant positively correlated with deep frying. This table indicates that there is a strong correlation present among the **raw state, open pan dry roasting, shallow frying and deep frying** in 15 days control preservation without preservative.

Table no 5.12.4.1.6 Correlation of cooking methods in 24 hours preservation with salt and turmeric

Condition	RS	B	OPDR	SF	DF
Raw State(R)	1	.961(S)	-.052	-.500	1.000**(S)
Boiling (B)	.961(S)	1	-.327	-.240	.961(S)
Open Pan Dry Roasting (OPDR)	-.052	-.327	1	-.839(S)	-.052
Shallow Frying (SF)	-.500	-.240	-.839(S)	1	-.500
Deep Frying (DF)	1.000**(S)	.961(S)	-.052	-.500	1

***.Correlation is highly significant at the 0.01 level (2-tailed)* Positive Negative *S= Significant*

This table shows the correlation of carbohydrate content of lobster with cooking methods. In 24 hours salt and turmeric preservation, there is significant positive correlation present between the raw state and boiling, and perfect positive correlation present between the raw state and deep frying, whereas boiling is significant positively correlated with deep frying. Open pan dry roasting is significant negatively correlated with shallow frying. This table indicates that there is a strong correlation present among the **raw state, boiling, open pan dry roasting, shallow frying and deep frying** in 24 hours salt and turmeric preservation.

Table no 5.12.4.1.7 Correlation of cooking methods in 48 hours preservation with salt and turmeric

Condition	RS	B	OPDR	SF	DF
Raw State (RS)	1	-.038	1.000**(S)	-.996(S)	.419
Boiling (B)	-.038	1	-.038	-.052	.891(S)
Open Pan Dry Roasting (OPDR)	1.000**(S)	-.038	1	-.996(S)	.419
Shallow Frying (SF)	-.996(S)	-.052	-.996(S)	1	-.500
Deep Frying (DF)	.419	.891(S)	.419	-.500	1

***.Correlation is highly significant at the 0.01 level (2-tailed)* ▭ Positive ▭ Negative *S= Significant*

This table shows the correlation of carbohydrate content of lobster with cooking methods. In 48 hours salt and turmeric preservation, there is significant negative correlation present between the raw state and shallow frying, and perfect positive correlation present between the raw state and open pan dry roasting, whereas boiling is significant positively correlated with deep frying. Open pan dry roasting is significant negatively correlated with shallow frying. This table indicates that there is a strong correlation present among the **raw state, boiling, open pan dry roasting, shallow frying and deep frying** in 48 hours salt and turmeric preservation.

Table no 5.12.4.1.8 Correlation of cooking methods in 14 days preservation with salt and turmeric

Condition	RS	B	OPDR	SF	DF
Raw State (RS)	1	-1.000**(S)	.961(S)	.993(S)	.982(S)
Boiling (B)	-1.000**(S)	1	-.961(S)	-.993(S)	-.982(S)
Open Pan Dry Roasting (OPDR)	.961(S)	-.961(S)	1	.986(S)	.996(S)
Shallow Frying (SF)	.993(S)	-.993(S)	.986(S)	1	.997*(S)
Deep Frying (DF)	.982(S)	-.982(S)	.996(S)	.997*(S)	1

***.Correlation is highly significant at the 0.01 level (2-tailed)* ▭ Positive ▭ Negative *S= Significant*
**.Correlation is highly significant at the 0.05 level (2-tailed)*

This table shows the correlation of carbohydrate content of lobster with cooking methods. In 14 days salt and turmeric preservation, there is significant positive correlation present between the raw state with open pan dry roasting, shallow frying and deep frying, and perfect negative correlation present between the raw state and boiling, whereas open pan dry roasting is significant positively correlated with shallow frying and deep frying. Shallow frying is highly significant positively correlated with deep frying. This table indicates that there is a strong correlation present among the **raw state, boiling, open pan dry roasting, shallow frying and deep frying** in 14 days salt and turmeric preservation.

Table no 5.12.4.1.9 Correlation of cooking methods in 15 days preservation with salt and turmeric

Condition	RS	B	OPDR	SF	DF
Raw State (RS)	1	-.371	.945(S)	.866(S)	-.371
Boiling (B)	-.371	1	-.655	.143	1.000**(S)
Open Pan Dry Roasting (OPDR)	.945(S)	-.655	1	.655	-.655
Shallow Frying (SF)	.866(S)	.143	.655	1	.143
Deep Frying (DF)	-.371	1.000**(S)	-.655	.143	1

***.Correlation is highly significant at the 0.01 level (2-tailed)* ▭ Positive *S= Significant*

This table shows the correlation of carbohydrate content of lobster with cooking methods. In 15 days salt and turmeric preservation, there is significant positive correlation present between the raw state with open pan dry roasting and shallow frying, whereas boiling is perfect positively correlated with deep frying. This table indicates that there is a strong correlation present among the **raw state, boiling, open pan dry roasting, shallow frying and deep frying** in 15 days salt and turmeric preservation.

Table no 5.12.4.1.10 Correlation of cooking methods in 24 hours preservation with KMS

Condition	RS	B	OPDR	SF	DF
Raw State (RS)	1	-.996(S)	.655	.434	.419
Boiling (B)	-.996(S)	1	-.721	-.350	-.500
Open Pan Dry Roasting (OPDR)	.655	-.721	1	-.397	.961(S)
Shallow Frying (SF)	.434	-.350	-.397	1	-.636
Deep Frying (DF)	.419	-.500	.961(S)	-.636	1

▭ Positive ▭ Negative *S= Significant*

This table shows the correlation of carbohydrate content of lobster with cooking methods. In 24 hours KMS preservation, there is significant negative correlation present between the raw state and boiling, whereas open pan dry roasting is significant positively correlated with deep frying. This table indicates that there is a strong correlation present between the **raw state and boiling and also between open pan dry roasting and deep frying** in 24 hours KMS preservation.

Table no 5.12.4.1.11 Correlation of cooking methods in 48 hours preservation with KMS

Condition	RS	B	OPDR	SF	DF
Raw State (RS)	1	.908(S)	1.000**(S)	.756	.866(S)
Boiling (B)	.908(S)	1	.908(S)	.961(S)	.577
Open Pan Dry Roasting (OPDR)	1.000**(S)	.908(S)	1	.756	.866(S)
Shallow Frying (SF	.756	.961(S)	.756	1	.327
Deep Frying (DF)	.866(S)	.577	.866(S)	.327	1

***.Correlation is highly significant at the 0.01 level (2-tailed)* ▭ Positive *S= Significant*

This table shows the correlation of carbohydrate content of lobster with cooking methods. In 48 hours KMS preservation, there is significant positive correlation present between the raw state with boiling and deep frying, and perfect positive correlation present between the raw state and open pan dry roasting, whereas open pan dry roasting is significant positively correlated with deep frying. Shallow frying is highly significant positively correlated with boiling. This table indicates that there is a strong correlation present among the **raw state, boiling, open pan dry roasting, shallow frying and deep frying** in 48 hours KMS preservation.

Table no 5.12.4.1.12 Correlation of cooking methods in 14 days preservation with KMS

Condition	RS	B	OPDR	SF	DF
Raw State (RS)	1	.500	.655	1.000**(S)	.500
Boiling (B)	.500	1	-.327	.500	1.000**(S)
Open Pan Dry Roasting (OPDR)	.655	-.327	1	.655	-.327
Shallow Frying (SF)	1.000**(S)	.500	.655	1	.500
Deep Frying (DF)	.500	1.000**(S)	-.327	.500	1

***.Correlation is highly significant at the 0.01 level (2-tailed)* Positive *S= Significant*

This table shows the correlation of carbohydrate content of lobster with cooking methods. In 14 days KMS preservation, there is perfect positive correlation present between the raw state and shallow frying, whereas perfect positive correlation present between boiling and deep frying. This table indicates that there is a strong correlation present between the **raw state and shallow frying and also between boiling and deep frying** in 14 days KMS preservation.

Table no 5.12.4.1.13 Correlation of cooking methods in 15 days preservation with KMS

Condition	RS	B	OPDR	SF	DF
Raw State (RS)	1	-.756	-.189	.866(S)	-.866(S)
Boiling (B)	-.756	1	.786	-.327	.327
Open Pan Dry Roasting (OPDR)	-.189	.786	1	.327	-.327
Shallow Frying (SF)	.866(S)	-.327	.327	1	-1.000**(S)
Deep Frying (DF)	-.866(S)	.327	-.327	-1.000**(S)	1

***.Correlation is highly significant at the 0.01 level (2-tailed)* Positive Negative *S= Significant*

This table shows the correlation of carbohydrate content of lobster with cooking methods. In 15 days KMS preservation, there is significant positive correlation present between the raw state and shallow frying and significant negative correlation present between the raw state and deep frying. Shallow frying is perfect negatively correlated with deep frying. This table indicates that there is a strong correlation present among the **raw state, shallow frying and deep frying** in 15 days KMS preservation.

Overall analysis reveals that the raw state is perfect negatively correlated with boiling in 14 days salt-turmeric preservation, whereas perfect positively correlated with open pan dry roasting in 48 hours preservation with KMS as well as 48 hours preservation with salt-turmeric, and perfect positively correlated with shallow frying and deep frying in 14 days KMS preservation and 24 hours salt and turmeric preservation respectively. Boiling is perfect positively correlated with open pan dry roasting in 48 hours preservation without preservative, whereas perfect positively correlated with shallow frying and deep frying in 24 hours control preservation without preservative and 15 days salt and turmeric preservation respectively. Open pan dry roasting is highly significant positively correlated with shallow frying in 24 hours control preservation without preservative, and significant positively correlated with deep frying in 14 days salt and turmeric preservation. Shallow frying is perfect negatively correlated with deep frying in 15 days KMS preservation. Most of the correlation of the carbohydrate content of lobster is found in **24 hours control preservation without preservative and 14 days salt-turmeric preservation** with respect to different cooking conditions.

5.12.4.2 Protein

Table no 5.12.4.2.1 Correlation of cooking methods in fresh condition

Condition	RS	B	OPDR	SF	DF
Raw State (RS)	1	.999*(S)	.619	-.240	.629
Boiling (B)	.999*(S)	1	.577	-.189	.587
Open Pan Dry Roasting (OPDR)	.619	.577	1	-.911(S)	1.000**(S)
Shallow Frying (SF)	-.240	-.189	-.911(S)	1	-.906(S)
Deep Frying (DF)	.629	.587	1.000**(S)	-.906(S)	1

***.Correlation is highly significant at the 0.01 level (2-tailed)* Positive Negative *S= Significant*
**.Correlation is highly significant at the 0.05 level (2-tailed)*

This table shows the correlation of protein content of lobster with cooking methods. In fresh condition, there is highly significant positive correlation present between the raw state and boiling, whereas open pan dry roasting is significant negatively correlated with shallow frying and perfect positive correlated with deep frying. Shallow frying is significant negatively correlated with deep frying This table indicates that there is a strong correlation present among the **raw state, boiling, open pan dry roasting, shallow frying and deep frying** in fresh condition.

Table no 5.12.4.2.2 Correlation of cooking methods in 24 hours preservation without preservative

Condition	RS	B	OPDR	SF	DF
Raw State (RS)	1	-.807(S)	1.000**(S)	.269	-.327
Boiling (B)	-.807(S)	1	-.807(S)	-.786	-.294
Open Pan Dry Roasting (OPDR)	1.000**(S)	-.807(S)	1	.269	-.327
Shallow Frying (SF)	.269	-.786	.269	1	.822(S)
Deep Frying (DF)	-.327	-.294	-.327	.822(S)	1

***.Correlation is highly significant at the 0.01 level (2-tailed)* Positive Negative *S= Significant*

This table shows the correlation of protein content of lobster with cooking methods. In 24 hours control preservation without preservative, there is significant negative correlation present between the raw state and boiling, and perfect positive correlation present between the raw state and open pan dry roasting, whereas open pan dry roasting is significant negatively correlated with boiling. Shallow frying is significant positively correlated with deep frying. This table indicates that there is a strong correlation present among the **raw state, boiling, open pan dry roasting, shallow frying and deep frying** in 24 hours control preservation.

Table no 5.12.4.2.3 Correlation of cooking methods in 48 hours preservation without preservative

Condition	RS	B	OPDR	SF	DF
Raw State (RS)	1	.362	.025	-.907(S)	.025
Boiling (B)	.362	1	.941(S)	-.721	.941(S)
Open Pan Dry Roasting (OPDR)	.025	.941(S)	1	-.444	1.000**(S)
Shallow Frying (SF)	-.907(S)	-.721	-.444	1	-.444
Deep Frying (DF)	.025	.941(S)	1.000**(S)	-.444	1

***.Correlation is highly significant at the 0.01 level (2-tailed)* Positive Negative *S= Significant*

This table shows the correlation of protein content of lobster with cooking methods. In 48 hours control preservation without preservative, there is significant negative correlation present between the raw state and shallow frying, whereas boiling is significant positively correlated with open pan dry roasting and deep frying. Open pan dry roasting is perfect positively correlated with deep frying. This table indicates that there is a strong correlation present between the **raw state, boiling, open pan dry roasting, shallow frying and deep frying** in 48 hours control preservation.

Table no 5.12.4.2.4 Correlation of cooking methods in 14 days preservation without preservative

Condition	RS	B	OPDR	SF	DF
Raw State (RS)	1	.829(S)	-.825(S)	.903(S)	-.119
Boiling (B)	.829(S)	1	-1.000**(S)	.509	-.654
Open Pan Dry Roasting (OPDR)	-.825(S)	-1.000**(S)	1	-.503	.659
Shallow Frying (SF)	.903(S)	.509	-.503	1	.319
Deep Frying (DF)	-.119	-.654	.659	.319	1

***.Correlation is highly significant at the 0.01 level (2-tailed)* Positive Negative *S= Significant*

This table shows the correlation of protein content of lobster with cooking methods. In 14 days control preservation without preservative, there is significant positive correlation present between the raw state with boiling and shallow frying, and significant negative correlation present between the raw state and open pan dry roasting, whereas boiling is perfect negatively correlated with open pan dry roasting. This table indicates that there is a strong correlation present between the **raw state, boiling, open pan dry roasting and shallow frying** in 14 days control preservation.

Table no 5.12.4.2.5 Correlation of cooking methods in 15 days preservation without preservative

Condition	RS	B	OPDR	SF	DF
Raw State (RS)	1	-.981(S)	-.500	.657	.495
Boiling (B)	-.981(S)	1	.324	-.790	-.653
Open Pan Dry Roasting (OPDR)	-.500	.324	1	.324	.505
Shallow Frying (SF)	.657	-.790	.324	1	.980(S)
Deep Frying (DF)	.495	-.653	.505	.980(S)	1

Positive Negative *S= Significant*

This table shows the correlation of protein content of lobster with cooking methods. In 15 days control preservation without preservative, there is significant negative correlation present between the raw state and boiling, whereas shallow frying is significant positively correlated with deep frying. This table indicates that there is a strong correlation present between the **raw state, boiling, shallow frying and deep frying** in 15 days control preservation.

Table no 5.12.4.2.6 Correlation of cooking methods in 24 hours preservation with salt and turmeric

Condition	R	B	OPDR	SF	DF
Raw State (RS)	1	-.916(S)	-.999*(S)	.310	-.814(S)
Boiling (B)	-.916(S)	1	.934(S)	.098	.513
Open Pan Dry Roasting (OPDR)	-.999*(S)	.934(S)	1	-.264	.786
Shallow Frying (SF)	.310	.098	-.264	1	-.804(S)
Deep Frying (DF)	-.814(S)	.513	.786	-.804(S)	1

**.Correlation is highly significant at the 0.05 level (2-tailed)* Positive Negative *S= Significant*

This table shows the correlation of protein content of lobster with cooking methods. In 24 hours salt and turmeric preservation, there is highly significant negative correlation present between the raw state and open pan dry roasting, and significant negative correlation present between the raw state with boiling and deep frying, whereas boiling is significant positively correlated with open pan dry roasting. Shallow frying is significant negatively correlated with deep frying. This table indicates that there is a strong correlation present between the **raw state, boiling, open pan dry roasting, shallow frying and deep frying** in 24 hours salt and turmeric preservation.

Table no 5.12.4.2.7 Correlation of cooking methods in 48 hours preservation with salt and turmeric

Condition	RS	B	OPDR	SF	DF
Raw State (R)S	1	1.000**(S)	-.999*(S)	.808(S)	.982(S)
Boiling (B)	1.000**(S)	1	-.999*(S)	.808(S)	.982(S)
Open Pan Dry Roasting (OPDR)	-.999*(S)	-.999*(S)	1	-.827(S)	-.988(S)
Shallow Frying (SF)	.808(S)	.808(S)	-.827(S)	1	.904(S)
Deep Frying (DF)	.982(S)	.982(S)	-.988(S)	.904(S)	1

**.Correlation is highly significant at the 0.05 level (2-tailed)* ▢ Positive ▢ Negative *S= Significant*
***.Correlation is highly significant at the 0.01 level (2-tailed)*

This table shows the correlation of protein content of lobster with cooking methods. In 48 hours salt and turmeric preservation, there is highly significant negative correlation present between the raw state and open pan dry roasting, and significant positive correlation present between the raw state with shallow frying and deep frying, and perfect positive correlation present between the raw state and boiling, whereas boiling is significant positively correlated with shallow frying and deep frying, and highly significant negatively correlated with open pan dry roasting. Open pan dry roasting is significant negatively correlated with shallow frying and deep frying. Shallow frying is significant positively correlated with deep frying. This table indicates that there is a strong correlation present among the **raw state, boiling, open pan dry roasting, shallow frying and deep frying** in 48 hours salt and turmeric preservation.

Table no 5.12.4.2.8 Correlation of cooking methods in 14 days preservation with salt and turmeric

Condition	RS	B	OPDR	SF	DF
Raw State (RS)	1	-1.000**(S)	-.912(S)	.493	.087
Boiling (B)	-1.000**(S)	1	.912(S)	-.493	-.087
Open Pan Dry Roasting (OPDR)	-.912(S)	.912(S)	1	-.806(S)	-.488
Shallow Frying (SF)	.493	-.493	-.806(S)	1	.909(S)
Deep Frying (DF)	.087	-.087	-.488	.909(S)	1

***.Correlation is highly significant at the 0.01 level (2-tailed)* ▢ Positive ▢ Negative *S= Significant*

This table shows the correlation of protein content of lobster with cooking methods. In 14 days salt and turmeric preservation, there is significant negative correlation present between the raw state and open pan dry roasting, and perfect negative correlation present between the raw state and boiling. Boiling is significant positively correlated with open pan dry roasting, whereas open pan dry roasting is significant negatively correlated with shallow frying. Shallow frying is significant positively correlated with deep frying. This table indicates that there is a strong correlation present among the **raw state, boiling, open pan dry roasting, shallow frying and deep frying** in 14 days salt and turmeric preservation.

Table no 5.12.4.2.9 Correlation of cooking methods in 15 days preservation with salt and turmeric

Condition	RS	B	OPDR	SF	DF
Raw State (RS)	1	.698	.619	.613	.710
Boiling (B)	.698	1	-.131	-.138	1.000*(S)
Open Pan Dry Roasting (OPDR)	.619	-.131	1	1.000**(S)	-.115
Shallow Frying (SF)	.613	-.138	1.000**(S)	1	-.122
Deep Frying (DF)	.710	1.000*(S)	-.115	-.122	1

***.Correlation is highly significant at the 0.01 level (2-tailed)* Positive *S= Significant*
**.Correlation is highly significant at the 0.05 level (2-tailed)*

This table shows the correlation of protein content of lobster with cooking methods. In 15 days salt and turmeric preservation, there is perfect positive correlation present between boiling and deep frying, whereas open pan dry roasting is perfect positively correlated with shallow frying. This table indicates that there is a strong correlation present between **boiling and deep frying and also between open pan dry roasting and shallow frying** in 15 days salt and turmeric preservation.

Table no 5.12.4.2.10 Correlation of cooking methods in 24 hours preservation with KMS

Condition	RS	B	OPDR	SF	DF
Raw State (RS)	1	.862(S)	.866(S)	-.257	-.848(S)
Boiling (B)	.862(S)	1	1.000**(S)	.268	-1.000*(S)
Open Pan Dry Roasting (OPDR)	.866(S)	1.000**(S)	1	.260	-.999*(S)
Shallow Frying (SF)	-.257	.268	.260	1	-.293
Deep Frying (DF)	-.848(S)	-1.000*(S)	-.999*(S)	-.293	1

***.Correlation is highly significant at the 0.01 level (2-tailed)* Positive Negative *S= Significant*
**.Correlation is highly significant at the 0.05 level (2-tailed)*

This table shows the correlation of protein content of lobster with cooking methods. In 24 hours KMS preservation, there is significant positive correlation present between the raw state with boiling and open pan dry roasting, and significant negative correlation present between the raw state and deep frying, whereas open pan dry roasting is perfect positively correlated with boiling and significant negatively correlated with deep frying. Boiling is perfect negatively correlated with deep frying. This table indicates that there is a strong correlation present among the **raw state, boiling, open pan dry roasting and deep frying** in 24 hours KMS preservation.

Table no 5.12.4.2.11 Correlation of cooking methods in 48 hours preservation with KMS

Condition	RS	B	OPDR	SF	DF
Raw State (RS)	1	.655	-.327	-.320	.322
Boiling (B)	.655	1	.500	.506	-.505
Open Pan Dry Roasting (OPDR)	-.327	.500	1	1.000**(S)	-1.000**(S)
Shallow Frying (SF)	-.320	.506	1.000**(S)	1	-1.000**(S)
Deep Frying (DF)	.322	-.505	-1.000**(S)	-1.000**(S)	1

***.Correlation is highly significant at the 0.01 level (2-tailed)* Positive Negative *S= Significant*

This table shows the correlation of protein content of lobster with cooking methods. In 48 hours KMS preservation, there is significant positive correlation present between open pan dry roasting and shallow frying, and perfect negative correlation present between open pan dry roasting and deep frying, whereas shallow frying is perfect negatively correlated with deep frying. This table indicates that there is a strong correlation present among **open pan dry roasting, shallow frying and deep frying** in 48 hours KMS preservation.

Table no 5.12.4.2.12 Correlation of cooking methods in 14 days preservation with KMS

Condition	RS	B	OPDR	SF	DF
Raw State (RS)	1	.900(S)	-.500	-.182	-.756
Boiling (B)	.900(S)	1	-.827(S)	.265	-.966(S)
Open Pan Dry Roasting (OPDR)	-.500	-.827(S)	1	-.761	.945(S)
Shallow Frying (SF)	-.182	.265	-.761	1	-.506
Deep Frying (DF)	-.756	-.966(S)	.945(S)	-.506	1

▢ Positive ▢ Negative *S= Significant*

This table shows the correlation of protein content of lobster with cooking methods. In 14 days KMS preservation, there is significant positive correlation present between the raw state and boiling, whereas boiling is significant negatively correlated with open pan dry roasting and deep frying, whereas open pan dry roasting is significant positively correlated with deep frying. This table indicates that there is a strong correlation present among the **raw state, boiling, open pan dry roasting and deep frying** in 14 days KMS preservation.

Table no 5.12.4.2.13 Correlation of cooking methods in 15 days preservation with KMS

Condition	RS	B	OPDR	SF	DF
Raw State (RS)	1	.983(S)	-1.000**(S)	-1.000**(S)	-.638
Boiling (B)	.983(S)	1	-.983(S)	-.985(S)	-.767
Open Pan Dry Roasting (OPDR)	-1.000**(S)	-.983(S)	1	1.000**(S)	.638
Shallow Frying (SF)	-1.000**(S)	-.985(S)	1.000**(S)	1	.643
Deep Frying (DF)	-.638	-.767	.638	.643	1

***.Correlation is highly significant at the 0.01 level (2-tailed)* ▢ Positive ▢ Negative *S= Significant*

This table shows the correlation of protein content of lobster with cooking methods. In 15 days KMS preservation, there is significant positive correlation present between the raw state and boiling, and perfect negative correlation present between the raw state with open pan dry roasting and shallow frying, whereas boiling is significant negatively correlated with open pan dry roasting and shallow frying. Open pan dry roasting is perfect positively correlated with shallow frying. This table indicates that there is a strong correlation present among the **raw state, boiling, open pan dry roasting and shallow frying** in 15 days KMS preservation.

Overall analysis reveals that the raw state is perfect positively correlated with boiling in 48 hours salt-turmeric preservation and perfect negatively correlated with boiling in 14 days salt-turmeric preservation, whereas perfect positively correlated with open pan dry roasting in 24 hours control preservation without preservative and perfect negatively correlated with open pan dry roasting in 15 days KMS preservation, perfect negatively correlated with shallow frying in 15 days KMS preservation, and significant positively correlated with deep frying in 48 hours salt-turmeric preservation. Boiling is perfect negatively correlated with open pan dry roasting in 14 days control preservation without preservative and perfect positively correlated with open pan dry roasting in 24 hours KMS preservation, whereas significant negatively correlated with shallow frying in 15 days KMS preservation, and perfect positively correlated with deep frying in 15 days salt-turmeric preservation, and perfect negatively correlated with deep frying in 24 hours KMS preservation. Open pan dry roasting is perfect positively correlated with shallow frying in 15 days salt and turmeric preservation and 48 hours KMS preservation, whereas perfect negatively correlated with deep frying in 48 hours KMS preservation and perfect positively correlated with deep frying in 48 hours control preservation without preservative. Shallow frying is perfect negatively correlated with deep frying in 48 hours KMS preservation. Most of the correlation of the protein content of lobster is found in **48 hours and 15 days KMS preservation** with respect to different cooking conditions.

5.12.4.3 Fat

Table no 5.12.4.3.1 Correlation of cooking methods in fresh condition

Condition	RS	B	OPDR	SF	DF
Raw State (RS)	1	.980(S)	-1.000*(S)	-.683	-.974(S)
Boiling (B)	.980(S)	1	-.976(S)	-.815(S)	-.909(S)
Open Pan Dry Roasting (OPDR)	-1.000*(S)	-.976(S)	1	.670	.978(S)
Shallow Frying (SF)	-.683	-.815(S)	.670	1	.500
Deep Frying (DF)	-.974(S)	-.909(S)	.978(S)	.500	1

***.Correlation is highly significant at the 0.01 level (2-tailed)* ▭ Positive ▭ Negative *S= Significant*

This table shows the correlation of fat content of lobster with cooking methods. In fresh condition, there is significant positive correlation present between the raw state and boiling, and perfect negative correlation present between the raw state and open pan dry roasting and significant negative correlation present between the raw state and deep frying, whereas boiling is significant negatively correlated with open pan dry roasting, shallow frying and deep frying. Open pan dry roasting is significant positively correlated with deep frying. This table indicates that there is a strong correlation present among the **raw state, boiling, open pan dry roasting, shallow frying and deep frying** in fresh condition.

Table no 5.12.4.3.2 Correlation of cooking methods in 24 hours preservation without preservative

Condition	RS	B	OPDR	SF	DF
Raw State (RS)	1	-.545	-.052	-.350	1.000**(S)
Boiling (B)	-.545	1	.866(S)	.976(S)	-.545
Open Pan Dry Roasting (OPDR)	-.052	.866(S)	1	.954(S)	-.052
Shallow Frying (SF)	-.350	.976(S)	.954(S)	1	-.350
Deep Frying (DF)	1.000**(S)	-.545	-.052	-.350	1

***.Correlation is highly significant at the 0.01 level (2-tailed)* ▭ Positive *S= Significant*

This table shows the correlation of fat content of lobster with cooking methods. In 24 hours control preservation without preservative, there is perfect positive correlation present between the raw state and deep frying, whereas boiling is significant positively correlated with open pan dry roasting and shallow frying. Open pan dry roasting is significant positively correlated with shallow frying. This table indicates that there is a strong correlation present among the **raw state, boiling, open pan dry roasting, shallow frying and deep frying** in 24 hours control preservation.

Table no 5.12.4.3.3 Correlation of cooking methods in 48 hours preservation without preservative

Condition	RS	B	OPDR	SF	DF
Raw State (RS)	1	.918(S)	.875(S)	.999*(S)	.899(S)
Boiling (B)	.918(S)	1	.995(S)	.899(S)	.999*(S)
Open Pan Dry Roasting (OPDR)	.875(S)	.995(S)	1	.851(S)	.999*(S)
Shallow Frying (SF)	.999*(S)	.899(S)	.851(S)	1	.877(S)
Deep Frying (DF)	.899(S)	.999*(S)	.999*(S)	.877(S)	1

**.Correlation is highly significant at the 0.05 level (2-tailed)* ▭ Positive *S= Significant*

This table shows the correlation of fat content of lobster with cooking methods. In 48 hours control preservation without preservative, there is significant positive correlation present between the raw state with boiling, open pan dry roasting, deep frying and highly significant positive correlation present between the raw state and shallow frying, whereas boiling is significant positively correlated with open pan dry roasting and shallow frying and highly significant positively correlated with deep frying. Open pan dry roasting is significant positively correlated with shallow frying and highly significant positively correlated with deep frying. This table indicates that there is a strong correlation present among the **raw state, boiling, open pan dry roasting, shallow frying and deep frying** in 48 hours control preservation.

Table no 5.12.4.3.4 Correlation of cooking methods in 14 days preservation without preservative

Condition	RS	B	OPDR	SF	DF
Raw State (RS)	1	.971(S)	1.000**(S)	.993(S)	.610
Boiling (B)	.971(S)	1	.971(S)	.992(S)	.782
Open Pan Dry Roasting (OPDR)	1.000**(S)	.971(S)	1	.993(S)	.610
Shallow Frying (SF)	.993(S)	.992(S)	.993(S)	1	.697
Deep Frying (DF)	.610	.782	.610	.697	1

***.Correlation is highly significant at the 0.01 level (2-tailed)* ▭ Positive *S= Significant*

This table shows the correlation of fat content of lobster with cooking methods. In 14 days control preservation without preservative, there is significant positive correlation present between the raw state with boiling and shallow frying, and highly significant positive correlation present between the raw state and open pan dry roasting, whereas boiling is significant positively correlated with open pan dry roasting and shallow frying. Open pan dry roasting is significant positively correlated with shallow frying. This table indicates that there is a strong correlation present among the **raw state, boiling, open pan dry roasting and shallow frying** in 14 days control preservation.

Table no 5.12.4.3.5 Correlation of cooking methods in 15 days preservation without preservative

Condition	RS	B	OPDR	SF	DF
Raw State (RS)	1	-1.000**(S)	-.832(S)	-.782	.606
Boiling (B)	-1.000**(S)	1	.832(S)	.782	-.606
Open Pan Dry Roasting (OPDR)	-.832(S)	.832(S)	1	.305	-.062
Shallow Frying (SF)	-.782	.782	.305	1	-.970(S)
Deep Frying (DF)	.606	-.606	-.062	-.970(S)	1

***.Correlation is highly significant at the 0.01 level (2-tailed)* ▭ Positive ▭ Negative *S= Significant*

This table shows the correlation of fat content of lobster with cooking methods. In 15 days control preservation without preservative, there is significant negative correlation present between the raw state and open pan dry roasting, and perfect negative correlation present between the raw state and boiling, whereas boiling is significant positively correlated with open pan dry roasting. Shallow frying is significant negatively correlated with deep frying. This table indicates that there is a strong correlation present among the **raw state, boiling, open pan dry roasting, shallow frying and deep frying** in 15 days control preservation.

Table no 5.12.4.3.6 Correlation of cooking methods in 24 hours preservation salt and turmeric

Condition	RS	B	OPDR	SF	DF
Raw State (RS)	1	.217	.655	.419	-.327
Boiling (B)	.217	1	-.596	-.795	-.993(S)
Open Pan Dry Roasting (OPDR)	.655	-.596	1	.961(S)	.500
Shallow Frying (SF)	.419	-.795	.961(S)	1	.721
Deep Frying (DF)	-.327	-.993(S)	.500	.721	1

Positive Negative *S= Significant*

This table shows the correlation of fat content of lobster with cooking methods. In 24 hours salt and turmeric preservation, there is significant negative correlation present between boiling and deep frying, whereas open pan dry roasting is significant positively correlated with shallow frying. This table indicates that there is a strong correlation present between **boiling and deep frying and also between open pan dry roasting and shallow frying** in 24 hours salt and turmeric preservation.

Table no 5.12.4.3.7 Correlation of cooking methods in 48 hours preservation with salt and turmeric

Condition	RS	B	OPDR	SF	DF
Raw State (RS)	1	-.700	-.911(S)	.756	.954(S)
Boiling (B)	-.700	1	.933(S)	-.062	-.882(S)
Open Pan Dry Roasting (OPDR)	-.911(S)	.933(S)	1	-.418	-.993(S)
Shallow Frying (SF)	.756	-.062	-.418	1	.524
Deep Frying (DF)	.954(S)	-.882(S)	-.993(S)	.524	1

Positive Negative *S= Significant*

This table shows the correlation of fat content of lobster with cooking methods. In 48 hours salt and turmeric preservation, there is significant negative correlation present between the raw state and open pan dry roasting, and significant positive correlation present between the raw state and deep frying, whereas open pan dry roasting is significant positively correlated with boiling and negatively correlated with shallow frying. Boiling is significant negatively correlated with deep frying. This table indicates that there is a strong correlation present among the **raw state, boiling, open pan dry roasting and deep frying** in 48 hours salt and turmeric preservation.

Table no 5.12.4.3.8 Correlation of cooking methods in 14 days preservation with salt and turmeric

Condition	RS	B	OPDR	SF	DF
Raw State(RS)	1	-.866(S)	.712	1.000**(S)	-.826(S)
Boiling (B)	-.866(S)	1	-.266	-.866(S)	.434
Open Pan Dry Roasting (OPDR)	.712	-.266	1	.712	-.984(S)
Shallow Frying (SF)	1.000**(S)	-.866(S)	.712	1	-.826(S)
Deep Frying (DF)	-.826(S)	.434	-.984(S)	-.826(S)	1

***.Correlation is highly significant at the 0.01 level (2-tailed)* Positive Negative *S= Significant*

This table shows the correlation of fat content of lobster with cooking methods. In 14 days salt and turmeric preservation, there is significant negative correlation present between the raw state with boiling and deep frying, and perfect positive correlation present between the raw state and shallow frying, whereas boiling is significant negatively correlated with shallow frying. Open pan dry roasting is significant negatively correlated with deep frying. Shallow frying is significant negatively correlated with deep frying. This table indicates that there is a strong correlation present among the **raw state, boiling, open pan dry roasting, shallow frying and deep frying** in 14 days salt and turmeric preservation.

Table no 5.12.4.3.9 Correlation of cooking methods in 15 days preservation with salt and turmeric

Condition	RS	B	OPDR	SF	DF
Raw State (RS)	1	.998* (S)	-.646	-.348	-.215
Boiling (B)	.998* (S)	1	-.596	-.407	-.277
Open Pan Dry Roasting (OPDR)	-.646	-.596	1	-.491	-.606
Shallow Frying (SF)	-.348	-.407	-.491	1	.990(S)
Deep Frying (DF)	-.215	-.277	-.606	.990(S)	1

**.Correlation is highly significant at the 0.05 level (2-tailed)* Positive *S= Significant*

This table shows the correlation of fat content of lobster with cooking methods. In 15 days salt and turmeric preservation, there is highly significant positive correlation present between the raw state and boiling, whereas shallow frying is significant positively correlated with deep frying. This table indicates that there is a strong correlation present between the **raw state and boiling and also between shallow frying and deep frying** in 15 days salt and turmeric preservation.

Table no 5.12.4.3.10 Correlation of cooking methods in 24 hours preservation with KMS

Condition	RS	B	OPDR	SF	DF
Raw State (RS)	1	-.763	.385	.675	.747
Boiling (B)	-.763	1	.302	-.038	-.141
Open Pan Dry Roasting (OPDR)	.385	.302	1	.941(S)	.901(S)
Shallow Frying (SF)	.675	-.038	.941(S)	1	.995(S)
Deep Frying (DF)	.747	-.141	.901(S)	.995(S)	1

Positive *S= Significant*

This table shows the correlation of fat content of lobster with cooking methods. In 24 hours KMS preservation, there is significant positive correlation present between open pan dry roasting with shallow frying and deep frying, whereas shallow frying is significant positively correlated with deep frying. This table indicates that there is a strong correlation present among **open pan dry roasting, shallow frying and deep frying** in 24 hours KMS preservation.

Table no 5.12.4.3.11 Correlation of cooking methods in 48 hours preservation with KMS

Condition	RS	B	OPDR	SF	DF
Raw State (RS)	1	-.327	-.171	-.721	.444
Boiling (B)	-.327	1	.987(S)	.891(S)	-.992(S)
Open Pan Dry Roasting (OPDR)	-.171	.987(S)	1	.806(S)	-.959(S)
Shallow Frying (SF)	-.721	.891(S)	.806(S)	1	-.941(S)
Deep Frying (DF)	.444	-.992(S)	-.959(S)	-.941(S)	1

Positive Negative *S= Significant*

This table shows the correlation of fat content of lobster with cooking methods. In 48 hours KMS preservation, there is significant negative correlation present between boiling and deep frying, and significant positive correlation present between boiling with open pan dry roasting and shallow frying, whereas open pan dry roasting is significant negatively correlated with deep frying and significant positively correlated with shallow frying. Shallow frying is significant negatively correlated with deep frying. This table indicates that there is a strong correlation present among **boiling, open pan dry roasting, shallow frying and deep frying** in 48 hours KMS preservation.

Table no 5.12.4.3.12 Correlation of cooking methods in 14 days preservation with KMS

Condition	RS	B	OPDR	SF	DF
Raw State (RS)	1	-.195	-.449	-.272	-.058
Boiling (B)	-.195	1	.964(S)	.997(S)	-.968(S)
Open Pan Dry Roasting (OPDR)	-.449	.964(S)	1	.982(S)	-.866(S)
Shallow Frying (SF)	-.272	.997(S)	.982(S)	1	-.945(S)
Deep Frying (DF)	-.058	-.968(S)	-.866(S)	-.945(S)	1

Positive Negative *S= Significant*

This table shows the correlation of fat content of lobster with cooking methods. In 14 days KMS preservation, there is significant negative correlation present between boiling and deep frying and significant positive correlation present between boiling with open pan dry roasting and shallow frying, whereas open pan dry roasting is significant negatively correlated with deep frying and significant positively correlated with shallow frying. Shallow frying is significant negatively correlated with deep frying. This table indicates that there is a strong correlation present among **boiling, open pan dry roasting, shallow frying and deep frying** in 14 days KMS preservation.

Table no 5.12.4.3.13 Correlation of cooking methods in 15 days preservation with KMS

Condition	RS	B	OPDR	SF	DF
Raw State (RS)	1	.778	.933(S)	-.461	-.820(S)
Boiling (B)	.778	1	.500	.200	-.277
Open Pan Dry Roasting (OPDR)	.933(S)	.500	1	-.749	-.971(S)
Shallow Frying (SF)	-.461	.200	-.749	1	.886(S)
Deep Frying (DF)	-.820(S)	-.277	-.971(S)	.886(S)	1

Positive Negative *S= Significant*

This table shows the correlation of fat content of lobster with cooking methods. In 15 days KMS preservation, there is significant positive correlation present between the raw state and open pan dry roasting, and significant negative correlation present between the raw state and deep frying. Open pan dry roasting is significant negatively correlated with deep frying. Shallow frying is significant positively correlated with deep frying. This table indicates that there is a strong correlation present among the **raw state, open pan dry roasting, shallow frying and deep frying** in 15 days KMS preservation.

Overall analysis reveals that the raw state is perfect negatively correlated with boiling in 15 days control preservation without preservative, whereas perfect positively correlated with open pan dry roasting in 14 days control preservation without preservative and perfect negatively correlated with open pan dry roasting in fresh condition, and perfect positively correlated with shallow frying and deep frying in 14 days salt and turmeric preservation and 24 hours control preservation without preservative respectively. Boiling is significant positively correlated with open pan dry roasting in 48 hours control preservation without preservative, whereas significant positively correlated with shallow frying in 14 days KMS preservation, and highly significant positively correlated with deep frying in 48 hours control preservation without preservative. Open pan dry roasting is significant positively correlated with shallow frying in 14 days control preservation without preservative, and highly significant positively correlated with deep frying in 48 hours control preservation without preservative. Shallow frying is significant positively correlated with deep frying in 24 hours KMS preservation. Most of the correlation of the fat content of lobster is found in **48 hours control preservation without preservative** with respect to different cooking conditions.

5.12.4.4 Moisture

Table no 5.12.4.4.1 Correlation of cooking methods in fresh condition

Condition	RS	B	OPDR	SF	DF
Raw State (RS)	1	-.834(S)	.999*(S)	-.878(S)	-.581
Boiling (B)	-.834(S)	1	-.811(S)	.996(S)	.933(S)
Open Pan Dry Roasting (OPDR)	.999*(S)	-.811(S)	1	-.858(S)	-.547
Shallow Frying (SF)	-.878(S)	.996(S)	-.858(S)	1	.899(S)
Deep Frying (DF)	-.581	.933(S)	-.547	.899(S)	1

**.Correlation is highly significant at the 0.05 level (2-tailed)* Positive Negative *S= Significant*

This table shows the correlation of moisture content of lobster with cooking methods. In fresh condition, there is highly significant positive correlation present between the raw state and open pan dry roasting, and significant negative correlation present between the raw state with boiling and shallow frying, whereas boiling is significant positively correlated with shallow frying and deep frying and significant negatively correlated with open pan dry roasting. Open pan dry roasting is significant negatively correlated with shallow frying. Shallow frying is significant positively correlated with deep frying. This table indicates that there is a strong correlation present among the **raw state, boiling, open pan dry roasting, shallow frying and deep frying** in fresh condition.

Table no 5.12.4.4.2 Correlation of cooking methods in 24 hours preservation without preservative

Condition	RS	B	OPDR	SF	DF
Raw State (RS)	1	.398	.772	.372	-.489
Boiling (B)	.398	1	-.276	-.704	.606
Open Pan Dry Roasting (OPDR)	.772	-.276	1	.877(S)	-.932(S)
Shallow Frying (SF)	.372	-.704	.877(S)	1	-.992(S)
Deep Frying (DF)	-.489	.606	-.932(S)	-.992(S)	1

Positive Negative *S= Significant*

This table shows the correlation of moisture content of lobster with cooking methods. In 24 hours control preservation without preservative, there is highly significant positive correlation present between open pan dry roasting with shallow frying, and significant negative correlation present between open pan dry roasting and deep frying, whereas shallow frying is significant negatively correlated with deep frying. This table indicates that there is a strong correlation present among **open pan dry roasting, shallow frying and deep frying** 24 hours control preservation.

Table no 5.12.4.4.3 Correlation of cooking methods in 48 hours preservation without preservative

Condition	RS	B	OPDR	SF	DF
Raw State (RS)	1	-.961(S)	-.596	.908(S)	.350
Boiling (B)	-.961(S)	1	.795	-.756	-.596
Open Pan Dry Roasting (OPDR)	-.596	.795	1	-.204	-.961(S)
Shallow Frying (SF)	.908(S)	-.756	-.204	1	-.075
Deep Frying (DF)	.350	-.596	-.961(S)	-.075	1

Positive Negative *S= Significant*

This table shows the correlation of moisture content of lobster with cooking methods. In 48 hours control preservation without preservative, there is significant positive correlation present between the raw state and shallow frying and significant negative correlation present between the raw state and boiling, whereas open pan dry roasting is significant negatively correlated with deep frying. This table indicates that there is a strong correlation present among the **raw state, boiling, open pan dry roasting, shallow frying and deep frying** 48 hours control preservation.

Table no 5.12.4.4.4 Correlation of cooking methods in 14 days preservation without preservative

Condition	RS	B	OPDR	SF	DF
Raw State (RS)	1	.961(S)	.999*(S)	.938(S)	-.996(S)
Boiling (B)	.961(S)	1	.947(S)	.997*(S)	-.982(S)
Open Pan Dry Roasting (OPDR)	.999*(S)	.947(S)	1	.920(S)	-.991(S)
Shallow Frying (SF)	.938(S)	.997*(S)	.920(S)	1	-.965(S)
Deep Frying (DF)	-.996(S)	-.982(S)	-.991(S)	-.965(S)	1

**.Correlation is highly significant at the 0.05 level (2-tailed)* Positive Negative *S= Significant*

This table shows the correlation of moisture content of lobster with cooking methods. In 14 days control preservation without preservative, there is highly significant positive correlation present between the raw state and open pan dry roasting, and significant positive correlation present between the raw state with boiling and shallow frying, and significant negative correlation present between the raw state and deep frying, whereas boiling is significant positively correlated with open pan dry roasting and shallow frying and significant negatively correlated with deep frying. Open pan dry roasting is significant negatively correlated with deep frying and significant positively correlated with shallow frying. Shallow frying is significant negatively correlated with deep frying. This table indicates that there is a strong correlation present among the **raw state, boiling, open pan dry roasting, shallow frying and deep frying** in 14 days control preservation.

Table no 5.122.4.4.5 Correlation of cooking methods in 15 days preservation without preservative

Condition	RS	B	OPDR	SF	DF
Raw State (RS)	1	.939(S)	.952(S)	.993(S)	.106
Boiling (B)	.939(S)	1	.999*(S)	.972(S)	-.244
Open Pan Dry Roasting (OPDR)	.952(S)	.999*(S)	1	.981(S)	-.203
Shallow Frying (SF)	.993(S)	.972(S)	.981(S)	1	-.011
Deep Frying (DF)	.106	-.244	-.203	-.011	1

**.Correlation is highly significant at the 0.05 level (2-tailed)* Positive *S= Significant*

This table shows the correlation of moisture content of lobster with cooking methods. In 15 days control preservation without preservative, there is significant positive correlation present between the raw state with boiling, open pan dry roasting and shallow frying, whereas boiling is highly significant positively correlated with open pan dry roasting and significant positively correlated with shallow frying. Open pan dry roasting is significant positively correlated with deep frying. This table indicates that there is a strong correlation present among the **raw state, boiling, open pan dry roasting and shallow frying** in 15 days control preservation.

Table no 5.12.4.4.6 Correlation of cooking methods in 24 hours preservation with salt and turmeric

Condition	RS	B	OPDR	SF	DF
Raw State (RS)	1	.350	.663	.447	.403
Boiling (B)	.350	1	-.470	.994(S)	.998*(S)
Open Pan Dry Roasting (OPDR)	.663	-.470	1	-.374	-.418
Shallow Frying (SF)	.447	.994(S)	-.374	1	.999*(S)
Deep Frying (DF)	.403	.998*(S)	-.418	.999*(S)	1

**.Correlation is highly significant at the 0.05 level (2-tailed)* Positive *S= Significant*

This table shows the correlation of moisture content of lobster with cooking methods. In 24 hours salt and turmeric preservation, there is highly significant positive correlation present between boiling and deep frying, and significant positive correlation present between boiling and shallow frying, whereas shallow frying is highly significant positively correlated with deep frying. This table indicates that there is a strong correlation present among **boiling, shallow frying and deep frying** in 24 hours salt and turmeric preservation.

Table no 5.12.4.4.7 Correlation of cooking methods in 48 hours preservation with salt and turmeric

Condition	RS	B	OPDR	SF	DF
Raw State (RS)	1	-.047	-.189	-.941(S)	.213
Boiling (B)	-.047	1	.990(S)	-.295	-.986(S)
Open Pan Dry Roasting (OPDR)	-.189	.990(S)	1	-.156	-1.000*(S)
Shallow Frying (SF)	-.941(S)	-.295	-.156	1	.132
Deep Frying (DF)	.213	-.986(S)	-1.000*(S)	.132	1

**.Correlation is highly significant at the 0.05 level (2-tailed)* Positive Negative *S= Significant*

This table shows the correlation of moisture content of lobster with cooking methods. In 48 hours salt and turmeric preservation, there is significant negative correlation present between the raw state and shallow frying, whereas significant positive correlation present between boiling and open pan dry roasting and significant negative correlation present between boiling and deep frying, whereas open pan dry roasting is perfect positively correlated with deep frying. This table indicates that there is a strong correlation present among the **raw state, boiling, open pan dry roasting, shallow frying and deep frying** in 48 hours salt and turmeric preservation.

Table no 5.12.4.4.8 Correlation of cooking methods in 14 days preservation with salt and turmeric

Condition	RS	B	OPDR	SF	DF
Raw State (RS)	1	-.821(S)	.973(S)	.551	-.062
Boiling (B)	-.821(S)	1	-.667	.024	.621
Open Pan Dry Roasting (OPDR)	.973(S)	-.667	1	.728	.170
Shallow Frying (SF)	.551	.024	.728	1	.799
Deep Frying (DF)	-.062	.621	.170	.799	1

**.Correlation is highly significant at the 0.05 level (2-tailed)* Positive Negative *S= Significant*

This table shows the correlation of moisture content of lobster with cooking methods. In 14 days salt and turmeric preservation, there is significant negative correlation present between the raw state and boiling, and significant positive correlation present between the raw state and open pan dry roasting. This table indicates that there is a strong correlation present among the **raw state, boiling and open pan dry roasting** in 14 days salt and turmeric preservation.

Table no 5.12.4.4.9 Correlation of cooking methods in 15 days preservation with salt and turmeric

Condition	RS	B	OPDR	SF	DF
Raw State (RS)	1	.999*(S)	.268	.981(S)	.994(S)
Boiling (B)	.999*(S)	1	.225	.972	.988
Open Pan Dry Roasting (OPDR)	.268	.225	1	.448	.374
Shallow Frying (SF)	.981(S)	.972(S)	.448	1	.997(S)
Deep Frying (DF)	.994(S)	.988(S)	.374	.997(S)	1

**.Correlation is highly significant at the 0.05 level (2-tailed)* Positive *S= Significant*

This table shows the correlation of moisture content of lobster with cooking methods. In 15 days salt and turmeric preservation, there is highly significant positive correlation present between the raw state and boiling and significant positive correlation present between the raw state and shallow frying and deep frying. Shallow frying is significant positively correlated with deep frying. This table indicates that there is a strong correlation present among the **raw state, boiling, shallow frying and deep frying** in 15 days salt and turmeric preservation.

Table no 5.12.4.4.10 Correlation of cooking methods in 24 hours preservation with KMS

Condition	RS	B	OPDR	SF	DF
Raw State (RS)	1	.995(S)	.664	.963(S)	1.000*(S)
Boiling (B)	.995(S)	1	.588	.985(S)	.997*(S)
Open Pan Dry Roasting (OPDR)	.664	.588	1	.437	.647
Shallow Frying (SF)	.963(S)	.985(S)	.437	1	.969(S)
Deep Frying (DF)	1.000*(S)	.997*(S)	.647	.969(S)	1

**.Correlation is highly significant at the 0.05 level (2-tailed)* Positive *S= Significant*

This table shows the correlation of moisture content of lobster with cooking methods. In 24 hours KMS preservation, there is highly significant positive correlation present between the raw state and boiling, and significant positive correlation present between the raw state and shallow frying and deep frying. Shallow frying is significant positively correlated with deep frying. This table indicates that there is a strong correlation present among the **raw state, boiling, shallow frying and deep frying** in 24 hours KMS preservation.

Table no 5.12.4.4.11 Correlation of cooking methods in 48 hours preservation with KMS

Condition	RS	B	OPDR	SF	DF
Raw State (RS)	1	-.313	-.022	-.970(S)	.134
Boiling (B)	-.313	1	.956(S)	.535	.899(S)
Open Pan Dry Roasting (OPDR)	-.022	.956(S)	1	.265	.988(S)
Shallow Frying (SF)	-.970(S)	.535	.265	1	.112
Deep Frying (DF)	.134	.899(S)	.988(S)	.112	1

**.Correlation is highly significant at the 0.05 level (2-tailed)* Positive Negative *S= Significant*

This table shows the correlation of moisture content of lobster with cooking methods. In 15 days salt and turmeric preservation, there is highly significant positive correlation present between the raw state and boiling, and significant positive correlation present between the raw state with shallow frying and deep frying. Shallow frying is significant positively correlated with deep frying. This table indicates that there is a strong correlation present among the **raw state, boiling, shallow frying and deep frying** in 15 days salt and turmeric preservation.

Table no 5.12.4.4.12 Correlation of cooking methods in 14 days preservation with KMS

Condition	RS	B	OPDR	SF	DF
Raw State (RS)	1	-.892(S)	.999*(S)	-.413	-.568
Boiling (B)	-.892(S)	1	-.908(S)	.780	.879(S)
Open Pan Dry Roasting (OPDR)	.999*(S)	-.908(S)	1	-.447	-.599
Shallow Frying (SF)	-.413	.780	-.447	1	.984(S)
Deep Frying (DF)	-.568	.879(S)	-.599	.984(S)	1

**.Correlation is highly significant at the 0.05 level (2-tailed)* Positive Negative *S= Significant*

This table shows the correlation of moisture content of lobster with cooking methods. In 14 days KMS preservation, there is highly significant positive correlation present between the raw state and open pan dry roasting, and significant negative correlation present between the raw state and boiling, whereas boiling is significant negatively correlated with open pan dry roasting and positively correlated with deep frying. Shallow frying is significant positively correlated with deep frying. This table indicates that there is a strong correlation present among the **raw state, boiling, open pan dry roasting, shallow frying and deep frying** in 14 days KMS preservation.

Table no 5.12.4.4.13 Correlation of cooking methods in 15 days preservation with KMS

Condition	RS	B	OPDR	SF	DF
Raw State (RS)	1	-.255	-.459	.982(S)	.936(S)
Boiling (B)	-.255	1	.976(S)	-.434	-.578
Open Pan Dry Roasting (OPDR)	-.459	.976(S)	1	-.619	-.741
Shallow Frying (SF)	.982(S)	-.434	-.619	1	.986(S)
Deep Frying (DF)	.936(S)	-.578	-.741	.986(S)	1

Positive *S= Significant*

This table shows the correlation of moisture content of lobster with cooking methods. In 15 days KMS preservation, there is significant positive correlation present between the raw state with shallow frying and deep frying, whereas boiling is significant positively correlated with open pan dry roasting. Shallow frying is significant positively correlated with deep frying. This table indicates that there is a strong correlation present among the **raw state, boiling, open pan dry roasting, shallow frying and deep frying** in 15 days KMS preservation.

Overall analysis reveals that the raw state is highly significant positively correlated with boiling in 15 days salt-turmeric preservation, whereas highly significant positively correlated with open pan dry roasting in fresh condition, 14 days control preservation without preservative and 14 days KMS preservation, significant positively correlated with shallow frying in 15 days control preservation without preservative, and perfect positively correlated with deep frying in 24 hours KMS preservation. Boiling is highly significant positively correlated with open pan dry roasting and shallow frying in 15 days control preservation without preservative, whereas highly significant positively correlated with deep frying in 24 hours salt and turmeric preservation. Open pan dry roasting is significant positively correlated with shallow frying in 15 days control preservation without preservative, and perfect positively correlated with deep frying in 48 hours salt and turmeric preservation. Shallow frying is highly significant positively correlated with deep frying in 24 hours salt-turmeric preservation. Most of the correlation of the moisture content of lobster is found in **15 days control preservation without preservative** with respect to different cooking conditions.

5.12.4.5 Ash

Table no 5.12.4.5.1 Correlation of cooking methods in fresh condition

Condition	RS	B	OPDR	SF	DF
Raw State (RS)	1	.836(S)	.980(S)	.058	-.991(S)
Boiling (B)	.836(S)	1	.929(S)	-.500	-.756
Open Pan Dry Roasting (OPDR)	.980(S)	.929(S)	1	-.143	-.945(S)
Shallow Frying (SF)	.058	-.500	-.143	1	-.189
Deep Frying (DF)	-.991(S)	-.756	-.945(S)	-.189	1

Positive Negative *S= Significant*

This table shows the correlation of ash content of lobster with cooking methods. In fresh condition, there is significant positive correlation present between the raw state with boiling and open pan dry roasting, and significant negative correlation present between the raw state and deep frying, whereas boiling is significant positively correlated with open pan dry roasting. This table indicates that there is a strong correlation present among the **raw state, boiling, open pan dry roasting and deep frying** in fresh condition.

Table no 5.12.4.5.2 Correlation of cooking methods in 24 hours preservation without preservative

Condition	RS	B	OPDR	SF	DF
Raw State (RS)	1	.189	-.327	-.596	.961(S)
Boiling (B)	.189	1	-.990(S)	-.901(S)	-.091
Open Pan Dry Roasting (OPDR)	-.327	-.990(S)	1	.954(S)	-.052
Shallow Frying (SF)	-.596	-.901(S)	.954(S)	1	-.350
Deep Frying (DF)	.961(S)	-.091	-.052	-.350	1

Positive Negative *S= Significant*

This table shows the correlation of ash content of lobster with cooking methods. In 24 hours control preservation without preservative, there is significant positive correlation present between the raw state and deep frying, whereas boiling is significant negatively correlated with open pan dry roasting and shallow frying. This table indicates that there is a strong correlation present among the **raw state, boiling, open pan dry roasting, shallow frying and deep frying** in 24 hours control preservation.

Table no 5.12.4.5.3 Correlation of cooking methods in 48 hours preservation without preservative

Condition	RS	B	OPDR	SF	DF
Raw State (RS)	1	.683	.227	.704	.277
Boiling (B)	.683	1	.866	1.000*(S)	.891(S)
Open Pan Dry Roasting (OPDR)	.227	.866(S)	1	.851(S)	.999*(S)
Shallow Frying (SF)	.704	1.000*(S)	.851(S)	1	.877(S)
Deep Frying (DF)	.277	.891(S)	.999*(S)	.877(S)	1

**.Correlation is highly significant at the 0.05 level (2-tailed)* Positive *S= Significant*

This table shows the correlation of ash content of lobster with cooking methods. In 48 hours control preservation without preservative, there is perfect positive correlation present between boiling and shallow frying, and significant positive correlation present between boiling and deep frying, whereas open pan dry roasting is significant positively correlated with deep frying and significant positively correlated with shallow frying. Shallow frying is significant positively correlated with deep frying. This table indicates that there is a strong correlation present among **boiling, open pan dry roasting, shallow frying and deep frying** in 48 hours control preservation.

Table no 5.12.4.5.4 Correlation of cooking methods in 14 days preservation without preservative

Condition	RS	B	OPDR	SF	DF
Raw State (RS)	1	.971(S)	1.000**(S)	.993(S)	.756
Boiling (B)	.971(S)	1	.971(S)	.992(S)	.891(S)
Open Pan Dry Roasting (OPDR)	1.000**(S)	.971(S)	1	.993(S)	.756
Shallow Frying (SF)	.993(S)	.992(S)	.993(S)	1	.826(S)
Deep Frying (DF)	.756	.891(S)	.756	.826(S)	1

**.Correlation is highly significant at the 0.05 level (2-tailed)* Positive *S= Significant*
***.Correlation is highly significant at the 0.01 level (2-tailed)*

This table shows the correlation of ash content of lobster with cooking methods. In 14 days control preservation without preservative, there is perfect positive correlation present between the raw state and open pan dry roasting, and significant positive correlation present between the raw state with boiling and shallow frying, whereas open pan dry roasting is significant positively correlated with boiling and shallow frying. Boiling is significant positively correlated with shallow frying and deep frying. Shallow frying is significant positively correlated with deep frying. This table shows that there is a strong correlation present among the **raw state, boiling, open pan dry roasting, shallow frying and deep frying** in 14 days control preservation.

Table no 5.12.4.5.5 Correlation of cooking methods in 15 days preservation without preservative

Condition	RS	B	OPDR	SF	DF
Raw State (RS)	1	-1.000**	-.832(S)	-.782	.606
Boiling (B)	-1.000**	1	.832(S)	.782	-.606
Open Pan Dry Roasting (OPDR)	-.832(S)	.832(S)	1	.305	-.062
Shallow Frying (SF)	-.782	.782	.305	1	-.970(S)
Deep Frying (DF)	.606	-.606	-.062	-.970(S)	1

***.Correlation is highly significant at the 0.01 level (2-tailed)* Positive Negative *S= Significant*

This table shows the correlation of ash content of lobster with cooking methods. In 15 days control preservation without preservative, there is perfect negative correlation present between the raw state and boiling, and significant negative correlation present between the raw state and open pan dry roasting, whereas open pan dry roasting is significant positively correlated with boiling. Shallow frying is significant negatively correlated with deep frying. This table indicates that there is a strong correlation present among the **raw state, boiling, open pan dry roasting, shallow frying and deep frying** in 15 days control preservation.

Table no 5.12.4.5.6 Correlation of cooking methods in 24 hours preservation with salt and turmeric

Condition	RS	B	OPDR	SF	DF
Raw State (RS)	1	.532	.996(S)	.495	.963(S)
Boiling (B)	.532	1	.456	.999*(S)	.740
Open Pan Dry Roasting (OPDR)	.996(S)	.456	1	.417	.936(S)
Shallow Frying (SF)	.495	.999*(S)	.417	1	.710
Deep Frying (DF)	.963(S)	.740	.936(S)	.710	1

**.Correlation is highly significant at the 0.05 level (2-tailed)* ▭ Positive *S= Significant*

This table shows the correlation of ash content of lobster with cooking methods. In 24 hours salt and turmeric preservation, there is significant positive correlation present between the raw state with open pan dry roasting and deep frying, whereas boiling is highly significant positively correlated with shallow frying. Open pan dry roasting is significant positively correlated with deep frying. This table indicates that there is a strong correlation present among the **raw state, boiling, open pan dry roasting, shallow frying and deep frying** in 24 hours salt and turmeric preservation.

Table no 5.12.4.5.7 Correlation of cooking methods in 48 hours preservation with salt and turmeric

Condition	RS	B	OPDR	SF	DF
Raw State (RS)	1	.458	.967(S)	.013	-.459
Boiling (B)	.458	1	.670	.895(S)	.579
Open Pan Dry Roasting (OPDR)	.967(S)	.670	1	.268	-.217
Shallow Frying (SF)	.013	.895(S)	.268	1	.882(S)
Deep Frying (DF)	-.459	.579	-.217	.882(S)	1

▭ Positive *S= Significant*

This table shows the correlation of ash content of lobster with cooking methods. In 48 hours salt and turmeric preservation, there is significant positive correlation present between the raw state and open pan dry roasting, whereas boiling is significant positively correlated with shallow frying. Shallow frying is significant positively correlated with deep frying. This table indicates that there is a strong correlation present among the **raw state, boiling, open pan dry roasting, shallow frying and deep frying** in 48 hours salt and turmeric preservation.

Table no 5.12.4.5.8 Correlation of cooking methods in 14 days preservation with salt and turmeric

Condition	RS	B	OPDR	SF	DF
Raw State (RS)	1	.104	.999*(S)	.062	.843(S)
Boiling (B)	.104	1	.059	-.986(S)	.623
Open Pan Dry Roasting (OPDR)	.999*(S)	.059	1	.107	.818(S)
Shallow Frying (SF)	.062	-.986(S)	.107	1	-.485
Deep Frying (DF)	.843(S)	.623	.818(S)	-.485	1

**.Correlation is highly significant at the 0.05 level (2-tailed)* Positive Negative *S= Significant*

This table shows the correlation of ash content of lobster with cooking methods. In 14 days salt and turmeric preservation, there is significant positive correlation present between the raw sate and deep frying and highly significant positive correlation present between the raw state and open pan dry roasting, whereas boiling is significant negatively correlated with shallow frying. Open pan dry roasting is significant positively correlated with deep frying. This table indicates that there is a strong correlation present among the **raw state, boiling, open pan dry roasting, shallow frying and deep frying** in 14 days salt and turmeric preservation.

Table no 5.12.4.5.9 Correlation of cooking methods in 15 days preservation with salt and turmeric

Condition	RS	B	OPDR	SF	DF
Raw State (RS)	1	.427	.427	-.484	.948(S)
Boiling (B)	.427	1	1.000**(S)	-.998*(S)	.693
Open Pan Dry Roasting (OPDR)	.427	1.000**(S)	1	-.998*(S)	.693
Shallow Frying (SF)	-.484	-.998*(S)	-.998*(S)	1	-.738
Deep Frying (DF)	.948(S)	.693	.693	-.738	1

**.Correlation is highly significant at the 0.05 level (2-tailed)* Positive Negative *S= Significant*
***.Correlation is highly significant at the 0.01 level (2-tailed)*

This table shows the correlation of ash content of lobster with cooking methods. In 15 days salt and turmeric preservation, there is significant positive correlation present between the raw state and deep frying, whereas boiling is significant negatively correlated with shallow frying and perfect positively correlated with open pan dry roasting . Open pan dry roasting is significant negatively correlated with shallow frying. This table indicates that there is a strong correlation present among the **raw state, boiling, open pan dry roasting, shallow frying and deep frying** in 15 days salt and turmeric preservation.

Table no 5.12.4.5.10 Correlation of cooking methods in 24 hours preservation with KMS

Condition	RS	B	OPDR	SF	DF
Raw State (RS)	1	.933(S)	.872(S)	.933(S)	.860(S)
Boiling (B)	.933(S)	1	.990(S)	1.000**(S)	.619
Open Pan Dry Roasting (OPDR)	.872(S)	.990(S)	1	.990(S)	.500
Shallow Frying (SF)	.933(S)	1.000**(S)	.990(S)	1	.619
Deep Frying (DF)	.860(S)	.619	.500	.619	1

***.Correlation is highly significant at the 0.01 level (2-tailed)* Positive *S= Significant*

This table shows the correlation of ash content of lobster with cooking methods. In 24 hours KMS preservation, there is significant positive correlation present between the raw state with boiling, open pan dry roasting, shallow frying and deep frying, whereas boiling is significant positively correlated with open pan dry roasting and perfect positively correlated with shallow frying. Open pan dry roasting is significant positively correlated with shallow frying. This table indicates that there is a strong correlation present among the **raw state, boiling, open pan dry roasting, shallow frying and deep frying** in 24 hours KMS preservation.

Table no 5.12.4.5.11 Correlation of cooking methods in 48 hours preservation with KMS

Condition	RS	B	OPDR	SF	DF
Raw State (RS)	1	-.230	.034	.579	.982(S)
Boiling (B)	-.230	1	.965(S)	.660	-.410
Open Pan Dry Roasting (OPDR)	.034	.965(S)	1	.834(S)	-.156
Shallow Frying (SF)	.579	.660	.834(S)	1	.415
Deep Frying (DF)	.982(S)	-.410	-.156	.415	1

***.Correlation is highly significant at the 0.01 level (2-tailed)* ▭ Positive *S= Significant*

This table shows the correlation of ash content of lobster with cooking methods. In 48 hours KMS preservation, there is significant positive correlation present between the raw state and deep frying, whereas boiling is significant positively correlated with open pan dry roasting. Open pan dry roasting is significant positively correlated with shallow frying. This table indicates that there is a strong correlation present among the **raw state, boiling, open pan dry roasting, shallow frying and deep frying** in 48 hours KMS preservation.

Table no 5.12.4.5.12 Correlation of cooking methods in 14 days preservation with salt and turmeric

Condition	RS	B	OPDR	SF	DF
Raw State (RS)	1	.962(S)	.984(S)	.962(S)	1.000*(S)
Boiling (B)	.962(S)	1	.898(S)	1.000**(S)	.957(S)
Open Pan Dry Roasting (OPDR)	.984(S)	.898(S)	1	.898(S)	.987(S)
Shallow Frying (SF)	.962(S)	1.000**(S)	.898(S)	1	.957(S)
Deep Frying (DF)	1.000*(S)	.957(S)	.987(S)	.957(S)	1

***.Correlation is highly significant at the 0.01 level (2-tailed)* ▭ Positive *S= Significant*
**.Correlation is highly significant at the 0.05 level (2-tailed)*

This table shows the correlation of ash content of lobster with cooking methods. In 14 days KMS preservation, there is significant positive correlation present between the raw state with boiling, open pan dry roasting, shallow frying and perfect positive correlation present with deep frying, whereas boiling is significant positively correlated with open pan dry roasting and deep frying, but perfect positive correlation present with shallow frying. Open pan dry roasting is significant positively correlated with shallow frying and deep frying. Shallow frying is significant positively correlated with deep frying. This table indicates that there is a strong correlation present among the **raw state, boiling, open pan dry roasting, shallow frying and deep frying** in 14 days KMS preservation.

Table no 5.12.4.5.13 Correlation of cooking methods in 15 days preservation with KMS

Condition	RS	B	OPDR	SF	DF
Raw State (RS)	1	.997(S)	.997(S)	.997(S)	.997(S)
Boiling (B)	.997(S)	1	1.000**(S)	1.000**(S)	1.000**(S)
Open Pan Dry Roasting (OPDR)	.997(S)	1.000**(S)	1	1.000**(S)	1.000**(S)
Shallow Frying (SF)	.997(S)	1.000**(S)	1.000**(S)	1	1.000**(S)
Deep Frying (DF)	.997(S)	1.000**(S)	1.000**(S)	1.000**(S)	1

***.Correlation is highly significant at the 0.01 level (2-tailed)* ▭ Positive *S= Significant*

This table shows the correlation of ash content of lobster with cooking methods. In 15 days KMS preservation, there is significant positive correlation present between the raw state with boiling, open pan dry roasting, shallow frying and deep frying, whereas boiling is perfect positively correlated with open pan dry roasting, shallow frying and deep frying. Open pan dry roasting is perfect positively correlated with shallow frying and deep frying. Shallow frying is perfect positively correlated with deep frying. This table indicates that there is a strong correlation present among the **raw state, boiling, open pan dry roasting, shallow frying and deep frying** in 15 days KMS preservation.

Overall analysis reveals that the raw state is perfect negatively correlated with boiling in 15 days control preservation without preservative, whereas perfect positively correlated with open pan dry roasting and deep frying in 14 days control preservation without preservative and 14 days KMS preservation, and significant positively correlated with shallow frying in 15 days KMS preservation. Boiling is perfect positively correlated with open pan dry roasting in 15 days salt-turmeric preservation and 15 days KMS preservation, whereas perfect positively correlated with shallow frying in 24 hours, 14 days and 15 days KMS preservation and 48 hours control preservation without preservative, and perfect positively correlated with deep frying in 15 days KMS preservation. Open pan dry roasting is perfect positively correlated with shallow frying in 15 days KMS preservation, and highly significant positively correlated with deep frying in 15 days KMS preservation. Shallow frying is perfect positively correlated with deep frying in 15 days KMS preservation. Most of the correlation of the ash content of lobster is found in **15 days KMS preservation** with respect to different cooking conditions.

5.12.4.6 Calcium

Table no 5.12.4.6.1 Correlation of cooking methods in fresh condition

Condition	RS	B	OPDR	SF	DF
Raw State (RS)	1	.929(S)	.982(S)	1.000**(S)	.929(S)
Boiling (B)	.929(S)	1	.982(S)	.929(S)	1.000**(S)
Open Pan Dry Roasting (OPDR)	.982(S)	.982(S)	1	.982(S)	.982(S)
Shallow Frying (SF)	1.000**(S)	.929(S)	.982(S)	1	.929(S)
Deep Frying (DF)	.929(S)	1.000**(S)	.982(S)	.929(S)	1

***.Correlation is highly significant at the 0.01 level (2-tailed)* ▭ Positive *S= Significant*

This table shows the correlation of calcium content of lobster with cooking methods. In fresh condition, there is significant positive correlation present between the raw state with boiling, open pan dry roasting and deep frying, but perfect positive correlation present between the raw state and shallow frying, whereas boiling is perfect positively correlated with deep frying and significant positively correlated with open pan dry roasting and shallow frying. Open pan dry roasting is significant positively correlated with shallow frying and deep frying. Shallow frying is significant positively correlated with deep frying. This table indicates that there is a strong correlation present among the **raw state, boiling, open pan dry roasting, shallow frying and deep frying** in fresh condition.

Table no 5.12.4.6.2 Correlation of cooking methods in 24 hours preservation without preservation

Condition	RS	B	OPDR	SF	DF
Raw State (RS)	1	.982(S)	.929(S)	-.143	.929(S)
Boiling (B)	.982(S)	1	.982(S)	-.327	.982(S)
Open Pan Dry Roasting (OPDR)	.929(S)	.982(S)	1	-.500	1.000**(S)
Shallow Frying (SF)	-.143	-.327	-.500	1	-.500
Deep Frying (DF)	.929(S)	.982(S)	1.000**(S)	-.500	1

***.Correlation is highly significant at the 0.01 level (2-tailed)* Positive *S= Significant*

This table shows the correlation of calcium content of lobster with cooking methods. In 24 hours control preservation without preservative, there is significant positive correlation present between the raw state with boiling, open pan dry roasting and deep frying, whereas boiling is significant positively correlated with deep frying and open pan dry roasting. Open pan dry roasting is perfect positively correlated with deep frying. This table indicates that there is a strong correlation present among the **raw state, boiling, open pan dry roasting and deep frying** in 24 hours control preservation without preservative.

Table no 5.12.4.6.3 Correlation of cooking methods in 48 hours preservation without preservation

Condition	RS	B	OPDR	SF	DF
Raw State (RS)	1	.749	.836(S)	.592	-.402
Boiling (B)	.749	1	.990(S)	-.091	-.908(S)
Open Pan Dry Roasting (OPDR)	.836(S)	.990(S)	1	.052	-.839(S)
Shallow Frying (SF)	.592	-.091	.052	1	.500
Deep Frying (DF)	-.402	-.908(S)	-.839(S)	.500	1

Positive Negative *S= Significant*

This table shows the correlation of calcium content of lobster with cooking methods. In 48 hours control preservation without preservative, there is significant positive correlation present between the raw state and open pan dry roasting, whereas boiling is significant positively correlated with open pan dry roasting. Open pan dry roasting is significant negatively correlated with deep frying. This table indicates that there is a strong correlation present among the **raw state, boiling, open pan dry roasting and deep frying** in 48 hours control preservation without preservative.

Table no 5.12.4.6.4 Correlation of cooking methods in 14 days preservation without preservation

Condition	RS	B	OPDR	SF	DF
Raw State (RS)	1	1.000**(S)	1.000**(S)	-.240	.982(S)
Boiling (B)	1.000**(S)	1	1.000**(S)	-.240	.982(S)
Open Pan Dry Roasting (OPDR)	1.000**(S)	1.000**(S)	1	-.240	.982(S)
Shallow Frying (SF)	-.240	-.240	-.240	1	-.052
Deep Frying (DF)	.982(S)	.982(S)	.982(S)	-.052	1

***.Correlation is highly significant at the 0.01 level (2-tailed)* Positive *S= Significant*

This table shows the correlation of calcium content of lobster with cooking methods. In 14 days control preservation without preservative, there is significant positive correlation present between the raw state with deep frying, and perfect positive correlation present between the raw state with boiling and open pan dry roasting, whereas boiling is significant positively correlated with deep frying and perfect positively correlated with open pan dry roasting. Open pan dry roasting is significant positively correlated with deep frying. This table indicates that there is a strong correlation present among the **raw**

state, boiling, open pan dry roasting and deep frying in 14 days control preservation without preservative.

Table no 5.12.4.6.5 Correlation of cooking methods in 15 days preservation without preservation

Condition	RS	B	OPDR	SF	DF
Raw State (RS)	1	.929(S)	.891(S)	-.500	-.052
Boiling (B)	.929(S)	1	.996(S)	-.786	-.419
Open Pan Dry Roasting (OPDR)	.891(S)	.996(S)	1	-.839(S)	-.500
Shallow Frying (SF)	-.500	-.786	-.839(S)	1	.891(S)
Deep Frying (DF)	-.052	-.419	-.500	.891(S)	1

Positive Negative *S= Significant*

This table shows the correlation of calcium content of lobster with cooking methods. In 15 days control preservation without preservative, there is significant positive correlation present between the raw state with boiling and open pan dry roasting, whereas boiling is significant positively correlated with open pan dry roasting. Open pan dry roasting is significant negatively correlated with shallow frying. Shallow frying is significant positively correlated with deep frying. This table indicates that there is a strong correlation present among the **raw state, boiling, open pan dry roasting, shallow frying and deep frying** in 15 days control preservation without preservative.

Table no 5.12.4.6.6 Correlation of cooking methods in 24 hours preservation with salt and turmeric

Condition	RS	B	OPDR	SF	DF
Raw State (RS)	1	.500	.397	.619	-.655
Boiling (B)	.500	1	-.596	-.371	.327
Open Pan Dry Roasting (OPDR)	.397	-.596	1	.967(S)	-.954(S)
Shallow Frying (SF)	.619	-.371	.967(S)	1	-.999*(S)
Deep Frying (DF)	-.655	.327	-.954(S)	-.999*(S)	1

**.Correlation is highly significant at the 0.05 level (2-tailed)* Positive Negative *S= Significant*

This table shows the correlation of calcium content of lobster with cooking methods. In 24 hours salt and turmeric preservation, there is significant positive correlation present between open pan dry roasting and shallow frying, and significant negative correlation present between open pan dry roasting and deep frying, whereas shallow frying is highly significant negatively correlated with deep frying. This table indicates that there is a strong correlation present among **open pan dry roasting, shallow frying and deep frying** in 24 hours salt and turmeric preservation.

Table no 5.12.4.6.7 Correlation of cooking methods in 48 hours preservation with salt and turmeric

Condition	RS	B	OPDR	SF	DF
Raw State (RS)	1	1.000**(S)	-.500	.737	.596
Boiling (B)	1.000**(S)	1	-.500	.737	.596
Open Pan Dry Roasting (OPDR)	-.500	-.500	1	.217	.397
Shallow Frying (SF)	.737	.737	.217	1	.982(S)
Deep Frying (DF)	.596	.596	.397	.982(S)	1

***.Correlation is highly significant at the 0.01 level (2-tailed)* Positive *S= Significant*

This table shows the correlation of calcium content of lobster with cooking methods. In 48 hours salt and turmeric preservation, there is perfect positive correlation present between the raw state and boiling, whereas shallow frying is significant positively correlated with deep frying. This table indicates that there is a strong correlation present between the **raw state and boiling and also between shallow frying and deep frying** in 48 hours salt and turmeric preservation.

Table no 5.12.4.6.8 Correlation of cooking methods in 14 days preservation with salt and turmeric

Condition	RS	B	OPDR	SF	DF
Raw State (RS)	1	.982(S)	.143	-.564	.655
Boiling (B)	.982(S)	1	.327	-.397	.500
Open Pan Dry Roasting (OPDR)	.143	.327	1	.737	-.655
Shallow Frying (SF)	-.564	-.397	.737	1	-.993(S)
Deep Frying (DF)	.655	.500	-.655	-.993(S)	1

Positive Negative *S= Significant*

This table shows the correlation of calcium content of lobster with cooking methods. In 14 days salt and turmeric preservation, there is significant positive correlation present between the raw state and boiling, whereas shallow frying is significant negatively correlated with deep frying. This table indicates that there is a strong correlation present between the **raw state and boiling and also between shallow frying and deep frying** in 14 days salt and turmeric preservation.

Table no 5.12.4.6.9 Correlation of cooking methods in 15 days preservation with salt and turmeric

Condition	RS	B	OPDR	SF	DF
Raw State (RS)	1	.954(S)	.974(S)	1.000**(S)	.993(S)
Boiling (B)	.954(S)	1	.997*(S)	.954(S)	.982(S)
Open Pan Dry Roasting (OPDR)	.974(S)	.997*(S)	1	.974(S)	.993(S)
Shallow Frying (SF)	1.000**(S)	.954(S)	.974(S)	1	.993(S)
Deep Frying (DF)	.993(S)	.982(S)	.993(S)	.993(S)	1

***.Correlation is highly significant at the 0.01 level (2-tailed)* Positive *S= Significant*
**.Correlation is highly significant at the 0.05 level (2-tailed)*

This table shows the correlation of calcium content of lobster with cooking methods. In 15 days salt and turmeric preservation, there is perfect positive correlation present between the raw state and shallow frying and significant positive correlation present between the raw state with boiling, open pan dry roasting and deep frying, whereas boiling is highly significant positively correlated with open pan dry roasting and significant positively correlated with shallow frying and deep frying. Open pan dry roasting is significant positively correlated with shallow frying and deep frying. Shallow frying is significant positively correlated with deep frying. This table shows that there is a strong correlation present among the **raw state, boiling, open pan dry roasting, shallow frying and deep frying** in 15 days salt and turmeric preservation.

Table no 5.12.4.6.10 Correlation of cooking methods in 24 hours preservation with KMS

Condition	RS	B	OPDR	SF	DF
Raw State (RS)	1	.655	.655	.655	1.000**(S)
Boiling (B)	.655	1	1.000**(S)	1.000**(S)	.655
Open Pan Dry Roasting (OPDR)	.655	1.000**(S)	1	1.000**(S)	.655
Shallow Frying (SF)	.655	1.000**(S)	1.000**(S)	1	.655
Deep Frying (DF)	1.000**(S)	.655	.655	.655	1

***.Correlation is highly significant at the 0.01 level (2-tailed)* Positive *S= Significant*

This table shows the correlation of calcium content of lobster with cooking methods. In 24 hours KMS preservation, there is perfect positive correlation present between the raw state and deep frying, whereas boiling is perfect positively correlated with open pan dry roasting and deep frying. Open pan dry roasting is perfect positively correlated with shallow frying. This table indicates that there is a strong correlation present among the **raw state, boiling, open pan dry roasting, shallow frying and deep frying** in 24 hours KMS preservation.

Table no 5.12.4.6.11 Correlation of cooking methods in 48 hours preservation with KMS

Condition	RS	B	OPDR	SF	DF
Raw State (RS)	1	.721	.721	-.419	.885(S)
Boiling (B)	.721	1	1.000**(S)	.327	.961(S)
Open Pan Dry Roasting (OPDR)	.721	1.000**(S)	1	.327	.961(S)
Shallow Frying (SF)	-.419	.327	.327	1	.052
Deep Frying (DF)	.885(S)	.961(S)	.961(S)	.052	1

***.Correlation is highly significant at the 0.01 level (2-tailed)* ▭ Positive *S= Significant*

This table shows the correlation of calcium content of lobster with cooking methods. In 48 hours KMS preservation, there is significant positive correlation present between the raw state and deep frying, whereas boiling is perfect positively correlated with open pan dry roasting and significant positively correlated with deep frying. Open pan dry roasting is significant positively correlated with deep frying. This table indicates that there is a strong correlation present among the **raw state, boiling, open pan dry roasting and deep frying** in 48 hours KMS preservation.

Table no 5.12.4.6.12 Correlation of cooking methods in 14 days preservation with KMS

Condition	RS	B	OPDR	SF	DF
Raw State (RS)	1	-.908(S)	-.350	.961(S)	-.240
Boiling (B)	-.908(S)	1	-.075	-.756	-.189
Open Pan Dry Roasting (OPDR)	-.350	-.075	1	-.596	.993(S)
Shallow Frying (SF)	.961(S)	-.756	-.596	1	-.500
Deep Frying (DF)	-.240	-.189	.993(S)	-.500	1

▭ Positive ▭ Negative *S= Significant*

This table shows the correlation of calcium content of lobster with cooking methods. In 14 days KMS preservation, there is significant negative correlation present between the raw state and boiling, and significant positive correlation present between the raw state and shallow frying, whereas open pan dry roasting is significant positively correlated with deep frying. This table indicates that there is a strong correlation present among the **raw state, boiling, open pan dry roasting, shallow frying and deep frying** in 14 days KMS preservation.

Table no 5.12.4.6.13 Correlation of cooking methods in 15 days preservation with KMS

Condition	RS	B	OPDR	SF	DF
Raw State (RS)	1	-.075	-.350	1.000**(S)	.993(S)
Boiling (B)	-.075	1	-.908(S)	-.075	-.189
Open Pan Dry Roasting (OPDR)	-.350	-.908(S)	1	-.350	-.240
Shallow Frying (SF)	1.000**(S)	-.075	-.350	1	.993(S)
Deep Frying (DF)	.993(S)	-.189	-.240	.993(S)	1

***.Correlation is highly significant at the 0.01 level (2-tailed)* ▭ Positive ▭ Negative *S= Significant*

This table shows the correlation of calcium content of lobster with cooking methods. In 15 days KMS preservation, there is significant positive correlation present between the raw state and deep frying, and perfect positive correlation present between the raw state and shallow frying, whereas boiling is significant negatively correlated with open pan dry roasting. Shallow frying is significant positively correlated with deep frying. This table indicates that there is a strong correlation present among the **raw state, boiling, open pan dry roasting, shallow frying and deep frying** in 15 days KMS preservation.

Overall analysis reveals that the raw state is perfect positively correlated with boiling in 14 days control preservation without preservative and 48 hours salt-turmeric preservation, whereas perfect positively correlated with open pan dry roasting and deep frying in 14 days control preservation without preservative and 24 hours KMS preservation respectively, and perfect positively correlated with shallow frying in 15 days salt and turmeric preservation, 15 days KMS preservation and in fresh condition. Boiling is perfect positively correlated with open pan dry roasting in 14 days control preservation without preservative, 24 hours and 48 hours KMS preservation, whereas perfect positively correlated with shallow frying and deep frying in 24 hours KMS preservation and in fresh condition respectively. Open pan dry roasting is perfect positively correlated with shallow frying and deep frying in 24 hours KMS preservation and 24 hours control preservation without preservative respectively. Shallow frying is highly significant negatively correlated with deep frying in 24 hours salt-turmeric preservation. Most of the correlation of the calcium content of lobster is found in **24 hours KMS preservation** with respect to different cooking conditions.

5.12.4.7 Iron

Table no 5.12.4.7.1 Correlation of cooking methods in fresh condition

Condition	RS	B	OPDR	SF	DF
Raw State (RS)	1	-.904(S)	.866(S)	.786	-.918(S)
Boiling (B)	-.904(S)	1	-.997(S)	-.975(S)	.999*(S)
Open Pan Dry Roasting (OPDR)	.866(S)	-.997(S)	1	.990(S)	-.993(S)
Shallow Frying (SF)	.786	-.975(S)	.990(S)	1	-.967(S)
Deep Frying (DF)	-.918(S)	.999*(S)	-.993(S)	-.967(S)	1

**.Correlation is highly significant at the 0.05 level (2-tailed)* ▭ Positive ▭ Negative *S= Significant*

This table shows the correlation of iron content of lobster with cooking methods. In fresh condition, there is significant positive correlation present between the raw state and open pan dry roasting, and significant negative correlation present between the raw state with boiling and deep frying, whereas boiling is significant negatively correlated with open pan dry roasting and shallow frying. Highly significant positive correlation present between boiling and deep frying. Open pan dry roasting is significant positively correlated with shallow frying and significant negatively correlated with deep frying. Shallow frying is significant negatively correlated with deep frying. This table indicates that there is a strong correlation present among the **raw state, boiling, open pan dry roasting, shallow frying and deep frying** in fresh condition.

Table no 5.12.4.7.2 Correlation of cooking methods in 24 hours preservation without preservative

Condition	RS	B	OPDR	SF	DF
Raw State (RS)	1	.997(S)	-.444	-.397	1.000**(S)
Boiling (B)	.997(S)	1	-.368	-.321	.997(S)
Open Pan Dry Roasting (OPDR)	-.444	-.368	1	.999*(S)	-.444
Shallow Frying (SF)	-.397	-.321	.999*(S)	1	-.397
Deep Frying (DF)	1.000**(S)	.997(S)	-.444	-.397	1

**.Correlation is highly significant at the 0.05 level (2-tailed)* Positive *S= Significant*
***.Correlation is highly significant at the 0.05 level (2-tailed)*

This table shows the correlation of iron content of lobster with cooking methods. In 24 hours control preservation without preservative, there is significant positive correlation present between the raw state and boiling, and perfect positive correlation present between the raw state and deep frying, whereas boiling is significant positively correlated with deep frying. Open pan dry roasting is highly significant positively correlated with shallow frying. This table indicates that there is a strong correlation present among the **raw state, boiling, open pan dry roasting, shallow frying and deep frying** in 24 hours control preservation.

Table no 5.12.4.7.3 Correlation of cooking methods in 48 hours preservation without preservative

Condition	RS	B	OPDR	SF	DF
Raw State (RS)	1	.961(S)	.397	-.554	-.240
Boiling (B)	.961(S)	1	.127	-.302	.038
Open Pan Dry Roasting (OPDR)	.397	.127	1	-.984(S)	-.986(S)
Shallow Frying (SF)	-.554	-.302	-.984(S)	1	.941(S)
Deep Frying (DF)	-.240	.038	-.986(S)	.941(S)	1

Positive *S= Significant*

This table shows the correlation of iron content of lobster with cooking methods. In 48 hours control preservation without preservative, there is significant positive correlation present between the raw state and boiling. Open pan dry roasting is significant negatively correlated with shallow frying and deep frying. Shallow frying is significant positively correlated with deep frying. This table indicates that there is a strong correlation present among the **raw state, boiling, open pan dry roasting, shallow frying and deep frying** in 48 hours control preservation.

Table no 5.12.4.7.4 Correlation of cooking methods in 14 days preservation without preservative

Condition	RS	B	OPDR	SF	DF
Raw State (RS)	1	.250	.751	.538	.631
Boiling (B)	.250	1	-.452	-.682	-.594
Open Pan Dry Roasting (OPDR)	.751	-.452	1	.961(S)	.986(S)
Shallow Frying (SF)	.538	-.682	.961(S)	1	.993(S)
Deep Frying (DF)	.631	-.594	.986(S)	.993(S)	1

Positive *S= Significant*

This table shows the correlation of iron content of lobster with cooking methods. In 14 days control preservation without preservative, there is significant positive correlation present between open pan dry roasting with shallow frying and deep frying. Shallow frying is significant positively correlated with deep frying. This table indicates that there is a strong correlation present among **open pan dry roasting, shallow frying and deep frying** in 14 days control preservation.

Table no 5.12.4.7.5 Correlation of cooking methods in 15 days preservation without preservative

Condition	RS	B	OPDR	SF	DF
Raw State (RS)	1	.684	.795	.737	.954(S)
Boiling (B)	.684	1	.986(S)	.997*(S)	.434
Open Pan Dry Roasting (OPDR)	.795	.986(S)	1	.996(S)	.577
Shallow Frying (SF)	.737	.997*(S)	.996(S)	1	.500
Deep Frying (DF)	.954(S)	.434	.577	.500	1

**.Correlation is highly significant at the 0.05 level (2-tailed)* Positive *S= Significant*

This table shows the correlation of iron content of lobster with cooking methods. In 15 days control preservation without preservative, there is significant positive correlation present between the raw state and deep frying. Boiling is significant positively correlated with open pan dry roasting and highly significant positively correlated with shallow frying. Shallow frying is significant positively correlated with open pan dry roasting. This table indicates that there is a strong correlation present among the **raw state, boiling, open pan dry roasting, shallow frying and deep frying** in 15 days control preservation.

Table no 5.12.4.7.6 Correlation of cooking methods in 24 hours preservation with salt and turmeric

Condition	RS	B	OPDR	SF	DF
Raw State (RS)	1	-.614	-.680	.999*(S)	.923(S)
Boiling (B)	-.614	1	-.161	-.655	-.262
Open Pan Dry Roasting (OPDR)	-.680	-.161	1	-.641	-.910(S)
Shallow Frying (SF)	.999*(S)	-.655	-.641	1	.901(S)
Deep Frying (DF)	.923(S)	-.262	-.910(S)	.901(S)	1

**.Correlation is highly significant at the 0.05 level (2-tailed)* Positive Negative *S= Significant*

This table shows the correlation of iron content of lobster with cooking methods. In 24 hours salt and turmeric preservation, there is highly significant positive correlation present between the raw state and shallow frying and significant positive correlation present between the raw state and deep frying. Open pan dry roasting is significant negatively correlated with deep frying. Shallow frying is significant positively correlated with deep frying. This table indicates that there is a strong correlation present among the **raw state, open pan dry roasting, shallow frying and deep frying in** 24 hours salt and turmeric preservation.

Table no 5.12.4.7.7 Correlation of cooking methods in 48 hours preservation with salt and turmeric

Condition	RS	B	OPDR	SF	DF
Raw State (RS)	1	1.000**(S)	-.721	.986(S)	.923(S)
Boiling (B)	1.000**(S)	1	-.721	.986(S)	.923(S)
Open Pan Dry Roasting (OPDR)	-.721	-.721	1	-.596	-.397
Shallow Frying (SF)	.986(S)	.986(S)	-.596	1	.974(S)
Deep Frying (DF)	.923(S)	.923(S)	-.397	.974(S)	1

***.Correlation is highly significant at the 0.01 level (2-tailed)* Positive *S= Significant*

This table shows the correlation of iron content of lobster with cooking methods. In 48 hours salt and turmeric preservation, there is perfect positive correlation present between the raw state and boiling, and significant positive correlation present between the raw state with shallow frying and deep frying. Boiling is significant positively correlated with shallow frying and deep frying. Shallow frying is significant positively correlated with deep frying. This table indicates that there is a strong correlation present among the **raw state, boiling, shallow frying and deep frying in** 48 hours salt and turmeric preservation.

Table no 5.12.4.7.8 Correlation of cooking methods in 14 days preservation with salt and turmeric

Condition	RS	B	OPDR	SF	DF
Raw State (RS)	1	.715	.500	.715	-1.000** (S)
Boiling (B)	.715	1	-.249	1.000** (S)	-.715
Open Pan Dry Roasting (OPDR)	.500	-.249	1	-.249	-.500
Shallow Frying (SF)	.715	1.000** (S)	-.249	1	-.715
Deep Frying (DF)	-1.000** (S)	-.715	-.500	-.715	1

***.Correlation is highly significant at the 0.01 level (2-tailed)* Positive Negative *S= Significant*

This table shows the correlation of iron content of lobster with cooking methods. In 14 days salt and turmeric preservation, there is perfect negative correlation present between the raw state and deep frying, whereas boiling is perfect positively correlated with shallow frying. This table indicates that there is a strong correlation present between the **raw state and deep frying and also between shallow frying and boiling** in 14 days salt and turmeric preservation.

Table no 5.12.4.7.9 Correlation of cooking methods in 15 days preservation with salt and turmeric

Condition	RS	B	OPDR	SF	DF
Raw State (RS)	1	-.327	.997(S)	1.000** (S)	.993(S)
Boiling (B)	-.327	1	-.249	-.327	-.217
Open Pan Dry Roasting (OPDR)	.997(S)	-.249	1	.997(S)	.999* (S)
Shallow Frying (SF)	1.000** (S)	-.327	.997(S)	1	.993(S)
Deep Frying (DF)	.993(S)	-.217	.999* (S)	.993(S)	1

***.Correlation is highly significant at the 0.01 level (2-tailed)* Positive *S= Significant*

This table shows the correlation of iron content of lobster with cooking methods. In 15 days salt and turmeric preservation, there is perfect positive correlation present between the raw state and shallow frying, and significant positive correlation present between the raw state with open pan dry roasting and deep frying. Open pan dry roasting is significant positively correlated with shallow frying and highly significant positively correlated with deep frying. Shallow frying is significant positively correlated with deep frying. This table indicates that there is a strong correlation present between the **raw state, open pan dry roasting, shallow frying and deep frying** in 15 days salt and turmeric preservation.

Table no 5.12.4.7.10 Correlation of cooking methods in 24 hours preservation with KMS

Condition	RS	B	OPDR	SF	DF
Raw State (RS)	1	.974(S)	.974(S)	1.000** (S)	1.000** (S)
Boiling (B)	.974(S)	1	1.000** (S)	.974(S)	.974(S)
Open Pan Dry Roasting (OPDR)	.974(S)	1.000** (S)	1	.974(S)	.974(S)
Shallow Frying (SF)	1.000** (S)	.974(S)	.974(S)	1	1.000** (S)
Deep Frying (DF)	1.000** (S)	.974(S)	.974(S)	1.000** (S)	1

***.Correlation is highly significant at the 0.01 level (2-tailed)* Positive *S= Significant*

This table shows the correlation of iron content of lobster with cooking methods. In 24 hours KMS preservation, there is perfect positive correlation present between the raw state with shallow frying and deep frying, and significant positive correlation present between the raw state with open pan dry roasting and boiling. Boiling is significant positively correlated with shallow frying and deep frying and perfect positively correlated with open pan dry roasting. Shallow frying is perfect positively correlated with deep frying. This table indicates that there is a strong correlation present between the **raw state, boiling, open pan dry roasting, shallow frying and deep frying** in 24 hours KMS preservation.

Table no 5.12.4.7.11 Correlation of cooking methods in 48 hours preservation with KMS

Condition	RS	B	OPDR	SF	DF
Raw State (RS)	1	.596	.636	-.262	-.500
Boiling (B)	.596	1	-.240	.619	-.993(S)
Open Pan Dry Roasting (OPDR)	.636	-.240	1	-.911(S)	.350
Shallow Frying (SF)	-.262	.619	-.911(S)	1	-.705
Deep Frying (DF)	-.500	-.993(S)	.350	-.705	1

☐ Negative *S= Significant*

This table shows the correlation of iron content of lobster with cooking methods. In 48 hours KMS preservation, there is significant negative correlation present between boiling and deep frying, whereas open pan dry roasting is significant negatively correlated with shallow frying. This table indicates that there is a strong correlation present between **boiling and deep frying and also present between open pan dry roasting and shallow frying** in 48 hours KMS preservation.

Table no 5.12.4.7.12 Correlation of cooking methods in 14 days preservation with KMS

Condition	RS	B	OPDR	SF	DF
Raw State (RS)	1	.974(S)	.771	.289	-.705
Boiling (B)	.974(S)	1	.606	.500	-.524
Open Pan Dry Roasting (OPDR)	.771	.606	1	-.386	-.995(S)
Shallow Frying (SF)	.289	.500	-.386	1	.475
Deep Frying (DF)	-.705	-.524	-.995(S)	.475	1

☐ Negative *S= Significant*

This table shows the correlation of iron content of lobster with cooking methods. In 14 days KMS preservation, there is significant positive correlation present between the raw state and boiling, whereas open pan dry roasting is significant negatively correlated with deep frying. This table indicates that there is a strong correlation present between the **raw state and boiling and also present between open pan dry roasting and deep frying** in 14 days KMS preservation.

Table no 5.12.4.7.13 Correlation of cooking methods in 15 days preservation with KMS

Condition	RS	B	OPDR	SF	DF
Raw State (RS)	1	-.684	-.500	-.500	-.500
Boiling (B)	-.684	1	.974(S)	.974(S)	.974(S)
Open Pan Dry Roasting (OPDR)	-.500	.974(S)	1	1.000**(S)	1.000**(S)
Shallow Frying (SF)	-.500	.974(S)	1.000**(S)	1	1.000**(S)
Deep Frying (DF)	-.500	.974(S)	1.000**(S)	1.000**(S)	1

***.Correlation is highly significant at the 0.01 level (2-tailed)* ☐ Positive *S= Significant*

This table shows the correlation of iron content of Lobster with cooking methods. In 15 days KMS preservation, there is significant positive correlation present between boiling and open pan dry roasting, shallow frying and deep frying, whereas open pan dry roasting is perfect positively correlated with shallow frying and deep frying. Shallow frying is perfect positively correlated with deep frying. This table indicates that there is a strong correlation present between **boiling, open pan dry roasting, shallow frying and deep frying** in 15 days KMS preservation.

Overall analysis reveals that the raw state is perfect positively correlated with boiling in 48 hours control preservation without preservative, whereas significant positively correlated with open pan dry roasting in 15 days salt-turmeric preservation, perfect positively correlated with shallow frying in 15 days salt and turmeric preservation and 24 hours KMS preservation, and perfect positively correlated with deep frying in 24 hours KMS preservation and 24 hours control preservation without preservative and perfect negatively correlated with deep frying in 15 days salt-turmeric preservation. Boiling is perfect positively correlated with open pan dry roasting and shallow frying in 24 hours KMS preservation and 24 hours salt-turmeric preservation respectively, whereas highly significant positively correlated with deep frying in fresh condition and 15 days salt and turmeric preservation. Open pan dry roasting is perfect positively correlated with shallow frying and deep frying in 15 days KMS preservation. Shallow frying is perfect positively correlated with deep frying in 24 hours and 15 days KMS preservation. Most of the correlation of the iron content of lobster is found in **24 hours KMS preservation** with respect to different cooking conditions.

5.12.4.8 Energy

Table no 5.12.4.8.1 Correlation of cooking methods in fresh condition

Condition	RS	B	OPDR	SF	DF
Raw State (RS)	1	.960(S)	.798	.803(S)	.693
Boiling (B)	.960(S)	1	.598	.604	.464
Open Pan Dry Roasting (OPDR)	.798	.598	1	1.000**(S)	.987(S)
Shallow Frying (SF)	.803(S)	.604	1.000**(S)	1	.986(S)
Deep Frying (DF)	.693	.464	.987(S)	.986(S)	1

***.Correlation is highly significant at the 0.01 level (2-tailed)* Positive *S= Significant*

This table shows the correlation of energy content of lobster with cooking methods. In fresh condition, there is significant positive correlation present between the raw state with boiling and shallow frying, whereas open pan dry roasting is perfect positively correlated with shallow frying and significant positively correlated with deep frying. Shallow frying is significant positively correlated with deep frying. This table indicates that there is a strong correlation present among the **raw state, boiling, open pan dry roasting, shallow frying and deep frying** in fresh condition.

Table no 5.12.4.8.2 Correlation of cooking methods in 24 hours preservation without preservative

Condition	RS	B	OPDR	SF	DF
Raw State (RS)	1	-.276	.185	-.520	-.136
Boiling (B)	-.276	1	.894(S)	.964(S)	-.915(S)
Open Pan Dry Roasting (OPDR)	.185	.894(S)	1	.743	-.999*(S)
Shallow Frying (SF)	-.520	.964(S)	.743	1	-.776
Deep Frying (DF)	-.136	-.915(S)	-.999*(S)	-.776	1

***.Correlation is highly significant at the 0.01 level (2-tailed)* Positive Negative *S= Significant*

This table shows the correlation of energy content of lobster with cooking methods. In 24 hours control preservation without preservative, there is significant positive correlation present between boiling with open pan dry roasting, shallow frying, and significant negative correlation present between boiling and deep frying, whereas open pan dry roasting is highly significant negatively correlated with deep frying. This table indicates that there is a strong correlation present among **boiling, open pan dry roasting, shallow frying and deep frying** in 24 hours control preservation.

Table no 5.12.4.8.3 Correlation of cooking methods in 48 hours preservation without preservative

Condition	RS	B	OPDR	SF	DF
Raw State (RS)	1	.137	-.144	-.930(S)	.158
Boiling (B)	.137	1	.961(S)	.237	1.000*(S)
Open Pan Dry Roasting (OPDR)	-.144	.961(S)	1	.497	.954(S)
Shallow Frying (SF)	-.930(S)	.237	.497	1	.216
Deep Frying (DF)	.158	1.000*(S)	.954(S)	.216	1

**.Correlation is highly significant at the 0.05 level (2-tailed)* ▭ Positive ▭ Negative *S= Significant*

This table shows the correlation of energy content of lobster with cooking methods. In 48 hours control preservation without preservative, there is significant negative correlation present between the raw state and boiling, whereas boiling is significant positively correlated with open pan dry roasting, and perfect positive correlation present between boiling and deep frying, whereas open pan dry roasting is significant positively correlated with deep frying. This table indicates that there is a strong correlation present among the **raw state, boiling, open pan dry roasting, shallow frying and deep frying** in 48 hours control preservation.

Table no 5.12.4.8.4 Correlation of cooking methods in 14 days preservation without preservative

Condition	RS	B	OPDR	SF	DF
Raw State (RS)	1	-.779	.570	.727	.923(S)
Boiling (B)	-.779	1	-.959(S)	-.997(S)	-.477
Open Pan Dry Roasting (OPDR)	.570	-.959(S)	1	.979(S)	.209
Shallow Frying (SF)	.727	-.997(S)	.979(S)	1	.406
Deep Frying (DF)	.923(S)	-.477	.209	.406	1

▭ Positive ▭ Negative *S= Significant*

This table shows the correlation of energy content of lobster with cooking methods. In 14 days control preservation without preservative, there is significant positive correlation present between the raw state and deep frying, whereas boiling is significant negatively correlated with open pan dry roasting and shallow frying. Open pan dry roasting is significant positively correlated with shallow frying. This table indicates that there is a strong correlation present among the **raw state, boiling, open pan dry roasting, shallow frying and deep frying** in 14 days control preservation.

Table no 5.12.4.8.5 Correlation of cooking methods in 15 days preservation without preservative

Condition	RS	B	OPDR	SF	DF
Raw State (RS)	1	-.845(S)	-.506	.701	.475
Boiling (B)	-.845(S)	1	-.033	-.974(S)	-.872(S)
Open Pan Dry Roasting (OPDR)	-.506	-.033	1	.260	.519
Shallow Frying (SF)	.701	-.974(S)	.260	1	.960(S)
Deep Frying (DF)	.475	-.872(S)	.519	.960(S)	1

▭ Positive ▭ Negative *S= Significant*

This table shows the correlation of energy content of lobster with cooking methods. In 15 days control preservation without preservative, there is significant negative correlation present between the raw state and boiling, whereas boiling is significant negatively correlated with shallow frying and deep frying. Shallow frying is significant positively correlated with deep frying. This table indicates that there is a strong correlation present among the **raw state, boiling, shallow frying and deep frying** in 15 days control preservation.

Table no 5.12.4.8.6 Correlation of cooking methods in 24 hours preservation with salt and turmeric

Condition	RS	B	OPDR	SF	DF
Raw State (RS)	1	-.997*(S)	-.977(S)	.486	-.913(S)
Boiling (B)	-.997*(S)	1	.959(S)	-.549	.941(S)
Open Pan Dry Roasting (OPDR)	-.977(S)	.959(S)	1	-.291	.806(S)
Shallow Frying (SF)	.486	-.549	-.291	1	-.800(S)
Deep Frying (DF)	-.913(S)	.941(S)	.806(S)	-.800(S)	1

**.Correlation is highly significant at the 0.05 level (2-tailed)* Positive Negative *S= Significant*

This table shows the correlation of energy content of lobster with cooking methods. In 24 hours salt and turmeric preservation, there is highly significant negative correlation present between the raw state and boiling, and significant negative correlation present between the raw state with open pan dry roasting and deep frying, whereas boiling is significant positively correlated with open pan dry roasting and deep frying. Open pan dry roasting is significant positively correlated with deep frying. Shallow frying is significant negatively correlated with deep frying. This table indicates that there is a strong correlation present among the **raw state, boiling, open pan dry roasting, shallow frying and deep frying** in 24 hours salt and turmeric preservation.

Table no 5.12.4.8.7 Correlation of cooking methods in 48 hours preservation with salt and turmeric

Condition	RS	B	OPDR	SF	DF
Raw State (RS)	1	.770	-.956(S)	.970(S)	.901(S)
Boiling (B)	.770	1	-.924(S)	.593	.970(S)
Open Pan Dry Roasting (OPDR)	-.956(S)	-.924(S)	1	-.856(S)	-.989(S)
Shallow Frying (SF)	.970(S)	.593	-.856(S)	1	.770
Deep Frying (DF)	.901(S)	.970(S)	-.989(S)	.770	1

Positive Negative *S= Significant*

This table shows the correlation of energy content of lobster with cooking methods. In 48 hours salt and turmeric preservation, there is significant negative correlation present between the raw state and open pan dry roasting, and significant positive correlation present between the raw state with shallow frying and deep frying, whereas boiling is significant negatively correlated with open pan dry roasting and significant positively correlated with deep frying. Open pan dry roasting is significant negatively correlated with shallow frying and deep frying. This table indicates that there is a strong correlation present among the **raw state, boiling, open pan dry roasting, shallow frying and deep frying** in 48 hours salt and turmeric preservation.

Table no 5.12.4.8.8 Correlation of cooking methods in 14 days preservation with salt and turmeric

Condition	RS	B	OPDR	SF	DF
Raw State (RS)	1	-.977(S)	-.839(S)	.546	-.852(S)
Boiling (B)	-.977(S)	1	.936(S)	-.354	.944(S)
Open Pan Dry Roasting (OPDR)	-.839(S)	.936(S)	1	-.001	1.000*(S)
Shallow Frying (SF)	.546	-.354	-.001	1	-.027
Deep Frying (DF)	-.852(S)	.944(S)	1.000*(S)	-.027	1

Positive Negative *S= Significant*

This table shows the correlation of energy content of lobster with cooking methods. In 14 days salt and turmeric preservation, there is significant negative correlation present between the raw state with boiling, open pan dry roasting and deep frying, whereas boiling is significant positively correlated with open pan dry roasting and deep frying. Open pan dry roasting is perfect positively correlated with deep frying. This table indicates that there is a strong correlation present among the **raw state, boiling, open pan dry roasting and deep frying** in 14 days salt and turmeric preservation.

Table no 5.12.4.8.9 Correlation of cooking methods in 15 days preservation with salt and turmeric

Condition	RS	B	OPDR	SF	DF
Raw State (RS)	1	.636	.533	.942(S)	.702
Boiling (B)	.636	1	-.314	.339	.996(S)
Open Pan Dry Roasting (OPDR)	.533	-.314	1	.786	-.229
Shallow Frying (SF)	.942(S)	.339	.786	1	.421
Deep Frying (DF)	.702	.996(S)	-.229	.421	1

Positive *S= Significant*

This table shows the correlation of energy content of lobster with cooking methods. In 15 days salt and turmeric preservation, there is significant positive correlation present between the raw state and shallow frying, whereas boiling is significant positively correlated with deep frying. This table indicates that there is a strong correlation present between the **raw state and shallow frying and also between boiling and deep frying** in 15 days salt and turmeric preservation.

Table no 5.12.4.8.10 Correlation of cooking methods in 24 hours preservation with KMS

Condition	RS	B	OPDR	SF	DF
Raw State (RS)	1	.839(S)	.968(S)	-.133	-.735
Boiling (B)	.839(S)	1	.949(S)	.427	-.986(S)
Open Pan Dry Roasting (OPDR)	.968(S)	.949(S)	1	.121	-.882(S)
Shallow Frying (SF)	-.133	.427	.121	1	-.574
Deep Frying (DF)	-.735	-.986(S)	-.882(S)	-.574	1

Positive Negative *S= Significant*

This table shows the correlation of energy content of lobster with cooking methods. In 24 hours KMS preservation, there is significant positive correlation present between the raw state with boiling and open pan dry roasting, whereas boiling is significant positively correlated with open pan dry roasting and significant negatively correlated with deep frying. Open pan dry roasting is significant negatively correlated with deep frying. This table indicates that there is a strong correlation present among the **raw state, boiling, open pan dry roasting and deep frying** in 24 hours KMS preservation.

Table no 5.12.4.8.11 Correlation of cooking methods in 48 hours preservation with KMS

Condition	RS	B	OPDR	SF	DF
Raw State (RS)	1	.817(S)	.114	-.272	-.753
Boiling (B)	.817(S)	1	.666	.333	-.995(S)
Open Pan Dry Roasting (OPDR)	.114	.666	1	.925(S)	-.740
Shallow Frying (SF)	-.272	.333	.925(S)	1	-.429
Deep Frying (DF)	-.753	-.995(S)	-.740	-.429	1

Positive Negative *S= Significant*

This table shows the correlation of energy content of lobster with cooking methods. In 48 hours KMS preservation, there is significant positive correlation present between the raw state and boiling, whereas boiling is significant negatively correlated with deep frying. Open pan dry roasting is significant positively correlated with shallow frying. This table indicates that there is a strong correlation present among the **raw state, boiling, open pan dry roasting, shallow frying and deep frying** in 48 hours KMS preservation.

Table no 5.12.4.8.12 Correlation of cooking methods in 14 days preservation with KMS

Condition	RS	B	OPDR	SF	DF
Raw State (RS)	1	.902(S)	-.497	-.732	-.716
Boiling (B)	.902(S)	1	-.822(S)	-.954(S)	-.947(S)
Open Pan Dry Roasting (OPDR)	-.497	-.822(S)	1	.955(S)	.962(S)
Shallow Frying (SF)	-.732	-.954(S)	.955(S)	1	1.000*(S)
Deep Frying (DF)	-.716	-.947(S)	.962(S)	1.000*(S)	1

**.Correlation is highly significant at the 0.05 level (2-tailed)* Positive Negative *S= Significant*

This table shows the correlation of energy content of lobster with cooking methods. In 14 days KMS preservation, there is significant positive correlation present between the raw state and boiling, whereas boiling is significant negatively correlated with open pan dry roasting, shallow frying and deep frying. Open pan dry roasting is significant positively correlated with shallow frying and deep frying. Shallow frying is perfect positively correlated with deep frying. This table indicates that there is a strong correlation present among the **raw state, boiling, open pan dry roasting, shallow frying and deep frying** in 14 days KMS preservation.

Table no 5.12.4.8.13 Correlation of cooking methods in 15 days preservation with KMS

Condition	RS	B	OPDR	SF	DF
Raw State (RS)	1	.997(S)	-.987(S)	-.999*(S)	-.711
Boiling (B)	.997(S)	1	-.971(S)	-.992(S)	-.650
Open Pan Dry Roasting (OPDR)	-.987(S)	-.971(S)	1	.993(S)	.813(S)
Shallow Frying (SF)	-.999*(S)	-.992(S)	.993(S)	1	.739
Deep Frying (DF)	-.711	-.650	.813(S)	.739	1

**.Correlation is highly significant at the 0.05 level (2-tailed)* Positive Negative *S= Significant*

This table shows the correlation of energy content of lobster with cooking methods. In 15 days KMS preservation, there is significant positive correlation present between the raw state and boiling, and significant negative correlation present between the raw state with open pan dry roasting and shallow frying, whereas boiling is significant negatively correlated with open pan dry roasting and shallow frying. Open pan dry roasting is significant positively correlated with shallow frying and deep frying.

This table indicates that there is a strong correlation present among the **raw state, boiling, open pan dry roasting, shallow frying and deep frying** in 15 days KMS preservation.

Overall analysis reveals that the raw state is highly significant negatively correlated with boiling in 24 hours salt-turmeric preservation and significant positively correlated with boiling in 15 days KMS preservation, whereas significant negatively correlated with open pan dry roasting in 15 days preservation with KMS, highly significant positively correlated with shallow frying in 15 days KMS preservation, and significant negatively correlated with deep frying in 48 hours KMS preservation. Boiling is significant negatively correlated with both open pan dry roasting and shallow frying in 15 days KMS preservation, whereas perfect positively correlated with deep frying in 48 hours control preservation without preservative. Open pan dry roasting is perfect positively correlated with shallow frying and deep frying in fresh condition and 14 days salt and turmeric preservation respectively. Shallow frying is perfect positively correlated with deep frying in 14 days KMS preservation. Most of the correlation of the energy content of lobster is found in **15 days KMS preservation** with respect to different cooking conditions.

5.12.5 Pomfret *(Pampus argenteus)*

5.12.5.1 Carbohydrate

Table no 5.12.5.1.1 Correlation of cooking methods in fresh condition

Condition	RS	B	OPDR	SF	DF
Raw State (RS)	1	.519	.998*(S)	.609	-.921(S)
Boiling (B)	.519	1	.468	-.362	-.146
Open Pan Dry Roasting (OPDR)	.998*(S)	.468	1	.655	-.943(S)
Shallow Frying (SF)	.609	-.362	.655	1	-.870(S)
Deep Frying (DF)	-.921(S)	-.146	-.943(S)	-.870(S)	1

**.Correlation is highly significant at the 0.05 level (2-tailed)* ▭ Positive ▭ Negative *S= Significant*

This table shows the correlation of carbohydrate content of pomfret with cooking methods. In fresh condition, there is significant positive correlation present between the raw state and open pan dry roasting, and significant negative correlation present between the raw state and deep frying, whereas both open pan dry roasting and shallow frying are significant negatively correlated with deep frying. This table indicates that there is a strong correlation present among the **raw state, open pan dry roasting, shallow frying and deep frying** in fresh condition.

Table no 5.12.5.1.2 Correlation of cooking methods in 24 hours preservation without preservative

Condition	RS	B	OPDR	SF	DF
Raw State (RS)	1	-.116	-.168	.916(S)	.137
Boiling (B)	-.116	1	.999*(S)	-.505	-1.000*(S)
Open Pan Dry Roasting (OPDR)	-.168	.999*(S)	1	-.550	-.999*(S)
Shallow Frying (SF)	.916(S)	-.505	-.550	1	.523
Deep Frying (DF)	.137	-1.000*(S)	-.999*(S)	.523	1

**.Correlation is highly significant at the 0.05 level (2-tailed)* ▭ Positive ▭ Negative *S= Significant*

This table shows the correlation of carbohydrate content of pomfret with cooking methods. In 24 hours control preservation without preservative, there is significant positive correlation present between the raw state and shallow frying, whereas boiling is highly significant positively correlated with open pan dry roasting and perfect negative correlation present with deep frying. Open pan dry roasting is highly significant negatively correlated with deep frying. This table indicates that there is a strong correlation present among the **raw state, boiling, open pan dry roasting, shallow frying and deep frying** in 24 hours control preservation.

Table no 5.12.5.1.3 Correlation of cooking methods in 48 hours preservation without preservative

Condition	RS	B	OPDR	SF	DF
Raw State (RS)	1	-.194	.945(S)	.381	.782
Boiling (B)	-.194	1	-.503	.833(S)	-.762
Open Pan Dry Roasting (OPDR)	.945(S)	-.503	1	.059	.943(S)
Shallow Frying (SF)	.381	.833(S)	.059	1	-.277
Deep Frying (DF)	.782	-.762	.943(S)	-.277	1

Positive *S= Significant*

This table shows the correlation of carbohydrate content of pomfret with cooking methods. In 48 hours control preservation without preservative, there is significant positive correlation present between the raw state and open pan dry roasting, whereas boiling is significant positively correlated with shallow frying. Open pan dry roasting is significant positively correlated with deep frying. This table indicates that there is a strong correlation present among the **raw state, boiling, open pan dry roasting, shallow frying and deep frying** in 48 hours control preservation.

Table no 5.12.5.1.4 Correlation of cooking methods in 14 days preservation without preservative

Condition	RS	B	OPDR	SF	DF
Raw State (RS)	1	.791	-.690	.921(S)	-.784
Boiling (B)	.791	1	-.102	.967(S)	-.240
Open Pan Dry Roasting (OPDR)	-.690	-.102	1	-.353	.990(S)
Shallow Frying (SF)	.921(S)	.967(S)	-.353	1	-.480
Deep Frying (DF)	-.784	-.240	.990(S)	-.480	1

Positive *S= Significant*

This table shows the correlation of carbohydrate content of pomfret with cooking methods. In 14 days control preservation without preservative, there is significant positive correlation present between the raw state and shallow frying, whereas boiling is also significant positively correlated with shallow frying. Open pan dry roasting is significant positively correlated with deep frying. This table indicates that there is a strong correlation present among the **raw state, boiling, open pan dry roasting, shallow frying and deep frying** in 14 days control preservation.

Table no 5.12.5.1.5 Correlation of cooking methods in 15 days preservation without preservative

Condition	RS	B	OPDR	SF	DF
Raw State (RS)	1	-.976(S)	.638	.912(S)	.927(S)
Boiling (B)	-.976(S)	1	-.455	-.979(S)	-.986(S)
Open Pan Dry Roasting (OPDR)	.638	-.455	1	.266	.302
Shallow Frying (SF)	.912(S)	-.979(S)	.266	1	.999*(S)
Deep Frying (DF)	.927(S)	-.986(S)	.302	.999*(S)	1

**.Correlation is highly significant at the 0.05 level (2-tailed)* Positive Negative *S= Significant*

This table shows the correlation of carbohydrate content of pomfret with cooking methods. In 15 days control preservation without preservative, there is significant positive correlation present between the raw state with shallow frying and deep frying, and significant negative correlation present between the raw state and boiling, whereas boiling is significant negatively correlated with shallow frying and deep frying. Shallow frying is highly significant positively correlated with deep frying. This table indicates that there is a strong correlation present among the **raw state, boiling, shallow frying and deep frying** in 15 days control preservation.

Table no 5.12.5.1.6 Correlation of cooking methods in 24 hours preservation with salt and turmeric

Condition	RS	B	OPDR	SF	DF
Raw State (RS)	1	-.982(S)	-.786	.929(S)	-.989(S)
Boiling (B)	-.982(S)	1	.655	-.982(S)	.999*(S)
Open Pan Dry Roasting (OPDR)	-.786	.655	1	-.500	.683
Shallow Frying (SF)	.929(S)	-.982(S)	-.500	1	-.974(S)
Deep Frying (DF)	-.989(S)	.999*(S)	.683	-.974(S)	1

**.Correlation is highly significant at the 0.05 level (2-tailed)* Positive Negative *S= Significant*

This table shows the correlation of carbohydrate content of pomfret with cooking methods. In 24 hours salt and turmeric preservation, there is significant positive correlation present between the raw state and shallow frying, and significant negative correlation present between the raw state with boiling and deep frying, whereas boiling is significant negatively correlated with shallow frying and highly significant positively correlated with deep frying. Shallow frying is significant negatively correlated with deep frying. This table indicates that there is a strong correlation present among the **raw state, boiling, shallow frying and deep frying** in 24 hours salt and turmeric preservation.

Table no 5.12.5.1.7 Correlation of cooking methods in 48 hours preservation with salt and turmeric

Condition	RS	B	OPDR	SF	DF
Raw State (RS)	1	-.500	.500	.240	-.610
Boiling (B)	-.500	1	.500	.721	.991(S)
Open Pan Dry Roasting (OPDR)	.500	.500	1	.961(S)	.381
Shallow Frying (SF)	.240	.721	.961(S)	1	.623
Deep Frying (DF)	-.610	.991(S)	.381	.623	1

Positive *S= Significant*

This table shows the correlation of carbohydrate content of pomfret with cooking methods. In 48 hours salt and turmeric preservation, there is significant positive correlation present between boiling and deep frying, whereas open pan dry roasting is significant positively correlated with shallow frying. This table indicates that there is a strong correlation present **between boiling and deep frying and also between open pan dry roasting and shallow frying** in 48 hours salt and turmeric preservation.

Table no 5.12.5.1.8 Correlation of cooking methods in 14 days preservation with salt and turmeric

Condition	RS	B	OPDR	SF	DF
Raw State (RS)	1	.982(S)	.500	-.655	.991(S)
Boiling (B)	.982(S)	1	.655	-.786	.948(S)
Open Pan Dry Roasting (OPDR)	.500	.655	1	-.982(S)	.381
Shallow Frying (SF)	-.655	-.786	-.982(S)	1	-.549
Deep Frying (DF)	.991(S)	.948(S)	.381	-.549	1

Positive Negative *S= Significant*

This table shows the correlation of carbohydrate content of pomfret with cooking methods. In 14 days salt and turmeric preservation, there is significant positive correlation present between the raw state with boiling and deep frying, whereas boiling is significant positively correlated with deep frying. Open pan dry roasting is significant negatively correlated with shallow frying. This table indicates that there is a strong correlation present among **boiling, open pan dry roasting, shallow frying and deep frying** in 14 days salt and turmeric preservation.

Table no 5.12.5.1.9 Correlation of cooking methods in 15 days preservation with salt and turmeric

Condition	RS	B	OPDR	SF	DF
Raw State (RS)	1	.929(S)	-.756	.866(S)	.956(S)
Boiling (B)	.929(S)	1	-.945(S)	.619	.780
Open Pan Dry Roasting (OPDR)	-.756	-.945(S)	1	-.327	-.532
Shallow Frying (SF)	.866(S)	.619	-.327	1	.974(S)
Deep Frying (DF)	.956(S)	.780	-.532	.974(S)	1

Positive Negative *S= Significant*

This table shows the correlation of carbohydrate content of pomfret with cooking methods. In 15 days salt and turmeric preservation, there is significant positive correlation present between the raw state with boiling, shallow frying and deep frying, whereas boiling is significant negatively correlated with open pan dry roasting. Shallow frying is significant positively correlated with deep frying. This table indicates that there is a strong correlation present among the **raw state, boiling, open pan dry roasting, shallow frying and deep frying** in 15 days salt and turmeric preservation.

Table no 5.12.5.1.10 Correlation of cooking methods in 24 hours preservation with KMS

Condition	RS	B	OPDR	SF	DF
Raw State (RS)	1	.655	-.655	.327	-.371
Boiling (B)	.655	1	-1.000**(S)	-.500	-.945(S)
Open Pan Dry Roasting (OPDR)	-.655	-1.000**(S)	1	.500	.945(S)
Shallow Frying (SF)	.327	-.500	.500	1	.756
Deep Frying (DF)	-.371	-.945(S)	.945(S)	.756	1

***.Correlation is highly significant at the 0.01 level (2-tailed)* Positive Negative *S= Significant*

This table shows the correlation of carbohydrate content of pomfret with cooking methods. In 24 hours KMS preservation, there is perfect negative correlation present between boiling and open pan dry roasting, and significant negative correlation present between boiling and deep frying, whereas open pan dry roasting is significant positively correlated with deep frying. This table indicates that there is a strong correlation present among **boiling, open pan dry roasting and deep frying** in 24 hours KMS preservation.

Table no 5.12.5.1.11 Correlation of cooking methods in 48 hours preservation with KMS

Condition	RS	B	OPDR	SF	DF
Raw State (RS)	1	-.500	.500	.327	-.500
Boiling (B)	-.500	1	.500	.655	1.000**(S)
Open Pan Dry Roasting (OPDR)	.500	.500	1	.982(S)	.500
Shallow Frying (SF)	.327	.655	.982(S)	1	.655
Deep Frying (DF)	-.500	1.000**(S)	.500	.655	1

***.Correlation is highly significant at the 0.01 level (2-tailed)* ▭ Positive *S= Significant*

This table shows the correlation of carbohydrate content of pomfret with cooking methods. In 48 hours KMS preservation, there is perfect positive correlation present between boiling and deep frying, whereas open pan dry roasting is significant positively correlated with shallow frying. This table indicates that there is a strong correlation present between **boiling and deep frying and also between open pan dry roasting and shallow frying** in 48 hours KMS preservation.

Table no 5.12.5.1.12 Correlation of cooking methods in 14 days preservation with KMS

Condition	RS	B	OPDR	SF	DF
Raw State (RS)	1	-.866(S)	.285	-.454	-.655
Boiling (B)	-.866(S)	1	.232	.839(S)	.945(S)
Open Pan Dry Roasting (OPDR)	.285	.232	1	.725	.538
Shallow Frying (SF)	-.454	.839(S)	.725	1	.971(S)
Deep Frying (DF)	-.655	.945(S)	.538	.971(S)	1

▭ Positive ▭ Negative *S= Significant*

This table shows the correlation of carbohydrate content of pomfret with cooking methods. In 14 days KMS preservation, there is significant negative correlation present between the raw state and boiling, whereas boiling is significant positively correlated with shallow frying and deep frying. Shallow frying is significant positively correlated with deep frying. This table indicates that there is a strong correlation present among the **raw state, boiling, shallow frying and deep frying** in 14 days KMS preservation.

Table no 5.12.5.1.13 Correlation of cooking methods in 15 days preservation with KMS

Condition	RS	B	OPDR	SF	DF
Raw State (RS)	1	-1.000**(S)	-.982(S)	-.655	-1.000**(S)
Boiling (B)	-1.000**(S)	1	.982(S)	.655	1.000**(S)
Open Pan Dry Roasting (OPDR)	-.982(S)	.982(S)	1	.786	.982(S)
Shallow Frying (SF)	-.655	.655	.786	1	.655
Deep Frying (DF)	-1.000**(S)	1.000**(S)	.982(S)	.655	1

***.Correlation is highly significant at the 0.01 level (2-tailed)* ▭ Positive ▭ Negative *S= Significant*

This table shows the correlation of carbohydrate content of pomfret with cooking methods. In 15 days KMS preservation, there is perfect negative correlation present between the raw state with boiling and deep frying, and significant negative correlation present between the raw state and open pan dry roasting, whereas boiling is significant positively correlated with open pan dry roasting and perfect positively correlated with deep frying. Open pan dry roasting is significant positively correlated with deep frying. This table indicates that there is a strong correlation present among the **raw state, boiling, open pan dry roasting and deep frying** in 15 days KMS preservation.

Overall analysis reveals that the raw state is perfect negatively correlated with boiling and deep frying in 15 days KMS preservation, whereas highly significant positively correlated with open pan dry roasting in fresh condition, and significant positively correlated with shallow frying in 24 hours salt and turmeric preservation. Boiling is perfect positively correlated with open pan dry roasting in 24 hours KMS preservation, whereas significant negatively correlated with shallow frying in 24 hours salt and turmeric preservation, and perfect positively correlated with deep frying in 48 hours and 15 days KMS preservation and perfect negatively correlated with deep frying in 24 hours control preservation without preservative. Open pan dry roasting is significant negatively correlated with shallow frying in 14 days salt and turmeric and significant positively correlated with shallow frying in 48 hours KMS preservation, and highly significant positively correlated with deep frying in 24 hours control preservation without preservative. Shallow frying is highly significant positively correlated with deep frying in 15 days control preservation without preservative. Most of the correlation of the carbohydrate content of pomfret is found in **15 days KMS preservation** with respect to different cooking conditions.

5.12.5.2 Protein

Table no 5.12.5.2.1 Correlation of cooking methods in fresh condition

Condition	RS	B	OPDR	SF	DF
Raw State (RS)	1	.874(S)	-.016	-.860(S)	.013
Boiling (B)	.874(S)	1	-.500	-1.000*(S)	-.475
Open Pan Dry Roasting (OPDR)	-.016	-.500	1	.524	1.000*(S)
Shallow Frying (SF)	-.860(S)	-1.000*(S)	.524	1	.500
Deep Frying (DF)	.013	-.475	1.000*(S)	.500	1

**.Correlation is highly significant at the 0.05 level (2-tailed)* ▭ Positive ▭ Negative *S= Significant*

This table shows the correlation of protein content of pomfret with cooking methods. In fresh condition, there is perfect negative correlation present between the raw state and shallow frying, and significant positive correlation present between the raw state and boiling, whereas boiling is perfect negatively correlated with shallow frying. Open pan dry roasting is perfect positively correlated with deep frying. This table indicates that there is a strong correlation present among the **raw state, boiling, open pan dry roasting, shallow frying and deep frying** in fresh condition.

Table no 5.12.5.2.2 Correlation of cooking methods in 24 hours preservation without preservative

Condition	RS	B	OPDR	SF	DF
Raw State (RS)	1	1.000**(S)	-.327	-.901(S)	-.200
Boiling (B)	1.000**(S)	1	-.327	-.901(S)	-.200
Open Pan Dry Roasting (OPDR)	-.327	-.327	1	-.115	.991(S)
Shallow Frying (SF)	-.901(S)	-.901(S)	-.115	1	-.245
Deep Frying (DF)	-.200	-.200	.991(S)	-.245	1

***.Correlation is highly significant at the 0.01 level (2-tailed)* ▭ Positive ▭ Negative *S= Significant*

This table shows the correlation of protein content of pomfret with cooking methods. In 24 hours control preservation without preservative, there is perfect positive correlation present between the raw state and boiling, and significant negative correlation present between the raw state and shallow frying, whereas boiling is significant negatively correlated with shallow frying. Open pan dry roasting is significant positively correlated with deep frying. This table indicates that there is a strong correlation present among the **raw state, boiling, open pan dry roasting, shallow frying and deep frying** in 24 hours control preservation.

Table no 5.12.5.2.3 Correlation of cooking methods in 48 hours preservation without preservative

Condition	RS	B	OPDR	SF	DF
Raw State (RS)	1	-.567	-.941(S)	-.958(S)	-.198
Boiling (B)	-.567	1	.812(S)	.780	.920(S)
Open Pan Dry Roasting (OPDR)	-.941(S)	.812(S)	1	.999*(S)	.518
Shallow Frying (SF)	-.958(S)	.780	.999*(S)	1	.471
Deep Frying (DF)	-.198	.920(S)	.518	.471	1

***.Correlation is highly significant at the 0.01 level (2-tailed)* ▭ Positive ▭ Negative *S= Significant*

This table shows the correlation of protein content of pomfret with cooking methods. In 48 hours control preservation without preservative, there is significant negative correlation present between the raw state with open pan dry roasting and shallow frying, whereas boiling is significant positively correlated with open pan dry roasting and deep frying. Open pan dry roasting is highly significant positively correlated with shallow frying. This table indicates that there is a strong correlation present among the **raw state, boiling, open pan dry roasting, shallow frying and deep frying** in 48 hours control preservation.

Table no 5.12.5.2.4 Correlation of cooking methods in 14 days preservation without preservative

Condition	RS	B	OPDR	SF	DF
Raw State (RS)	1	-.507	-.330	.506	.504
Boiling (B)	-.507	1	.981(S)	.487	-1.000**(S)
Open Pan Dry Roasting (OPDR)	-.330	.981(S)	1	.648	-.981(S)
Shallow Frying (SF)	.506	.487	.648	1	-.490
Deep Frying (DF)	.504	-1.000**(S)	-.981(S)	-.490	1

***.Correlation is highly significant at the 0.01 level (2-tailed)* ▭ Positive ▭ Negative *S= Significant*

This table shows the correlation of protein content of pomfret with cooking methods. In 14 days control preservation without preservative, there is significant positive correlation present between boiling and open pan dry roasting, and perfect negative correlation present between boiling and deep frying, whereas open pan dry roasting is significant negatively correlated with deep frying. This table indicates that there is a strong correlation present among **boiling, open pan dry roasting and deep frying** in 14 days control preservation.

Table no 5.12.5.2.5 Correlation of cooking methods in 15 days preservation without preservative

Condition	RS	B	OPDR	SF	DF
Raw State (RS)	1	.493	-1.000**(S)	.500	.504
Boiling (B)	.493	1	-.488	1.000**(S)	1.000**(S)
Open Pan Dry Roasting (OPDR)	-1.000** (S)	-.488	1	-.495	-.500
Shallow Frying (SF)	.500	1.000**(S)	-.495	1	1.000**(S)
Deep Frying (DF)	.504	1.000** (S)	-.500	1.000**(S)	1

***.Correlation is highly significant at the 0.01 level (2-tailed)* ▭ Positive ▭ Negative *S= Significant*

This table shows the correlation of protein content of pomfret with cooking methods. In 15 days control preservation without preservative, there is perfect negative correlation present between the raw state and open pan dry roasting, whereas boiling is perfect positively correlated with shallow frying and deep frying. Shallow frying is perfect positively correlated with deep frying. This table indicates that there is a strong correlation present among **boiling, open pan dry roasting and deep frying** in 15 days control preservation.

Table no 5.12.5.2.6 Correlation of cooking methods in 24 hours preservation with salt and turmeric

Condition	RS	B	OPDR	SF	DF
Raw State (RS)	1	-.327	-.382	.660	-.994(S)
Boiling (B)	-.327	1	-.748	.494	.222
Open Pan Dry Roasting (OPDR)	-.382	-.748	1	-.947(S)	.481
Shallow Frying (SF)	.660	.494	-.947(S)	1	-.738
Deep Frying (DF)	-.994(S)	.222	.481	-.738	1

☐ Negative *S= Significant*

This table shows the correlation of protein content of pomfret with cooking methods. In 24 hours salt and turmeric preservation, there is significant negative correlation present between the raw state and deep frying, whereas open pan dry roasting is significant negatively correlated with shallow frying. This table indicates that there is a strong correlation present **between the raw state and deep frying and also between open pan dry roasting and shallow frying** in 24 hours salt and turmeric preservation.

Table no 5.12.5.2.7 Correlation of cooking methods in 48 hours preservation with salt and turmeric

Condition	RS	B	OPDR	SF	DF
Raw State (RS)	1	-.983(S)	.995(S)	.994(S)	.393
Boiling (B)	-.983(S)	1	-.959(S)	-.997*(S)	-.553
Open Pan Dry Roasting (OPDR)	.995(S)	-.959(S)	1	.978(S)	.295
Shallow Frying (SF)	.994(S)	-.997*(S)	.978(S)	1	.490
Deep Frying (DF)	.393	-.553	.295	.490	1

***.Correlation is highly significant at the 0.01 level (2-tailed)* ☐ Positive ☐ Negative *S= Significant*

This table shows the correlation of protein content of pomfret with cooking methods. In 48 hours salt and turmeric preservation, there is significant positive correlation present between the raw state with open pan dry roasting and shallow frying, and significant negative correlation present between the raw state and boiling, whereas boiling is significant negatively correlated with deep frying and significant negatively correlated with open pan dry roasting. Shallow frying is significant positively correlated with open pan dry roasting. This table indicates that there is a strong correlation present among the **raw state, boiling, open pan dry roasting and shallow frying** in 48 hours salt and turmeric preservation.

Table no 5.12.5.2.8 Correlation of cooking methods in 14 days preservation with salt and turmeric

Condition	RS	B	OPDR	SF	DF
Raw State (RS)	1	1.000**(S)	.495	.506	-.982(S)
Boiling (B)	1.000**(S)	1	.503	.513	-.984(S)
Open Pan Dry Roasting (OPDR)	.495	.503	1	1.000**(S)	-.649
Shallow Frying (SF)	.506	.513	1.000**(S)	1	-.658
Deep Frying (DF)	-.982(S)	-.984(S)	-.649	-.658	1

***.Correlation is highly significant at the 0.01 level (2-tailed)* ☐ Positive ☐ Negative *S= Significant*

This table shows the correlation of protein content of pomfret with cooking methods. In 14 days salt and turmeric preservation, there is perfect positive correlation present between the raw state and boiling, and significant negative correlation present between the raw state and deep frying, whereas boiling is significant negatively correlated with deep frying. Shallow frying is perfect positively correlated with open pan dry roasting. This table indicates that there is a strong correlation present among the **raw state, boiling, open pan dry roasting, shallow frying and deep frying** in 14 days salt and turmeric preservation.

Table no 5.12.5.2.9 Correlation of cooking methods in 15 days preservation with salt and turmeric

Condition	RS	B	OPDR	SF	DF
Raw State (RS)	1	-.500	-1.000*(S)	1.000**(S)	-1.000**(S)
Boiling (B)	-.500	1	.472	-.494	.500
Open Pan Dry Roasting (OPDR)	-1.000* (S)	.472	1	-1.000*(S)	1.000*(S)
Shallow Frying (SF)	1.000**(S)	-.494	-1.000*(S)	1	-1.000**(S)
Deep Frying (DF)	-1.000**(S)	.500	1.000*(S)	-1.000**(S)	1

***.Correlation is highly significant at the 0.01 level (2-tailed)* Positive Negative *S= Significant*

This table shows the correlation of protein content of pomfret with cooking methods. In 15 days salt and turmeric preservation, there is perfect negative correlation present between the raw state with open pan dry roasting, shallow frying and deep frying, whereas open pan dry roasting is perfect negatively correlated with shallow frying and perfect positively correlated with deep frying. Shallow frying is perfect positively correlated with deep frying. This table indicates that there is a strong correlation present among the **raw state, open pan dry roasting, shallow frying and deep frying** in 15 days salt and turmeric preservation.

Table no 5.12.5.2.10 Correlation of cooking methods in 24 hours preservation with KMS

Condition	RS	B	OPDR	SF	DF
Raw State (RS)	1	-.983(S)	.505	-1.000**(S)	.495
Boiling (B)	-.983(S)	1	-.653	.985(S)	-.645
Open Pan Dry Roasting (OPDR)	.505	-.653	1	-.510	1.000**(S)
Shallow Frying (SF)	-1.000**(S)	.985(S)	-.510	1	-.501
Deep Frying (DF)	.495	-.645	1.000**(S)	-.501	1

***.Correlation is highly significant at the 0.01 level (2-tailed)* Positive Negative *S= Significant*

This table shows the correlation of protein content of pomfret with cooking methods. In 24 hours KMS preservation, there is perfect negative correlation present between the raw state and shallow frying, and significant negative correlation present between the raw state and boiling, whereas boiling is significant positively correlated with shallow frying. Open pan dry roasting is perfect positively correlated with deep frying. This table indicates that there is a strong correlation present among the **raw state, boiling, open pan dry roasting, shallow frying and deep frying** in 24 hours KMS preservation.

Table no 5.12.5.2.11 Correlation of cooking methods in 48 hours preservation with KMS

Condition	RS	B	OPDR	SF	DF
Raw State (RS)	1	-.953(S)	-.994(S)	-.403	-.336
Boiling (B)	-.953(S)	1	.980(S)	.662	.034
Open Pan Dry Roasting (OPDR)	-.994(S)	.980(S)	1	.501	.231
Shallow Frying (SF)	-.403	.662	.501	1	-.726
Deep Frying (DF)	-.336	.034	.231	-.726	1

Positive Negative *S= Significant*

This table shows the correlation of protein content of pomfret with cooking methods. In 48 hours KMS preservation, there is significant negative correlation present between the raw state with boiling and open pan dry roasting, whereas boiling is significant positively correlated with open pan dry roasting. This table indicates that there is a strong correlation present among the **raw state, boiling and open pan dry roasting** in 48 hours KMS preservation.

Table no 5.12.5.2.12 Correlation of cooking methods in 14 days preservation with KMS

Condition	RS	B	OPDR	SF	DF
Raw State (R)	1	1.000**(S)	1.000**(S)	.494	1.000**(S)
Boiling (B)	1.000**(S)	1	1.000**(S)	.494	1.000**(S)
Open Pan Dry Roasting (OPDR)	1.000**(S)	1.000**(S)	1	.494	1.000**(S)
Shallow Frying (SF)	.494	.494	.494	1	.499
Deep Frying (DF)	1.000**(S)	1.000**(S)	1.000**(S)	.499	1

***.Correlation is highly significant at the 0.01 level (2-tailed)* Positive *S= Significant*

This table shows the correlation of protein content of pomfret with cooking methods. In 14 days KMS preservation, there is perfect positive correlation present between the raw state with boiling, open pan dry roasting and deep frying, whereas boiling is perfect positively correlated with open pan dry roasting and deep frying. Open pan dry roasting is perfect positively correlated with deep frying. This table indicates that there is a strong correlation present among the **raw state, boiling, open pan dry roasting and deep frying** in 14 days KMS preservation.

Table no 5.12.5.2.13 Correlation of cooking methods in 15 days preservation with KMS

Condition	RS	B	OPDR	SF	DF
Raw State (RS)	1	.657	.495	.506	.422
Boiling (B)	.657	1	.980(S)	-.318	-.406
Open Pan Dry Roasting (OPDR)	.495	.980(S)	1	-.499	-.579
Shallow Frying (SF)	.506	-.318	-.499	1	.996(S)
Deep Frying (DF)	.422	-.406	-.579	.996(S)	1

Positive *S= Significant*

This table shows the correlation of protein content of pomfret with cooking methods. In 15 days KMS preservation, there is significant positive correlation present between boiling and open pan dry roasting, whereas shallow frying is significant positively correlated with deep frying. This table indicates that there is a strong correlation present between **boiling and open pan dry roasting and also between shallow frying and deep frying** in 15 days KMS preservation.

Overall analysis reveals that the raw state is perfect positively correlated with boiling in 24 hours control preservation without preservative, 14 days salt-turmeric preservation and 14 days KMS preservation, whereas perfect positively correlated with open pan dry roasting in 14 days preservation with KMS and perfect negatively correlated with open pan dry roasting in 15 days salt-turmeric preservation, 15 days control preservation, perfect positively correlated with shallow frying in 15 days salt and turmeric preservation and perfect negatively correlated with shallow frying in 24 hours KMS preservation, and perfect positively correlated with deep frying in 14 days KMS preservation and perfect negatively correlated with deep frying in 15 days salt-turmeric preservation. Boiling is perfect positively correlated with open pan dry roasting in 14 days preservation with KMS, whereas highly perfect positively correlated with shallow frying in 15 days control preservation without preservative and in fresh condition, and perfect positively correlated with deep frying in 48 hours KMS preservation and 15 days control preservation without preservative and perfect negatively correlated with deep frying in 14 days control preservation without preservative. Open pan dry roasting is perfect negatively correlated with shallow frying in 14 days and 15 days salt and turmeric preservation, and perfect positively correlated with deep frying in fresh condition, 15 days salt and turmeric preservation and 24 hours and 14 days KMS preservation. Shallow frying is perfect positively correlated with deep frying in 15 days control preservation without preservative and perfect positively correlated with deep frying in 15 days salt-turmeric preservation. Most of the correlation of the protein content of pomfret is found in **15 days salt and turmeric preservation and 14 days KMS preservation** with respect to different cooking conditions.

5.12.5.3 Fat

Table no 5.12.5.3.1 Correlation of cooking methods in fresh condition

Condition	RS	B	OPDR	SF	DF
Raw State (RS)	1	.403	-.702	.763	.675
Boiling (B)	.403	1	.369	-.283	.948(S)
Open Pan Dry Roasting (OPDR)	-.702	.369	1	-.996(S)	.052
Shallow Frying (SF)	.763	-.283	-.996(S)	1	.038
Deep Frying (DF)	.675	.948(S)	.052	.038	1

Positive Negative *S= Significant*

This table shows the correlation of fat content of pomfret with cooking methods. In fresh condition, there is significant positive correlation present between boiling and deep frying, whereas open pan dry roasting is significant negatively correlated with shallow frying. This table indicates that there is a strong correlation present between **boiling and deep frying and also between shallow frying and open pan dry roasting** in fresh condition.

Table no 5.12.5.3.2 Correlation of cooking methods in 24 hours preservation without preservative

Condition	RS	B	OPDR	SF	DF
Raw State (RS)	1	-.756	-.945(S)	-.999*(S)	-.189
Boiling (B)	-.756	1	.500	.721	-.500
Open Pan Dry Roasting (OPDR)	-.945(S)	.500	1	.961(S)	.500
Shallow Frying (SF)	-.999*(S)	.721	.961(S)	1	.240
Deep Frying (DF)	-.189	-.500	.500	.240	1

***.Correlation is highly significant at the 0.01 level (2-tailed)* Positive Negative *S= Significant*

This table shows the correlation of fat content of pomfret with cooking methods. In 24 hours control preservation without preservative, there is significant negative correlation present between the raw state and open pan dry roasting, and highly significant negative correlation present between the raw state and shallow frying, whereas open pan dry roasting is significant positively correlated with shallow frying. This table indicates that there is a strong correlation present among the **raw state, open pan dry roasting and shallow frying** in 24 hours control preservation.

Table no 5.12.5.3.3 Correlation of cooking methods in 48 hours preservation without preservative

Condition	RS	B	OPDR	SF	DF
Raw State (RS)	1	.684	.993(S)	.737	.500
Boiling (B)	.684	1	.596	.997*(S)	.974(S)
Open Pan Dry Roasting (OPDR)	.993(S)	.596	1	.655	.397
Shallow Frying (SF)	.737	.997*(S)	.655	1	.954(S)
Deep Frying (DF)	.500	.974	.397	.954(S)	1

**.Correlation is highly significant at the 0.05 level (2-tailed)* ▭ Positive *S= Significant*

This table shows the correlation of fat content of pomfret with cooking methods. In 48 hours control preservation without preservative, there is significant positive correlation present between the raw state and open pan dry roasting, whereas boiling is highly significant positively correlated with shallow frying and significant positively correlated with deep frying. Shallow frying is significant positively correlated with deep frying. This table indicates that there is a strong correlation present among the **raw state, boiling, open pan dry roasting, shallow frying and deep frying** in 48 hours control preservation.

Table no 5.12.5.3.4 Correlation of cooking methods in 14 days preservation without preservative

Condition	RS	B	OPDR	SF	DF
Raw State (RS)	1	-.308	-.268	-.483	-.540
Boiling (B)	-.308	1	.999*(S)	-.684	.967(S)
Open Pan Dry Roasting (OPDR)	-.268	.999*(S)	1	-.714	.955(S)
Shallow Frying (SF)	-.483	-.684	-.714	1	-.475
Deep Frying (DF)	-.540	.967(S)	.955(S)	-.475	1

**.Correlation is highly significant at the 0.05 level (2-tailed)* ▭ Positive *S= Significant*

This table shows the correlation of fat content of pomfret with cooking methods. In 14 days control preservation without preservative, there is highly significant positive correlation present between boiling and open pan dry roasting, and significant positive correlation present between boiling and deep frying, whereas open pan dry roasting is significant positively correlated with deep frying. This table indicates that there is a strong correlation present among **boiling, open pan dry roasting and deep frying** in 14 days control preservation.

Table no 5.12.5.3.5 Correlation of cooking methods in 15 days preservation without preservative

Condition	RS	B	OPDR	SF	DF
Raw State (RS)	1	-.996(S)	-.524	.982(S)	.590
Boiling (B)	-.996(S)	1	.445	-.961(S)	-.661
Open Pan Dry Roasting (OPDR)	-.524	.445	1	-.676	.378
Shallow Frying (SF)	.982(S)	-.961(S)	-.676	1	.427
Deep Frying (DF)	.590	-.661	.378	.427	1

▭ Positive ▭ Negative *S= Significant*

This table shows the correlation of fat content of pomfret with cooking methods. In 15 days control preservation without preservative, there is significant positive correlation present between the raw state and shallow frying, and significant negative correlation present between the raw state and boiling, whereas boiling is significant negatively correlated with shallow frying. This table indicates that there is a strong correlation present among the **raw state, boiling and shallow frying** in 15 days control preservation.

Table no 5.12.5.3.6 Correlation of cooking methods in 24 hours preservation with salt and turmeric

Condition	RS	B	OPDR	SF	DF
Raw State (RS)	1	.756	-.371	.993(S)	-.596
Boiling (B)	.756	1	-.888(S)	.676	-.976(S)
Open Pan Dry Roasting (OPDR)	-.371	-.888(S)	1	-.262	.967(S)
Shallow Frying (SF)	.993(S)	.676	-.262	1	-.500
Deep Frying (DF)	-.596	-.976(S)	.967(S)	-.500	1

Positive Negative *S= Significant*

This table shows the correlation of fat content of pomfret with cooking methods. In 24 hours salt and turmeric preservation, there is significant positive correlation present between the raw state and shallow frying, whereas boiling is significant negatively correlated with open pan dry roasting and deep frying. Open pan dry roasting is significant positively correlated with deep frying. This table indicates that there is a strong correlation present among the **raw state, boiling, open pan dry roasting, shallow frying and deep frying** in 24 hours salt and turmeric preservation.

Table no 5.12.5.3.7 Correlation of cooking methods in 48 hours preservation with salt and turmeric

Condition	RS	B	OPDR	SF	DF
Raw State (RS)	1	.764	-.756	.976(S)	.786
Boiling (B)	.764	1	-.156	.886(S)	.999*(S)
Open Pan Dry Roasting (OPDR)	-.756	-.156	1	-.596	-.189
Shallow Frying (SF)	.976(S)	.886(S)	-.596	1	.901(S)
Deep Frying (DF)	.786	.999*(S)	-.189	.901(S)	1

**.Correlation is highly significant at the 0.05 level (2-tailed)* Positive *S= Significant*

This table shows the correlation of fat content of pomfret with cooking methods. In 48 hours salt and turmeric preservation, there is significant positive correlation present between the raw state and shallow frying, whereas boiling is significant positively correlated with shallow frying and highly significant positively correlated with deep frying. Shallow frying is significant positively correlated with deep frying. This table indicates that there is a strong correlation present among the **raw state, boiling, shallow frying and deep frying** in 48 hours salt and turmeric preservation.

Table no 5.12.5.3.8 Correlation of cooking methods in 14 days preservation with salt and turmeric

Condition	RS	B	OPDR	SF	DF
Raw State (RS)	1	1.000**(S)	.918(S)	-.500	.993(S)
Boiling (B)	1.000**(S)	1	.918(S)	-.500	.993(S)
Open Pan Dry Roasting (OPDR)	.918(S)	.918(S)	1	-.803(S)	.866(S)
Shallow Frying (SF)	-.500	-.500	-.803(S)	1	-.397
Deep Frying (DF)	.993(S)	.993(S)	.866(S)	-.397	1

**.Correlation is highly significant at the 0.05 level (2-tailed)* Positive Negative *S= Significant*

This table shows the correlation of fat content of pomfret with cooking methods. In 14 days salt and turmeric preservation, there is significant positive correlation present between the raw state with open pan dry roasting and deep frying, and perfect positive correlation present between the raw state and boiling, whereas boiling is significant positively correlated with deep frying. Open pan dry roasting is significant positively correlated with deep frying and significant negatively correlated with shallow frying. This table indicates that there is a strong correlation present among the **raw state, boiling, open pan dry roasting, shallow frying and deep frying** in 14 days salt and turmeric preservation.

Table no 5.12.5.3.9 Correlation of cooking methods in 15 days preservation with salt and turmeric

Condition	RS	B	OPDR	SF	DF
Raw state (RS)	1	.491	.540	.990(S)	.655
Boiling (B)	.491	1	.998*(S)	.610	.980(S)
Open Pan Dry Roasting (OPDR)	.540	.998*(S)	1	.655	.990(S)
Shallow Frying (SF)	.990(S)	.610	.655	1	.756
Deep Frying (DF)	.655	.980(S)	.990(S)	.756	1

**.Correlation is highly significant at the 0.05 level (2-tailed)* Positive *S= Significant*

This table shows the correlation of fat content of pomfret with cooking methods. In 15 days salt and turmeric preservation, there is significant positive correlation present between the raw state and shallow frying, whereas boiling is highly significant positively correlated with open pan dry roasting and significant positively correlated with deep frying. Open pan dry roasting is significant positively correlated with deep frying. This table indicates that there is a strong correlation present among the **raw state, boiling, open pan dry roasting, shallow frying and deep frying** in 15 days salt and turmeric preservation.

Table no 5.12.5.3.10 Correlation of cooking methods in 24 hours preservation with KMS

Condition	RS	B	OPDR	SF	DF
Raw State (RS)	1	-1.000**(S)	-.923(S)	-.818(S)	.015
Boiling (B)	-1.000**(S)	1	.920(S)	.813(S)	-.023
Open Pan Dry Roasting (OPDR)	-.923(S)	.920(S)	1	.976(S)	.371
Shallow Frying (SF)	-.818(S)	.813(S)	.976(S)	1	.564
Deep Frying (DF)	.015	-.023	.371	.564	1

**.Correlation is highly significant at the 0.05 level (2-tailed)* Positive Negative *S= Significant*

This table shows the correlation of fat content of pomfret with cooking methods. In 24 hours KMS preservation, there is significant negative correlation present between the raw state with open pan dry roasting and shallow frying, and perfect negative correlation present between the raw state and boiling, whereas boiling is significant positively correlated with open pan dry roasting and shallow frying. Open pan dry roasting is significant positively correlated with shallow frying. This table indicates that there is a strong correlation present among the **raw state, boiling, open pan dry roasting and shallow frying** in 24 hours KMS preservation.

Table no 5.12.5.3.11 Correlation of cooking methods in 48 hours preservation with KMS

Condition	RS	B	OPDR	SF	DF
Raw State (RS)	1	1.000**(S)	.619	.995(S)	.610
Boiling (B)	1.000**(S)	1	.619	.995(S)	.610
Open Pan Dry Roasting (OPDR)	.619	.619	1	.540	1.000**(S)
Shallow Frying (SF)	.995(S)	.995(S)	.540	1	.531
Deep Frying (DF)	.610	.610	1.000**(S)	.531	1

***.Correlation is highly significant at the 0.01 level (2-tailed)* Positive *S= Significant*

This table shows the correlation of fat content of pomfret with cooking methods. In 48 hours KMS preservation, there is significant positive correlation present between the raw state and shallow frying, and perfect positive correlation present between the raw state and boiling, whereas boiling is significant positively correlated with shallow frying. Open pan dry roasting is perfect positively correlated with deep frying. This table indicates that there is a strong correlation present among the **raw state, boiling, open pan dry roasting, shallow frying and deep frying** in 48 hours KMS preservation.

Table no 5.12.5.3.12 Correlation of cooking methods in 14 days preservation with KMS

Condition	RS	B	OPDR	SF	DF
Raw State (RS)	1	.581	.189	-.500	.995(S)
Boiling (B)	.581	1	.909(S)	.415	.500
Open Pan Dry Roasting (OPDR)	.189	.909(S)	1	.756	.094
Shallow Frying (SF)	-.500	.415	.756	1	-.581
Deep Frying (DF)	.995(S)	.500	.094	-.581	1

Positive *S= Significant*

This table shows the correlation of fat content of pomfret with cooking methods. In 14 days KMS preservation, there is significant positive correlation present between the raw state and deep frying, whereas boiling is significant positively correlated with open pan dry roasting. This table indicates that there is a strong correlation present between the **raw state and deep frying and also between boiling and open pan dry roasting** in 14 days KMS preservation.

Table no 5.12.5.3.13 Correlation of cooking methods in 15 days preservation with KMS

Condition	RS	B	OPDR	SF	DF
Raw State (RS)	1	.992(S)	-.906(S)	.926(S)	.000
Boiling (B)	.992(S)	1	-.845(S)	.967(S)	.127
Open Pan Dry Roasting (OPDR)	-.906(S)	-.845(S)	1	-.680	.423
Shallow Frying (SF)	.926(S)	.967(S)	-.680	1	.376
Deep Frying (DF)	.000	.127	.423	.376	1

Positive Negative *S= Significant*

This table shows the correlation of fat content of pomfret with cooking methods. In 15 days KMS preservation, there is significant positive correlation present between the raw state with boiling and shallow frying, and significant negative correlation present between the raw state and open pan dry roasting, whereas boiling is significant negatively correlated with open pan dry roasting and significant positively correlated with shallow frying. This table indicates that there is a strong correlation present among the **raw state, boiling, open pan dry roasting, shallow frying and deep frying** in 15 days KMS preservation.

Overall analysis reveals that the raw state is perfect positively correlated with boiling in 14 days salt-turmeric preservation and 48 hours KMS preservation and perfect negatively correlated with boiling in 24 hours KMS preservation, whereas significant positively correlated with open pan dry roasting and deep frying in 48 hours control preservation without preservation and 14 days KMS preservation respectively, and highly significant positively correlated with shallow frying in 24 hours control preservation without preservative. Boiling is highly significant positively correlated with open pan dry roasting, shallow frying and deep frying in 14 days, 48 hours control preservation without preservative and 48 hours salt-turmeric preservation respectively. Open pan dry roasting is positively correlated with shallow frying in 24 hours KMS preservation, and perfect positively correlated with deep frying in 48 hours KMS preservation. Shallow frying is significant positively correlated with deep frying in fresh condition. Most of the correlation of the fat content of pomfret is found in **24 hours and 48 hours control preservation without preservative and 48 hours KMS preservation** with respect to different cooking conditions.

5.12.5.4 Moisture

Table no 5.12.5.4.1 Correlation of cooking methods in fresh condition

Condition	RS	B	OPDR	SF	DF
Raw State (RS)	1	.426	-.862(S)	-.836(S)	-.682
Boiling (B)	.426	1	-.826(S)	-.852(S)	.371
Open Pan Dry Roasting (OPDR)	-.862(S)	-.826(S)	1	.999*(S)	.217
Shallow Frying (SF)	-.836(S)	-.852(S)	.999*(S)	1	.169
Deep Frying (DF)	-.682	.371	.217	.169	1

**.Correlation is highly significant at the 0.05 level (2-tailed)* ▭ Positive ▭ Negative *S= Significant*

This table shows the correlation of moisture content of pomfret with cooking methods. In fresh condition, there is significant negative correlation present between the raw state with open pan dry roasting and shallow frying, whereas boiling is also significant positively correlated with open pan dry roasting and shallow frying. Open pan dry roasting is highly significant positively correlated with shallow frying. This table indicates that there is a strong correlation present among the **raw state, boiling, open pan dry roasting and shallow frying** in fresh condition.

Table no 5.12.5.4.2 Correlation of cooking methods in 24 hours preservation without preservative

Condition	RS	B	OPDR	SF	DF
Raw State (RS)	1	-.998*(S)	.805(S)	.917(S)	.876(S)
Boiling (B)	-.998*(S)	1	-.762	-.887(S)	-.907(S)
Open Pan Dry Roasting (OPDR)	.805(S)	-.762	1	.975(S)	.418
Shallow Frying (SF)	.917(S)	-.887(S)	.975(S)	1	.611
Deep Frying (DF)	.876(S)	-.907(S)	.418	.611	1

**.Correlation is highly significant at the 0.05 level (2-tailed)* ▭ Positive ▭ Negative *S= Significant*

This table shows the correlation of moisture content of pomfret with cooking methods. In 24 hours control preservation without preservative, there is highly significant negative correlation present between the raw state and boiling, and significant positive correlation present between the raw state with open pan dry roasting, shallow frying and deep frying, whereas boiling is significant negatively correlated with shallow frying and deep frying. Open pan dry roasting is significant positively correlated with shallow frying. This table indicates that there is a strong correlation present among the **raw state, boiling, open pan dry roasting, shallow frying and deep frying** in 24 hours control preservation.

Table no 5.12.5.4.3 Correlation of cooking methods in 48 hours preservation without preservative

Condition	RS	B	OPDR	SF	DF
Raw State (RS)	1	-.434	.886(S)	.564	.181
Boiling (B)	-.434	1	.034	.500	.808(S)
Open Pan Dry Roasting (OPDR)	.886(S)	.034	1	.882(S)	.616
Shallow Frying (SF)	.564	.500	.882(S)	1	.914(S)
Deep Frying (DF)	.181	.808(S)	.616	.914(S)	1

Positive *S= Significant*

This table shows the correlation of moisture content of pomfret with cooking methods. In 48 hours control preservation without preservative, there is significant positive correlation present between the raw state and open pan dry roasting, whereas boiling is significant positively correlated with deep frying. Open pan dry roasting is significant positively correlated with shallow frying. Shallow frying is significant positively correlated with deep frying. This table shows that there is a strong correlation present among the **raw state, boiling, open pan dry roasting, shallow frying and deep frying** in 48 hours control preservation.

Table no 5.12.5.4.4 Correlation of cooking methods in 14 days preservation without preservative

Condition	RS	B	OPDR	SF	DF
Raw State (RS)	1	.968(S)	.982(S)	.605	.866(S)
Boiling (B)	.968(S)	1	.998*(S)	.385	.964(S)
Open Pan Dry Roasting (OPDR)	.982(S)	.998*(S)	1	.444	.945(S)
Shallow Frying (SF)	.605	.385	.444	1	.126
Deep Frying (DF)	.866(S)	.964	.945(S)	.126	1

**.Correlation is highly significant at the 0.05 level (2-tailed)* Positive *S= Significant*

This table shows the correlation of moisture content of pomfret with cooking methods. In 14 days control preservation without preservative, there is significant positive correlation present between the raw state with boiling, open pan dry roasting and deep frying, whereas boiling is highly significant positively correlated with open pan dry roasting, and significant positively correlated with deep frying. Open pan dry roasting is significant positively correlated with deep frying. This table indicates that there is a strong correlation present among the **raw state, boiling, open pan dry roasting and deep frying** in 14 days control preservation.

Table no 5.12.5.4.5 Correlation of cooking methods in 15 days preservation without preservative

Condition	RS	B	OPDR	SF	DF
Raw State (RS)	1	-.755	.996(S)	.736	-.146
Boiling (B)	-.755	1	-.811(S)	-.112	.759
Open Pan Dry Roasting (OPDR)	.996(S)	-.811(S)	1	.672	-.235
Shallow Frying (SF)	.736	-.112	.672	1	.562
Deep Frying (DF)	-.146	.759	-.235	.562	1

Positive *S= Significant*

This table shows the correlation of moisture content of pomfret with cooking methods. In 15 days control preservation without preservative, there is significant positive correlation present between the raw state and open pan dry roasting, whereas boiling is significant negatively correlated with open pan dry roasting. This table indicates that there is a strong correlation present among the **raw state, boiling and open pan dry roasting** in 15 days control preservation.

Table no 5.12.5.4.6 Correlation of cooking methods in 24 hours preservation with salt and turmeric

Condition	RS	B	OPDR	SF	DF
Raw State (RS)	1	.982(S)	-.982(S)	-.877(S)	-.891(S)
Boiling (B)	.982(S)	1	-1.000**(S)	-.952(S)	-.961(S)
Open Pan Dry Roasting (OPDR)	-.982(S)	-1.000**(S)	1	.952(S)	.961(S)
Shallow Frying (SF)	-.877(S)	-.952(S)	.952(S)	1	1.000*(S)
Deep Frying (DF)	-.891(S)	-.961(S)	.961(S)	1.000*(S)	1

***.Correlation is highly significant at the 0.01 level (2-tailed)* Positive Negative *S= Significant*

This table shows the correlation of moisture content of pomfret with cooking methods. In 24 hours salt and turmeric preservation, there is significant positive correlation present between the raw state and boiling, and significant negative correlation present between the raw state with open pan dry roasting, shallow frying and deep frying, whereas boiling is perfect negatively correlated with open pan dry roasting, and significant negatively correlated with shallow frying and deep frying. Open pan dry roasting is significant positively correlated with shallow frying and deep frying. Shallow frying is perfect positively correlated with deep frying. This table indicates that there is a strong correlation present among the **raw state, boiling, open pan dry roasting, shallow frying and deep frying** in 24 hours salt and turmeric preservation.

Table no 5.12.5.4.7 Correlation of cooking methods in 48 hours preservation with salt and turmeric

Condition	RS	B	OPDR	SF	DF
Raw State (RS)	1	-1.000**(S)	.392	-.924(S)	-.507
Boiling (B)	-1.000**(S)	1	-.385	.927(S)	.500
Open Pan Dry Roasting (OPDR)	.392	-.385	1	-.011	-.992(S)
Shallow Frying (SF)	-.924(S)	.927(S)	-.011	1	.139
Deep Frying (DF)	-.507	.500	-.992(S)	.139	1

***.Correlation is highly significant at the 0.01 level (2-tailed)* Positive Negative *S= Significant*

This table shows the correlation of moisture content of pomfret with cooking methods. In 48 hours salt and turmeric preservation, there is perfect negative correlation present between the raw state and boiling, and significant negative correlation present between the raw state and shallow frying, whereas boiling is significant positively correlated with shallow frying. Open pan dry roasting is significant negatively correlated with deep frying. This table indicates that there is a strong correlation present among the **raw state, boiling, open pan dry roasting, shallow frying and deep frying** in 48 hours salt and turmeric preservation.

Table no 5.12.5.4.8 Correlation of cooking methods in 14 days preservation with salt and turmeric

Condition	RS	B	OPDR	SF	DF
Raw State (RS)	1	.932(S)	.802(S)	.948(S)	-.011
Boiling (B)	.932(S)	1	.530	.999*(S)	-.374
Open Pan Dry Roasting (OPDR)	.802(S)	.530	1	.572	.588
Shallow Frying (SF)	.948(S)	.999*(S)	.572	1	-.327
Deep Frying (DF)	-.011	-.374	.588	-.327	1

**.Correlation is highly significant at the 0.05 level (2-tailed)* Positive *S= Significant*

This table shows the correlation of moisture content of pomfret with cooking methods. In 14 days salt and turmeric preservation, there is significant positive correlation present between the raw state with boiling, open pan dry roasting and shallow frying, whereas boiling is highly significant positively correlated with shallow frying. This table indicates that there is a strong correlation present among the **raw state, boiling, open pan dry roasting and shallow frying** in 14 days salt and turmeric preservation.

Table no 5.12.5.4.9 Correlation of cooking methods in 15 days preservation with salt and turmeric

Condition	RS	B	OPDR	SF	DF
Raw State (RS)	1	1.000*(S)	.885(S)	.877(S)	.998*(S)
Boiling (B)	1.000*(S)	1	.894(S)	.886(S)	.999*(S)
Open Pan Dry Roasting (OPDR)	.885(S)	.894(S)	1	1.000*(S)	.915(S)
Shallow Frying (SF)	.877(S)	.886(S)	1.000*(S)	1	.908(S)
Deep Frying (DF)	.998*(S)	.999*(S)	.915(S)	.908(S)	1

**.Correlation is highly significant at the 0.05 level (2-tailed)* Positive *S= Significant*

This table shows the correlation of moisture content of pomfret with cooking methods. In 15 days salt and turmeric preservation, there is highly significant positive correlation present between the raw state and deep frying, and significant positive correlation present between the raw state with open pan dry roasting and shallow frying, and perfect positive correlation present between the raw state and boiling. Boiling is highly significant positively correlated with deep frying and significant positively correlated with open pan dry roasting and shallow frying. Open pan dry roasting is perfect positively correlated shallow frying and significant positively correlate with deep frying. Shallow frying is significant positively correlated with deep frying. This table indicates that there is a strong correlation present among the **raw state, boiling, open pan dry roasting, shallow frying and deep frying** in 15 days salt and turmeric preservation.

Table no 5.12.5.4.10 Correlation of cooking methods in 24 hours preservation with KMS

Condition	RS	B	OPDR	SF	DF
Raw State (RS)	1	.980(S)	.998*(S)	.617	.957(S)
Boiling (B)	.980(S)	1	.966(S)	.763	.996(S)
Open Pan Dry Roasting (OPDR)	.998*(S)	.966(S)	1	.569	.938(S)
Shallow Frying (SF)	.617	.763	.569	1	.818(S)
Deep Frying (DF)	.957(S)	.996(S)	.938(S)	.818(S)	1

**.Correlation is highly significant at the 0.05 level (2-tailed)* Positive *S= Significant*

This table shows the correlation of moisture content of pomfret with cooking methods. In 24 hours KMS preservation, there is highly significant positive correlation present between the raw state and open pan dry roasting, and significant positive correlation present between the raw state with boiling and deep frying, whereas boiling is significant positively correlated with open pan dry roasting and deep frying. Open pan dry roasting is significant positively correlated with deep frying. Shallow frying is significant positively correlated with deep frying. This table indicates that there is a strong correlation present among the **raw state, boiling, open pan dry roasting, shallow frying and deep frying** in 24 hours KMS preservation.

Table no 5.12.5.4.11 Correlation of cooking methods in 48 hours preservation with KMS

Condition	RS	B	OPDR	SF	DF
Raw State (RS)	1	.933(S)	-1.000**(S)	-.781	.982(S)
Boiling (B)	.933(S)	1	-.933(S)	-.505	.849(S)
Open Pan Dry Roasting (OPDR)	-1.000**(S)	-.933(S)	1	.781	-.982(S)
Shallow Frying (SF)	-.781	-.505	.781	1	-.885(S)
Deep Frying (DF)	.982(S)	.849(S)	-.982(S)	-.885(S)	1

***.Correlation is highly significant at the 0.01 level (2-tailed)* Positive Negative *S= Significant*

This table shows the correlation of moisture content of pomfret with cooking methods. In 48 hours KMS preservation, there is significant positive correlation present between the raw state with boiling and deep frying, and perfect negative correlation present between the raw state with open pan dry roasting, whereas boiling is significant positively correlated with deep frying, and significant negative correlation present between boiling and open pan dry roasting. Open pan dry roasting is significant negatively correlated with deep frying. Shallow frying is significant negatively correlated with deep frying. This table indicates that there is a strong correlation present among the **raw state, boiling, open pan dry roasting, shallow frying and deep frying** in 48 hours KMS preservation.

Table no 5.12.5.4.12 Correlation of cooking methods in 14 days preservation with KMS

Condition	RS	B	OPDR	SF	DF
Raw State (RS)	1	.834(S)	.942(S)	.924(S)	-.821(S)
Boiling (B)	.834(S)	1	.971(S)	.558	-.369
Open Pan Dry Roasting (OPDR)	.942(S)	.971(S)	1	.742	-.582
Shallow Frying (SF)	.924(S)	.558	.742	1	-.977(S)
Deep Frying (DF)	-.821(S)	-.369	-.582	-.977(S)	1

Positive Negative *S= Significant*

This table shows the correlation of moisture content of pomfret with cooking methods. In 14 days KMS preservation, there is significant positive correlation present between the raw state with boiling, open pan dry roasting and shallow frying, and significant negative correlation present between the raw state and deep frying, whereas boiling is significant positively correlated with open pan dry roasting. Shallow frying is significant negatively correlated with deep frying. This table indicates that there is a strong correlation present among the **raw state, boiling, open pan dry roasting, shallow frying and deep frying** in 14 days KMS preservation.

Table no 5.12.5.4.13 Correlation of cooking methods in 15 days preservation with KMS

Condition	RS	B	OPDR	SF	DF
Raw State (RS)	1	.854(S)	.989(S)	.999*(S)	.724
Boiling (B)	.854(S)	1	.767	.879(S)	.977(S)
Open Pan Dry Roasting (OPDR)	.989(S)	.767	1	.980(S)	.614
Shallow Frying (SF)	.999*(S)	.879(S)	.980(S)	1	.758
Deep Frying (DF)	.724	.977(S)	.614	.758	1

***.Correlation is highly significant at the 0.01 level (2-tailed)* Positive *S= Significant*

This table shows the correlation of moisture content of pomfret with cooking methods. In 15 days KMS preservation, there is significant positive correlation present between the raw state with boiling, open pan dry roasting, and highly significant positive correlation present between the raw state and shallow frying, whereas boiling is significant positively correlated with shallow frying and deep frying. Shallow frying is significant positively correlated with open pan dry roasting. This table indicates that there is a strong correlation present among the **raw state, boiling, open pan dry roasting, shallow frying and deep frying** in 15 days KMS preservation.

Overall analysis reveals that the raw state is perfect negatively correlated with boiling in 48 hours salt-turmeric preservation and perfect positively correlated with boiling in 15 days salt-turmeric preservation, whereas perfect negatively correlated with open pan dry roasting in 48 hours preservation with KMS, highly significant positively correlated with shallow frying and deep frying in 15 days KMS preservation and 15 days salt-turmeric preservation respectively. Boiling is perfect negatively correlated with open pan dry roasting in 24 hours salt-turmeric preservation, whereas highly significant positively correlated with shallow frying and deep frying in 14 days and 15 days salt and turmeric preservation respectively. Open pan dry roasting is perfect positively correlated with shallow frying in 15 days salt and turmeric, and significant negatively correlated with deep frying in 48 hours salt and turmeric preservation. Shallow frying is perfect positively correlated with deep frying in 24 hours salt-turmeric preservation. Most of the correlation of the moisture content of pomfret is found in **15 days salt and turmeric preservation** with respect to different cooking conditions.

5.12.5.5 Ash

Table no 5.12.5.5.1 Correlation of cooking methods in fresh condition

Condition	RS	B	OPDR	SF	DF
Raw State (RS)	1	.908(S)	.996(S)	.795	.908(S)
Boiling (B)	.908(S)	1	.866(S)	.976(S)	1.000**(S)
Open Pan Dry Roasting (OPDR)	.996(S)	.866(S)	1	.737	.866(S)
Shallow Frying (SF)	.795	.976(S)	.737	1	.976(S)
Deep Frying (DF)	.908(S)	1.000**(S)	.866(S)	.976(S)	1

***.Correlation is highly significant at the 0.01 level (2-tailed)* Positive *S= Significant*

This table shows the correlation of ash content of pomfret with cooking methods. In fresh condition, there is significant positive correlation present between the raw state with boiling, open pan dry roasting and deep frying, whereas boiling is significant positively correlated with open pan dry roasting and shallow frying, and perfect positive correlation present between boiling and deep frying. Open pan dry roasting is significant positively correlated with deep frying. Shallow frying is significant positively correlated with deep frying. This table indicates that there is a strong correlation present among the **raw state, boiling, open pan dry roasting, shallow frying and deep frying** in fresh condition.

Table no 5.12.5.5.2 Correlation of cooking methods in 24 hours preservation without preservative

Condition	RS	B	OPDR	SF	DF
Raw State (RS)	1	1.000**(S)	.990(S)	-.540	-.990(S)
Boiling (B)	1.000**(S)	1	.990(S)	-.540	-.990(S)
Open Pan Dry Roasting (OPDR)	.990(S)	.990(S)	1	-.655	-1.000**(S)
Shallow Frying (SF)	-.540	-.540	-.655	1	.655
Deep Frying (DF)	-.990(S)	-.990(S)	-1.000**(S)	.655	1

***.Correlation is highly significant at the 0.01 level (2-tailed)* Positive Negative *S= Significant*

This table shows the correlation of ash content of pomfret with cooking methods. In 24 hours control preservation without preservative, there is significant positive correlation present between the raw state and open pan dry roasting, and significant negative correlation present between the raw state and deep frying, and perfect positive correlation present between the raw state and boiling. Boiling is significant positively correlated with open pan dry roasting and significant negatively correlated with deep frying. Open pan dry roasting is perfect negatively correlated with deep frying. This table indicates that there is a strong correlation present among the **raw state, boiling, open pan dry roasting and deep frying in** 24 hours control preservation.

Table no 5.12.5.5.3 Correlation of cooking methods in 48 hours preservation without preservative

Condition	RS	B	OPDR	SF	DF\
Raw State (RS)	1	-.912(S)	-.971(S)	-.596	-.945(S)
Boiling (B)	-.912(S)	1	.787	.873(S)	.728
Open Pan Dry Roasting (OPDR)	-.971(S)	.787	1	.386	.996(S)
Shallow Frying (SF)	-.596	.873(S)	.386	1	.300
Deep Frying (DF)	-.945(S)	.728	.996(S)	.300	1

Positive Negative *S= Significant*

This table shows the correlation of ash content of pomfret with cooking methods. In 48 hours control preservation without preservative, there is significant negative correlation present between the raw state with boiling, open pan dry roasting and deep frying, whereas boiling is significant positively correlated with shallow frying. Open pan dry roasting is significant positively correlated with deep frying. This table indicates that there is a strong correlation present among the **raw state, boiling, open pan dry roasting, shallow frying and deep frying in** 48 hours control preservation.

Table no 5.12.5.5.4 Correlation of cooking methods in 14 days preservation without preservative

Condition	RS	B	OPDR	SF	DF
Raw State (RS)	1	.540	.540	.472	.690
Boiling (B)	.540	1	1.000**(S)	.997(S)	.982(S)
Open Pan Dry Roasting (OPDR)	.540	1.000**(S)	1	.997(S)	.982(S)
Shallow Frying (SF)	.472	.997(S)	.997(S)	1	.964(S)
Deep Frying (DF)	.690	.982(S)	.982(S)	.964(S)	1

***.Correlation is highly significant at the 0.01 level (2-tailed)* Positive *S= Significant*

This table shows the correlation of ash content of pomfret with cooking methods. In 14 days control preservation without preservative, there is significant positive correlation present between boiling with shallow frying and deep frying, and perfect positive correlation present between boiling and open pan dry roasting, whereas open pan dry roasting is significant positively correlated with shallow frying and deep frying. Shallow frying is significant positively correlated with deep frying. This table indicates that there is a strong correlation present among **boiling, open pan dry roasting, shallow frying and deep frying** in 14 days control preservation.

Table no 5.12.5.5.5 Correlation of cooking methods in 15 days preservation without preservative

Condition	RS	B	OPDR	SF	DF
Raw State (RS)	1	-.792	-.971(S)	-.952(S)	1.000**(S)
Boiling (B)	-.792	1	.623	.568	-.792
Open Pan Dry Roasting (OPDR)	-.971(S)	.623	1	.998*(S)	-.971(S)
Shallow Frying (SF)	-.952(S)	.568	.998*(S)	1	-.952(S)
Deep Frying (DF)	1.000**(S)	-.792	-.971(S)	-.952(S)	1

**.Correlation is highly significant at the 0.05 level (2-tailed)* Positive Negative *S= Significant*
***.Correlation is highly significant at the 0.01 level (2-tailed)*

This table shows the correlation of ash content of pomfret with cooking methods. In 15 days control preservation without preservative, there is significant negative correlation present between the raw state with open pan dry roasting and shallow frying, and perfect positive correlation present between the raw state and deep frying, whereas open pan dry roasting is highly significant positively correlated with shallow frying and significant negatively correlated with deep frying. Shallow frying is significant negatively correlated with deep frying. This table indicates that there is a strong correlation present among the **raw state, open pan dry roasting, shallow frying and deep frying in** 15 days control preservation.

Table no 5.12.5.5.6 Correlation of cooking methods in 24 hours preservation with salt and turmeric

Condition	RS	B	OPDR	SF	DF
Raw State (RS)	1	.990(S)	.836(S)	.866(S)	.884(S)
Boiling (B)	.990(S)	1	.749	.786	.808(S)
Open Pan Dry Roasting (OPDR)	.836(S)	.749	1	.998*(S)	.996(S)
Shallow Frying (SF)	.866(S)	.786	.998*(S)	1	.999*(S)
Deep Frying (DF)	.884(S)	.808(S)	.996(S)	.999*(S)	1

**.Correlation is highly significant at the 0.05 level (2-tailed)* ▭ Positive *S= Significant*

This table shows the correlation of ash content of pomfret with cooking methods. In 24 hours salt and turmeric preservation, there is significant positive correlation present between the raw state with boiling, open pan dry roasting, shallow frying and deep frying, whereas boiling is significant positively correlated with deep frying. Open pan dry roasting is significant positively correlated with deep frying. Shallow frying is highly significant positively correlated with open pan dry roasting and deep frying. This table indicates that there is a strong correlation present among the **raw state, boiling, open pan dry roasting, shallow frying and deep frying** in 24 hours salt and turmeric preservation.

Table no 5.12.5.5.7 Correlation of cooking methods in 48 hours preservation with salt and turmeric

Condition	RS	B	OPDR	SF	DF
Raw State (RS)	1	-.485	-1.000**(S)	-.676	-.434
Boiling (B)	-.485	1	.485	-.317	.998*(S)
Open Pan Dry Roasting (OPDR)	-1.000** (S)	.485	1	.676	.434
Shallow Frying (SF)	-.676	-.317	.676	1	-.371
Deep Frying (DF)	-.434	.998*(S)	.434	-.371	1

***.Correlation is highly significant at the 0.01 level (2-tailed)* ▭ Positive ▭ Negative *S= Significant*
**.Correlation is highly significant at the 0.0 5 level (2-tailed)*

This table shows the correlation of ash content of pomfret with cooking methods. In 48 hours salt and turmeric preservation, there is perfect negative correlation present between the raw state and open pan dry roasting, whereas boiling is highly significant positively correlated with deep frying. This table indicates that there is a strong correlation present **between the raw state and open pan dry roasting and also between boiling and deep frying** in 48 hours salt and turmeric preservation.

Table no 5.12.5.5.8 Correlation of cooking methods in 14 days preservation with salt and turmeric

Condition	RS	B	OPDR	SF	DF
Raw State (RS)	1	-.959(S)	-.672	-.800(S)	.800(S)
Boiling (B)	-.959(S)	1	.434	.596	-.596
Open Pan Dry Roasting (OPDR)	-.672	.434	1	.982(S)	-.982(S)
Shallow Frying (SF)	-.800(S)	.596	.982(S)	1	-1.000**(S)
Deep Frying (DF)	.800(S)	-.596	-.982(S)	-1.000**(S)	1

***.Correlation is highly significant at the 0.01 level (2-tailed)* ▭ Positive ▭ Negative *S= Significant*

This table shows the correlation of ash content of pomfret with cooking methods. In 14 days salt and turmeric preservation, there is significant negative correlation present between the raw state with boiling and shallow frying, and significant positive correlation present between the raw state and deep frying, whereas open pan dry roasting is significant positively correlated with shallow frying and significant negatively correlated with deep frying. Shallow frying is perfect negatively correlated with deep frying. This table indicates that there is a strong correlation present among the **raw state, boiling, open pan dry roasting, shallow frying and deep frying** in 14 days salt and turmeric preservation.

Table no 5.12.5.5.9 Correlation of cooking methods in 15 days preservation with salt and turmeric

Condition	RS	B	OPDR	SF	DF
Raw State (RS)	1	.945(S)	1.000**(S)	.596	.990(S)
Boiling (B)	.945(S)	1	.945	.300	.982(S)
Open Pan Dry Roasting (OPDR)	1.000**(S)	.945(S)	1	.596	.990(S)
Shallow Frying (SF)	.596	.300	.596	1	.475
Deep Frying (DF)	.990(S)	.982(S)	.990(S)	.475	1

***.Correlation is highly significant at the 0.01 level (2-tailed)* Positive *S= Significant*

This table shows the correlation of ash content of pomfret with cooking methods. In 15 days salt and turmeric preservation, there is significant positive correlation present between the raw state with boiling and deep frying, and perfect positive correlation present between the raw state and open pan dry roasting, whereas boiling is significant positively correlated with deep frying. Open pan dry roasting is significant positively correlated with deep frying. This table indicates that there is a strong correlation present among the **raw state, boiling, open pan dry roasting and deep frying** in 15 days salt and turmeric preservation.

Table no 5.12.5.5.10 Correlation of cooking methods in 24 hours preservation with KMS

Condition	RS	B	OPDR	SF	DF
Raw State (RS)	1	.998*(S)	.929(S)	1.000**(S)	1.000**(S)
Boiling (B)	.998*(S)	1	.948(S)	.998*(S)	.998*(S)
Open Pan Dry Roasting (OPDR)	.929(S)	.948(S)	1	.929(S)	.929(S)
Shallow Frying (SF)	1.000**(S)	.998*(S)	.929(S)	1	1.000**(S)
Deep Frying (DF)	1.000**(S)	.998*(S)	.929(S)	1.000**(S)	1

***.Correlation is highly significant at the 0.01 level (2-tailed)* Positive *S= Significant*

This table shows the correlation of ash content of pomfret with cooking methods. In 24 hours KMS preservation, there is highly significant positive correlation present between the raw state and boiling, and perfect positive correlation present between the raw state with shallow frying and deep frying, and significant positive correlation present between the raw state and open pan dry roasting. Boiling is highly significant positively correlated with shallow frying and deep frying. Open pan dry roasting is significant positively correlated with shallow frying and deep frying. Shallow frying is perfect positively correlated with deep frying. This table indicates that there is a strong correlation present among the **raw state, boiling, open pan dry roasting, shallow frying and deep frying** in 24 hours KMS preservation.

Table no 5.12.5.5.11 Correlation of cooking methods in 48 hours preservation with KMS

Condition	RS	B	OPDR	SF	DF
Raw State (RS)	1	.697	-.901(S)	-.217	-.362
Boiling (B)	.697	1	-.317	.549	.417
Open Pan Dry Roasting (OPDR)	-.901(S)	-.317	1	.619	.730
Shallow Frying (SF)	-.217	.549	.619	1	.989(S)
Deep Frying (DF)	-.362	.417	.730	.989(S)	1

Positive Negative *S= Significant*

This table shows the correlation of ash content of pomfret with cooking methods. In 48 hours KMS preservation, there is significant negative correlation present between the raw state and open pan dry roasting, whereas shallow frying is significant positively correlated with deep frying. This table indicates that there is a strong correlation present between the **raw state and open pan dry roasting and also between shallow frying and deep frying** in 48 hours KMS preservation.

Table no 5.12.5.5.12 Correlation of cooking methods in 14 days preservation with KMS

Condition	RS	B	OPDR	SF	DF
Raw State (RS)	1	.999*(S)	.941(S)	.929(S)	.975(S)
Boiling (B)	.999*(S)	1	.929 (S)	.916(S)	.982(S)
Open Pan Dry Roasting (OPDR)	.941(S)	.929(S)	1	.999*(S)	.842(S)
Shallow Frying (SF)	.929(S)	.916(S)	.999*(S)	1	.824(S)
Deep Frying (DF)	.975(S)	.982(S)	.842(S)	.824(S)	1

**.Correlation is highly significant at the 0.05 level (2-tailed)* ▭ Positive *S= Significant*

This table shows the correlation of ash content of pomfret with cooking methods. In 14 days KMS preservation, there is highly significant positive correlation present between the raw state and boiling, and significant positive correlation present between the raw state with open pan dry roasting, shallow frying and deep frying. Boiling is significant positively correlated with open pan dry roasting, shallow frying and deep frying. Open pan dry roasting is highly significant positively correlated with shallow frying and significant positively correlated with deep frying. Shallow frying is significant positively correlated with deep frying. This table indicates that there is a strong correlation present among the **raw state, boiling, open pan dry roasting, shallow frying and deep frying** in 14 days KMS preservation.

Table no 5.12.5.5.13 Correlation of cooking methods in 15 days preservation with KMS

Condition	RS	B	OPDR	SF	DF
Raw State (RS)	1	-.041	-.075	-.217	-.923(S)
Boiling (B)	-.041	1	.999*(S)	.984(S)	.423
Open Pan Dry Roasting (OPDR)	-.075	.999*(S)	1	.990(S)	.454
Shallow Frying (SF)	-.217	.984(S)	.990(S)	1	.577
Deep Frying (DF)	-.923(S)	.423	.454	.577	1

**.Correlation is highly significant at the 0.05 level (2-tailed)* ▭ Positive ▭ Negative *S= Significant*

This table shows the correlation of ash content of pomfret with cooking methods. In 15 days KMS preservation, there is significant negative correlation present between the raw state and deep frying, whereas boiling is highly significant positively correlated with open pan dry roasting and significant positively correlated with shallow frying. Open pan dry roasting is significant positively correlated with shallow frying. This table indicates that there is a strong correlation present among the **raw state, boiling, open pan dry roasting, shallow frying and deep frying** in 15 days KMS preservation.

Overall analysis reveals that the raw state is perfect positively correlated with boiling and shallow frying in 24 hours control preservation without preservative and 24 hours KMS preservation respectively, whereas perfect negatively correlated with open pan dry roasting in 48 hours preservation with salt-turmeric and perfect positively correlated with open pan dry roasting in 15 days salt-turmeric preservation, and perfect positively correlated with deep frying in 24 hours KMS preservation and 15 days control preservation without preservative. Boiling is perfect positively correlated with open pan dry roasting and deep frying in 14 days preservation without preservative and in fresh condition respectively, whereas highly significant positively correlated with shallow frying in 24 hours KMS preservation. Open pan dry roasting is highly positively correlated with shallow frying in 14 days KMS preservation, and perfect positively correlated with deep frying in 24 hours control preservation without preservative. Shallow frying is perfect positively correlated with deep frying in 14 days salt-turmeric preservation. Most of the correlation of the ash content of pomfret is found in **24 hours KMS preservation** with respect to different cooking conditions.

5.12.5.6 Calcium

Table no 5.12.5.6.1 Correlation of cooking methods in fresh condition

Condition	RS	B	OPDR	SF	DF
Raw State (RS)	1	.500	.929(S)	.786	.786
Boiling (B)	.500	1	.143	.929(S)	.929(S)
Open Pan Dry Roasting (OPDR)	.929(S)	.143	1	.500	.500
Shallow Frying (SF)	.786	.929(S)	.500	1	1.000**(S)
Deep Frying (DF)	.786	.929(S)	.500	1.000**(S)	1

***.Correlation is highly significant at the 0.01 level (2-tailed)* ▭ Positive *S= Significant*

This table shows the correlation of calcium content of pomfret with cooking methods. In fresh condition, there is significant positive correlation present between the raw state and open pan dry roasting, whereas boiling is significant positively correlated with shallow frying and deep frying. Shallow frying is perfect positively correlated with deep frying. This table indicates that there is a strong correlation present among the **raw state, boiling, open pan dry roasting, shallow frying and deep frying** in fresh condition.

Table no 5.12.5.6.2 Correlation of cooking methods in 24 hours preservation without preservative

Condition	RS	B	OPDR	SF	DF
Raw State (RS)	1	.993(S)	.115	.993	.993
Boiling (B)	.993(S)	1	.000	1.000**(S)	1.000**(S)
Open Pan Dry Roasting (OPDR)	.115	.000	1	.000	.000
Shallow Frying (SF)	.993(S)	1.000**(S)	.000	1	1.000**(S)
Deep Frying (DF)	.993(S)	1.000**(S)	.000	1.000**(S)	1

***.Correlation is highly significant at the 0.01 level (2-tailed)* ▭ Positive *S= Significant*

This table shows the correlation of calcium content of pomfret with cooking methods. In 24 hours control preservation without preservative, there is significant positive correlation present between the raw state and boiling, whereas boiling is perfect positively correlated with shallow frying and deep frying. Shallow frying is perfect positively correlated with deep frying. This table indicates that there is a strong correlation present among the **raw state, boiling, shallow frying and deep frying** in 24 hours control preservation.

Table no 5.12.5.6.3 Correlation of cooking methods in 48 hours preservation without preservative

Condition	RS	B	OPDR	SF	DF
Raw State (RS)	1	1.000**(S)	.923(S)	.564	-.596
Boiling (B)	1.000**(S)	1	.923(S)	.564	-.596
Open Pan Dry Roasting (OPDR)	.923(S)	.923(S)	1	.839(S)	-.240
Shallow Frying (SF)	.564	.564	.839(S)	1	.327
Deep Frying (DF)	-.596	-.596	-.240	.327	1

***.Correlation is highly significant at the 0.01 level (2-tailed)* ▭ Positive *S= Significant*

This table shows the correlation of calcium content of pomfret with cooking methods. In 48 hours control preservation without preservative, there is significant positive correlation present between the raw state and open pan dry roasting, and perfect positive correlation present between the raw state and boiling, whereas boiling is significant positively correlated with open pan dry roasting. Shallow frying is significant positively correlated with open pan dry roasting. This table indicates that there is a strong correlation present among the **raw state, boiling, open pan dry roasting and shallow frying** in 48 hours control preservation.

Table no 5.12.5.6.4 Correlation of cooking methods in 14 days preservation without preservative

Condition	RS	B	OPDR	SF	DF
Raw State (RS)	1	-.240	-.397	1.000**(S)	-.693
Boiling (B)	-.240	1	.986(S)	-.240	.866(S)
Open Pan Dry Roasting (OPDR)	-.397	.986(S)	1	-.397	.937(S)
Shallow Frying (SF)	1.000**(S)	-.240	-.397	1	-.693
Deep Frying (DF)	-.693	.866(S)	.937(S)	-.693	1

***.Correlation is highly significant at the 0.01 level (2-tailed)* ▭ Positive *S= Significant*

This table shows the correlation of calcium content of pomfret with cooking methods. In 14 days control preservation without preservative, there is perfect positive correlation present between the raw state and shallow frying, whereas boiling is significant positively correlated with open pan dry roasting and deep frying. Open pan dry roasting is significant positively correlated with deep frying. This table indicates that there is a strong correlation present among the **raw state, boiling, open pan dry roasting, shallow frying and deep frying** in 14 days control preservation.

Table no 5.12.5.6.5 Correlation of cooking methods in 15 days preservation without preservative

Condition	RS	B	OPDR	SF	DF
Raw State (RS)	1	.564	.655	.882(S)	.882(S)
Boiling (B)	.564	1	.993(S)	.886(S)	.886(S)
Open Pan Dry Roasting (OPDR)	.655	.993(S)	1	.933(S)	.933(S)
Shallow Frying (SF)	.882(S)	.886(S)	.933(S)	1	1.000**(S)
Deep Frying (DF)	.882(S)	.886(S)	.933(S)	1.000**(S)	1

***.Correlation is highly significant at the 0.01 level (2-tailed)* ▭ Positive *S= Significant*

This table shows the correlation of calcium content of pomfret with cooking methods. In 15 days control preservation without preservative, there is significant positive correlation present between the raw state with shallow frying and deep frying, whereas boiling is significant positively correlated with open pan dry roasting, shallow frying and deep frying. Open pan dry roasting is significant positively correlated with shallow frying and deep frying. Shallow frying is perfect positively correlated with deep frying.

This table indicates that there is a strong correlation present among the **raw state, boiling, open pan dry roasting, shallow frying and deep frying** in 15 days control preservation.

Table no 5.12.5.6.6 Correlation of cooking methods in 24 hours preservation with salt and turmeric

Condition	RS	B	OPDR	SF	DF
Raw State (RS)	1	-.923(S)	.961(S)	.911(S)	.795
Boiling (B)	-.923(S)	1	-.993(S)	-1.000*(S)	-.500
Open Pan Dry Roasting (OPDR)	.961(S)	-.993(S)	1	.990(S)	.596
Shallow Frying (SF)	.911(S)	-1.000*(S)	.990(S)	1	.475
Deep Frying (DF)	.795	-.500	.596	.475	1

*.Correlation is highly significant at the 0.05 level (2-tailed) Positive Negative S= Significant

This table shows the correlation of calcium content of pomfret with cooking methods. In 24 hours salt and turmeric preservation, there is significant positive correlation present between the raw state with shallow frying and deep frying, and significant negative correlation present between the raw state and boiling, whereas boiling is significant negatively correlated with open pan dry roasting, and perfect negatively correlated with shallow frying. Open pan dry roasting is significant positively correlated with shallow frying. This table indicates that there is a strong correlation present among the **raw state, boiling, open pan dry roasting and shallow frying** in 24 hours salt and turmeric preservation.

Table no 5.12.5.6.7 Correlation of cooking methods in 48 hours preservation with salt and turmeric

Condition	RS	B	OPDR	SF	DF
Raw State (RS)	1	.923(S)	1.000**(S)	.676	1.000**(S)
Boiling (B)	.923(S)	1	.923(S)	.908(S)	.923(S)
Open Pan Dry Roasting (OPDR)	1.000**(S)	.923(S)	1	.676	1.000**(S)
Shallow Frying (SF)	.676	.908(S)	.676	1	.676
Deep Frying (DF)	1.000**(S)	.923(S)	1.000**(S)	.676	1

*.Correlation is highly significant at the 0.05 level (2-tailed) Positive S= Significant

This table shows the correlation of calcium content of pomfret with cooking methods. In 48 hours salt and turmeric preservation, there is significant positive correlation present between the raw state and boiling, and perfect positive correlation present between the raw state with open pan dry roasting and deep frying, whereas boiling is significant positively correlated with open pan dry roasting, shallow frying and deep frying. Open pan dry roasting is perfect positively correlated with deep frying. This table indicates that there is a strong correlation present among the **raw state, boiling, open pan dry roasting, shallow frying and deep frying** in 48 hours salt and turmeric preservation.

Table no 5.12.5.6.8 Correlation of cooking methods in 14 days preservation with salt and turmeric

Condition	RS	B	OPDR	SF	DF
Raw State (RS)	1	.993(S)	-.500	.982(S)	-.993(S)
Boiling (B)	.993(S)	1	-.596	.997*(S)	-.974(S)
Open Pan Dry Roasting (OPDR)	-.500	-.596	1	-.655	.397
Shallow Frying (SF)	.982(S)	.997*(S)	-.655	1	-.954(S)
Deep Frying (DF)	-.993(S)	-.974(S)	.397	-.954(S)	1

*.Correlation is highly significant at the 0.05 level (2-tailed) Positive Negative S= Significant

This table shows the correlation of calcium content of pomfret with cooking methods. In 14 days salt and turmeric preservation, there is significant positive correlation present between the raw state with boiling and shallow frying, and significant negative correlation present between the raw state and deep frying, whereas boiling is highly significant positively correlated with shallow frying and significant negatively correlated with deep frying. Shallow frying is significant negatively correlated with deep frying. This table indicates that there is a strong correlation present among the **raw state, boiling, shallow frying and deep frying** in 14 days salt and turmeric preservation.

Table no 5.12.5.6.9 Correlation of cooking methods in 15 days preservation with salt and turmeric

Condition	RS	B	OPDR	SF	DF
Raw State (RS)	1	.500	-.982(S)	-.500	-.655
Boiling (B)	.500	1	-.327	.500	.327
Open Pan Dry Roasting (OPDR)	-.982(S)	-.327	1	.655	.786
Shallow Frying (SF)	-.500	.500	.655	1	.982(S)
Deep Frying (DF)	-.655	.327	.786	.982(S)	1

Positive Negative correlation *S= Significant*

This table shows the correlation of calcium content of pomfret with cooking methods. In 15 days salt and turmeric preservation, there is significant negative correlation present between the raw state and open pan dry roasting, whereas shallow frying is significant positively correlated with deep frying. This table indicates that there is a strong correlation present **between the raw state and open pan dry roasting and also between shallow frying and deep frying** in 15 days salt and turmeric preservation.

Table no 5.12.5.6.10 Correlation of cooking methods in 24 hours preservation with KMS

Condition	RS	B	OPDR	SF	DF
Raw State (RS)	1	-.327	-.655	-.327	.839(S)
Boiling (B)	-.327	1	-.500	1.000**(S)	.240
Open Pan Dry Roasting (OPDR)	-.655	-.500	1	-.500	-.961(S)
Shallow Frying (SF)	-.327	1.000**(S)	-.500	1	.240
Deep Frying (DF)	.839(S)	.240	-.961(S)	.240	1

***.Correlation is highly significant at the 0.01 level (2-tailed)* Positive Negative *S= Significant*

This table shows the correlation of calcium content of pomfret with cooking methods. In 24 hours KMS preservation, there is significant positive correlation present between the raw state and deep frying, whereas boiling is perfect positively correlated with shallow frying. Open pan dry roasting is significant negatively correlated with deep frying. This table indicates that there is a strong correlation present among the **raw state, boiling, open pan dry roasting, shallow frying and deep frying** in 24 hours KMS preservation.

Table no 5.12.5.6.11 Correlation of cooking methods in 48 hours preservation with KMS

Condition	RS	B	OPDR	SF	DF
Raw state (RS)	1	.289	.993(S)	.397	.217
Boiling (B)	.289	1	.397	.993(S)	.997*(S)
Open Pan Dry Roasting (OPDR)	.993(S)	.397	1	.500	.327
Shallow Frying (SF)	.397	.993(S)	.500	1	.982(S)
Deep Frying (DF)	.217	.997*(S)	.327	.982(S)	1

Positive *S= Significant*

This table shows the correlation of calcium content of pomfret with cooking methods. In 48 hours KMS preservation, there is significant positive correlation present between the raw state and open pan dry roasting, whereas boiling is significant positively correlated with shallow frying and highly significant positively correlated with deep frying. Shallow frying is significant positively correlated with deep frying. This table indicates that there is a strong correlation present among the **raw state, boiling, open pan dry roasting, shallow frying and deep frying** in 48 hours KMS preservation.

Table no 5.12.5.6.12 Correlation of cooking methods in 14 days preservation with KMS

Condition	RS	B	OPDR	SF	DF
Raw State (RS)	1	.217	.327	-.327	1.000**(S)
Boiling (B)	.217	1	.993(S)	-.993(S)	.217
Open Pan Dry Roasting (OPDR)	.327	.993(S)	1	-1.000**(S)	.327
Shallow Frying (SF)	-.327	-.993(S)	-1.000**(S)	1	-.327
Deep Frying (DF)	1.000**(S)	.217	.327	-.327	1

***.Correlation is highly significant at the 0.01 level (2-tailed)* Positive Negative *S= Significant*

This table shows the correlation of calcium content of pomfret with cooking methods. In 14 days KMS preservation, there is perfect positive correlation present between the raw state and deep frying, whereas boiling is significant positively correlated with open pan dry roasting and significant negatively correlated with shallow frying. Shallow frying is perfect negatively correlated with open pan dry roasting. This table indicates that there is a strong correlation present among the **raw state, boiling, open pan dry roasting, shallow frying and deep frying** in 14 days KMS preservation.

Table no 5.12.5.6.13 Correlation of cooking methods in 15 days preservation with KMS

Condition	RS	B	OPDR	SF	DF
Raw State (RS)	1	-.500	-.954(S)	-.705	-.684
Boiling (B)	-.500	1	.217	.967(S)	.974(S)
Open Pan Dry Roasting (OPDR)	-.954(S)	.217	1	.459	.434
Shallow Frying (SF)	-.705	.967(S)	.459	1	1.000*(S)
Deep Frying (DF)	-.684	.974(S)	.434	1.000*(S)	1

**.Correlation is highly significant at the 0.05 level (2-tailed)* Positive Negative *S= Significant*

This table shows the correlation of calcium content of pomfret with cooking methods. In 15 days KMS preservation, there is significant negative correlation present between the raw state and open pan dry roasting, whereas boiling is significant positively correlated with shallow frying and deep frying. Shallow frying is perfect positively correlated with deep frying. This table shows that there is a strong correlation present among the **raw state, boiling, open pan dry roasting, shallow frying and deep frying** in 15 days KMS preservation.

Overall analysis reveals that the raw state is perfect positively correlated with boiling, open pan dry roasting and deep frying in 48 hours control preservation without preservative, 48 hours salt-turmeric preservation and 14 days KMS preservation respectively, whereas highly significant positively correlated with shallow frying in 14 days control preservation without preservative. Boiling is significant positively correlated with open pan dry roasting in 15 days control preservation without preservative and significant negatively correlated with open pan dry roasting in 24 hours salt-turmeric preservation, whereas highly significant negatively correlated with shallow frying in 24 hours salt and turmeric preservation, and perfect positively correlated with deep frying in 24 hours KMS preservation and 24 hours control preservation without preservative. Open pan dry roasting is perfect negatively correlated with shallow frying in 14 days KMS preservation, and perfect positively correlated with deep frying in 48 hours salt and turmeric preservation. Shallow frying is perfect positively correlated with deep frying in fresh condition and 24 hours control preservation without preservative. Most of the correlation of the calcium content of pomfret is found in **24 hours control preservation without preservative** with respect to different cooking conditions.

5.12.5.7 Iron

Table no 5.12.5.7.1 Correlation of cooking methods in fresh condition

Condition	RS	B	OPDR	SF	DF
Raw State (RS)	1	.971(S)	.721	.327	.991(S)
Boiling (B)	.971(S)	1	.866(S)	.545	.994(S)
Open Pan Dry Roasting (OPDR)	.721	.866(S)	1	.891(S)	.806(S)
Shallow Frying (SF)	.327	.545	.891(S)	1	.449
Deep Frying (DF)	.991(S)	.994(S)	.806(S)	.449	1

Positive *S= Significant*

This table shows the correlation of iron content of pomfret with cooking methods. In fresh condition, there is significant positive correlation present between the raw state with boiling and deep frying, whereas boiling is significant positively correlated with open pan dry roasting and deep frying. Open pan dry roasting is significant positively correlated with shallow frying and deep frying. This table indicates that there is a strong correlation present among the **raw state, boiling, open pan dry roasting, shallow frying and deep frying** in fresh condition.

Table no 5.12.5.7.2 Correlation of cooking methods in 24 hours preservation without preservative

Condition	RS	B	OPDR	SF	DF
Raw state (RS)	1	-.550	-.676	.994(S)	-.676
Boiling (B)	-.550	1	.987(S)	-.454	.987(S)
Open Pan Dry Roasting (OPDR)	-.676	.987(S)	1	-.590	1.000**(S)
Shallow Frying (SF)	.994(S)	-.454	-.590	1	-.590
Deep Frying (DF)	-.676	.987(S)	1.000**(S)	-.590	1

***.Correlation is highly significant at the 0.01 level (2-tailed)* Positive *S= Significant*

This table shows the correlation of iron content of pomfret with cooking methods. In 24 hours control preservation without preservative, there is significant positive correlation present between the raw state and shallow frying, whereas boiling is significant positively correlated with open pan dry roasting and deep frying. Open pan dry roasting is perfect positively correlated with deep frying. This table indicates that there is a strong correlation present among the **raw state, boiling, open pan dry roasting, shallow frying and deep frying** in 24 hours control preservation.

Table no 5.12.5.7.3 Correlation of cooking methods in 48 hours preservation without preservative

Condition	RS	B	OPDR	SF	DF
Raw State (RS)	1	.999*(S)	-.262	.911(S)	.967(S)
Boiling (B)	.999*(S)	1	-.311	.931(S)	.979(S)
Open Pan Dry Roasting (OPDR)	-.262	-.311	1	-.637	-.500
Shallow Frying (SF)	.911(S)	.931(S)	-.637	1	.986(S)
Deep Frying (DF)	.967(S)	.979(S)	-.500	.986(S)	1

**.Correlation is highly significant at the 0.05 level (2-tailed)* ▭ Positive *S= Significant*

This table shows the correlation of iron content of pomfret with cooking methods. In 48 hours control preservation without preservative, there is significant positive correlation present between the raw state with shallow frying and deep frying, and highly significant positive correlation present between the raw state and boiling, whereas boiling is significant positively correlated with shallow frying and deep frying. Shallow frying is significant positively correlated with deep frying. This table indicates that there is a strong correlation present among the **raw state, boiling, shallow frying and deep frying** in 48 hours control preservation.

Table no 5.12.5.7.4 Correlation of cooking methods in 14 days preservation without preservative

Condition	RS	B	OPDR	SF	DF
Raw State (RS)	1	.715	.982(S)	.996(S)	.967(S)
Boiling (B)	.715	1	.569	.775	.870(S)
Open Pan Dry Roasting (OPDR)	.982(S)	.569	1	.961(S)	.901(S)
Shallow Frying (SF)	.996(S)	.775	.961(S)	1	.986(S)
Deep Frying (DF)	.967(S)	.870(S)	.901(S)	.986(S)	1

▭ Positive *S= Significant*

This table shows the correlation of iron content of pomfret with cooking methods. In 14 days control preservation without preservative, there is significant positive correlation present between the raw state with open pan dry roasting, shallow frying and deep frying, whereas boiling is significant positively correlated with deep frying. Open pan dry roasting is significant positively correlated with shallow frying and deep frying. Shallow frying is significant positively correlated with deep frying. This table indicates that there is a strong correlation present among the **raw state, boiling, open pan dry roasting, shallow frying and deep frying** in 14 days control preservation.

Table no 5.12.5.7.5 Correlation of cooking methods in 15 days preservation without preservative

Condition	RS	B	OPDR	SF	DF
Raw State (RS)	1	-.500	.945(S)	.596	.993(S)
Boiling (B)	-.500	1	-.189	.397	-.596
Open Pan Dry Roasting (OPDR)	.945(S)	-.189	1	.826(S)	.901(S)
Shallow Frying (SF)	.596	.397	.826(S)	1	.500
Deep Frying (DF)	.993(S)	-.596	.901(S)	.500	1

▭ Positive *S= Significant*

This table shows the correlation of iron content of pomfret with cooking methods. In 15 days control preservation without preservative, there is significant positive correlation present between the raw state with open pan dry roasting and deep frying, whereas open pan dry roasting is significant positively correlated with shallow frying and deep frying. This table indicates that there is a strong correlation present among the **raw state, open pan dry roasting, shallow frying and deep frying** in 15 days control preservation.

Table no 5.12.5.7.6 Correlation of cooking methods in 24 hours preservation with salt and turmeric

Condition	R	B	OPDR	SF	DF
Raw (R)	1	1.000**(S)	.993(S)	.993(S)	.961(S)
Boiling (B)	1.000**(S)	1	.993(S)	.993(S)	.961(S)
Open Pan Dry Roasting (OPDR)	.993(S)	.993(S)	1	1.000**(S)	.923(S)
Shallow Frying (SF)	.993(S)	.993(S)	1.000**(S)	1	.923(S)
Deep Frying (DF)	.961(S)	.961(S)	.923(S)	.923(S)	1

***.Correlation is highly significant at the 0.01 level (2-tailed)* Positive *S= Significant*

This table shows the correlation of iron content of pomfret with cooking methods. In 24 hours salt and turmeric preservation, there is significant positive correlation present between the raw state with open pan dry roasting, shallow frying and deep frying, and perfect positive correlation present between the raw state and boiling, whereas boiling is significant positively correlated with open pan dry roasting, shallow frying and deep frying. Open pan dry roasting is significant positively correlated with deep frying and perfect positively correlated with shallow frying. Shallow frying is significant positively correlated with deep frying. This table indicates that there is a strong correlation present among the **raw state, boiling, open pan dry roasting, shallow frying and deep frying** in 24 hours salt and turmeric preservation.

Table no 5.12.5.7.7 Correlation of cooking methods in 48 hours preservation with salt and turmeric

Condition	RS	B	OPDR	SF	DF
Raw state (RS)	1	-.596	.596	.596	-1.000**(S)
Boiling (B)	-.596	1	.289	.289	.596
Open Pan Dry Roasting (OPDR)	.596	.289	1	1.000**(S)	-.596
Shallow Frying (SF)	.596	.289	1.000**(S)	1	-.596
Deep Frying (DF)	-1.000**(S)	.596	-.596	-.596	1

***.Correlation is highly significant at the 0.01 level (2-tailed)* Positive Negative *S= Significant*

This table shows the correlation of iron content of pomfret with cooking methods. In 48 hours salt and turmeric preservation, there is perfect negative correlation present between the raw state and deep frying, whereas shallow frying is perfect positively correlated with open pan dry roasting. This table indicates that there is a strong correlation present **between the raw state and deep frying and also between open pan dry roasting and shallow frying** in 48 hours salt and turmeric preservation.

Table no 5.12.5.7.8 Correlation of cooking methods in 14 days preservation with salt and turmeric

Condition	RS	B	OPDR	SF	DF
Raw State (RS)	1	.961(S)	.038	1.000**(S)	-.986(S)
Boiling (B)	.961(S)	1	-.240	.961(S)	-.993(S)
Open Pan Dry Roasting (OPDR)	.038	-.240	1	.038	.127
Shallow Frying (SF)	1.000**(S)	.961(S)	.038	1	-.986(S)
Deep Frying (DF)	-.986(S)	-.993(S)	.127	-.986(S)	1

***.Correlation is highly significant at the 0.01 level (2-tailed)* Positive Negative *S= Significant*

This table shows the correlation of iron content of pomfret with cooking methods. In 14 days salt and turmeric preservation, there is perfect positive correlation present between the raw state and shallow frying, and significant positive correlation present between the raw state and boiling, and significant negative correlation present between the raw state and deep frying. Boiling is significant positively correlated with shallow frying and significant negatively correlated with deep frying. Shallow frying is significant negatively correlated with deep frying. This table indicates that there is a strong correlation present among the **raw state, boiling, shallow frying and deep frying** in 14 days salt and turmeric preservation.

Table no 5.12.5.7.9 Correlation of cooking methods in 15 days preservation with salt and turmeric

Condition	R	B	OPDR	SF	DF
Raw State (RS)	1	-.993(S)	-.596	.684	-.500
Boiling (B)	-.993(S)	1	.500	-.596	.397
Open Pan Dry Roasting (OPDR)	-.596	.500	1	-.993(S)	.993(S)
Shallow Frying (SF)	.684	-.596	-.993(S)	1	-.974(S)
Deep Frying (DF)	-.500	.397	.993(S)	-.974(S)	1

Positive Negative *S= Significant*

This table shows the correlation of iron content of pomfret with cooking methods. In 15 days salt and turmeric preservation, there is significant negative correlation present between the raw state and boiling, whereas open pan dry roasting is significant positively correlated with deep frying and significant negatively correlated with shallow frying. Shallow frying is significant negatively correlated with deep frying. This table indicates that there is a strong correlation present among the **raw state, boiling, open pan dry roasting, shallow frying and deep frying** in 15 days salt and turmeric preservation

Table no 5.12.5.7.10 Correlation of cooking methods in 24 hours preservation with KMS

Condition	RS	B	OPDR	SF	DF
Raw State (RS)	1	-.974(S)	-.500	-.974(S)	-.705
Boiling (B)	-.974(S)	1	.684	1.000**(S)	.524
Open Pan Dry Roasting (OPDR)	-.500	.684	1	.684	-.262
Shallow Frying (SF)	-.974(S)	1.000**(S)	.684	1	.524
Deep Frying (DF)	-.705	.524	-.262	.524	1

***.Correlation is highly significant at the 0.01 level (2-tailed)* Positive Negative *S= Significant*

This table shows the correlation of iron content of pomfret with cooking methods. In 24 hours KMS preservation, there is significant negative correlation present between the raw state with boiling and shallow frying, whereas boiling is perfect positively correlated with shallow frying. This table indicates that there is a strong correlation present among the **raw state, boiling and shallow frying** in 24 hours KMS preservation.

Table no 5.12.5.7.11 Correlation of cooking methods in 48 hours preservation with KMS

Condition	RS	B	OPDR	SF	DF
Raw State (RS)	1	.289	.289	.684	.993(S)
Boiling (B)	.289	1	1.000**(S)	-.500	.397
Open Pan Dry Roasting (OPDR)	.289	1.000**(S)	1	-.500	.397
Shallow Frying (SF)	.684	-.500	-.500	1	.596
Deep Frying (DF)	.993(S)	.397	.397	.596	1

***.Correlation is highly significant at the 0.01 level (2-tailed)* Positive *S= Significant*

This table shows the correlation of iron content of pomfret with cooking methods. In 48 hours KMS preservation, there is significant positive correlation present between the raw state and deep frying, whereas boiling is perfect positively correlated with open pan dry roasting. This table indicates that there is a strong correlation present **between the raw state and deep frying and also between boiling and open pan dry roasting** in 48 hours KMS preservation.

Table no 5.12.5.7.12 Correlation of cooking methods in 14 days preservation with KMS

Condition	RS	B	OPDR	SF	DF
Raw State (RS)	1	.974(S)	1.000**(S)	1.000**(S)	-.826(S)
Boiling (B)	.974(S)	1	.974(S)	.974(S)	-.676
Open Pan Dry Roasting (OPDR)	1.000**(S)	.974(S)	1	1.000**(S)	-.826(S)
Shallow Frying (SF)	1.000**(S)	.974(S)	1.000**(S)	1	-.826(S)
Deep Frying (DF)	-.826(S)	-.676	-.826(S)	-.826(S)	1

***.Correlation is highly significant at the 0.01 level (2-tailed)* Positive Negative *S= Significant*

This table shows the correlation of iron content of pomfret with cooking methods. In 14 days KMS preservation, there is significant positive correlation present between the raw state and boiling, and perfect positive correlation present between the raw state with open pan dry roasting and shallow frying, and significant negative correlation present between the raw state and deep frying. Boiling is significant positively correlated with open pan dry roasting and shallow frying. Open pan dry roasting is significant negatively correlated with deep frying and perfect positively correlated with shallow frying. Shallow frying is significant negatively correlated with deep frying. This table indicates that there is a strong correlation present among the **raw state, boiling, open pan dry roasting, shallow frying and deep frying** in 14 days KMS preservation.

Table no 5.12.5.7.13 Correlation of cooking methods in 15 days preservation with KMS

Condition	RS	B	OPDR	SF	DF
Raw State (RS)	1	1.000**(S)	.923(S)	-.524	-.976(S)
Boiling (B)	1.000**(S)	1	.923(S)	-.524	-.976(S)
Open Pan Dry Roasting (OPDR)	.923(S)	.923(S)	1	-.812(S)	-.817(S)
Shallow Frying (SF)	-.524	-.524	-.812(S)	1	.327
Deep Frying (DF)	-.976(S)	-.976(S)	-.817(S)	.327	1

***.Correlation is highly significant at the 0.01 level (2-tailed)* Positive Negative *S= Significant*

This table shows the correlation of iron content of pomfret with cooking methods. In 15 days KMS preservation, there is significant positive correlation present between the raw state and open pan dry roasting, and perfect positive correlation present between the raw state and boiling, and significant negative correlation present between the raw state and deep frying. Boiling is significant negatively correlated with deep frying. Open pan dry roasting is significant negatively correlated with shallow frying and deep frying. This table indicates that there is a strong correlation present among the **raw state, boiling, open pan dry roasting, shallow frying and deep frying** in 15 days KMS preservation.

Overall analysis reveals that the raw state is perfect positively correlated with boiling and open pan dry roasting in 24 hours salt-turmeric preservation, 14 days KMS preservation respectively, whereas perfect positively correlated with shallow frying in 14 days KMS preservation as well as 14 days salt-turmeric preservation, and perfect negatively correlated with deep frying in 48 hours salt-turmeric preservation. Boiling is perfect positively correlated with open pan dry roasting in 48 hours and 24 hours KMS preservation respectively, whereas significant negatively correlated with deep frying in 14 days salt and turmeric preservation. Open pan dry roasting is perfect positively correlated with shallow frying in 24 hours and 48 hours salt and turmeric preservation and 14 days KMS preservation, and perfect positively correlated with deep frying in 24 hours control preservation without preservative. Shallow frying is significant positively correlated with deep frying in 48 hours control preservation without preservative and 14 days salt-turmeric preservation respectively. Most of the correlation of the iron content of pomfret is found in **14 days salt and turmeric preservation and 14 days KMS preservation** with respect to different cooking conditions.

5.12.5.8 Energy

Table no 5.12.5.8.1 Correlation of cooking methods in fresh condition

Condition	RS	B	OPDR	SF	DF
Raw State (RS)	1	-.152	.867(S)	.142	.640
Boiling (B)	-.152	1	.360	-1.000**(S)	-.857(S)
Open Pan Dry Roasting (OPDR)	.867(S)	.360	1	-.369	.173
Shallow Frying (SF)	.142	-1.000**(S)	-.369	1	.852(S)
Deep Frying (DF)	.640	-.857(S)	.173	.852(S)	1

***.Correlation is highly significant at the 0.01 level (2-tailed)* Positive Negative *S= Significant*

This table shows the correlation of energy content of pomfret with cooking methods. In fresh condition, there is significant positive correlation present between the raw state and open pan dry roasting, whereas boiling is significant negatively correlated with deep frying and perfect negatively correlated with shallow frying. Shallow frying is significant positively correlated with deep frying. This table indicates that there is a strong correlation present among the **raw state, boiling, open pan dry roasting, shallow frying and deep frying** in fresh condition.

Table no 5.12.5.8.2 Correlation of cooking methods in 24 hours preservation without preservative

Condition	RS	B	OPDR	SF	DF
Raw state (RS)	1	-.983(S)	-.541	-.214	.412
Boiling (B)	-.983(S)	1	.688	.391	-.236
Open Pan Dry Roasting (OPDR)	-.541	.688	1	.937(S)	.543
Shallow Frying (SF)	-.214	.391	.937(S)	1	.802(S)
Deep Frying (DF)	.412	-.236	.543	.802(S)	1

Positive Negative *S= Significant*

This table shows the correlation of energy content of pomfret with cooking methods. In 24 hours control preservation without preservative, there is significant negative correlation present between the raw state and boiling, whereas open pan dry roasting is significant positively correlated with shallow frying. Shallow frying is significant positively correlated with deep frying. This table indicates that there is a strong correlation present among the **raw state, boiling, open pan dry roasting, shallow frying and deep frying** in 24 hours control preservation.

Table no 5.12.5.8.3 Correlation of cooking methods in 48 hours preservation without preservative

Condition	RS	B	OPDR	SF	DF
Raw state (RS)	1	-.710	-.849(S)	-.745	.102
Boiling (B)	-.710	1	.231	.999*(S)	.628
Open Pan Dry Roasting (OPDR)	-.849(S)	.231	1	.280	-.612
Shallow Frying (SF)	-.745	.999*(S)	.280	1	.587
Deep Frying (DF)	.102	.628	-.612	.587	1

**.Correlation is highly significant at the 0.05 level (2-tailed0* Positive Negative *S= Significant*

This table shows the correlation of energy content of pomfret with cooking methods. In 48 hours control preservation without preservative, there is significant negative correlation present between the raw state and open pan dry roasting, whereas boiling is highly significant positively correlated with shallow frying. This table indicates that there is a strong correlation present **between the raw state and open pan dry roasting and also between boiling and shallow frying** in 48 hours control preservation.

Table no 5.12.5.8.4 Correlation of cooking methods in 14 days preservation without preservative

Condition	RS	B	OPDR	SF	DF
Raw State (RS)	1	-.898(S)	-.576	.542	.475
Boiling (B)	-.898(S)	1	.877(S)	-.118	-.814(S)
Open Pan Dry Roasting (OPDR)	-.576	.877(S)	1	.374	-.993(S)
Shallow Frying (SF)	.542	-.118	.374	1	-.481
Deep Frying (DF)	.475	-.814(S)	-.993(S)	-.481	1

**.Correlation is highly significant at the 0.05 level (2-tailed)* Positive Negative *S= Significant*

This table shows the correlation of energy content of pomfret with cooking methods. In 14 days control preservation without preservative, there is significant negative correlation present between the raw state and open pan dry roasting, whereas boiling is highly significant positively correlated with shallow frying. This table indicates that there is a strong correlation present **between the raw state and open pan dry roasting and also between boiling and shallow frying** in 48 hours control preservation.

Table no 5.12.5.8.5 Correlation of cooking methods in 15 days preservation without preservative

Condition	RS	B	OPDR	SF	DF
Raw state (RS)	1	.521	-1.000**(S)	-.179	-.375
Boiling (B)	.521	1	-.523	.747	-.987(S)
Open Pan Dry Roasting (OPDR)	-1.000**(S)	-.523	1	.176	.378
Shallow Frying (SF)	-.179	.747	.176	1	-.845(S)
Deep Frying (DF)	-.375	-.987(S)	.378	-.845(S)	1

***.Correlation is highly significant at the 0.01 level (2-tailed)* Negative *S= Significant*

This table shows the correlation of energy content of pomfret with cooking methods. In 15 days control preservation without preservative, there is perfect negative correlation present between the raw state and open pan dry roasting, whereas boiling is significant negatively correlated with deep frying. Shallow frying is significant negatively correlated with deep frying. This table indicates that there is a strong correlation present among the **raw state, boiling, open pan dry roasting, shallow frying and deep frying** in 15 days control preservation.

Table no 5.12.5.8.6 Correlation of cooking methods in 24 hours preservation with salt and turmeric

Condition	RS	B	OPDR	SF	DF
Raw State (RS)	1	-.849(S)	.263	.409	-.829(S)
Boiling (B)	-.849(S)	1	-.733	.135	.408
Open Pan Dry Roasting (OPDR)	.263	-.733	1	-.773	.321
Shallow Frying (SF)	.409	.135	-.773	1	-.849(S)
Deep Frying (DF)	-.829(S)	.408	.321	-.849(S)	1

Negative *S= Significant*

This table shows the correlation of energy content of pomfret with cooking methods. In 24 hours salt and turmeric preservation, there is significant negative correlation present between the raw state with boiling and deep frying, whereas shallow frying is significant negatively correlated with deep frying. This table indicates that there is a strong correlation present among the **raw state, boiling, shallow frying and deep frying** in 24 hours salt and turmeric preservation.

Table no 5.12.5.8.7 Correlation of cooking methods in 48 hours preservation with salt and turmeric

Condition	RS	B	OPDR	SF	DF
Raw State (RS)	1	-.600	.675	.676	-.425
Boiling (B)	-.600	1	-.995(S)	-.995(S)	-.469
Open Pan Dry Roasting (OPDR)	.675	-.995(S)	1	1.000**(S)	.381
Shallow Frying (SF)	.676	-.995(S)	1.000**(S)	1	.380
Deep Frying (DF)	-.425	-.469	.381	.380	1

***.Correlation is highly significant at the 0.01 level (2-tailed)* Positive Negative *S= Significant*

This table shows the correlation of energy content of pomfret with cooking methods. In 48 hours salt and turmeric preservation, there is significant negative correlation present between boiling with open pan dry roasting and shallow frying, whereas shallow frying is perfect positively correlated with open pan dry roasting. This table indicates that there is a strong correlation present among **boiling, open pan dry roasting and shallow frying** in 48 hours salt and turmeric preservation.

Table no 5.12.5.8.8 Correlation of cooking methods in 14 days preservation with salt and turmeric

Condition	RS	B	OPDR	SF	DF
Raw State (RS)	1	.986(S)	.273	.441	-.859(S)
Boiling (B)	.986(S)	1	.432	.586	-.933(S)
Open Pan Dry Roasting (OPDR)	.273	.432	1	.984(S)	-.727
Shallow Frying (SF)	.441	.586	.984(S)	1	-.838(S)
Deep Frying (DF)	-.859(S)	-.933(S)	-.727	-.838(S)	1

Positive Negative *S= Significant*

This table shows the correlation of energy content of pomfret with cooking methods. In 14 days salt and turmeric preservation, there is significant negative correlation present between the raw state and deep frying, and significant positive correlation present between the raw state and boiling, whereas boiling is significant negatively correlated with deep frying. Open pan dry roasting is significant positively correlated with shallow frying. Shallow frying is significant negatively correlated with deep frying. This table indicates that there is a strong correlation present among the **raw state, boiling, open pan dry roasting, shallow frying and deep frying** in 14 days salt and turmeric preservation.

Table no 5.12.5.8.9 Correlation of cooking methods in 15 days preservation with salt and turmeric

Condition	RS	B	OPDR	SF	DF
Raw state (RS)	1	-.123	-.918(S)	.998*(S)	-.855(S)
Boiling (B)	-.123	1	.506	-.179	.619
Open Pan Dry Roasting (OPDR)	-.918(S)	.506	1	-.939(S)	.991(S)
Shallow Frying (SF)	.998*(S)	-.179	-.939(S)	1	-.883(S)
Deep Frying (DF)	-.855(S)	.619	.991(S)	-.883(S)	1

**.Correlation is highly significant at the 0.05 level (2-tailed)* ▢ Positive ▢ Negative *S= Significant*

This table shows the correlation of energy content of pomfret with cooking methods. In 15 days salt and turmeric preservation, there is significant negative correlation present between the raw state with open pan dry roasting and deep frying, and highly significant positive correlation present between the raw state and shallow frying, whereas open pan dry roasting is significant negatively correlated with shallow frying and significant positively correlated with deep frying. Shallow frying is significant negatively correlated with deep frying. This table indicates that there is a strong correlation present among the **raw state, open pan dry roasting, shallow frying and deep frying** in 15 days salt and turmeric preservation.

Table no 5.12.5.8.10 Correlation of cooking methods in 24 hours preservation with KMS

Condition	RS	B	OPDR	SF	DF
Raw state (RS)	1	-1.000**(S)	.531	-.998*(S)	.857(S)
Boiling (B)	-1.000**(S)	1	-.533	.998*(S)	-.858(S)
Open Pan Dry Roasting (OPDR)	.531	-.533	1	-.588	.892(S)
Shallow Frying (SF)	-.998*(S)	.998*(S)	-.588	1	-.890(S)
Deep Frying (DF)	.857(S)	-.858(S)	.892(S)	-.890(S)	1

***.Correlation is highly significant at the 0.01 level (2-tailed)* ▢ Positive ▢ Negative *S= Significant*

This table shows the correlation of energy content of pomfret with cooking methods. In 24 hours KMS preservation, there is highly significant negative correlation present between the raw state and shallow frying, and perfect negative correlation present between the raw state and boiling, and significant positive correlation present between the raw state and deep frying, whereas boiling is significant negatively correlated with deep frying and highly significant positively correlated with shallow frying. Open pan dry roasting is significant positively correlated with deep frying. Shallow frying is significant negatively correlated with deep frying. This table indicates that there is a strong correlation present among the **raw state, boiling, open pan dry roasting, shallow frying and deep frying** in 24 hours KMS preservation.

Table no 5.12.5.8.11 Correlation of cooking methods in 48 hours preservation with KMS

Condition	RS	B	OPDR	SF	DF
Raw state (RS)	1	-.951(S)	-1.000*(S)	-.552	-.580
Boiling (B)	-.951(S)	1	.957(S)	.782	.301
Open Pan Dry Roasting (OPDR)	-1.000*(S)	.957(S)	1	.568	.564
Shallow Frying (SF)	-.552	.782	.568	1	-.359
Deep Frying (DF)	-.580	.301	.564	-.359	1

**.Correlation is highly significant at the 0.05 level (2-tailed)* ▢ Positive ▢ Negative *S= Significant*

This table shows the correlation of energy content of pomfret with cooking methods. In 48 hours KMS preservation, there is significant negative correlation present between the raw state and boiling, and perfect negative correlation present between the raw state and open pan dry roasting, whereas boiling is significant positively correlated with open pan dry roasting. This table indicates that there is a strong correlation present among the **raw state, boiling and open pan dry roasting** in 48 hours KMS preservation.

Table no 5.12.5.8.12 Correlation of cooking methods in 14 days preservation with KMS

Condition	RS	B	OPDR	SF	DF
Raw State (RS)	1	1.000**(S)	1.000*(S)	.836(S)	1.000**(S)
Boiling (B)	1.000**(S)	1	1.000*(S)	.843(S)	1.000*(S)
Open Pan Dry Roasting (OPDR)	1.000*(S)	1.000*(S)	1	.827(S)	1.000**(S)
Shallow Frying (SF)	.836(S)	.843(S)	.827(S)	1	.829(S)
Deep Frying (DF)	1.000**(S)	1.000*(S)	1.000**(S)	.829(S)	1

**.Correlation is highly significant at the 0.05 level (2-tailed)* ▭ Positive *S= Significant*
***.Correlation is highly significant at the 0.01 level (2-tailed)*

This table shows the correlation of energy content of pomfret with cooking methods. In 14 days KMS preservation, there is perfect positive correlation present between the raw state with boiling, open pan dry roasting and deep frying, and significant positive correlation present between the raw state and shallow frying, whereas boiling is perfect positively correlated with open pan dry roasting and deep frying and significant positively correlated with shallow frying. Open pan dry roasting is perfect positively correlated with deep frying and significant positively correlated with shallow frying. Shallow frying is significant positively correlated with deep frying. This table indicates that there is a strong correlation present among the **raw state, boiling, open pan dry roasting, shallow frying and deep frying** in 14 days KMS preservation.

Table no 5.12.5.8.13 Correlation of cooking methods in 15 days preservation with KMS

Condition	RS	B	OPDR	SF	DF
Raw State (RS)	1	.910(S)	.982(S)	.136	.134
Boiling (B)	.910(S)	1	.973(S)	-.286	-.288
Open Pan Dry Roasting (OPDR)	.982(S)	.973(S)	1	-.055	-.057
Shallow Frying (SF)	.136	-.286	-.055	1	1.000**(S)
Deep Frying (DF)	.134	-.288	-.057	1.000**(S)	1

***.Correlation is highly significant at the 0.01 level (2-tailed)* ▭ Positive *S= Significant*

This table shows the correlation of energy content of pomfret with cooking methods. In 15 days KMS preservation, there is significant positive correlation present between the raw state with boiling and open pan dry roasting, whereas boiling is significant positively correlated with open pan dry roasting. Shallow frying is perfect positively correlated with deep frying. This table indicates that there is a strong correlation present among the **raw state, boiling, open pan dry roasting, shallow frying and deep frying** in 15 days KMS preservation.

Overall analysis reveals that the raw state is perfect negatively correlated with boiling in 24 hours KMS preservation and perfect positively correlated with boiling in 14 days KMS preservation, whereas perfect positively correlated with open pan dry roasting in 14 days preservation with KMS and perfect negatively correlated with open pan dry roasting in 48 hours KMS preservation and 15 days control preservation without preservative, highly significant positively correlated with shallow frying in 15 days salt and turmeric preservation and highly significant negatively correlated with shallow frying in 24 hours KMS preservation, and perfect positively correlated with deep frying in 14 days KMS preservation. Boiling is perfect positively correlated with open pan dry roasting and deep frying in 14 days KMS preservation, whereas perfect negatively correlated with shallow frying in fresh condition. Open pan dry roasting is perfect positively correlated with shallow frying and deep frying in 48 hours salt and turmeric preservation and 14 days KMS preservation respectively. Shallow frying is significant negatively correlated with deep frying in 24 hours KMS preservation. Most of the correlation of the energy content of pomfret is found in **14 days KMS preservation** with respect to different cooking conditions.

5.12.6 *Hilsa (Tenualosa ilisha)*

5.12.6.1 Carbohydrate

Table no 5.12.6.1.1 Correlation of cooking methods in fresh condition

Condition	RS	B	OPDR	SF	DF
Raw state (RS)	1	.755	.972(S)	-.900(S)	-.072
Boiling (B)	.755	1	.579	-.966(S)	-.708
Open Pan Dry Roasting (OPDR)	.972(S)	.579	1	-.771	.165
Shallow Frying (SF)	-.900(S)	-.966(S)	-.771	1	.500
Deep Frying (DF)	-.072	-.708	.165	.500	1

Positive Negative *S= Significant*

This table shows the correlation of carbohydrate content of *hilsa* with cooking methods. In fresh condition, there is significant positive correlation present between the raw state and open pan dry roasting, and significant negative correlation present between the raw state and shallow frying, whereas boiling is significant negatively correlated with shallow frying. This table indicates that there is a strong correlation present among the **raw state, boiling, open pan dry roasting and shallow frying** in fresh condition.

Table no 5.12.6.1.2 Correlation of cooking methods in 24 hours preservation without preservative

Condition	RS	B	OPDR	SF	DF
Raw State (RS)	1	-.636	.445	-.127	.808(S)
Boiling (B)	-.636	1	-.974(S)	.846(S)	-.059
Open Pan Dry Roasting (OPDR)	.445	-.974(S)	1	-.945(S)	-.169
Shallow Frying (SF)	-.127	.846(S)	-.945(S)	1	.482
Deep Frying (DF)	.808(S)	-.059	-.169	.482	1

Positive Negative *S= Significant*

This table shows the correlation of carbohydrate content of *hilsa* with cooking methods. In 24 hours control preservation without preservative, there is significant positive correlation present between the raw state and deep frying, whereas boiling is significant negatively correlated with open pan dry roasting and significant positively correlated with shallow frying. Open pan dry roasting is significant negatively correlated with shallow frying. This table indicates that there is a strong correlation present among the **raw state, boiling, open pan dry roasting, shallow frying and deep frying** in 24 hours control preservation.

Table no 5.12.6.1.3 Correlation of cooking methods in 48 hours preservation without preservative

Condition	RS	B	OPDR	SF	DF
Raw State (RS)	1	.951	.733	.670	.798
Boiling (B)	.951	1	.907	.866	.945
Open Pan Dry Roasting (OPDR)	.733	.907	1	.996	.995
Shallow Frying (SF)	.670	.866	.996	1	.982
Deep Frying (DF)	.798	.945	.995	.982	1

▭ Positive *S= Significant*

This table shows the correlation of carbohydrate content of *hilsa* with cooking methods. In 48 hours control preservation without preservative, there is significant positive correlation present between the raw state and boiling, whereas boiling is significant positively correlated with open pan dry roasting, shallow and deep frying. Open pan dry roasting is significant positively correlated with shallow frying and deep frying. Shallow frying is significant positively correlated with deep frying. This table indicates that there is a strong correlation present among the **raw state, boiling, open pan dry roasting, shallow frying and deep frying** in 48 hours control preservation.

Table no 5.12.6.1.4 Correlation of cooking methods in 14 days preservation without preservative

Condition	RS	B	OPDR	SF	DF
Raw State (RS)	1	.235	-.176	.416	.974(S)
Boiling (B)	.235	1	-.998*(S)	-.786	.449
Open Pan Dry Roasting (OPDR)	-.176	-.998* (S)	1	.822(S)	-.394
Shallow Frying (SF)	.416	-.786	.822(S)	1	.200
Deep Frying (DF)	.974(S)	.449	-.394	.200	1

**.Correlation is highly significant at the 0.05 level (2-tailed)* ▭ Positive ▭ Negative *S= Significant*

This table shows the correlation of carbohydrate content of *hilsa* with cooking methods. In 14 days control preservation without preservative, there is significant positive correlation present between the raw state and deep frying, whereas boiling is highly significant negatively correlated with open pan dry roasting. Open pan dry roasting is significant positively correlated with shallow frying. This table indicates that there is a strong correlation present among the **raw state, boiling, open pan dry roasting, shallow frying and deep frying** in 14 days control preservation.

Table no 5.12.6.1.5 Correlation of cooking methods in 15 days preservation without preservative

Condition	RS	B	OPDR	SF	DF
Raw state (RS)	1	.982(S)	.143	.982(S)	.982(S)
Boiling (B)	.982(S)	1	.327	1.000**(S)	1.000**(S)
Open Pan Dry Roasting (OPDR)	.143	.327	1	.327	.327
Shallow Frying (SF)	.982(S)	1.000**(S)	.327	1	1.000**(S)
Deep Frying (DF)	.982(S)	1.000**(S)	.327	1.000**(S)	1

***.Correlation is highly significant at the 0.01 level (2-tailed)* ▭ Positive *S= Significant*

This table shows the correlation of carbohydrate content of *hilsa* with cooking methods. In 15 days control preservation without preservative, there is significant positive correlation present between the raw state with boiling, shallow frying and deep frying, whereas boiling is perfect positively correlated with shallow frying and deep frying. Shallow frying is perfect positively correlated with deep frying. This table indicates that there is a strong correlation present among the **raw state, boiling, shallow frying and deep frying** in 15 days control preservation.

Table no 5.12.6.1.6 Correlation of cooking methods in 24 hours preservation with salt and turmeric

Condition	RS	B	OPDR	SF	DF
Raw State (RS)	1	-.915(S)	-.904(S)	.108	-.807(S)
Boiling (B)	-.915(S)	1	.655	-.500	.500
Open Pan Dry Roasting (OPDR)	-.904(S)	.655	1	.327	.982(S)
Shallow Frying (SF)	.108	-.500	.327	1	.500
Deep Frying (DF)	-.807(S)	.500	.982(S)	.500	1

Positive Negative *S= Significant*

This table shows the correlation of carbohydrate content of *hilsa* with cooking methods. In 24 hours salt and turmeric preservation, there is significant negative correlation present between the raw state with boiling, open pan dry roasting and deep frying, whereas open pan dry roasting is significant positively correlated with deep frying. This table indicates that there is a strong correlation present among the **raw state, boiling, open pan dry roasting and deep frying** in 24 hours salt and turmeric preservation.

Table no 5.12.6.1.7 Correlation of cooking methods in 48 hours preservation with salt and turmeric

Condition	RS	B	OPDR	SF	DF
Raw State (RS)	1	-.569	-.427	.404	.569
Boiling (B)	-.569	1	-.500	-.982(S)	-1.000**(S)
Open Pan Dry Roasting (OPDR)	-.427	-.500	1	.655	.500
Shallow Frying (SF)	.404	-.982(S)	.655	1	.982(S)
Deep Frying (DF)	.569	-1.000**(S)	.500	.982(S)	1

***.Correlation is highly significant at the 0.01 level (2-tailed)* Positive Negative *S= Significant*

This table shows the correlation of carbohydrate content of *hilsa* with cooking methods. In 48 hours salt and turmeric preservation, there is significant negative correlation present between boiling and shallow frying, and perfect negative correlation present between boiling and deep frying, whereas shallow frying is significant positively correlated with deep frying. This table indicates that there is a strong correlation present among **boiling, shallow frying and deep frying** in 48 hours salt and turmeric preservation.

Table no 5.12.6.1.8 Correlation of cooking methods in 14 days preservation with salt and turmeric

Condition	RS	B	OPDR	SF	DF
Raw State (RS)	1	.982(S)	.419	-.982(S)	.500
Boiling (B)	.982(S)	1	.240	-1.000**(S)	.327
Open Pan Dry Roasting (OPDR)	.419	.240	1	-.240	.996(S)
Shallow Frying (SF)	-.982(S)	-1.000**(S)	-.240	1	-.327
Deep Frying (DF)	.500	.327	.996(S)	-.327	1

***.Correlation is highly significant at the 0.01 level (2-tailed)* Positive Negative *S= Significant*

This table shows the correlation of carbohydrate content of *hilsa* with cooking methods. In 14 days salt and turmeric preservation, there is significant negative correlation present between the raw state and boiling, and significant negative correlation present between the raw state and shallow frying, whereas boiling is perfect negatively correlated with shallow frying. Open pan dry roasting is significant positively correlated with deep frying. This table indicates that there is a strong correlation present among the **raw state, boiling, open pan dry roasting, shallow frying and deep frying** in 14 days salt and turmeric preservation.

Table no 5.12.6.1.9 Correlation of cooking methods in 15 days preservation with salt and turmeric

Condition	RS	B	OPDR	SF	DF
Raw State (RS)	1	.500	-1.000**(S)	-1.000**(S)	-.993(S)
Boiling (B)	.500	1	-.500	-.500	-.596
Open Pan Dry Roasting (OPDR)	-1.000**(S)	-.500	1	1.000**(S)	.993(S)
Shallow Frying (SF)	-1.000**(S)	-.500	1.000**(S)	1	.993(S)
Deep Frying (DF)	-.993	-.596	.993(S)	.993(S)	1

***.Correlation is highly significant at the 0.01 level (2-tailed)* Positive Negative *S= Significant*

This table shows the correlation of carbohydrate content of *hilsa* with cooking methods. In 15 days salt and turmeric preservation, there is significant negative correlation present between the raw state and deep frying, and perfect negative correlation present between the raw state with open pan dry roasting and shallow frying, whereas open pan dry roasting is perfect positively correlated with shallow frying and significant positively correlated with deep frying. Shallow frying is significant positively correlated with deep frying. This table indicates that there is a strong correlation present among the **raw state, open pan dry roasting, shallow frying and deep frying** in 15 days salt and turmeric preservation.

Table no 5.12.6.1.10 Correlation of cooking methods in 24 hours preservation with KMS

Condition	RS	B	OPDR	SF	DF
Raw State (RS)	1	-.500	-1.000**(S)	-.655	.982(S)
Boiling (B)	-.500	1	.500	.982(S)	-.655
Open Pan Dry Roasting (OPDR)	-1.000**(S)	.500	1	.655	-.982(S)
Shallow Frying (SF)	-.655	.982(S)	.655	1	-.786
Deep Frying (DF)	.982(S)	-.655	-.982(S)	-.786	1

***.Correlation is highly significant at the 0.01 level (2-tailed)* Positive Negative *S= Significant*

This table shows the correlation of carbohydrate content of *hilsa* with cooking methods. In 24 hours KMS preservation, there is perfect negative correlation present between the raw state and open pan dry roasting, and significant positive correlation present between the raw state and deep frying, whereas boiling is significant positively correlated with shallow frying. Open pan dry roasting is significant negatively correlated with deep frying. This table indicates that there is a strong correlation present among the **raw state, boiling, open pan dry roasting, shallow frying and deep frying** in 24 hours KMS preservation.

Table no 5.12.6.1.11 Correlation of cooking methods in 48 hours preservation with KMS

Condition	RS	B	OPDR	SF	DF
Raw State (RS)	1	-.982(S)	1.000**(S)	-.327	.327
Boiling (B)	-.982(S)	1	-.982(S)	.143	-.500
Open Pan Dry Roasting (OPDR)	1.000**(S)	-.982(S)	1	-.327	.327
Shallow Frying (SF)	-.327	.143	-.327	1	.786
Deep Frying (DF)	.327	-.500	.327	.786	1

***.Correlation is highly significant at the 0.01 level (2-tailed)* Positive Negative *S= Significant*

This table shows the correlation of carbohydrate content of *hilsa* with cooking methods. In 48 hours KMS preservation, there is perfect positive correlation present between the raw state and open pan dry roasting, and significant negative correlation present between the raw state and boiling, whereas boiling is significant negatively correlated with open pan dry roasting. This table indicates that there is a strong correlation present among the **raw state, boiling and open pan dry roasting** in 48 hours KMS preservation.

Table no 5.12.6.1.12 Correlation of cooking methods in 14 days preservation with KMS

Condition	RS	B	OPDR	SF	DF
Raw State (RS)	1	1.000** (S)	1.000** (S)	-1.000** (S)	1.000** (S)
Boiling (B)	1.000** (S)	1	1.000** (S)	-1.000** (S)	1.000** (S)
Open Pan Dry Roasting (OPDR)	1.000** (S)	1.000** (S)	1	-1.000** (S)	1.000** (S)
Shallow Frying (SF)	-1.000** (S)	-1.000** (S)	-1.000** (S)	1	-1.000** (S)
Deep Frying (DF)	1.000** (S)	1.000** (S)	1.000** (S)	-1.000** (S)	1

***.Correlation is highly significant at the 0.01 level (2-tailed)* Positive Negative *S= Significant*

This table shows the correlation of carbohydrate content of *hilsa* with cooking methods. In 14 days KMS preservation, there is perfect positive correlation present between the raw state with boiling, open pan dry roasting and deep frying, and perfect negative correlation present between the raw state and shallow frying, whereas both boiling and open pan dry roasting are perfect negatively correlated with shallow frying and perfect positively correlated with deep frying. Shallow frying is perfect negatively correlated with deep frying. This table indicates that there is a strong correlation present among the **raw state, boiling, open pan dry roasting, shallow frying and deep frying** in 14 days KMS preservation.

Table no 5.12.6.1.13 Correlation of cooking methods in 15 days preservation with KMS

Condition	RS	B	OPDR	SF	DF
Raw State (RS)	1	-1.000** (S)	-1.000** (S)	-.500	1.000** (S)
Boiling (B)	-1.000** (S)	1	1.000** (S)	.500	-1.000** (S)
Open Pan Dry Roasting (OPDR)	-1.000** (S)	1.000** (S)	1	.500	-1.000** (S)
Shallow Frying (SF)	-.500	.500	.500	1	-.500
Deep Frying (DF)	1.000** (S)	-1.000** (S)	-1.000** (S)	-.500	1

***.Correlation is highly significant at the 0.01 level (2-tailed)* Positive Negative *S= Significant*

This table shows the correlation of carbohydrate content of *hilsa* with cooking methods. In 15 days KMS preservation, there is perfect negative correlation present between the raw state with boiling and open pan dry roasting, and perfect positive correlation present between the raw state and deep frying, whereas boiling is perfect negatively correlated with deep frying and perfect positively correlated with open pan dry roasting. Open pan dry roasting is perfect negatively correlated with deep frying. This table indicates that there is a strong correlation present among the **raw state, boiling, open pan dry roasting and deep frying** in 15 days KMS preservation.

Overall analysis reveals that the raw state is perfect positively correlated with boiling in 14 days KMS preservation and perfect negatively correlated with boiling in 15 days KMS preservation, whereas perfect positively correlated with open pan dry roasting in 48 hours and 14 days preservation with KMS and perfect negatively correlated with open pan dry roasting in 15 days salt-turmeric preservation and 24 hours and 15 days KMS preservation, perfect negatively correlated with shallow frying in 15 days salt and turmeric preservation and 14 days KMS preservation, and perfect positively correlated with deep frying in 14 days and 15 days KMS preservation. Boiling is perfect positively correlated with open pan dry roasting in 14 days KMS preservation, whereas perfect negatively correlated with shallow frying in 14 days salt-turmeric preservation and 14 days KMS preservation, and perfect positively correlated with deep frying in 15 days control preservation without preservative and 14 days KMS preservation and perfect negatively correlated with deep frying in 48 hours salt-turmeric preservation. Open pan dry roasting is perfect positively correlated with shallow frying in 15 days salt and turmeric preservation and 14 days KMS preservation, and perfect positively correlated with deep frying in 15 days control preservation without preservative and 14 days KMS preservation. Shallow frying is perfect negatively correlated with deep frying in 14 days KMS preservation. Most of the correlation of the carbohydrate content of pomfret is found in **14 days KMS preservation** with respect to different cooking conditions.

5.12.6.2 Protein

Table no 5.12.6.2.1 Correlation of cooking methods in fresh condition

Condition	RS	B	OPDR	SF	DF
Raw State (RS)	1	-.515	.992(S)	-.984(S)	.500
Boiling (B)	-.515	1	-.621	.355	-1.000*(S)
Open Pan Dry Roasting (OPDR)	.992(S)	-.621	1	-.953(S)	.607
Shallow Frying (SF)	-.984(S)	.355	-.953(S)	1	-.338
Deep Frying (DF)	.500	-1.000*(S)	.607	-.338	1

**.Correlation is highly significant at the 0.05 level (2-tailed)* Positive Negative *S= Significant*

This table shows the correlation of protein content of *hilsa* with cooking methods. In fresh condition, there is significant positive correlation present between the raw state and open pan dry roasting, and significant negative correlation present between the raw state and shallow frying, whereas boiling is perfect negatively correlated with deep frying. Shallow frying is significant negatively correlated with open pan dry roasting. This table indicates that there is a strong correlation present among the **raw state, boiling, open pan dry roasting, shallow frying and deep frying** in fresh condition.

Table no 5.12.6.2.2 Correlation of cooking methods in 24 hours preservation without preservative

Condition	RS	B	OPDR	SF	DF
Raw State (RS)	1	.009	.721	.775	-.602
Boiling (B)	.009	1	.700	-.625	.793
Open Pan Dry Roasting (OPDR)	.721	.700	1	.120	.120
Shallow Frying (SF)	.775	-.625	.120	1	-.971(S)
Deep Frying (DF)	-.602	.793	.120	-.971(S)	1

Negative *S= Significant*

This table shows the correlation of protein content of *hilsa* with cooking methods. In 24 hours control preservation without preservative, there is significant negative correlation present between shallow frying and deep frying. This table indicates that there is a strong correlation present between **shallow frying and deep frying** in 24 hours control preservation without preservative.

Table no 5.12.6.2.3 Correlation of cooking methods in 48 hours preservation without preservative

Condition	RS	B	OPDR	SF	DF
Raw State (RS)	1	-.999*(S)	-.536	.886(S)	-.749
Boiling (B)	-.999*(S)	1	.500	-.866(S)	.721
Open Pan Dry Roasting (OPDR)	-.536	.500	1	-.866(S)	.961(S)
Shallow Frying (SF)	.886(S)	-.866(S)	-.866(S)	1	-.971(S)
Deep Frying (DF)	-.749	.721	.961(S)	-.971(S)	1

**.Correlation is highly significant at the 0.05 level (2-tailed)* Positive Negative *S= Significant*

This table shows the correlation of protein content of *hilsa* with cooking methods. In 48 hours control preservation without preservative, there is significant positive correlation present between the raw state and shallow frying, and highly significant negative correlation present between the raw state and boiling, whereas boiling is significant negatively correlated with shallow frying. Open pan dry roasting is significant negatively correlated with shallow frying and significant positively correlated with deep frying. Shallow frying is significant negatively correlated with deep frying This table indicates that there is a strong correlation present among the **raw state, boiling, open pan dry roasting, shallow frying and deep frying** in 48 hours control preservation without preservative.

Table no 5.12.6.2.4 Correlation of cooking methods in 14 days preservation without preservative

Condition	RS	B	OPDR	SF	DF
Raw State (RS)	1	-.537	-.508	.931(S)	-1.000**(S)
Boiling (B)	-.537	1	.999*(S)	-.191	.537
Open Pan Dry Roasting (OPDR)	-.508	.999*(S)	1	-.157	.508
Shallow Frying (SF)	.931(S)	-.191	-.157	1	-.931(S)
Deep Frying (DF)	-1.000**(S)	.537	.508	-.931(S)	1

**.Correlation is highly significant at the 0.05 level (2-tailed)* Positive Negative *S= Significant*
***.Correlation is highly significant at the 0.01 level (2-tailed)*

This table shows the correlation of protein content of *hilsa* with cooking methods. In 14 days control preservation without preservative, there is significant positive correlation present between the raw state and shallow frying, and perfect negative correlation present between the raw state and deep frying, whereas boiling is highly significant positively correlated with open pan dry roasting. Shallow frying is significant negatively correlated with deep frying. This table indicates that there is a strong correlation present among the **raw state, boiling, open pan dry roasting, shallow frying and deep frying** in 14 days control preservation without preservative

Table no 5.12.6.2.5 Correlation of cooking methods in 15 days preservation without preservative

Condition	RS	B	OPDR	SF	DF
Raw State (RS)	1	.985(S)	-.159	.569	-.866(S)
Boiling (B)	.985(S)	1	.013	.420	-.939(S)
Open Pan Dry Roasting (OPDR)	-.159	.013	1	-.902(S)	-.356
Shallow Frying (SF)	.569	.420	-.902(S)	1	-.082
Deep Frying (DF)	-.866(S)	-.939(S)	-.356	-.082	1

Positive Negative *S= Significant*

This table shows the correlation of protein content of *hilsa* with cooking methods. In 15 days control preservation without preservative, there is significant positive correlation present between the raw state and boiling, and significant negative correlation present between the raw state and deep frying, whereas boiling is significant positively correlated with deep frying. Shallow frying is significant negatively correlated with open pan dry roasting. This table indicates that there is a strong correlation present among the **raw state, boiling, open pan dry roasting, shallow frying and deep frying** in 15 days control preservation without preservative.

Table no 5.12.6.2.6 Correlation of cooking methods in 24 hours preservation with salt and turmeric

Condition	RS	B	OPDR	SF	DF
Raw State (RS)	1	.885(S)	.423	.505	.240
Boiling (B)	.885(S)	1	-.049	.044	-.240
Open Pan Dry Roasting (OPDR)	.423	-.049	1	.996(S)	.981(S)
Shallow Frying (SF)	.505	.044	.996(S)	1	.959(S)
Deep Frying (DF)	.240	-.240	.981(S)	.959(S)	1

Positive *S= Significant*

This table shows the correlation of protein content of *hilsa* with cooking methods. In 24 hours salt and turmeric preservation, there is significant positive correlation present between the raw state and boiling, whereas open pan dry roasting is significant positively correlated with shallow frying and deep frying. Shallow frying is significant positively correlated with deep frying. This table indicates that there is a strong correlation present among the **raw state, boiling, open pan dry roasting, shallow frying and deep frying** in 24 hours salt and turmeric preservation.

Table no 5.12.6.2.7 Correlation of cooking methods in 48 hours preservation with salt and turmeric

Condition	RS	B	OPDR	SF	DF
Raw State (RS)	1	-.786	.653	.982(S)	.327
Boiling (B)	-.786	1	-.044	-.655	.327
Open Pan Dry Roasting (OPDR)	.653	-.044	1	.784	.929(S)
Shallow Frying (SF)	.982(S)	-.655	.784	1	.500
Deep Frying (DF)	.327	.327	.929(S)	.500	1

Positive *S= Significant*

This table shows the correlation of protein content of *hilsa* with cooking methods. In 48 hours salt and turmeric preservation, there is significant positive correlation present between the raw state and shallow frying, whereas open pan dry roasting is significant positively correlated with deep frying. This table indicates that there is a strong correlation present **between the raw state and shallow frying and also between open pan dry roasting and deep frying** in 48 hours salt and turmeric preservation.

Table no 5.12.6.2.8 Correlation of cooking methods in 14 days preservation with salt and turmeric

Condition	RS	B	OPDR	SF	DF
Raw State (RS)	1	.564	-.296	-.397	.596
Boiling (B)	.564	1	-.956(S)	-.982(S)	-.327
Open Pan Dry Roasting (OPDR)	-.296	-.956(S)	1	.994(S)	.590
Shallow Frying (SF)	-.397	-.982(S)	.994(S)	1	.500
Deep Frying (DF)	.596	-.327	.590	.500	1

Positive Negative *S= Significant*

This table shows the correlation of protein content of *hilsa* with cooking methods. In 14 days salt and turmeric preservation, there is significant negative correlation present between boiling with open pan dry roasting and shallow frying, whereas open pan dry roasting is significant positively correlated with shallow frying. This table indicates that there is a strong correlation present among **boiling, open pan dry roasting and shallow frying** in 14 days salt and turmeric preservation.

Table no 5.12.6.2.9 Correlation of cooking methods in 15 days preservation with salt and turmeric

Condition	RS	B	OPDR	SF	DF
Raw State (RS)	1	.500	.364	-1.000**(S)	-.500
Boiling (B)	.500	1	.989(S)	-.494	.500
Open Pan Dry Roasting (OPDR)	.364	.989(S)	1	-.357	.625
Shallow Frying (SF)	-1.000**(S)	-.494	-.357	1	.506
Deep Frying (DF)	-.500	.500	.625	.506	1

***.Correlation is highly significant at the 0.01 level (2-tailed)* Positive Negative *S= Significant*

This table shows the correlation of protein content of *hilsa* with cooking methods. In 15 days salt and turmeric preservation, there is perfect positive correlation present between the raw state and shallow frying, whereas boiling is significant positively correlated with open pan dry roasting. This table indicates that there is a strong correlation present **between the raw state and shallow frying and also between boiling and open pan dry roasting** in 15 days salt and turmeric preservation.

Table no 5.12.6.2.10 Correlation of cooking methods in 24 hours preservation with KMS

Condition	RS	B	OPDR	SF	DF
Raw State (RS)	1	-.549	.000	.500	.500
Boiling (B)	-.549	1	-.836(S)	.449	.449
Open Pan Dry Roasting (OPDR)	.000	-.836(S)	1	-.866(S)	-.866(S)
Shallow Frying (SF)	.500	.449	-.866(S)	1	1.000**(S)
Deep Frying (DF)	.500	.449	-.866(S)	1.000**(S)	1

***.Correlation is highly significant at the 0.01 level (2-tailed)* Positive Negative *S= Significant*

This table shows the correlation of protein content of *hilsa* with cooking methods. In 24 hours KMS preservation, there is significant negative correlation present between boiling and open pan dry roasting, whereas open pan dry roasting is significant negatively correlated with shallow frying and deep frying. Shallow frying is perfect positively correlated with deep frying. This table indicates that there is a strong correlation present among **boiling, open pan dry roasting, shallow frying and deep frying** in 24 hours KMS preservation.

Table no 5.12.6.2.11 Correlation of cooking methods in 48 hours preservation with KMS

Condition	RS	B	OPDR	SF	DF
Raw State (RS)	1	1.000*(S)	-.500	.670	.974(S)
Boiling (B)	1.000*(S)	1	-.525	.691	.980(S)
Open Pan Dry Roasting (OPDR)	-.500	-.525	1	-.978(S)	-.682
Shallow Frying (SF)	.670	.691	-.978(S)	1	.820(S)
Deep Frying (DF)	.974(S)	.980(S)	-.682	.820(S)	1

**.Correlation is highly significant at the 0.05 level (2-tailed)* Positive Negative *S= Significant*

This table shows the correlation of protein content of *hilsa* with cooking methods. In 48 hours KMS preservation, there is significant positive correlation present between the raw state and deep frying, and perfect positive correlation present between the raw state and boiling, whereas boiling is significant positively correlated with deep frying. Open pan dry roasting is significant negatively correlated with shallow frying. Shallow frying is significant positively correlated with deep frying. This table indicates that there is a strong correlation present among the **raw state, boiling, open pan dry roasting, shallow frying and deep frying** in 48 hours KMS preservation.

Table no 5.12.6.2.12 Correlation of cooking methods in 14 days preservation with KMS

Condition	RS	B	OPDR	SF	DF
Raw State (RS)	1	.500	-.975(S)	-.982(S)	-.345
Boiling (B)	.500	1	-.297	-.655	.640
Open Pan Dry Roasting (OPDR)	-.975(S)	-.297	1	.916(S)	.543
Shallow Frying (SF)	-.982(S)	-.655	.916(S)	1	.161
Deep Frying (DF)	-.345	.640	.543	.161	1

Positive Negative *S= Significant*

This table shows the correlation of protein content of *hilsa* with cooking methods. In 14 days KMS preservation, there is significant negative correlation present between the raw state with open pan dry roasting and shallow frying, whereas open pan dry roasting is significant positively correlated with shallow frying. This table indicates that there is a strong correlation present among the **raw state, open pan dry roasting and shallow frying** in 14 days KMS preservation.

Table no 5.12.6.2.13 Correlation of cooking methods in 15 days preservation with KMS

Condition	RS	B	OPDR	SF	DF
Raw State (RS)	1	.993(S)	.094	.853(S)	.993(S)
Boiling (B)	.993(S)	1	.208	.907(S)	1.000**(S)
Open Pan Dry Roasting (OPDR)	.094	.208	1	.601	.208
Shallow Frying (SF)	.853(S)	.907(S)	.601	1	.907(S)
Deep Frying (DF)	.993(S)	1.000**(S)	.208	.907(S)	1

***.Correlation is highly significant at the 0.01 level (2-tailed)* Positive *S= Significant*

This table shows the correlation of protein content of *hilsa* with cooking methods. In 15 days KMS preservation, there is significant positive correlation present between the raw state with boiling, shallow frying and deep frying, whereas boiling is significant positively correlated with shallow frying and perfect positively correlated with deep frying. Shallow frying is significant positively correlated with deep frying. This table indicates that there is a strong correlation present among the **raw state, boiling, shallow frying and deep frying** in 15 days KMS preservation.

Overall analysis reveals that the raw state is highly significant positively correlated with boiling in 48 hours KMS preservation, whereas significant positively correlated with open pan dry roasting in fresh condition, perfect negatively correlated with shallow frying in 15 days salt-turmeric preservation, and perfect positively correlated with deep frying in 15 days KMS preservation and perfect negatively correlated with deep frying in 14 days control preservation without preservative. Boiling is highly significant positively correlated with open pan dry roasting in 14 days control preservation without preservative, whereas significant negatively correlated with shallow frying in 14 days salt and turmeric preservation, and perfect positively correlated with deep frying in fresh condition. Open pan dry roasting is significant positively correlated with shallow frying and deep frying in 24 hours salt and turmeric preservation. Shallow frying is highly significant positively correlated with deep frying in 24 hours KMS preservation. Most of the correlation of the protein content of *hilsa* is found in **fresh condition, 14 days control preservation without preservative and 24 hours salt-turmeric preservation** with respect to different cooking conditions.

5.12.6.3 Fat

Table no 5.12.6.3.1 Correlation of cooking methods in fresh condition

Condition	RS	B	OPDR	SF	DF
Raw State (RS)	1	-.649	.892(S)	.949(S)	-.894(S)
Boiling (B)	-.649	1	-.923(S)	-.376	.240
Open Pan Dry Roasting (OPDR)	.892(S)	-.923(S)	1	.705	-.596
Shallow Frying (SF)	.949(S)	-.376	.705	1	-.990(S)
Deep Frying (DF)	-.894(S)	.240	-.596	-.990(S)	1

Positive Negative *S= Significant*

This table shows the correlation of fat content of *hilsa* with cooking methods. In fresh condition, there is significant positive correlation present between the raw state with open pan dry roasting and shallow frying, and negative correlation present between the raw state and deep frying, whereas boiling is significant negatively correlated with open pan dry roasting. Shallow frying is significant negatively correlated with deep frying. This table indicates that there is a strong correlation present among the **raw state, boiling, open pan dry roasting, shallow frying and deep frying** in fresh condition.

Table no 5.12.6.3.2 Correlation of cooking methods in 24 hours preservation without preservative

Condition	RS	B	OPDR	SF	DF
Raw State (RS)	1	.661(S)	.994(S)	.475	-.020
Boiling (B)	.661	1	.738	.974(S)	-.763
Open Pan Dry Roasting (OPDR)	.994(S)	.738	1	.567	-.127
Shallow Frying (SF)	.475	.974(S)	.567	1	-.889(S)
Deep Frying (DF)	-.020	-.763	-.127	-.889(S)	1

Positive Negative *S= Significant*

This table shows the correlation of fat content of *hilsa* with cooking methods. In 24 hours control preservation without preservative, there is significant positive correlation present between the raw state with boiling and open pan dry roasting, whereas boiling is significant positively correlated with shallow frying. Shallow frying is significant negatively correlated with deep frying. This table indicates that there is a strong correlation present among the **raw state, boiling, open pan dry roasting, shallow frying and deep frying** in 24 hours control preservation.

Table no 5.12.6.3.3 Correlation of cooking methods in 48 hours preservation without preservative

Condition	RS	B	OPDR	SF	DF
Raw State (RS)	1	.993(S)	.866(S)	-.243	-.553
Boiling (B)	.993(S)	1	.803(S)	-.352	-.454
Open Pan Dry Roasting (OPDR)	.866(S)	.803(S)	1	.275	-.896(S)
Shallow Frying (SF)	-.243	-.352	.275	1	-.674
Deep Frying (DF)	-.553	-.454	-.896(S)	-.674	1

Positive Negative *S= Significant*

This table shows the correlation of fat content of *hilsa* with cooking methods. In 48 hours control preservation without preservative, there is significant positive correlation present between the raw state with boiling and open pan dry roasting, whereas boiling is significant positively correlated with open pan dry roasting. Open pan dry roasting is significant negatively correlated with deep frying. This table indicates that there is a strong correlation present among the **raw state, boiling, open pan dry roasting and deep frying** in 48 hours control preservation.

Table no 5.12.6.3.4 Correlation of cooking methods in 14 days preservation without preservative

Condition	RS	B	OPDR	SF	DF
Raw State (RS)	1	-1.000**(S)	.445	.086	-.204
Boiling (B)	-1.000**(S)	1	-.434	-.098	.217
Open Pan Dry Roasting (OPDR)	.445	-.434	1	-.854(S)	.786
Shallow Frying (SF)	.086	-.098	-.854(S)	1	-.993(S)
Deep Frying (DF)	-.204	.217	.786	-.993(S)	1

***.Correlation is highly significant at the 0.01 level (2-tailed)* ☐ Negative *S= Significant*

This table shows the correlation of fat content of *hilsa* with cooking methods. In 14 days control preservation without preservative, there is perfect negative correlation present between the raw state and boiling, whereas open pan dry roasting is significant negatively correlated with open pan dry roasting. Open pan dry roasting is significant negatively correlated with shallow frying. Shallow frying is significant negatively correlated with deep frying. This table indicates that there is a strong correlation present among the **raw state, boiling, open pan dry roasting, shallow frying and deep frying** in 14 days control preservation.

Table no 5.12.6.3.5 Correlation of cooking methods in 15 days preservation without preservative

Condition	RS	B	OPDR	SF	DF
Raw State (RS)	1	-.397	-.554	-.945(S)	.264
Boiling (B)	-.397	1	-.543	.075	-.990(S)
Open Pan Dry Roasting (OPDR)	-.554	-.543	1	.796	.657
Shallow Frying (SF)	-.945(S)	.075	.796	1	.066
Deep Frying (DF)	.264	-.990(S)	.657	.066	1

☐ Negative *S= Significant*

This table shows the correlation of fat content of *hilsa* with cooking methods. In 14 days control preservation without preservative, there is perfect negative correlation present between the raw state and boiling, whereas open pan dry roasting is significant negatively correlated with open pan dry roasting. Open pan dry roasting is significant negatively correlated with shallow frying. Shallow frying is significant negatively correlated with deep frying. This table indicates that there is a strong correlation present among the **raw state, boiling, open pan dry roasting, shallow frying and deep frying** in 14 days control preservation.

Table no 5.12.6.3.6 Correlation of cooking methods in 24 hours preservation with salt and turmeric

Condition	RS	B	OPDR	SF	DF
Raw State (RS)	1	.462	.596	.684	.596
Boiling (B)	.462	1	-.436	-.330	-.436
Open Pan Dry Roasting (OPDR)	.596	-.436	1	.993(S)	1.000**(S)
Shallow Frying (SF)	.684	-.330	.993(S)	1	.993(S)
Deep Frying (DF)	.596	-.436	1.000**(S)	.993(S)	1

***.Correlation is highly significant at the 0.01 level (2-tailed)* ☐ Positive *S= Significant*

This table shows the correlation of fat content of *hilsa* with cooking methods. In 24 hours salt and turmeric preservation, there is perfect positive correlation present between open pan dry roasting and deep frying, and significant positive correlation present between open pan dry roasting and shallow frying, whereas shallow frying is significant positively correlated with deep frying. This table indicates that there is a strong correlation present among **open pan dry roasting, shallow frying and deep frying** in 24 hours salt and turmeric preservation.

Table no 5.12.6.3.7 Correlation of cooking methods in 48 hours preservation with salt and turmeric

Condition	RS	B	OPDR	SF	DF
Raw State (RS)	1	.189	.990(S)	-.371	-.888(S)
Boiling (B)	.189	1	.327	-.982(S)	-.619
Open Pan Dry Roasting (OPDR)	.990(S)	.327	1	-.500	-.945(S)
Shallow Frying (SF)	-.371	-.982(S)	-.500	1	.756
Deep Frying (DF)	-.888(S)	-.619	-.945(S)	.756	1

Positive Negative *S= Significant*

This table shows the correlation of fat content of *hilsa* with cooking methods. In 48 hours salt and turmeric preservation, there is significant positive correlation present between the raw state and open pan dry roasting, and significant negative correlation present between the raw state and deep frying, whereas boiling is significant negatively correlated with shallow frying. open pan dry roasting is significant negatively correlated with deep frying. This table indicates that there is a strong correlation present among the **raw state, boiling, open pan dry roasting, shallow frying and deep frying** in 48 hours salt and turmeric preservation.

Table no 5.12.6.3.8 Correlation of cooking methods in 14 days preservation with salt and turmeric

Condition	RS	B	OPDR	SF	DF
Raw State (RS)	1	-.327	.655	-.737	-.982(S)
Boiling (B)	-.327	1	.500	-.397	.500
Open Pan Dry Roasting (OPDR)	.655	.500	1	-.993(S)	-.500
Shallow Frying (SF)	-.737	-.397	-.993(S)	1	.596
Deep Frying (DF)	-.982(S)	.500	-.500	.596	1

***.Correlation is highly significant at the 0.01 level (2-tailed)* Negative *S= Significant*

This table shows the correlation of fat content of *hilsa* with cooking methods. In 14 days salt and turmeric preservation, there is significant negative correlation present between the raw state and deep frying, whereas open pan dry roasting is significant negatively correlated with shallow frying. This table indicates that there is a strong correlation present **between the raw state and deep frying and also between open pan dry roasting and shallow frying** in 14 days salt and turmeric preservation.

Table no 5.12.6.3.9 Correlation of cooking methods in 15 days preservation with salt and turmeric

Condition	RS	B	OPDR	SF	DF
Raw State (RS)	1	-.034	-.327	.982(S)	-.997*(S)
Boiling (B)	-.034	1	-.933(S)	.156	-.041
Open Pan Dry Roasting (OPDR)	-.327	-.933(S)	1	-.500	.397
Shallow Frying (SF)	.982(S)	.156	-.500	1	-.993(S)
Deep Frying (DF)	-.997*(S)	-.041	.397	-.993(S)	1

***.Correlation is highly significant at the 0.01 level (2-tailed)* Positive Negative *S= Significant*

This table shows the correlation of fat content of *hilsa* with cooking methods. In 15 days salt and turmeric preservation, there is significant positive correlation present between the raw state and shallow frying, and highly significant correlation present between the raw state and deep frying. Open pan dry roasting is significant negatively correlated with boiling. Shallow frying is significant negatively correlated with deep frying. This table indicates that there is a strong correlation present among the **raw state, boiling, open pan dry roasting, shallow frying and deep frying** in 15 days salt and turmeric preservation.

Table no 5.12.6.3.10 Correlation of cooking methods in 24 hours preservation with KMS

Condition	RS	B	OPDR	SF	DF
Raw State (RS)	1	.998*(S)	1.000**(S)	.954(S)	-.597
Boiling (B)	.998*(S)	1	.998*(S)	.933(S)	-.545
Open Pan Dry Roasting (OPDR)	1.000**(S)	.998*(S)	1	.954(S)	-.597
Shallow Frying (SF)	.954(S)	.933(S)	.954(S)	1	-.810(S)
Deep Frying (DF)	-.597	-.545	-.597	-.810(S)	1

***.Correlation is highly significant at the 0.01 level (2-tailed)* ▭ Positive *S= Significant*

**.Correlation is highly significant at the 0.05 level (2-tailed)*

This table shows the correlation of fat content of *hilsa* with cooking methods. In 24 hours KMS preservation, there is highly significant positive correlation present between the raw state and boiling, and perfect positive correlation present between the raw state and open pan dry roasting, and significant positive correlation present between the raw state and shallow frying, whereas boiling is significant positively correlated with open pan dry roasting and shallow frying. Shallow frying is significant positively correlated with open pan dry roasting and deep frying. This table indicates that there is a strong correlation present among the **raw state, boiling, open pan dry roasting, shallow frying and deep frying** in 24 hours KMS preservation.

Table no 5.12.6.3.11 Correlation of cooking methods in 48 hours preservation with KMS

Condition	RS	B	OPDR	SF	DF
Raw State (RS)	1	.998*(S)	.956(S)	-.597	.995(S)
Boiling (B)	.998*(S)	1	.973(S)	-.545	.999*(S)
Open Pan Dry Roasting (OPDR)	.956(S)	.973(S)	1	-.336	.981(S)
Shallow Frying (SF)	-.597	-.545	-.336	1	-.512
Deep Frying (DF)	.995(S)	.999*(S)	.981(S)	-.512	1

**.Correlation is highly significant at the 0.05 level (2-tailed)* ▭ Positive *S= Significant*

This table shows the correlation of fat content of *hilsa* with cooking methods. In 48 hours KMS preservation, there is highly significant positive correlation present between the raw state and boiling, and significant positive correlation present between the raw state with open pan dry roasting and deep frying. Boiling is significant positively correlated with open pan dry roasting and highly significant positively correlated with deep frying. Open pan dry roasting is significant positively correlated with deep frying. This table indicates that there is a strong correlation present among the **raw state, boiling, open pan dry roasting and deep frying** in 48 hours KMS preservation.

Table no 5.12.6.3.12 Correlation of cooking methods in 14 days preservation with KMS

Condition	RS	B	OPDR	SF	DF
Raw State (RS)	1	.945(S)	.397	-.545	-.545
Boiling (B)	.945(S)	1	.075	-.240	-.240
Open Pan Dry Roasting (OPDR)	.397	.075	1	-.986(S)	-.986(S)
Shallow Frying (SF)	-.545	-.240	-.986(S)	1	1.000**(S)
Deep Frying (DF)	-.545	-.240	-.986(S)	1.000**(S)	1

***.Correlation is highly significant at the 0.01 level (2-tailed)* Positive Negative *S= Significant*

This table shows the correlation of fat content of *hilsa* with cooking methods. In 14 days KMS preservation, there is significant positive correlation present between the raw state and boiling, whereas open pan dry roasting is significant negatively correlated with shallow frying and deep frying. Shallow frying is significant negatively correlated with open pan dry roasting and perfect positively correlated with deep frying. This table indicates that there is a strong correlation present among the **raw state, boiling, open pan dry roasting, shallow frying and deep frying** in 14 days KMS preservation.

Table no 5.12.6.3.13 Correlation of cooking methods in 15 days preservation with KMS

Condition	Rs	B	OPDR	SF	DF
Raw State (RS)	1	.350	-.977(S)	-.361	-.869(S)
Boiling (B)	.350	1	-.543	-1.000**(S)	-.768
Open Pan Dry Roasting (OPDR)	-.977(S)	-.543	1	.553	.955(S)
Shallow Frying (SF)	-.361	-1.000**(S)	.553	1	.775
Deep Frying (DF)	-.869(S)	-.768	.955(S)	.775	1

***.Correlation is highly significant at the 0.01 level (2-tailed)* Positive Negative *S= Significant*

This table shows the correlation of fat content of *hilsa* with cooking methods. In 15 days KMS preservation, there is significant negative correlation present between the raw state with open pan dry roasting and deep frying, whereas boiling is perfect negatively correlated with shallow frying. Open pan dry roasting is significant positively correlated with deep frying. This table indicates that there is a strong correlation present among the **raw state, boiling, open pan dry roasting, shallow frying and deep frying** in 15 days KMS preservation.

Overall analysis reveals that the raw state is perfect negatively correlated with boiling in 14 days control preservation without preservative, whereas perfect positively correlated with open pan dry roasting in 24 hours preservation with KMS, significant positively correlated with shallow frying in 15 days salt and turmeric preservation, and highly significant negatively correlated with deep frying in 15 days salt-turmeric preservation. Boiling is highly significant positively correlated with open pan dry roasting and deep frying in 24 hours and 48 hours KMS preservation respectively, whereas perfect positively correlated with shallow frying in 15 days KMS preservation. Open pan dry roasting is significant positively correlated with shallow frying in 24 hours salt and turmeric and significant negatively correlated with shallow frying in 14 days salt-turmeric preservation, and perfect positively correlated with deep frying in 24 hours salt and turmeric preservation. Shallow frying is perfect positively correlated with deep frying in 14 days KMS preservation. Most of the correlation of the fat content of *hilsa* is found in **24 hours and 15 days salt and turmeric preservation and 24 hours KMS preservation** with respect to different cooking conditions.

5.12.6.4 Moisture

Table no 5.12.5.4.1 Correlation of cooking methods in fresh condition

Condition	RS	B	OPDR	SF	DF
Raw State (RS)	1	.976(S)	.974(S)	-.041	.659
Boiling (B)	.976(S)	1	.901(S)	.176	.480
Open Pan Dry Roasting (OPDR)	.974(S)	.901(S)	1	-.268	.813(S)
Shallow Frying (SF)	-.041	.176	-.268	1	-.779
Deep Frying (DF)	.659	.480	.813(S)	-.779	1

□ Positive *S= Significant*

This table shows the correlation of moisture content of *hilsa* with cooking methods. In fresh condition, there is significant positive correlation present between the raw state with boiling and open pan dry roasting, whereas boiling is significant positively correlated with open pan dry roasting. Open pan dry roasting is significant positively correlated with deep frying. This table indicates that there is a strong correlation present among the **raw state, boiling, open pan dry roasting and deep frying** in fresh condition.

Table no 5.12.6.4.2 Correlation of cooking methods in 24 hours preservation without preservative

Condition	RS	B	OPDR	SF	DF
Raw State (RS)	1	-.343	-.581	-.590	.460
Boiling (B)	-.343	1	.964(S)	.961(S)	.676
Open Pan Dry Roasting (OPDR)	-.581	.964(S)	1	1.000**(S)	.455
Shallow Frying (SF)	-.590	.961(S)	1.000**(S)	1	.445
Deep Frying (DF)	.460	.676	.455	.445	1

***.Correlation is highly significant at the 0.01 level (2-tailed)* □ Positive *S= Significant*

This table shows the correlation of moisture content of *hilsa* with cooking methods. In 24 hours control preservation without preservative, there is significant positive correlation present between boiling with open pan dry roasting and shallow frying, whereas open pan dry roasting is perfect positively correlated with shallow frying. This table indicates that there is a strong correlation present among **boiling, open pan dry roasting and shallow frying** in 24 hours control preservation.

Table no 5.12.6.4.3 Correlation of cooking methods in 48 hours preservation without preservative

Condition	RS	B	OPDR	SF	DF
Raw State (RS)	1	1.000*(S)	.471	.963(S)	.321
Boiling (B)	1.000*(S)	1	.445	.971(S)	.349
Open Pan Dry Roasting (OPDR)	.471	.445	1	.217	-.684
Shallow Frying (SF)	.963(S)	.971(S)	.217	1	.564
Deep Frying (DF)	.321	.349	-.684	.564	1

**.Correlation is highly significant at the 0.05 level (2-tailed)* □ Positive *S= Significant*

This table shows the correlation of moisture content of *hilsa* with cooking methods. In 48 hours control preservation without preservative, there is significant positive correlation present between the raw state and shallow frying, and perfect positive correlation present between the raw state and boiling, whereas boiling is significant positively correlated with shallow frying. This table indicates that there is a strong correlation present among the **raw state, boiling and shallow frying** in 48 hours control preservation.

Table no 5.12.6.4.4 Correlation of cooking methods in 14 days preservation without preservative

Condition	RS	B	OPDR	SF	DF
Raw State (RS)	1	-.250	.156	.156	.742
Boiling (B)	-.250	1	.918(S)	.918(S)	.464
Open Pan Dry Roasting (OPDR)	.156	.918(S)	1	1.000**(S)	.778
Shallow Frying (SF)	.156	.918(S)	1.000**(S)	1	.778
Deep Frying (DF)	.742	.464	.778	.778	1

***.Correlation is highly significant at the 0.01 level (2-tailed)* ▭ Positive *S= Significant*

This table shows the correlation of moisture content of *hilsa* with cooking methods. In 14 days control preservation without preservative, there is significant positive correlation present between the raw state and shallow frying, and perfect positive correlation present between the raw state and boiling, whereas boiling is significant positively correlated with shallow frying. This table indicates that there is a strong correlation present among **boiling, open pan dry roasting and shallow frying** in 14 days control preservation.

Table no 5.12.6.4.5 Correlation of cooking methods in 15 days preservation without preservative

Condition	RS	B	OPDR	SF	DF
Raw State (RS)	1	-.059	-.995(S)	-.999*(S)	-.813(S)
Boiling (B)	-.059	1	-.040	.012	.629
Open Pan Dry Roasting (OPDR)	-.995(S)	-.040	1	.999*(S)	.751
Shallow Frying (SF)	-.999*(S)	.012	.999*(S)	1	.785
Deep Frying (DF)	-.813(S)	.629	.751	.785	1

**.Correlation is highly significant at the 0.05 level (2-tailed)* ▭ Positive ▭ Negative *S= Significant*

This table shows the correlation of moisture content of *hilsa* with cooking methods. In 15 days control preservation without preservative, there is significant negative correlation present between the raw state with open pan dry roasting and deep frying, and highly significant negative correlation present between the raw state and shallow frying, whereas open pan dry roasting is highly significant positively correlated with shallow frying. This table indicates that there is a strong correlation present among the **raw state, open pan dry roasting, shallow frying and deep frying** in 15 days control preservation.

Table no 5.12.6.4.6 Correlation of cooking methods in 24 hours preservation with salt and turmeric

Condition	RS	B	OPDR	SF	DF
Raw State (RS)	1	-.387	-.538	.936(S)	.956(S)
Boiling (B)	-.387	1	.986(S)	-.038	-.100
Open Pan Dry Roasting (OPDR)	-.538	.986(S)	1	-.207	-.267
Shallow Frying (SF)	.936(S)	-.038	-.207	1	.998*(S)
Deep Frying (DF)	.956(S)	-.100	-.267	.998*(S)	1

**.Correlation is highly significant at the 0.05 level (2-tailed)* ▭ Positive *S= Significant*

This table shows the correlation of moisture content of *hilsa* with cooking methods. In 24 hours salt and turmeric preservation, there is significant positive correlation present between the raw state with shallow frying and deep frying, whereas shallow frying is highly significant positively correlated with deep frying. This table indicates that there is a strong correlation present among the **raw state**, **boiling, open pan dry roasting, shallow frying and deep frying** in 24 hours salt and turmeric preservation.

Table no 5.12.6.4.7 Correlation of cooking methods in 48 hours preservation with salt and turmeric

Condition	RS	B	OPDR	SF	DF
Raw State (RS)	1	.993(S)	.636	1.000**(S)	.613
Boiling (B)	.993(S)	1	.541	.995(S)	.515
Open Pan Dry Roasting (OPDR)	.636	.541	1	.625	1.000*(S)
Shallow Frying (SF)	1.000**(S)	.995(S)	.625	1	.601
Deep Frying (DF)	.613	.515	1.000*(S)	.601	1

**.Correlation is highly significant at the 0.05 level (2-tailed)* ▭ Positive *S= Significant*
***.Correlation is highly significant at the 0.05 level (2-tailed)*

This table shows the correlation of moisture content of *hilsa* with cooking methods. In 48 hours salt and turmeric preservation, there is significant positive correlation present between the raw state and boiling, and perfect positive correlation present between the raw state and shallow frying, whereas boiling is significant positively correlated with shallow frying. Open pan dry roasting is perfect positively correlated with deep frying. This table indicates that there is a strong correlation present among the **raw state, boiling, open pan dry roasting, shallow frying and deep frying** in 48 hours salt and turmeric preservation.

Table no 5.12.6.4.8 Correlation of cooking methods in 14 days preservation with salt and turmeric

Condition	RS	B	OPDR	SF	DF
Raw State (RS)	1	.075	-.640	-.320	-.612
Boiling (B)	.075	1	.718	.921(S)	.743
Open Pan Dry Roasting (OPDR)	-.640	.718	1	.933(S)	.999*(S)
Shallow Frying (SF)	-.320	.921(S)	.933(S)	1	.945(S)
Deep Frying (DF)	-.612	.743	.999*(S)	.945(S)	1

**.Correlation is highly significant at the 0.05 level (2-tailed)* ▭ Positive *S= Significant*

This table shows the correlation of moisture content of *hilsa* with cooking methods. In 14 days salt and turmeric preservation, there is significant positive correlation present between boiling and shallow frying, whereas open pan dry roasting is significant positively correlated with shallow frying and highly significant positively correlated with deep frying. Shallow frying is significant positively correlated with deep frying. This table indicates that there is a strong correlation present among **boiling, open pan dry roasting, shallow frying and deep frying** in 14 days salt and turmeric preservation.

Table no 5.12.6.4.9 Correlation of cooking methods in 15 days preservation with salt and turmeric

Condition	RS	B	OPDR	SF	DF
Raw State (RS)	1	-.514	.381	.967(S)	.756
Boiling (B)	-.514	1	-.989(S)	-.279	.173
Open Pan Dry Roasting (OPDR)	.381	-.989(S)	1	.132	-.317
Shallow Frying (SF)	.967(S)	-.279	.132	1	.898(S)
Deep Frying (DF)	.756	.173	-.317	.898(S)	1

▭ Positive *S= Significant*

This table shows the correlation of moisture content of *hilsa* with cooking methods. In 15 days salt and turmeric preservation, there is significant positive correlation present between the raw state and shallow frying, whereas open pan dry roasting is significant negatively correlated with boiling. Shallow frying is significant positively correlated with deep frying. This table indicates that there is a strong correlation present among the **raw state, boiling, open pan dry roasting, shallow frying and deep frying** in 15 days salt and turmeric preservation.

Table no 5.12.6.4.10 Correlation of cooking methods in 24 hours preservation with KMS

Condition	RS	B	OPDR	SF	DF
Raw State (RS)	1	-.321	-.404	-.946(S)	.521
Boiling (B)	-.321	1	-.736	.611	.641
Open Pan Dry Roasting (OPDR)	-.404	-.736	1	.086	-.991(S)
Shallow Frying (SF)	-.946(S)	.611	.086	1	-.217
Deep Frying (DF)	.521	.641	-.991(S)	-.217	1

Negative *S= Significant*

This table shows the correlation of moisture content of *hilsa* with cooking methods. In 24 hours KMS preservation, there is significant negative correlation present between the raw state and shallow frying, whereas open pan dry roasting is significant negatively correlated with deep frying. This table indicates that there is a strong correlation present **between the raw state and shallow frying and also between open pan dry roasting and deep frying** in 24 hours KMS preservation.

Table no 5.12.6.4.11 Correlation of cooking methods in 48 hours preservation with KMS

Condition	RS	B	OPDR	SF	DF
Raw State (RS)	1	.393	.350	.732	.911(S)
Boiling (B)	.393	1	-.724	.914(S)	-.020
Open Pan Dry Roasting (OPDR)	.350	-.724	1	-.382	.705
Shallow Frying (SF)	.732	.914(S)	-.382	1	.387
Deep Frying (DF)	.911(S)	-.020	.705	.387	1

Positive *S= Significant*

This table shows the correlation of moisture content of *hilsa* with cooking methods. In 48 hours KMS preservation, there is significant positive correlation present between the raw state and deep frying, whereas boiling is significant positively correlated with shallow frying. This table indicates that there is a strong correlation present **between the raw state and deep frying and also between boiling and shallow frying** in 48 hours KMS preservation.

Table no 5.12.6.4.12 Correlation of cooking methods in 14 days preservation with KMS

Condition	RS	B	OPDR	SF	DF
Raw State (RS)	1	.905(S)	.605	-.715	-.750
Boiling (B)	.905(S)	1	.886(S)	-.349	-.397
Open Pan Dry Roasting (OPDR)	.605	.886(S)	1	.125	.073
Shallow Frying (SF)	-.715	-.349	.125	1	.999*(S)
Deep Frying (DF)	-.750	-.397	.073	.999*(S)	1

**.Correlation is highly significant at the 0.05 level (2-tailed)* Positive *S= Significant*

This table shows the correlation of moisture content of *hilsa* with cooking methods. In 14 days KMS preservation, there is significant positive correlation present between the raw state and boiling, whereas open pan dry roasting is significant positively correlated with boiling. Shallow frying is highly significant positively correlated with deep frying. This table indicates that there is a strong correlation present among the **raw state, boiling, open pan dry roasting, shallow frying and deep frying** in 14 days KMS preservation.

Table no 5.12.6.4.13 Correlation of cooking methods in 15 days preservation with KMS

Condition	RS	B	OPDR	SF	DF
Raw State (RS)	1	.806(S)	1.000**(S)	-.994(S)	.884(S)
Boiling (B)	.806(S)	1	.802(S)	-.736	.989(S)
Open Pan Dry Roasting (OPDR)	1.000**(S)	.802(S)	1	-.995(S)	.881(S)
Shallow Frying (SF)	-.994(S)	-.736	-.995(S)	1	-.827(S)
Deep Frying (DF)	.884(S)	.989(S)	.881(S)	-.827(S)	1

***.Correlation is highly significant at the 0.01 level (2-tailed)* Positive Negative *S= Significant*

This table shows the correlation of moisture content of *hilsa* with cooking methods. In 15 days KMS preservation, there is significant negative correlation present between the raw state and shallow frying, and significant positive correlation present between the raw state with boiling and deep frying, and perfect positive correlation present between the raw state and open pan dry roasting. Boiling is significant positively correlated with open pan dry roasting and deep frying. Open pan dry roasting is significant positively correlated with deep frying and significant negatively correlated with shallow frying. Shallow frying is significant negatively correlated with deep frying. This table indicates that there is a strong correlation present among the **raw state, boiling, open pan dry roasting, shallow frying and deep frying** in 15 days KMS preservation.

Overall analysis reveals that the raw state is perfect positively correlated with boiling, open pan dry roasting and shallow frying in 48 hours control preservation without preservative, 15 days KMS preservation and 48 hours salt-turmeric preservation respectively, whereas significant positively correlated with deep frying in 24 hours salt and turmeric preservation. Boiling is significant negatively correlated with open pan dry roasting in 15 days salt-turmeric preservation, and significant positively correlated with shallow frying and deep frying in 48 salt-turmeric preservation and 15 days KMS preservation respectively. Open pan dry roasting is perfect positively correlated with shallow frying in 24 hours and 14 days control preservation without preservative, and perfect positively correlated with deep frying in 48 hours salt and turmeric preservation. Shallow frying is highly significant positively correlated with deep frying in 24 hours salt-turmeric preservation. Most of the correlation of the moisture content of *hilsa* is found in **48 hours salt and turmeric preservation** with respect to different cooking conditions.

5.12.6.5 Ash

Table no 5.12.6.5.1 Correlation of cooking methods in fresh condition

Condition	RS	B	OPDR	SF	DF
Raw State (RS)	1	.969(S)	.953(S)	.822(S)	.953(S)
Boiling (B)	.969(S)	1	.998*(S)	.655	.998*(S)
Open Pan Dry Roasting (OPDR)	.953(S)	.998*(S)	1	.610	1.000**(S)
Shallow Frying (SF)	.822(S)	.655	.610	1	.610
Deep Frying (DF)	.953(S)	.998*(S)	1.000**(S)	.610	1

***.Correlation is highly significant at the 0.01 level (2-tailed)*

**.Correlation is highly significant at the 0.05 level (2-tailed)* Positive *S= Significant*

This table shows the correlation of ash content of *hilsa* with cooking methods. In fresh condition, there is significant positive correlation present between the raw state with boiling, open pan dry roasting, shallow frying and deep frying, whereas boiling is highly significant positively correlated with open pan dry roasting and deep frying. Open pan dry roasting is perfect positively correlated with deep frying. This table indicates that there is a strong correlation present among the **raw state, boiling, open pan dry roasting, shallow frying and deep frying** in fresh condition

Table no 5.12.6.5.2 Correlation of cooking methods in 24 hours preservation without preservative

Condition	RS	B	OPDR	SF	DF
Raw State (RS)	1	.961(S)	.993(S)	.371	.945(S)
Boiling (B)	.961(S)	1	.986(S)	.099	.817(S)
Open Pan Dry Roasting (OPDR)	.993(S)	.986(S)	1	.262	.901(S)
Shallow Frying (SF)	.371	.099	.262	1	.655
Deep Frying (DF)	.945(S)	.817(S)	.901(S)	.655	1

Positive *S= Significant*

This table shows the correlation of ash content of *hilsa* with cooking methods. In 24 hours control preservation without preservative, there is significant positive correlation present between the raw state with boiling, open pan dry roasting and deep frying, whereas boiling is significant positively correlated with open pan dry roasting and deep frying. Open pan dry roasting is significant positively correlated with deep frying. This table indicates that there is a strong correlation present among the **raw state, boiling, open pan dry roasting and deep frying** in 24 hours control preservation.

Table no 5.12.6.5.3 Correlation of cooking methods in 48 hours preservation without preservative

Condition	RS	B	OPDR	SF	DF
Raw State (RS)	1	.986(S)	-.903(S)	.454	-.454
Boiling (B)	.986(S)	1	-.962(S)	.596	-.596
Open Pan Dry Roasting (OPDR)	-.903(S)	-.962(S)	1	-.792	.792
Shallow Frying (SF)	.454	.596	-.792	1	-1.000**(S)
Deep Frying (DF)	-.454	-.596	.792	-1.000**(S)	1

***.Correlation is highly significant at the 0.01 level (2-tailed)* Positive Negative *S= Significant*

This table shows the correlation of ash content of *hilsa* with cooking methods. In 48 hours control preservation without preservative, there is significant positive correlation present between the raw state and boiling, and significant negative correlation present between the raw state and open pan dry roasting. Boiling is significant negatively correlated with open pan dry roasting. Shallow frying is perfect negatively correlated with deep frying. This table indicates that there is a strong correlation present among the **raw state, boiling, open pan dry roasting, shallow frying and deep frying** in 48 hours control preservation.

Table no 5.12.6.5.4 Correlation of cooking methods in 14 days preservation without preservative

Condition	RS	B	OPDR	SF	DF
Raw State (RS)	1	.999*(S)	.911(S)	-.127	.350
Boiling (B)	.999*(S)	1	.888(S)	-.075	.300
Open Pan Dry Roasting (OPDR)	.911(S)	.888(S)	1	-.524	.705
Shallow Frying (SF)	-.127	-.075	-.524	1	-.974(S)
Deep Frying (DF)	.350	.300	.705	-.974(S)	1

**.Correlation is highly significant at the 0.05 level (2-tailed)* Positive Negative *S= Significant*

This table shows the correlation of ash content of *hilsa* with cooking methods. In 14 days control preservation without preservative, there is highly significant positive correlation present between the raw state and boiling, and significant positive correlation present between the raw state and open pan dry roasting, whereas boiling is significant positively correlated with open pan dry roasting. Shallow frying is significant negatively correlated with deep frying. This table indicates that there is a strong correlation present among the **raw state, boiling, open pan dry roasting, shallow frying and deep frying** in 14 days control preservation.

Table no 5.12.6.5.5 Correlation of cooking methods in 15 days preservation without preservative

Condition	RS	B	OPDR	SF	DF
Raw State (RS)	1	-.862(S)	-.528	.603	-.157
Boiling (B)	-.862(S)	1	.886(S)	-.115	.636
Open Pan Dry Roasting (OPDR)	-.528	.886(S)	1	.359	.922(S)
Shallow Frying (SF)	.603	-.115	.359	1	.693
Deep Frying (DF)	-.157	.636	.922(S)	.693	1

**.Correlation is highly significant at the 0.05 level (2-tailed)* Positive Negative *S= Significant*

This table shows the correlation of ash content of *hilsa* with cooking methods. In 15 days control preservation without preservative, there is significant negative correlation present between the raw state and boiling, whereas boiling is significant positively correlated with open pan dry roasting. Open pan dry roasting is significant positively correlated with deep frying. This table indicates that there is a strong correlation present among the **raw state, boiling, open pan dry roasting and deep frying** in 15 days control preservation.

Table no 5.12.6.5.6 Correlation of cooking methods in 24 hours preservation with salt and turmeric

Condition	RS	B	OPDR	SF	DF
Raw State (RS)	1	.982(S)	.988(S)	.984(S)	.988(S)
Boiling (B)	.982(S)	1	.999*(S)	.933(S)	.941(S)
Open Pan Dry Roasting (OPDR)	.988(S)	.999*(S)	1	.945(S)	.952(S)
Shallow Frying (SF)	.984(S)	.933(S)	.945(S)	1	1.000*(S)
Deep Frying (DF)	.988(S)	.941(S)	.952(S)	1.000*(S)	1

**.Correlation is highly significant at the 0.05 level (2-tailed)* Positive *S= Significant*

This table shows the correlation of ash content of *hilsa* with cooking methods. In 24 hours salt and turmeric preservation, there is highly significant positive correlation present between the raw state with boiling, open pan dry roasting, shallow frying and deep frying, whereas boiling is highly significant positively correlated with open pan dry roasting and significant positively correlated with shallow frying and deep frying. Open pan dry roasting is significant positively correlated with shallow frying and deep frying. Shallow frying is perfect positively correlated with deep frying. This table indicates that there is a strong correlation present among the **raw state, boiling, open pan dry roasting, shallow frying and deep frying** in 24 hours salt and turmeric preservation.

Table no 5.12.6.5.7 Correlation of cooking methods in 48 hours preservation with salt and turmeric

Condition	RS	B	OPDR	SF	DF
Raw State (RS)	1	.143	-.240	.000	.693
Boiling (B)	.143	1	.926(S)	.990(S)	.812(S)
Open Pan Dry Roasting (OPDR)	-.240	.926(S)	1	.971(S)	.533
Shallow Frying (SF)	.000	.990(S)	.971(S)	1	.721
Deep Frying (DF)	.693	.812(S)	.533	.721	1

Positive *S= Significant*

This table shows the correlation of ash content of *hilsa* with cooking methods. In 48 hours salt and turmeric preservation, there is significant positive correlation present between boiling with open pan dry roasting, shallow frying and deep frying, whereas open pan dry roasting is significant positively correlated with shallow frying. This table indicates that there is a strong correlation present among **boiling, open pan dry roasting, shallow frying and deep frying** in 48 hours salt and turmeric preservation.

Table no 5.12.6.5.8 Correlation of cooking methods in 14 days preservation with salt and turmeric

Condition	RS	B	OPDR	SF	DF
Raw State (RS)	1	.475	.872(S)	-.475	.975(S)
Boiling (B)	.475	1	.845(S)	-1.000**(S)	.268
Open Pan Dry Roasting (OPDR)	.872(S)	.845(S)	1	-.845(S)	.742
Shallow Frying (SF)	-.475	-1.000**(S)	-.845(S)	1	-.268
Deep Frying (DF)	.975(S)	.268	.742	-.268	1

***.Correlation is highly significant at the 0.01 level (2-tailed)* Positive Negative *S= Significant*

This table shows the correlation of ash content of *hilsa* with cooking methods. In 14 days salt and turmeric preservation, there is significant positive correlation present between the raw state with open pan dry roasting and deep frying, whereas boiling is significant positively correlated with open pan dry roasting and perfect negatively correlated with shallow frying. Open pan dry roasting is significant negatively correlated with shallow frying. This table indicates that there is a strong correlation present among the **raw state, boiling, open pan dry roasting, shallow frying and deep frying** in 14 days salt and turmeric preservation.

Table no 5.12.6.5.9 Correlation of cooking methods in 15 days preservation with salt and turmeric

Condition	RS	B	OPDR	SF	DF
Raw State (RS)	1	-.327	-.929(S)	-.052	-.929(S)
Boiling (B)	-.327	1	.655	.961(S)	.655
Open Pan Dry Roasting (OPDR)	-.929(S)	.655	1	.419	1.000**(S)
Shallow Frying (SF)	-.052	.961(S)	.419	1	.419
Deep Frying (DF)	-.929(S)	.655	1.000**(S)	.419	1

***.Correlation is highly significant at the 0.01 level (2-tailed)* Positive Negative *S= Significant*

This table shows the correlation of ash content of *hilsa* with cooking methods. In 15 days salt and turmeric preservation, there is significant negative correlation present between the raw state with open pan dry roasting and deep frying, whereas boiling is significant positively correlated with shallow frying. Open pan dry roasting is perfect positively correlated with deep frying. This table indicates that there is a strong correlation present among the **raw state, boiling, open pan dry roasting, shallow frying and deep frying** in 15 days salt and turmeric preservation.

Table no 5.12.6.5.10 Correlation of cooking methods in 24 hours preservation with KMS

Condition	RS	B	OPDR	SF	DF
Raw State (RS)	1	.792	-.991(S)	.991(S)	-.673
Boiling (B)	.792	1	-.866(S)	.866(S)	-.082
Open Pan Dry Roasting (OPDR)	-.991(S)	-.866(S)	1	-1.000**(S)	.569
Shallow Frying (SF)	.991(S)	.866(S)	-1.000**(S)	1	-.569
Deep Frying (DF)	-.673	-.082	.569	-.569	1

***.Correlation is highly significant at the 0.01 level (2-tailed)* Positive Negative *S= Significant*

This table shows the correlation of ash content of *hilsa* with cooking methods. In 24 hours KMS preservation, there is significant negative correlation present between the raw state and open pan dry roasting, and significant positive correlation present between the raw state and deep frying, whereas boiling is significant positively correlated with shallow frying and significant negatively correlated with open pan dry roasting. Open pan dry roasting is perfect negatively correlated with shallow frying. This table indicates that there is a strong correlation present among the **raw state, boiling, open pan dry roasting and shallow frying** in 24 hours KMS preservation.

Table no 5.12.6.5.11 Correlation of cooking methods in 48 hours preservation with KMS

Condition	RS	B	OPDR	SF	DF
Raw State (RS)	1	.866(S)	.468	.866(S)	.945(S)
Boiling (B)	.866(S)	1	.847(S)	1.000**(S)	.982(S)
Open Pan Dry Roasting (OPDR)	.468	.847	1	.847(S)	.731
Shallow Frying (SF)	.866(S)	1.000**(S)	.847(S)	1	.982(S)
Deep Frying (DF)	.945(S)	.982(S)	.731	.982(S)	1

***.Correlation is highly significant at the 0.01 level (2-tailed)* Positive *S= Significant*

This table shows the correlation of ash content of *hilsa* with cooking methods. In 48 hours KMS preservation, there is significant positive correlation present between the raw state with boiling, shallow frying and deep frying, whereas boiling is significant positively correlated with open pan dry roasting and deep frying and perfect positively correlated with shallow frying. Open pan dry roasting is significant positively correlated with shallow frying. Shallow frying is significant positively correlated with deep frying. This table indicates that there is a strong correlation present among the **raw state, boiling, open pan dry roasting, shallow frying and deep frying** in 48 hours KMS preservation.

Table no 5.12.6.5.12 Correlation of cooking methods in 14 days preservation with KMS

Condition	RS	B	OPDR	SF	DF
Raw State (RS)	1	.945(S)	.990(S)	.997*(S)	.982(S)
Boiling (B)	.945(S)	1	.888(S)	.967(S)	.866(S)
Open Pan Dry Roasting (OPDR)	.990(S)	.888(S)	1	.976(S)	.999*(S)
Shallow Frying (SF)	.997*(S)	.967(S)	.976(S)	1	.965(S)
Deep Frying (DF)	.982(S)	.866(S)	.999*(S)	.965(S)	1

**.Correlation is highly significant at the 0.05 level (2-tailed)* Positive *S= Significant*

This table shows the correlation of ash content of *hilsa* with cooking methods. In 14 days KMS preservation, there is significant positive correlation present between the raw state with boiling, open pan dry roasting and deep frying, and highly significant positive correlation present between the raw state and shallow frying. Boiling is significant positively correlated with open pan dry roasting, shallow frying and deep frying. Open pan dry roasting is significant positively correlated with shallow frying and highly significant positively correlated with deep frying. Shallow frying is significant positively correlated with deep frying. This table indicates that there is a strong correlation present among the **raw state, boiling, open pan dry roasting, shallow frying and deep frying** in 14 days KMS preservation.

Table no 5.12.6.5.13 Correlation of cooking methods in 15 days preservation with KMS

Condition	RS	B	OPDR	SF	DF
Raw State (RS)	1	1.000**(S)	.990(S)	.945(S)	1.000**(S)
Boiling (B)	1.000**(S)	1	.990(S)	.945(S)	1.000**(S)
Open Pan Dry Roasting (OPDR)	.990(S)	.990(S)	1	.982(S)	.990(S)
Shallow Frying (SF)	.945(S)	.945(S)	.982(S)	1	.945(S)
Deep Frying (DF)	1.000**(S)	1.000**(S)	.990(S)	.945(S)	1

***.Correlation is highly significant at the 0.01 level (2-tailed)* ▭ Positive *S= Significant*

This table shows the correlation of ash content of *hilsa* with cooking methods. In 15 days KMS preservation, there is significant positive correlation present between the raw state with open pan dry roasting and shallow frying, and perfect positive correlation present between the raw state with boiling and deep frying. Boiling is significant positively correlated with open pan dry roasting and shallow frying and perfect positively correlated with deep frying. Open pan dry roasting is significant positively correlated with shallow frying and deep frying. Shallow frying is significant positively correlated with deep frying. This table indicates that there is a strong correlation present among the **raw state, boiling, open pan dry roasting, shallow frying and deep frying** in 15 days KMS preservation.

Overall analysis reveals that the raw state is perfect positively correlated with boiling in 15 days KMS preservation, whereas significant positively correlated with open pan dry roasting in 24 hours control preservation without preservative, highly significant positively correlated with shallow frying in 14 days KMS preservation, and perfect positively correlated with deep frying in 15 days KMS preservation. Boiling is highly significant positively correlated with open pan dry roasting in 24 hours salt-turmeric preservation, whereas perfect negatively correlated with shallow frying in 14 days salt and turmeric preservation and perfect positively correlated with shallow frying in 48 hours KMS preservation, and perfect positively correlated with deep frying in 15 days KMS preservation. Open pan dry roasting is perfect negatively correlated with shallow frying in 24 hours KMS preservation, and perfect positively correlated with deep frying in fresh condition and 15 days salt and turmeric preservation. Shallow frying is perfect positively correlated with deep frying in 24 hours salt-turmeric preservation. Most of the correlation of the ash content of *hilsa* is found in **15 days KMS preservation** with respect to different cooking conditions.

5.12.6.6 Calcium

Table no 5.12.6.6.1 Correlation of cooking methods in fresh condition

Condition	RS	B	OPDR	SF	DF
Raw State (RS)	1	.891(S)	.982(S)	.982(S)	.929(S)
Boiling (B)	.891(S)	1	.961(S)	.961(S)	.996(S)
Open Pan Dry Roasting (OPDR)	.982(S)	.961(S)	1	1.000**(S)	.982(S)
Shallow Frying (SF)	.982(S)	.961(S)	1.000**(S)	1	.982(S)
Deep Frying (DF)	.929(S)	.996(S)	.982(S)	.982(S)	1

***.Correlation is highly significant at the 0.01 level (2-tailed)* ▭ Positive *S= Significant*

This table shows the correlation of calcium content of *hilsa* with cooking methods. In fresh condition, there is significant positive correlation present between the raw state with boiling, open pan dry roasting, shallow frying and deep frying, whereas boiling is significant positively correlated with open pan dry roasting, shallow frying and deep frying. Open pan dry roasting is significant positively correlated with deep frying and perfect positively correlated with shallow frying. Shallow frying is significant positively correlated with deep frying. This table indicates that there is a strong correlation present among the **raw state, boiling, open pan dry roasting, shallow frying and deep frying** in fresh condition.

Table no 5.12.6.6.2 Correlation of cooking methods in 24 hours preservation without preservative

Condition	RS	B	OPDR	SF	DF
Raw State (RS)	1	.500	.929(S)	.982(S)	.996(S)
Boiling (B)	.500	1	.786	.655	.419
Open Pan Dry Roasting (OPDR)	.929(S)	.786	1	.982(S)	.891(S)
Shallow Frying (SF)	.982(S)	.655	.982(S)	1	.961(S)
Deep Frying (DF)	.996(S)	.419	.891(S)	.961(S)	1

▭ Positive *S= Significant*

This table shows the correlation of calcium content of *hilsa* with cooking methods. In 24 hours control preservation without preservative, there is significant positive correlation present between the raw state with open pan dry roasting, shallow frying and deep frying, whereas open pan dry roasting is significant positively correlated with shallow frying and deep frying. Shallow frying is significant positively correlated with deep frying. This table indicates that there is a strong correlation present among the **raw state, open pan dry roasting, shallow frying and deep frying** in 24 hours control preservation.

Table no 5.12.6.6.3 Correlation of cooking methods in 48 hours preservation without preservative

Condition	RS	B	OPDR	SF	DF
Raw State (RS)	1	.982(S)	-.655	1.000**(S)	.993(S)
Boiling (B)	.982(S)	1	-.786	.982(S)	.997*(S)
Open Pan Dry Roasting (OPDR)	-.655	-.786	1	-.655	-.737
Shallow Frying (SF)	1.000**(S)	.982(S)	-.655	1	.993(S)
Deep Frying (DF)	.993(S)	.997*(S)	-.737	.993(S)	1

***.Correlation is highly significant at the 0.01 level (2-tailed)* ▭ Positive *S= Significant*

This table shows the correlation of calcium content of *hilsa* with cooking methods. In 48 hours control preservation without preservative, there is significant positive correlation present between the raw state with boiling, open pan dry roasting, shallow frying and deep frying, whereas boiling is significant positively correlated with open pan dry roasting, shallow frying and deep frying. Open pan dry roasting is significant positively correlated with deep frying and perfect positively correlated with shallow frying.

Shallow frying is significant positively correlated with deep frying. This table indicates that there is a strong correlation present among the **raw state, boiling, open pan dry roasting, shallow frying and deep frying** in 48 hours control preservation.

Table no 5.12.6.6.4 Correlation of cooking methods in 14 days preservation without preservative

Condition	RS	B	OPDR	SF	DF
Raw State (RS)	1	.961(S)	1.000**(S)	1.000**(S)	-.240
Boiling (B)	.961(S)	1	.961(S)	.961(S)	-.500
Open Pan Dry Roasting (OPDR)	1.000**(S)	.961(S)	1	1.000**(S)	-.240
Shallow Frying (SF)	1.000**(S)	.961(S)	1.000**(S)	1	-.240
Deep Frying (DF)	-.240	-.500	-.240	-.240	1

***.Correlation is highly significant at the 0.01 level (2-tailed)* Positive *S= Significant*

This table shows the correlation of calcium content of *hilsa* with cooking methods. In 14 days control preservation without preservative, there is significant positive correlation present between the raw state and boiling, and perfect positive correlation present between the raw state with open pan dry roasting, and shallow frying, whereas boiling is significant positively correlated with open pan dry roasting and shallow frying. Open pan dry roasting is perfect positively correlated with shallow frying. This table indicates that there is a strong correlation present among the **raw state, boiling, open pan dry roasting and shallow frying** in 14 days control preservation.

Table no 5.12.6.6.5 Correlation of cooking methods in 15 days preservation without preservative

Condition	RS	B	OPDR	SF	DF
Raw State (RS)	1	.961(S)	.982(S)	.993(S)	.982(S)
Boiling (B)	.961(S)	1	.891(S)	.923(S)	.996(S)
Open Pan Dry Roasting (OPDR)	.982(S)	.891(S)	1	.997*(S)	.929(S)
Shallow Frying (SF)	.993(S)	.923(S)	.997*(S)	1	.954(S)
Deep Frying (DF)	.982(S)	.996(S)	.929(S)	.954(S)	1

**.Correlation is highly significant at the 0.05 level (2-tailed)* Positive *S= Significant*

This table shows the correlation of calcium content of *hilsa* with cooking methods. In 15 days control preservation without preservative, there is significant positive correlation present between the raw state with boiling, open pan dry roasting, shallow frying and deep frying, whereas boiling is significant positively correlated with open pan dry roasting, shallow frying and deep frying. Open pan dry roasting is highly significant positively correlated with shallow frying and significant positively correlated with deep frying. Shallow frying is significant positively correlated with deep frying. This table indicates that there is a strong correlation present among the **raw state, boiling, open pan dry roasting, shallow frying and deep frying** in 15 days control preservation.

Table no 5.12.6.6.6 Correlation of cooking methods in 24 hours preservation with salt and turmeric

Condition	RS	B	OPDR	SF	DF
Raw State (RS)	1	-.676	.967(S)	.986(S)	.636
Boiling (B)	-.676	1	-.842(S)	-.545	-.999*(S)
Open Pan Dry Roasting (OPDR)	.967(S)	-.842(S)	1	.911(S)	.812(S)
Shallow Frying (SF)	.986(S)	-.545	.911(S)	1	.500
Deep Frying (DF)	.636	-.999*(S)	.812(S)	.500	1

**.Correlation is highly significant at the 0.05 level (2-tailed)* Positive Negative *S= Significant*

This table shows the correlation of calcium content of *hilsa* with cooking methods. In 24 hours salt and turmeric preservation, there is significant positive correlation present between the raw state with open pan dry roasting and shallow frying, whereas boiling is significant negatively correlated with open pan dry roasting and highly significant negatively correlated with deep frying. Open pan dry roasting is significant positively correlated with shallow frying and deep frying. This table indicates that there is a strong correlation present among the **raw state, boiling, open pan dry roasting, shallow frying and deep frying** in 24 hours salt and turmeric preservation.

Table no 5.12.6.6.7 Correlation of cooking methods in 48 hours preservation with salt and turmeric

Condition	RS	B	OPDR	SF	DF
Raw State (RS)	1	-.524	.596	.993(S)	.596
Boiling (B)	-.524	1	.371	-.619	.371
Open Pan Dry Roasting (OPDR)	.596	.371	1	.500	1.000**(S)
Shallow Frying (SF)	.993(S)	-.619	.500	1	.500
Deep Frying (DF)	.596	.371	1.000**(S)	.500	1

***.Correlation is highly significant at the 0.01 level (2-tailed)* ▭ Positive *S= Significant*

This table shows the correlation of calcium content of *hilsa* with cooking methods. In 48 hours salt and turmeric preservation, there is significant positive correlation present between the raw state and shallow frying, whereas open pan dry roasting is significant positively correlated with deep frying. This table indicates that there is a strong correlation present between the **raw state and shallow frying and also between open pan dry roasting and deep frying** in 48 hours salt and turmeric preservation.

Table no 5.12.6.6.8 Correlation of cooking methods in 14 days preservation with salt and turmeric

Condition	RS	B	OPDR	SF	DF
Raw State (RS)	1	.993(S)	.795	1.000**(S)	.596
Boiling (B)	.993(S)	1	.721	.993(S)	.500
Open Pan Dry Roasting (OPDR)	.795	.721	1	.795	.961(S)
Shallow Frying (SF)	1.000**(S)	.993(S)	.795	1	.596
Deep Frying (DF)	.596	.500	.961(S)	.596	1

***.Correlation is highly significant at the 0.01 level (2-tailed)* ▭ Positive *S= Significant*

This table shows the correlation of calcium content of *hilsa* with cooking methods. In 14 days salt and turmeric preservation, there is significant positive correlation present between the raw state and boiling, and perfect positively correlated with shallow frying, whereas boiling is significant positively correlated with shallow frying. This table indicates that there is a strong correlation present among the **raw state, boiling, open pan dry roasting, shallow frying and deep frying** in 14 days salt and turmeric preservation.

Table no 5.12.6.6.9 Correlation of cooking methods in 15 days preservation with salt and turmeric

Condition	RS	B	OPDR	SF	DF
Raw State (RS)	1	1.000**(S)	.993(S)	.986(S)	.596
Boiling (B)	1.000**(S)	1	.993(S)	.986(S)	.596
Open Pan Dry Roasting (OPDR)	.993(S)	.993(S)	1	.961(S)	.500
Shallow Frying (SF)	.986(S)	.986(S)	.961(S)	1	.721
Deep Frying (DF)	.596	.596	.500	.721	1

***.Correlation is highly significant at the 0.01 level (2-tailed)* ▭ Positive *S= Significant*

This table shows the correlation of calcium content of *hilsa* with cooking methods. In 15 days salt and turmeric preservation, there is significant positive correlation present between the raw state with open pan dry roasting and shallow frying, and perfect positively correlated with boiling, whereas boiling is significant positively correlated with open pan dry roasting and shallow frying. This table indicates that there is a strong correlation present among the **raw state, boiling, open pan dry roasting and shallow frying** in 15 days salt and turmeric preservation.

Table no 5.12.6.6.10 Correlation of cooking methods in 24 hours preservation with KMS

Condition	RS	B	OPDR	SF	DF
Raw State (RS)	1	.982(S)	.997*(S)	.577	.996(S)
Boiling (B)	.982(S)	1	.993(S)	.721	.961(S)
Open Pan Dry Roasting (OPDR)	.997*(S)	.993(S)	1	.636	.986(S)
Shallow Frying (SF)	.577	.721	.636	1	.500
Deep Frying (DF)	.996(S)	.961(S)	.986(S)	.500	1

***.Correlation is highly significant at the 0.01 level (2-tailed)* Positive *S= Significant*

This table shows the correlation of calcium content of *hilsa* with cooking methods. In 24 hours KMS preservation, there is significant positive correlation present between the raw state with boiling and deep frying and highly significant positively correlated with open pan dry roasting, whereas boiling is significant positively correlated with open pan dry roasting and shallow frying. Open pan dry roasting is significant positively correlated with deep frying. This table indicates that there is a strong correlation present among the **raw state, boiling, open pan dry roasting and deep frying** in 24 hours KMS preservation.

Table no 5.12.6.6.11 Correlation of cooking methods in 48 hours preservation with KMS

Condition	RS	B	OPDR	SF	DF
Raw State (RS)	1	.945(S)	.945(S)	-.842(S)	-.091
Boiling (B)	.945(S)	1	1.000**(S)	-.619	.240
Open Pan Dry Roasting (OPDR)	.945(S)	1.000**(S)	1	-.619	.240
Shallow Frying (SF)	-.842(S)	-.619	-.619	1	.614
Deep Frying (DF)	-.091	.240	.240	.614	1

***.Correlation is highly significant at the 0.01 level (2-tailed)* Positive Negative *S= Significant*

This table shows the correlation of calcium content of *hilsa* with cooking methods. In 48 hours KMS preservation, there is significant positive correlation present between the raw state with boiling and open pan dry roasting and significant negatively correlated with shallow frying, whereas boiling is perfect positively correlated with open pan dry roasting. This table indicates that there is a strong correlation present among the **raw state, boiling, open pan dry roasting and shallow frying** in 48 hours KMS preservation.

Table no 5.12.6.6.12 Correlation of cooking methods in 14 days preservation with KMS

Condition	RS	B	OPDR	SF	DF
Raw State (RS)	1	.911(S)	-.419	-.350	-.240
Boiling (B)	.911(S)	1	-.756	-.705	-.619
Open Pan Dry Roasting (OPDR)	-.419	-.756	1	.997*(S)	.982(S)
Shallow Frying (SF)	-.350	-.705	.997*(S)	1	.993(S)
Deep Frying (DF)	-.240	-.619	.982(S)	.993(S)	1

**.Correlation is highly significant at the 0.05 level (2-tailed)* Positive *S= Significant*

This table shows the correlation of calcium content of *hilsa* with cooking methods. In 14 days KMS preservation, there is significant positive correlation present between the raw state and boiling, whereas open pan dry roasting is highly significant positively correlated with shallow frying. Deep frying is significant positively correlated with open pan dry roasting and shallow frying. This table indicates that there is a strong correlation present among the **raw state, boiling, open pan dry roasting, shallow frying and deep frying** in 14 days KMS preservation.

Table no 5.12.6.6.13 Correlation of cooking methods in 15 days preservation with KMS

Condition	RS	B	OPDR	SF	DF
Raw State (RS)	1	-.240	-.500	.993(S)	1.000**(S)
Boiling (B)	-.240	1	.961(S)	-.350	-.240
Open Pan Dry Roasting (OPDR)	-.500	.961(S)	1	-.596	-.500
Shallow Frying (SF)	.993(S)	-.350	-.596	1	.993(S)
Deep Frying (DF)	1.000**(S)	-.240	-.500	.993(S)	1

***.Correlation is highly significant at the 0.01 level (2-tailed)* Positive *S= Significant*

This table shows the correlation of calcium content of *hilsa* with cooking methods. In 15 days KMS preservation, there is significant positive correlation present between the raw state and shallow frying and perfect positively correlated with deep frying, whereas open pan dry roasting is significant positively correlated with boiling. Deep frying is significant positively correlated with shallow frying. This table indicates that there is a strong correlation present among the **raw state, boiling, open pan dry roasting, shallow frying and deep frying** in 15 days KMS preservation.

Overall analysis reveals that the raw state is perfect positively correlated with boiling, open pan dry roasting and deep frying in 15 days salt-turmeric preservation, 14 days control preservation without preservative and 15 days KMS preservation respectively, whereas perfect positively correlated with shallow frying in 14 days preservation with salt-turmeric and 14 days control preservation without preservative. Boiling is perfect positively correlated with open pan dry roasting in 48 hours KMS preservation, whereas significant positively correlated with shallow frying in 14 days salt and turmeric preservation, and highly significant negatively correlated with deep frying in 24 hours salt-turmeric preservation. Open pan dry roasting is perfect positively correlated with shallow frying in fresh condition and 14 days control preservation without preservative, and perfect positively correlated with deep frying in 48 hours salt and turmeric preservation. Shallow frying is significant positively correlated with deep frying in 48 hours control preservation without preservative, 14 days and 15 days KMS preservation. Most of the correlation of the calcium content of *hilsa* is found in **14 days control preservation without preservative** with respect to different cooking conditions.

5.12.6.7 Iron

Table no 5.12.6.7.1 Correlation of cooking methods in fresh condition

Condition	RS	B	OPDR	SF	DF
Raw State (RS)	1	.596	.756	.569	.756
Boiling (B)	.596	1	.976(S)	.999*(S)	-.075
Open Pan Dry Roasting (OPDR)	.756	.976(S)	1	.969(S)	.143
Shallow Frying (SF)	.569	.999*(S)	.969(S)	1	-.108
Deep Frying (DF)	.756	-.075	.143	-.108	1

***.Correlation is highly significant at the 0.01 level (2-tailed)* ▭ Positive *S= Significant*

This table shows the correlation of iron content of *hilsa* with cooking methods. In fresh condition, there is significant positive correlation present between boiling and open pan dry roasting and highly significant positively correlated with deep frying, whereas open pan dry roasting is significant positively correlated with boiling. Deep frying is significant positively correlated with shallow frying. This table indicates that there is a strong correlation present among **boiling, open pan dry roasting, shallow frying** in fresh condition.

Table no 5.12.6.7.2 Correlation of cooking methods in 24 hours preservation without preservative

Condition	RS	B	OPDR	SF	DF
Raw State (RS)	1	.702	-.964(S)	-1.000*(S)	-.922(S)
Boiling (B)	.702	1	-.866(S)	-.715	-.371
Open Pan Dry Roasting (OPDR)	-.964(S)	-.866(S)	1	.969(S)	.786
Shallow Frying (SF)	-1.000*(S)	-.715	.969(S)	1	.915(S)
Deep Frying (DF)	-.922(S)	-.371	.786	.915(S)	1

**.Correlation is highly significant at the 0.05 level (2-tailed)* ▭ Positive ▭ Negative *S= Significant*

This table shows the correlation of iron content of *hilsa* with cooking methods. In 24 hours control preservation without preservative, there is significant negative correlation present between the raw state with open pan dry roasting and deep frying and perfect negatively correlated with shallow frying, whereas open pan dry roasting is significant negatively correlated with boiling and significant positively correlated with shallow frying. Deep frying is significant positively correlated with shallow frying. This table indicates that there is a strong correlation present among the **raw state, boiling, open pan dry roasting, shallow frying and deep frying** in 24 hours control preservation.

Table no 5.12.6.7.3 Correlation of cooking methods in 48 hours preservation without preservative

Condition	RS	B	OPDR	SF	DF
Raw State (RS)	1	-.636	.038	.091	.775
Boiling (B)	-.636	1	-.795	-.826(S)	-.981(S)
Open Pan Dry Roasting (OPDR)	.038	-.795	1	.999*(S)	.661
Shallow Frying (SF)	.091	-.826	.999*(S)	1	.700
Deep Frying (DF)	.775	-.981(S)	.661	.700	1

**.Correlation is highly significant at the 0.05 level (2-tailed)* ▭ Positive ▭ Negative *S= Significant*

This table shows the correlation of iron content of *hilsa* with cooking methods. In 48 hours control preservation without preservative, there is significant negative correlation present between boiling with shallow frying and deep frying, whereas open pan dry roasting is highly significant positively correlated with shallow frying. This table indicates that there is a strong correlation present among **boiling, open pan dry roasting, shallow frying and deep frying** in 48 hours control preservation.

Table no 5.12.6.7.4 Correlation of cooking methods in 14 days preservation without preservative

Condition	RS	B	OPDR	SF	DF
Raw state (RS)	1	.540	.899(S)	.999*(S)	-.998*(S)
Boiling (B)	.540	1	.854(S)	.500	-.590
Open Pan Dry Roasting (OPDR)	.899(S)	.854(S)	1	.877(S)	-.924(S)
Shallow Frying (SF)	.999*(S)	.500	.877	1	-.994(S)
Deep Frying (DF)	-.998*(S)	-.590	-.924(S)	-.994(S)	1

**.Correlation is highly significant at the 0.05level (2-tailed)* Positive Negative *S= Significant*

This table shows the correlation of iron content of *hilsa* with cooking methods. In 14 days control preservation without preservative, there is significant positive correlation present between the raw state and open pan dry roasting, and highly significant positive correlation present between the raw state and shallow frying, and highly negative correlation present between the raw state and deep frying. Open pan dry roasting is significant positively correlated with boiling and shallow frying and significant negatively correlated with deep frying. Shallow frying is significant negatively correlated with deep frying. This table indicates that there is a strong correlation present among the **raw state, boiling, open pan dry roasting, shallow frying and deep frying** in 14 days control preservation.

Table no 5.12.6.7.5 Correlation of cooking methods in 15 days preservation without preservative

Condition	RS	B	OPDR	SF	DF
Raw State (RS)	1	-.327	.993(S)	-.132	.554
Boiling (B)	-.327	1	-.217	.980(S)	.605
Open Pan Dry Roasting (OPDR)	.993(S)	-.217	1	-.017	.646
Shallow Frying (SF)	-.132	.980(S)	-.017	1	.752
Deep Frying (DF)	.554	.605	.646	.752	1

Positive *S= Significant*

This table shows the correlation of iron content of *hilsa* with cooking methods. In 15 days control preservation without preservation, there is significant positive correlation present between the raw state and open pan dry roasting, whereas boiling is significant positively correlated with shallow frying. This table indicates that there is a strong correlation present between the **raw state and open pan dry roasting and also between boiling and shallow frying** in 15 days control preservation.

Table no 5.12.6.7.6 Correlation of cooking methods in 24 hours salt and turmeric preservation

Condition	RS	B	OPDR	SF	DF
Raw State (RS)	1	.954(S)	-.974(S)	-.974(S)	1.000**(S)
Boiling (B)	.954(S)	1	-.997*(S)	-.997*(S)	.954(S)
Open Pan Dry Roasting (OPDR)	-.974(S)	-.997*(S)	1	1.000**(S)	-.974(S)
Shallow Frying (SF)	-.974(S)	-.997*(S)	1.000**(S)	1	-.974(S)
Deep Frying (DF)	1.000**(S)	.954(S)	-.974(S)	-.974(S)	1

***.Correlation is highly significant at the 0.01 level (2-tailed)* Positive Negative *S= Significant*
**.Correlation is highly significant at the 0.05 level (2-tailed)*

This table shows the correlation of iron content of *hilsa* with cooking methods. In 24 hours salt and turmeric preservation, there is significant positive correlation present between the raw state with boiling, and significant negative correlation present between the raw state with open pan dry roasting and shallow frying, and perfect positive correlation present between the raw state and deep frying. Boiling is significant positively correlated deep frying and highly significant negatively correlated with open pan dry roasting and shallow frying. Open pan dry roasting is perfect positively correlated with shallow frying and significant negatively correlated with deep frying. Deep frying is significant negatively correlated with shallow frying. This table indicates that there is a strong correlation present among the **raw state, boiling, open pan dry roasting, shallow frying and deep frying** in 24 hours salt and turmeric preservation.

Table no 5.12.6.7.7 Correlation of cooking methods in 48 hours salt and turmeric preservation

Condition	RS	B	OPDR	SF	DF
Raw State (RS)	1	-.262	-.500	-.596	-.596
Boiling (B)	-.262	1	-.705	-.619	-.619
Open Pan Dry Roasting (OPDR)	-.500	-.705	1	.993(S)	.993(S)
Shallow Frying (SF)	-.596	-.619	.993(S)	1	1.000**(S)
Deep Frying (DF)	-.596	-.619	.993(S)	1.000**(S)	1

***.Correlation is highly significant at the 0.01 level (2-tailed)* ▭ Positive *S= Significant*

This table shows the correlation of iron content of *hilsa* with cooking methods. In 48 hours salt and turmeric preservation, there is significant positive correlation present between the open pan dry roasting and shallow frying and deep frying, whereas shallow frying is perfect positively correlated with deep frying. This table indicates that there is a strong correlation present among **open pan dry roasting, shallow frying and deep frying** in 48 hours salt and turmeric preservation.

Table no 5.12.6.7.8 Correlation of cooking methods in 14 days salt and turmeric preservation

Condition	RS	B	OPDR	SF	DF
Raw State (RS)	1	.235	.475	.524	.524
Boiling (B)	.235	1	.967(S)	-.705	-.705
Open Pan Dry Roasting (OPDR)	.475	.967(S)	1	-.500	-.500
Shallow Frying (SF)	.524	-.705	-.500	1	1.000**(S)
Deep Frying (DF)	.524	-.705	-.500	1.000**(S)	1

***.Correlation is highly significant at the 0.01 level (2-tailed)* ▭ Positive *S= Significant*

This table shows the correlation of iron content of *hilsa* with cooking methods. In 14 days salt and turmeric preservation, there is significant positive correlation present between boiling and open pan dry roasting, whereas deep frying is significant positively correlated with shallow frying. This table indicates that there is a strong correlation present between **boiling and open pan dry roasting and also between shallow frying and deep frying** in 14 days salt and turmeric preservation.

Table no 5.12.6.7.9 Correlation of cooking methods in 15 days salt and turmeric preservation

Condition	RS	B	OPDR	SF	DF
Raw State (RS)	1	-1.000**(S)	1.000**(S)	1.000**(S)	1.000**(S)
Boiling (B)	-1.000**(S)	1	-1.000**(S)	-1.000**(S)	-1.000**(S)
Open Pan Dry Roasting (OPDR)	1.000**(S)	-1.000**(S)	1	1.000**(S)	1.000**(S)
Shallow Frying (SF)	1.000**(S)	-1.000**(S)	1.000**(S)	1	1.000**(S)
Deep Frying (DF)	1.000**(S)	-1.000**(S)	1.000**(S)	1.000**(S)	1

***.Correlation is highly significant at the 0.01 level (2-tailed)* ▭ Positive ▭ Negative *S= Significant*

This table shows the correlation of iron content of *hilsa* with cooking methods. In 15 days salt and turmeric preservation, there is perfect positive correlation present between the raw state with open pan dry roasting, shallow frying and deep frying, and perfect negative correlation present between the raw state and boiling. Boiling is perfect positively correlated with open pan dry roasting and deep frying. Open pan dry roasting is perfect positively correlated with shallow frying and deep frying. Deep frying is perfect positively correlated with shallow frying. This table indicates that there is a strong correlation present among the **raw state, boiling, open pan dry roasting, shallow frying and deep frying** in 15 days salt and turmeric preservation.

Table no 5.12.6.7.10 Correlation of cooking methods in 24 hours KMS preservation

Condition	RS	B	OPDR	SF	DF
Raw State (RS)	1	1.000**(S)	-.992(S)	.923(S)	-1.000**(S)
Boiling (B)	1.000**(S)	1	-.992(S)	.923(S)	-1.000**(S)
Open Pan Dry Roasting (OPDR)	-.992(S)	-.992(S)	1	-.866(S)	.992(S)
Shallow Frying (SF)	.923(S)	.923(S)	-.866(S)	1	-.923(S)
Deep Frying (DF)	-1.000** (S)	-1.000**(S)	.992(S)	-.923(S)	1

***.Correlation is highly significant at the 0.01 level (2-tailed)* Positive Negative *S= Significant*

This table shows the correlation of iron content of *hilsa* with cooking methods. In 24 hours KMS preservation, there is significant positive correlation present between the raw state and boiling, whereas boiling is significant positively correlated with open pan dry roasting. Open pan dry roasting is significant negatively correlated with the raw state and shallow frying and significant positively correlated with deep frying. Shallow frying is significant positively correlated with the raw state and boiling and significant negatively correlated with deep frying. Deep frying is perfect negatively correlated with the raw state and boiling and significant positively correlated with open pan dry roasting. This table indicates that there is a strong correlation present among the **raw state, boiling, open pan dry roasting, shallow frying and deep frying** in 24 hours KMS preservation.

Table no 5.12.6.7.11 Correlation of cooking methods in 48 hours KMS preservation

Condition	RS	B	OPDR	SF	DF
Raw State (RS)	1	.974(S)	1.000**(S)	.986(S)	.986(S)
Boiling (B)	.974(S)	1	.974(S)	.923(S)	.923(S)
Open Pan Dry Roasting (OPDR)	1.000**(S)	.974(S)	1	.986(S)	.986(S)
Shallow Frying (SF)	.986(S)	.923(S)	.986(S)	1	1.000**(S)
Deep Frying (DF)	.986(S)	.923(S)	.986(S)	1.000**(S)	1

***.Correlation is highly significant at the 0.01 level (2-tailed)* Positive *S= Significant*

This table shows the correlation of iron content of *hilsa* with cooking methods. In 48 hours KMS preservation, there is significant positive correlation present between the raw state with boiling, shallow frying and deep frying, and perfect positive correlation present between the raw state and open pan dry roasting. Boiling is significant positively correlated with open pan dry roasting, shallow frying and deep frying. Open pan dry roasting is significant positively correlated with shallow frying and deep frying. Deep frying is perfect positively correlated with shallow frying. This table indicates that there is a strong correlation present among the **raw state, boiling, open pan dry roasting, shallow frying and deep frying** in 48 hours KMS preservation.

Table no 5.12.6.7.12 Correlation of cooking methods in 14 days KMS preservation

Condition	RS	B	OPDR	SF	DF
Raw state (RS)	1	1.000**(S)	.974(S)	-.705	.986(S)
Boiling (B)	1.000**(S)	1	.974(S)	-.705	.986(S)
Open Pan Dry Roasting (OPDR)	.974(S)	.974(S)	1	-.524	.923(S)
Shallow Frying (SF)	-.705	-.705	-.524	1	-.812(S)
Deep Frying (DF)	.986(S)	.986(S)	.923(S)	-.812(S)	1

***.Correlation is highly significant at the 0.01 level (2-tailed)* Positive Negative *S= Significant*

This table shows the correlation of iron content of *hilsa* with cooking methods. In 14 days KMS preservation, there is significant positive correlation present between the raw state with open pan dry roasting and deep frying, and perfect positively correlated with boiling. Boiling is significant positively correlated with open pan dry roasting and deep frying. Open pan dry roasting is significant positively correlated with deep frying. Deep frying is significant negatively correlated with shallow frying. This table indicates that there is a strong correlation present among the **raw state, boiling, open pan dry roasting, shallow frying and deep frying** in 14 days KMS preservation.

Table no 5.12.6.7.13 Correlation of cooking methods in 15 days KMS preservation

Condition	RS	B	OPDR	SF	DF
Raw State (RS)	1	-.705	.974(S)	-.705	.901(S)
Boiling (B)	-.705	1	-.524	1.000**(S)	-.327
Open Pan Dry Roasting (OPDR)	.974(S)	-.524	1	-.524	.976(S)
Shallow Frying (SF)	-.705	1.000**(S)	-.524	1	-.327
Deep Frying (DF)	.901(S)	-.327	.976(S)	-.327	1

***.Correlation is highly significant at the 0.01 level (2-tailed)* Positive *S= Significant*

This table shows the correlation of iron content of *hilsa* with cooking methods. In 15 days KMS preservation, there is significant positive correlation present between the raw state with open pan dry roasting and deep frying, whereas boiling is perfect positively correlated with shallow frying. Open pan dry roasting is significant positively correlated with deep frying. This table indicates that there is a strong correlation present among the **raw state, boiling, open pan dry roasting, shallow frying and deep frying** in 15 days KMS preservation.

Overall analysis reveals that the raw state is perfect positively correlated with boiling in 24 hours and 14 days KMS preservation and perfect negatively correlated with boiling in 15 days salt-turmeric preservation, whereas perfect positively correlated with open pan dry roasting in 48 hours preservation with KMS and 15 days salt-turmeric preservation, perfect positively correlated with shallow frying in 15 days salt and turmeric preservation and perfect negatively correlated with shallow frying in 24 hours control preservation without preservative, and perfect negatively correlated with deep frying in 24 hours KMS preservation and 15 days salt-turmeric preservation and perfect positively correlated with deep frying in 24 hours salt-turmeric preservation. Boiling is perfect positively correlated with open pan dry roasting in 15 days salt-turmeric preservation, whereas perfect positively correlated with shallow frying in 15 days KMS preservation and perfect negatively correlated with shallow frying in 15 days salt-turmeric preservation, and perfect positively correlated with deep frying in 24 hours KMS preservation and 15 days salt-turmeric preservation. Open pan dry roasting is perfect positively correlated with shallow frying and deep frying in 15 days salt and turmeric. Shallow frying is perfect positively correlated with deep frying in 48 hours KMS preservation, 48 hours, 14 days and 15 days salt-turmeric preservation. Most of the correlation of the iron content of *hilsa* is found in **15 days salt-turmeric preservation** with respect to different cooking conditions.

5.12.6.8 Energy

Table no 5.12.6.8.1 Correlation of cooking methods in fresh condition

Condition	RS	B	OPDR	SF	DF
Raw State (RS)	1	.561	.879(S)	.517	-.632
Boiling (B)	.561	1	.887(S)	-.419	.287
Open Pan Dry Roasting (OPDR)	.879(S)	.887(S)	1	.046	-.186
Shallow Frying (SF)	.517	-.419	.046	1	-.990(S)
Deep Frying (DF)	-.632	.287	-.186	-.990(S)	1

Positive Negative *S= Significant*

This table shows the correlation of energy content of *hilsa* with cooking methods. In fresh condition, there is significant positive correlation present between the raw state and open pan dry roasting, whereas open pan dry roasting is significant positively correlated with boiling. Deep frying is significant negatively correlated with shallow frying. This table indicates that there is a strong correlation present among the **raw state, boiling, open pan dry roasting, shallow frying and deep frying** in fresh condition.

Table no 5.12.6.8.2 Correlation of cooking methods in 24 hours preservation without preservative

Condition	RS	B	OPDR	SF	DF
Raw State (RS)	1	.716	-.781	.779	-.975(S)
Boiling (B)	.716	1	-.123	.120	-.543
Open Pan Dry Roasting (OPDR)	-.781	-.123	1	-1.000**	.900(S)
Shallow Frying (SF)	.779	.120	-1.000**(S)	1	-.899(S)
Deep Frying (DF)	-.975(S)	-.543	.900(S)	-.899(S)	1

***.Correlation is highly significant at the 0.01 level (2-tailed)* Positive Negative *S= Significant*

This table shows the correlation of energy content of *hilsa* with cooking methods. In 24 hours control preservation without preservative, there is significant negative correlation present between the raw state and deep frying, whereas open pan dry roasting is perfect negatively correlated with shallow frying and significant positively correlated with deep frying. Deep frying is significant negatively correlated with shallow frying. This table indicates that there is a strong correlation present among the **raw state, boiling, open pan dry roasting, shallow frying and deep frying** in 24 hours control preservation.

Table no 5.12.6.8.3 Correlation of cooking methods in 48 hours preservation without preservative

Condition	RS	B	OPDR	SF	DF
Raw State (RS)	1	-.199	.137	1.000**(S)	-.978(S)
Boiling (B)	-.199	1	.943(S)	-.186	.400
Open Pan Dry Roasting (OPDR)	.137	.943(S)	1	.151	.073
Shallow Frying (SF)	1.000**(S)	-.186	.151	1	-.975(S)
Deep Frying (DF)	-.978(S)	.400	.073	-.975(S)	1

***.Correlation is highly significant at the 0.01 level (2-tailed)* Positive Negative *S= Significant*

This table shows the correlation of energy content of *hilsa* with cooking methods. In 48 hours control preservation without preservative, there is perfect positive correlation present between the raw state and shallow frying and significant negatively correlated with deep frying, whereas open pan dry roasting is significant positively correlated with boiling. Deep frying is significant negatively correlated with shallow frying. This table indicates that there is a strong correlation present among the **raw state, boiling, open pan dry roasting, shallow frying and deep frying** in 48 hours control preservation.

Table no 5.12.6.8.4 Correlation of cooking methods in 14 days preservation without preservative

Condition	RS	B	OPDR	SF	DF
Raw State (RS)	1	-.910(S)	-.952(S)	.494	-.818(S)
Boiling (B)	-.910(S)	1	.738	-.089	.505
Open Pan Dry Roasting (OPDR)	-.952(S)	.738	1	-.737	.955(S)
Shallow Frying (SF)	.494	-.089	-.737	1	-.904(S)
Deep Frying (DF)	-.818(S)	.505	.955(S)	-.904(S)	1

***.Correlation is highly significant at the 0.01 level (2-tailed)* Positive Negative *S= Significant*

This table shows the correlation of energy content of *hilsa* with cooking methods. In 14 days control preservation, there is significant negative correlation present between the raw state with boiling, open pan dry roasting and deep frying, whereas open pan dry roasting is significant positively correlated with deep frying. Deep frying is significant positively correlated with open pan dry roasting and significant negatively correlated with shallow frying. This table indicates that there is a strong correlation present among the **raw state, boiling, open pan dry roasting, shallow frying and deep frying** in 14 days control preservation.

Table no 5.12.6.8.5 Correlation of cooking methods in 15 days preservation without preservative

Condition	RS	B	OPDR	SF	DF
Raw State (RS)	1	.932(S)	-.845(S)	.075	-.993(S)
Boiling (B)	.932(S)	1	-.981(S)	.431	-.968(S)
Open Pan Dry Roasting (OPDR)	-.845(S)	-.981(S)	1	-.596	.903(S)
Shallow Frying (SF)	.075	.431	-.596	1	-.193
Deep Frying (DF)	-.993(S)	-.968(S)	.903(S)	-.193	1

Positive *S= Significant*

This table shows the correlation of energy content of *hilsa* with cooking methods. In 15 days control preservation without preservative, there is significant positive correlation present between the raw state with boiling, and significant negative correlation present between the raw state with open pan dry roasting and deep frying. Boiling is significant negatively correlated with open pan dry roasting and deep frying. Open pan dry roasting is significant positively correlated with deep frying. This table indicates that there is a strong correlation present among the **raw state, boiling, open pan dry roasting and deep frying** in 15 days control preservation.

Table no 5.12.6.8.6 Correlation of cooking methods in 24 hours salt and turmeric preservation

Condition	RS	B	OPDR	SF	DF
Raw State (RS)	1	.640	.589	-.395	.032
Boiling (B)	.640	1	-.244	-.959(S)	-.748
Open Pan Dry Roasting (OPDR)	.589	-.244	1	.509	.826(S)
Shallow Frying (SF)	-.395	-.959(S)	.509	1	.906(S)
Deep Frying (DF)	.032	-.748	.826(S)	.906(S)	1

Positive Negative *S= Significant*

This table shows the correlation of energy content of *hilsa* with cooking methods. In 24 hours salt and turmeric preservation, there is significant negative correlation present between boiling and shallow frying, whereas both open pan dry roasting and shallow frying are significant positively correlated with deep frying. This table indicates that there is a strong correlation present among **boiling, open pan dry roasting, shallow frying and deep frying** in 24 hours salt and turmeric preservation.

Table no 5.12.6.8.7 Correlation of cooking methods in 48 hours salt and turmeric preservation

Condition	RS	B	OPDR	SF	DF
Raw State (RS)	1	.996(S)	-.021	.989(S)	.591
Boiling (B)	.996(S)	1	-.106	.972(S)	.519
Open Pan Dry Roasting (OPDR)	-.021	-.106	1	.131	.795
Shallow Frying (SF)	.989(S)	.972(S)	.131	1	.706
Deep Frying (DF)	.591	.519	.795	.706	1

Positive *S= Significant*

This table shows the correlation of energy content of *hilsa* with cooking methods. In 48 hours salt and turmeric preservation, there is significant positive correlation present between the raw state with boiling and shallow frying, whereas boiling is significant positively correlated with shallow frying. This table indicates that there is a strong correlation present among the **raw state, boiling and shallow frying** in 48 hours salt and turmeric preservation.

Table no 5.12.6.8.8 Correlation of cooking methods in 14 days salt and turmeric preservation

Condition	RS	B	OPDR	SF	DF
Raw State (RS)	1	.490	-.947(S)	-.346	.032
Boiling (B)	.490	1	-.184	-.987(S)	-.856(S)
Open Pan Dry Roasting (OPDR)	-.947(S)	-.184	1	.027	-.351
Shallow Frying (SF)	-.346	-.987(S)	.027	1	.927(S)
Deep Frying (DF)	.032	-.856(S)	-.351	.927(S)	1

Positive Negative *S= Significant*

This table shows the correlation of energy content of *hilsa* with cooking methods. In 14 days salt and turmeric preservation, there is significant negative correlation present between the raw state and open pan dry roasting, whereas boiling is significant negatively correlated with shallow frying and deep frying. Deep frying is significant positively correlated with shallow frying. This table indicates that there is a strong correlation present among the **raw state, boiling, open pan dry roasting, shallow frying and deep frying** in 14 days salt and turmeric preservation.

Table no 5.12.6.8.9 Correlation of cooking methods in 15 days salt and turmeric preservation

Condition	RS	B	OPDR	SF	DF
Raw State (RS)	1	.383	.842(S)	-.622	-.588
Boiling (B)	.383	1	.821(S)	.485	.521
Open Pan Dry Roasting (OPDR)	.842(S)	.821(S)	1	-.101	-.059
Shallow Frying (SF)	-.622	.485	-.101	1	.999*(S)
Deep Frying (DF)	-.588	.521	-.059	.999*(S)	1

**.Correlation is highly significant at the 0.05 level (2-tailed)* Positive *S= Significant*

This table shows the correlation of energy content of *hilsa* with cooking methods. In 15 days salt and turmeric preservation, there is significant positive correlation present between the raw state and open pan dry roasting, whereas open pan dry roasting is significant positively correlated with boiling. Deep frying is highly significant positively correlated with shallow frying. This table indicates that there is a strong correlation present among the **raw state, boiling, open pan dry roasting, shallow frying and deep frying** in 15 days salt and turmeric preservation.

Table no 5.12.6.8.10 Correlation of cooking methods in 24 hours KMS preservation

Condition	RS	B	OPDR	SF	DF
Raw State (RS)	1	-.271	.735	-.787	-.239
Boiling (B)	-.271	1	.454	-.381	-.870(S)
Open Pan Dry Roasting (OPDR)	.735	.454	1	-.997(S)	-.835(S)
Shallow Frying (SF)	-.787	-.381	-.997(S)	1	.787
Deep Frying (DF)	-.239	-.870(S)	-.835(S)	.787	1

***.Correlation is highly significant at the 0.01 level (2-tailed)* Negative *S= Significant*

This table shows the correlation of energy content of *hilsa* with cooking methods. In 24 hours KMS preservation, there is significant negative correlation present between boiling and deep frying, whereas open pan dry roasting is significant negatively correlated with shallow frying and deep frying. This table indicates that there is a strong correlation present among **boiling, open pan dry roasting, shallow frying and deep frying** in 24 hours KMS preservation.

Table no 5.12.6.8.11 Correlation of cooking methods in 48 hours KMS preservation

Condition	RS	B	OPDR	SF	DF
Raw State (RS)	1	.992(S)	.122	-.493	.951(S)
Boiling (B)	.992(S)	1	-.003	-.381	.982(S)
Open Pan Dry Roasting (OPDR)	.122	-.003	1	-.923(S)	-.190
Shallow Frying (SF)	-.493	-.381	-.923(S)	1	-.202
Deep Frying (DF)	.951(S)	.982(S)	-.190	-.202	1

Positive Negative *S= Significant*

This table shows the correlation of energy content of *hilsa* with cooking methods. In 48 hours KMS preservation, there is significant positive correlation present between the raw state with boiling and deep frying, whereas boiling is significant positively correlated with deep frying. Open pan dry roasting is significant positively correlated with shallow frying. This table indicates that there is a strong correlation present among the **raw state, boiling, open pan dry roasting, shallow frying and deep frying** in 48 hours KMS preservation.

Table no 5.12.6.8.12 Correlation of cooking methods in 14 days KMS preservation

Condition	RS	B	OPDR	SF	DF
Raw State (RS)	1	.985(S)	-.174	.502	.993(S)
Boiling (B)	.985(S)	1	-.344	.343	.998*(S)
Open Pan Dry Roasting (OPDR)	-.174	-.344	1	.764	-.286
Shallow Frying (SF)	.502	.343	.764	1	.399
Deep Frying (DF)	.993(S)	.998*(S)	-.286	.399	1

**.Correlation is highly significant at the 0.05 level (2-tailed)* Positive *S= Significant*

This table shows the correlation of energy content of *hilsa* with cooking methods. In 14 days KMS preservation, there is significant positive correlation present between the raw state with boiling and deep frying, whereas boiling is highly significant positively correlated with deep frying. This table indicates that there is a strong correlation present among the **raw state, boiling and deep frying** in 15 days KMS preservation.

Table no 5.12.6.8.13 Correlation of cooking methods in 15 days KMS preservation

Condition	RS	B	OPDR	SF	DF
Raw State (RS)	1	-.960(S)	-.945(S)	-.134	-.444
Boiling (B)	-.960(S)	1	.999*(S)	.406	.677
Open Pan Dry Roasting (OPDR)	-.945(S)	.999*(S)	1	.451	.713
Shallow Frying (SF)	-.134	.406	.451	1	.948(S)
Deep Frying (DF)	-.444	.677	.713	.948(S)	1

**.Correlation is highly significant at the 0.05 level (2-tailed)* Positive Negative *S= Significant*

This table shows the correlation of energy content of *hilsa* with cooking methods. In 15 days KMS preservation, there is significant negative correlation present between the raw state with boiling and open pan dry roasting, whereas open pan dry roasting is highly significant positively correlated with boiling. Deep frying is significant positively correlated with shallow frying. This table indicates that there is a strong correlation present among the **raw state, boiling, open pan dry roasting, shallow frying and deep frying** in 15 days KMS preservation.

Overall analysis reveals that the raw state is significant positively correlated with boiling in 48 hours salt-turmeric preservation, whereas significant negatively correlated with open pan dry roasting in 14 days control preservation without preservative, perfect positively correlated with shallow frying in 48 hours control preservation without preservative, and significant positively correlated with deep frying in 14 days KMS preservation and significant negatively correlated with deep frying in 15 days control preservation without preservative. Boiling is highly significant positively correlated with open pan dry roasting in 15 days preservation with KMS, whereas significant negatively correlated with shallow frying in 15 days salt and turmeric preservation, and highly significant positively correlated with deep frying in 14 days KMS preservation. Open pan dry roasting is perfect negatively correlated with shallow frying in 24 hours control preservation without preservative, and significant positively correlated with deep frying in 14 days control preservation without preservative. Shallow frying is highly significant positively correlated with deep frying in 15 days salt-turmeric preservation. Most of the correlation of the energy content of *hilsa* is found in **14 days control preservation without preservative and 14 days KMS preservation** with respect to different cooking conditions.

Finally, the overall correlation matrix analyses reveal that most of the correlation of the nutrient contents present in *rohu*, prawn and *hilsa* in 48 hours, 24 hours and 14 days control preservation without preservative respectively, whereas in *katla* in 48 hours KMS preservation as well as in 48 hours salt-turmeric preservation, and in lobster and pomfret in 15 days and 14 days KMS preservation respectively. Significant correlations mainly take place in control preservation without preservative and KMS preservation for all the samples. *Rohu* and prawn response mostly in control preservation without preservative, whereas *hilsa* responses in salt-turmeric preservation, and pomfret and lobster response in KMS preservation. Highest number of correlations found in prawn among the other samples. Most of the cooking methods are significant positively correlated with each other under different preservation conditions along with the fresh condition for all the nutrient contents in *rohu*, *katla*, lobster, pomfret and *hilsa*, whereas significant negative correlation present in prawn only.

5.13 Comparative Index

This statistical analysis is carried out to estimate the best cooking method for restoring nutrient content among the different studied conventional cooking methods, the best preservation day among the studied preservation days up to which fish and other edible aquatic species can be preserved, the best preservation methods among the studied different preservation methods for preserving the nutritional quality and lastly the best fish among the studied samples from the point of nutritional aspect.

Table no 5.13.1 Best cooking method

Conditions	*Rohu*	*Katla*	Prawn	Lobster	Pomfret	*Hilsa*
Raw	0.863	0.829	0.855	0.763	1.246	0.882
Boiling	0.953	1.185	1.00	0.653	1.415	0.980
Open pan dry roasting	0.965	0.918	0.974	0.732	1.347	0.859
Shallow frying	0.851	0.913	1.372	0.759	1.514	1.021
Deep frying	0.867	1.094	1.572	0.907	1.126	1.074

Highlighted colour represents the highest value for each sample.

This table shows the best cooking method to restore the nutritional quality among all the studied conventional cooking methods with respect to the raw condition for all fish and other edible aquatic species. The highlighted colours represent the highest values that indicate the best cooking method for different fish and other edible aquatic species. The table indicates that open pan dry roasting can restore the nutritive value of *rohu*, whereas boiling can restore the nutritive value of *katla*, and shallow frying can restore the nutrient content of pomfret, and deep frying can restore the nutritive value of prawn, lobster *and hilsa*. Comparative index number indicates that deep frying shows the highest value to restore the nutrient content for prawn. Hence overall analysis reveals that deep frying can mostly restore nutrient content among the studied methods for most of the samples. Cooking methods can be graded in the following manner- deep frying> shallow frying> boiling> open pan dry roasting.

Table no 5.13.2 Best preservation day

Duration	*Rohu*	*Katla*	Prawn	Lobster	Pomfret	*Hilsa*
Fresh	0.908	1.021	1.204	0.758	1.343	0.980
24 hours	0.999	0.984	1.592	0.878	0.874	0.542
48 hours	0.791	0.810	1.367	0.741	0.808	0.630
14 days	1.030	0.779	1.660	0.948	1.030	0.622
15 days	0.958	0.693	**1.775**	1.180	1.010	0.471

Highlighted colour represents the highest value for each sample.

This table shows the best preservation days to preserve the nutrient content among all the studied conventional preservation days up to which the samples are preserved with respect to fresh condition for all fish and other edible aquatic species. The highlighted colours represent the highest values that indicate the best preservation day of different samples with respect to fresh condition. 24 hours preserves *katla*, whereas 48 hours preserves *hilsa*, 14 days preserves *rohu* and pomfret, and 15 days preserves prawn and lobster to the maximum nutrient restoration phase. The comparative index number indicates that the 15 days preservation shows the highest value to restore nutrient content of prawn. Thus overall analysis reveals that 15 days is the best preservation day to preserve the crustaceans and 14 days is the best preservation day to preserve other studied fish, but *katla* cannot be preserved for prolonged period as the nutritional quality deteriorates. Preservation days can be graded in the following manner- 15 days>14 days>24 hours>48 hours.

Table no 5.13.3 Best preservation method

method	*Rohu*	*Katla*	Prawn	Lobster	Pomfret	*Hilsa*
Without preservative	0.865	1.112	1.091	0.713	1.276	0.948
Combination of salt and turmeric	1.039	0.982	1.094	0.804	1.403	1.026
KMS	0.807	0.860	1.191	0.762	1.293	0.908

Highlighted colour represents the highest value for each sample.

This table shows the best preservation method to preserve the nutrient content among all the studied conventional preservation methods for all fish and other edible aquatic species. The highlighted colours represent the highest values that indicate the effect of preservative on different samples. Combination of salt and turmeric preservation is effective for preserving *rohu*, lobster, pomfret, *hilsa*, whereas KMS preservation is effective to preserve prawn, and without preservative preservation is effective to preserve *katla*. The comparative index number indicates that the combination of salt and turmeric preservation shows the highest value to preserve pomfret. Thus overall analysis reveals that the combination of salt and turmeric preservation is most effective among the other preservation methods.

Table no 5.13.4 the Best fish / edible aquatic species

sample	Carbohydrate	Protein	Fat	Moisture	Ash	Ca	Fe	Energy	Overall Nutrient content
Rohu	0.774	1.115	1.312	1.218	0.977	0.508	0.593	1.134	0.908
Katla	0.585	1.047	1.159	1.200	2.060	1.583	0.407	1.044	1.021
Prawn	1.921	1.579	0.531	1.279	0.949	1.518	1.411	1.054	1.204
Lobster	0.692	0.975	0.593	1.251	0.505	0.770	0.653	0.855	0.758
Pomfret	1.066	1.009	2.644	1.439	1.244	1.367	0.741	2.048	1.343
Hilsa	0.626	0.434	2.132	1.282	0.798	1.202	0.868	1.374	0.980

Highlighted colour represents the highest value for each sample.

This table shows the best fish/ edible aquatic species depending on the nutrient content among all the studied fish and other edible aquatic species. The highlighted colours represent the highest values that indicate the highest nutrient contents of different samples. The comparative index number shows the overall comparison of nutrient content among different samples and results indicate that prawn is rich in carbohydrate, protein and iron, pomfret contains the highest amount of fat, energy and moisture while *katla* is rich in ash and calcium. Hence overall analysis reveals that pomfret is highly nutritious amongst all samples.

The gradation of fish and other edible aquatic species according to the nutrient content analysis shows Pomfret>Prawn>*Katla*>*Hilsa*>*Rohu*>Lobster.

Part – B Survey Result

A survey was carried out to determine the fish consumption pattern and nutrition awareness among the adult women of Kolkata city. In total, 100 samples were selected by snowball sampling technique from 4 zones of Kolkata city, *viz*. North, South, East and West. A self-structured questionnaire was used for the data collection. The graphical representation of the survey data is shown below.

5.13. Graphical representation

Fig. 5.13.1 Occupations of the surveyed sample

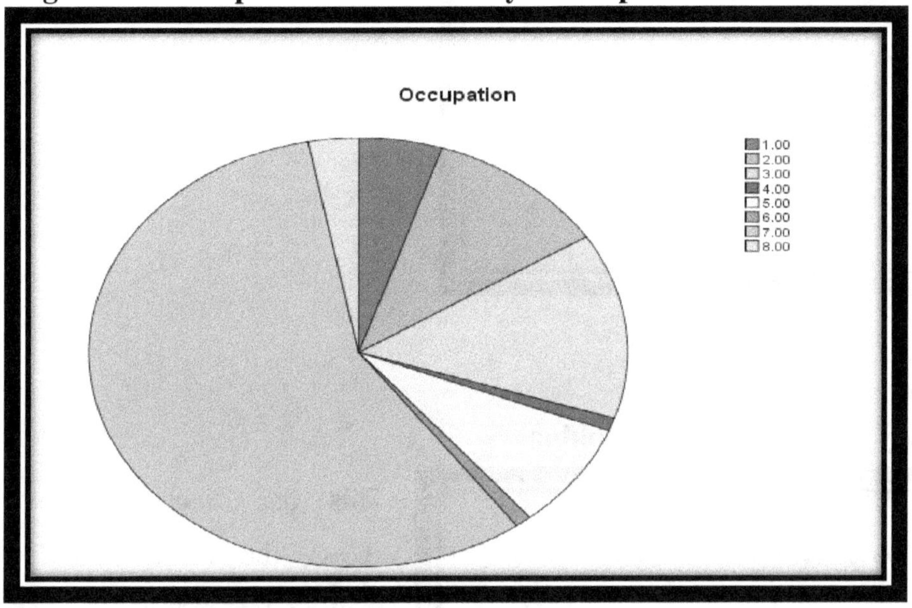

This pie chart represents the occupational variation of the surveyed women. The survey report indicates that most of the women are home-makers.

1= government employee, 2=private sector, 3= teacher, 4=doctor, 5= self-employed, 6= business, 7= home-maker, 8=others.

Fig. 5.13.2 Monthly family income levels

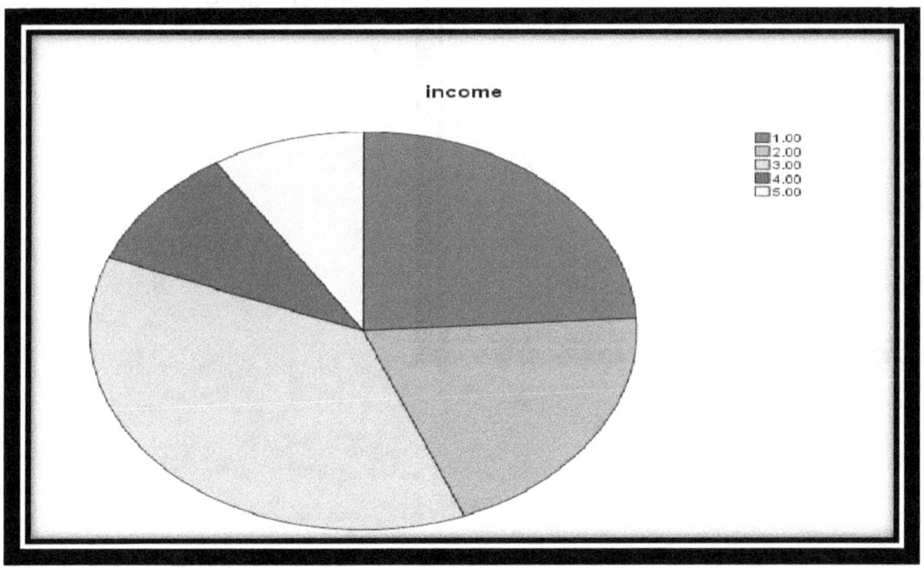

This pie chart represents the income variation of the surveyed women. The survey data shows that most of the surveyed people are from Rs. 30,000-79,999/- monthly family income group.

1= less than Rs.20,000/-, 2= Rs.20,000- 29,999/-, 3= Rs.30,000 - 79,999/-, 4= Rs. 80,000-1, 50,000/-, 5= more than Rs. 1,50,000/- .

Fig. 5.13.3 Frequency of fish consumption in a week

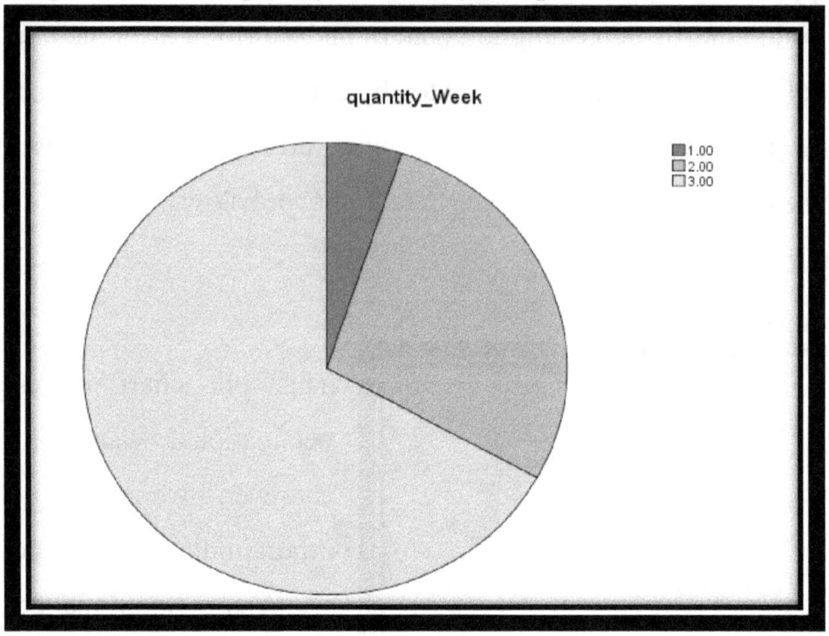

1 = 0-1 days, 2 = 2-4 days, 3 = 5 or more days.

This pie chart representation shows the frequency of fish consumption of the surveyed people in a week. The survey data shows that most people consume fish **5 or more times in a week**.

Fig. 5.13.4 Most frequently used method for cooking

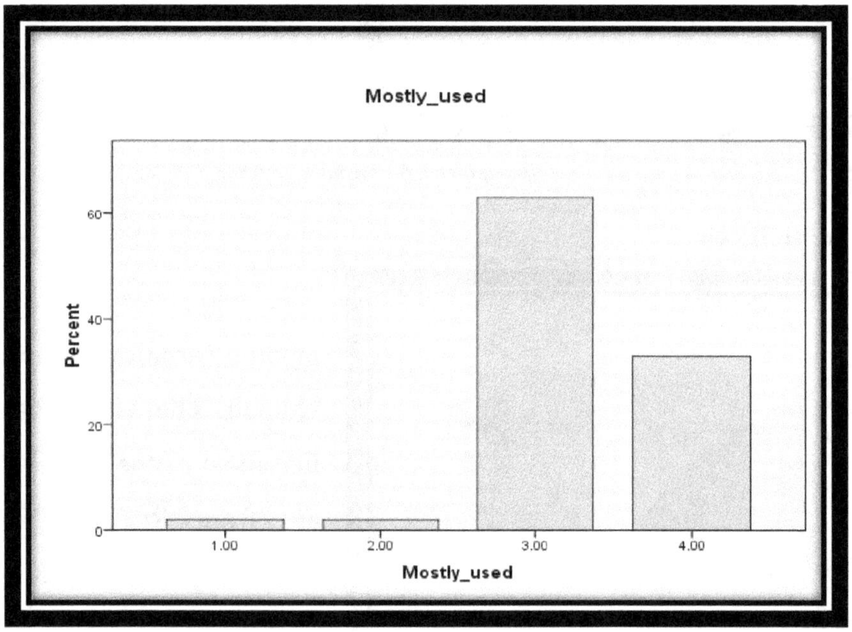

1= Boiling, 2= Open pan dry roasting, 3= Shallow frying, 4= Deep frying.

This bar diagram representation shows the most frequently used method for cooking fish and other edible aquatic species by the women surveyed. Data shows that most women use the **shallow frying** method for cooking.

Fig. 5.13.5 Most nutritious method for cooking according to the surveyed population

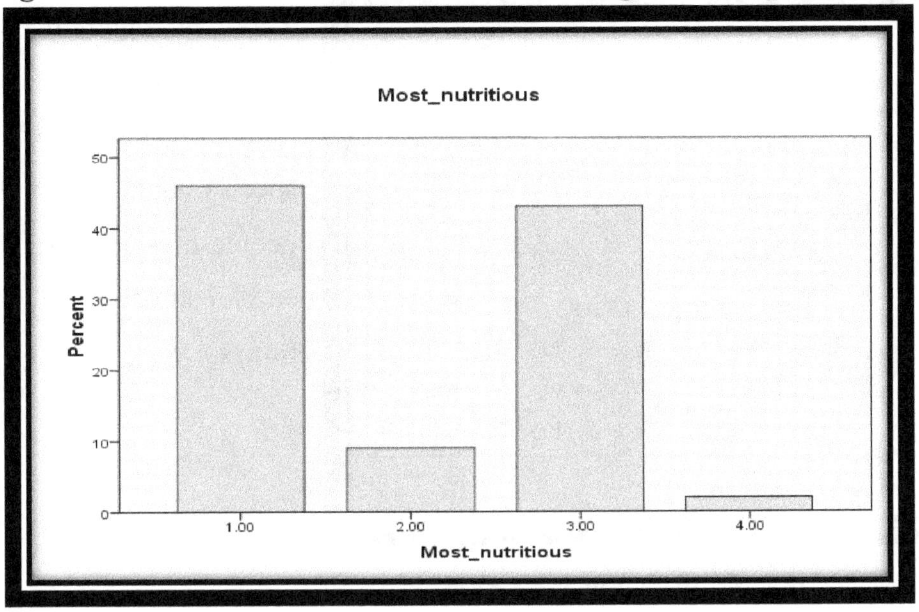

1= Boiling, 2= Open pan dry roasting, 3= Shallow frying, 4= Deep frying.

This bar diagram represents the most nutritious method for cooking fish and other edible aquatic species. Data shows that most women surveyed, think that **boiling** is the most nutritious method for cooking.

Fig. 5.13.6 Preservation pattern of fish according to the surveyed population

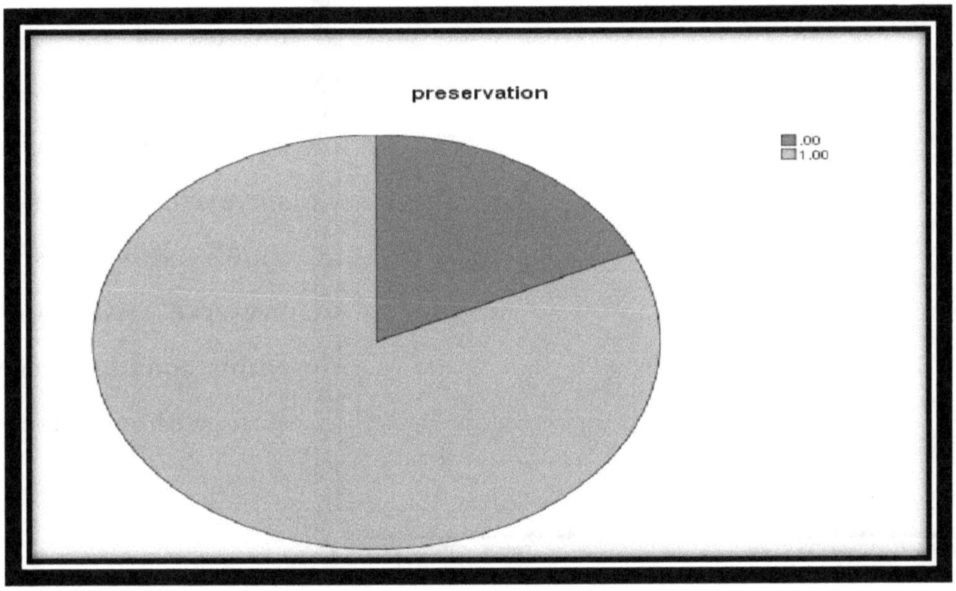

0= No preservation, 1= preservation.

This pie chart represents the preservation pattern of fish and other edible aquatic species. Data shows that most people preserve fish in **deep freezer**.

Fig. 5.13.7 Duration of fish preservation according to the surveyed population

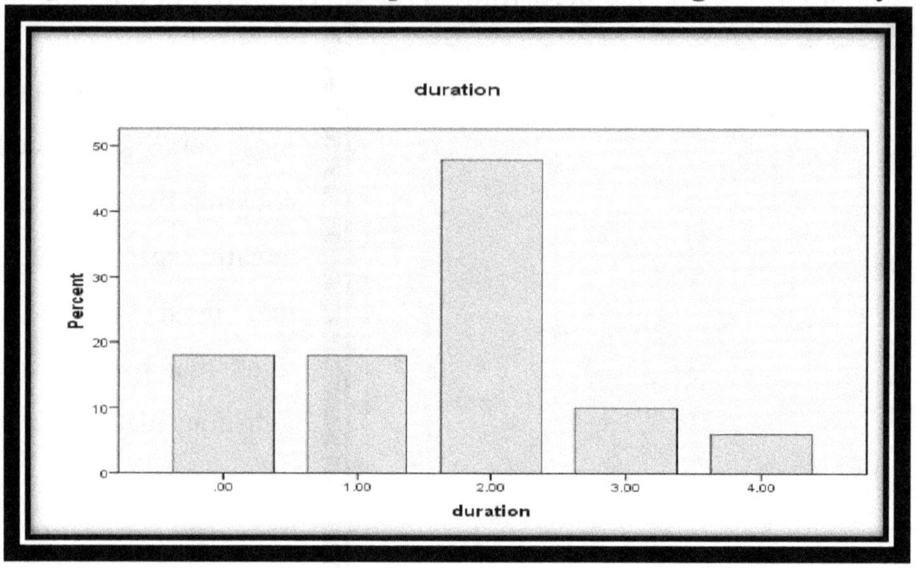

This bar diagram represents the duration of preservation of fish and other edible aquatic species. Data shows that most people preserve fish and other edible aquatic species for **48 hours**.

0= No preservation, 1= 24 hours, 2= 48 hours, 3= 14 days, 4=15 days.

Fig.5.13.8 Use of preservatives by the surveyed population

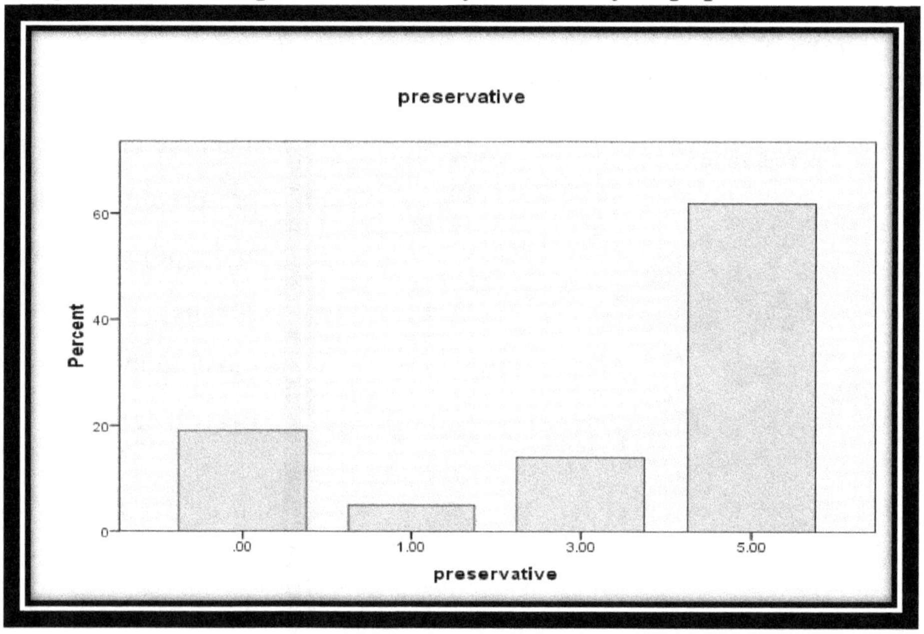

This bar diagram represents the use of preservatives to preserve fish and other edible aquatic species by the women surveyed. The survey report shows that most women **preserve fish and other edible aquatic species in raw state, without preservative**.

0= No preservation, 1= only salt, 3= salt and turmeric, 5= raw fish preservation without preservatives.

Fig. 5.13.9 Percentage of consumption of fish

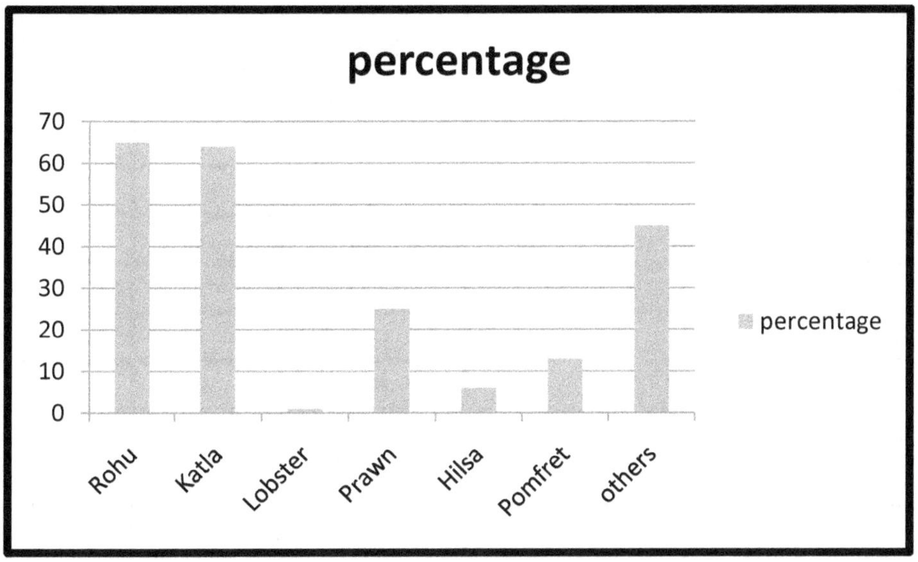

This bar diagram represents the percentage of consumption of fish and other edible aquatic species by the women surveyed. Data shows that most people **consume *rohu* and *katla* and other small fish. They consume *hilsa*, prawn, and pomfret occasionally.**

Fig. 5.13.10 Percentage of using methods of cooking by the surveyed population

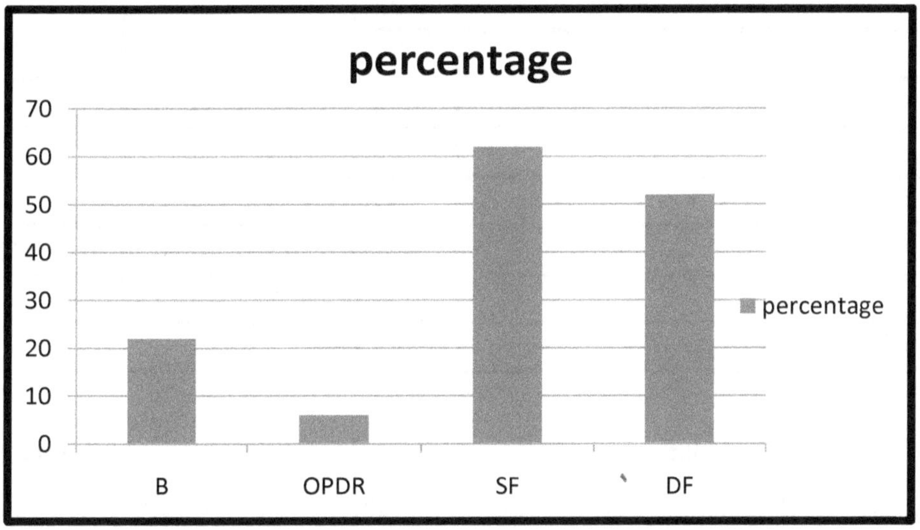

B= Boiling, OPDR= Open pan dry roasting, SF= Shallow frying, DF= Deep frying

This bar diagram represents the percentage of using methods of cooking of fish and other edible aquatic species by the women surveyed. The survey report shows that most people use **shallow frying** method for cooking.

5.14 Chi square test

Survey results are analysed by chi square test to estimate the level of significance and the degree of association between the independent and the dependent variables. The independent variables are age, zone, economic status and occupation and the dependent variables are fish consumption pattern, preservation pattern and cooking pattern of the surveyed population. This survey is the supporting study of the experimental study to determine the nutritional awareness and cooking practices of the women of Kolkata. Significance level is tallied with the tabular chi square value. If the observed value is greater than the tabular value, then there is a significant association present between the two variables.

5.14.1 Association of age with the dependent variables

Serial number	Dependent variable	Pearson Chi-Square	df	Asymp. Sig. (2-sided)
1.	Quantity of fish consumed per week	5.494(S)	8	.704
2.	Quantity of fish consumed per meal	7.506(S)	4	.111
3.	Mostly used method of cooking	7.962(S)	12	.788
4.	Most nutritious method	14.149(S)	12	.291
5.	Preservation of fish	2.375(S)	4	.667
6.	Duration of fish preservation	20.330(S)	16	.206
7.	Marination of fish before cooking	.948(S)	4	.918
8.	Use of preservative	5.414(S)	12	.943
9.	Use of marinate	7.456(S)	12	.826
10.	Method of cooking -1 (Boiling)	6.798(S)	4	.147
11.	Method of cooking -2 (Open pan dry roasting)	.308(NS)*	4	.989
12.	Method of cooking -3 (Shallow frying)	6.055(S)	4	.195
13.	Method of cooking - 4 (Deep frying)	4.063(S)	4	.397
14.	Consumption of *Rohu*	6.317(S)	4	.177
15.	Consumption of *katla*	7.605(S)	4	.107
16.	Consumption of *Hilsa*	2.594(S)	4	.628
17.	Consumption of Pomfret	7.167(S)	4	.127
18.	Consumption of prawn	3.907(S)	4	.419
19.	Consumption of lobster	6.760(S)	4	.149
20.	Consumption of other fish	10.792(S)	4	.029

*S= Significant *NS= Non-Significant*

This table shows that the observed chi square value is greater than the table value, which means all the values are statistically significant. It indicates that dependent variables have association with the age of the surveyed population except the use of cooking method open pan dry roasting is statistically non-significant that means there is no relation present between the age group and the use of cooking method open pan dry roasting. The data reveals that there is no age group variation present regarding the use of open pan method for cooking.

5.14.2 Association of zone with the dependent variables

Serial number	Dependent variable	Pearson Chi-Square	df	Asymp. Sig. (2-sided)
1.	Quantity of fish consumed per week	12.270(S)	6	.056
2.	Quantity of fish consumed per meal	2.745(S)	3	.433
3.	Mostly used method of cooking	8.560(S)	9	.479
4.	Most nutritious method	7.184(S)	9	.618
5.	Preservation of fish	.271(NS)*	3	.965
6.	Duration of fish preservation	5.456(S)	12	.941
7.	Marination of fish before cooking	.973(S)	3	.808
8.	Use of preservative	5.709(S)	9	.769
9.	Use of marinate	12.446(S)	9	.189
10.	Method of cooking -1 (Boiling)	44.988(S)	3	.000
11.	Method of cooking -2 (Open pan dry roasting)	6.383(S)	3	.094
12.	Method of cooking -3 (Shallow frying)	3.226(S)	3	.358
13.	Method of cooking - 4 (Deep frying)	.641(NS)*	3	.887
14.	Consumption of *Rohu*	.835(NS)*	3	.841
15.	Consumption of *katla*	3.819(S)	3	.282
16.	Consumption of *Hilsa*	3.546(S)	3	.315
17.	Consumption of Pomfret	7.339(S)	3	.062
18.	Consumption of prawn	.587(NS)*	3	.899
19.	Consumption of lobster	3.030(S)	3	.387
20.	Consumption of other fish	9.818(S)	3	.020

*S= Significant *NS= Non-Significant*

This table shows that the observed chi square value is greater than the table value, which means all the values are statistically significant. It indicates that dependent variables have association with the zone of the surveyed population except the preservation pattern of fish, use of deep frying as the cooking method, consumption of *rohu* and prawn are statistically non-significant, which means there is no relation present between the zone with the preservation pattern, use of deep frying as the cooking method and the consumption of *rohu* and prawn. The data reveals that there is no zonal difference present regarding preservation pattern, use of deep frying method for cooking and the consumption of *rohu* and prawn.

5.14.3 Association of economic status with the dependent variables

Serial number	Dependent variable	Pearson Chi-Square	df	Asymp. Sig. (2-sided)
1.	Quantity of fish consumed per week	15.029(S)	8	.059
2.	Quantity of fish consumed per meal	5.786(S)	4	.216
3.	Mostly used method of cooking	12.361(S)	12	.417
4.	Most nutritious method	10.693(S)	12	.555
5.	Preservation of fish	3.517(S)	4	.475
6.	Duration of fish preservation	9.596(S)	16	.887
7.	Marination of fish before cooking	1.800(S)	4	.773
8.	Use of preservative	8.582(S)	12	.738
9.	Use of marinate	10.099(S)	12	.607
10.	Method of cooking -1 (Boiling)	8.059(S)	4	.089
11.	Method of cooking -2 (Open pan dry roasting)	5.483(S)	4	.241
12.	Method of cooking -3 (Shallow frying)	7.415(S)	4	.116
13.	Method of cooking - 4 (Deep frying)	4.334(S)	4	.363
14.	Consumption of *Rohu*	3.833(S)	4	.429
15.	Consumption of *katla*	4.493(S)	4	.343
16.	Consumption of *Hilsa*	6.549(S)	4	.162
17.	Consumption of Pomfret	9.587(S)	4	.048
18.	Consumption of prawn	10.608(S)	4	.031
19.	Consumption of lobster	10.213(S)	4	.037
20.	Consumption of other fish	4.695(S)	4	.320

*S= Significant *NS= Non-Significant*

This table shows that the observed chi square value is greater than the table value, which means all the values are statistically significant. It indicates that dependent variables have an association with the economic status of the surveyed population. The data reveals that there is economic status difference present regarding consumption pattern, preservation pattern, the use of conventional method for cooking fish and crustaceans.

5.14.4 Association of occupation with the dependent variables

Serial number	Dependent variable	Pearson Chi-Square	df	Asymp. Sig. (2-sided)
1.	Quantity of fish consumed per week	31.085(S)	14	.005
2.	Quantity of fish consumed per meal	5.242(S)	7	.630
3.	Mostly used method of cooking	24.963(S)	21	.249
4.	Most nutritious method	25.666(S)	21	.219
5.	Preservation of fish	2.831(S)	7	.900
6.	Duration of fish preservation	35.503(S)	28	.156
7.	Marination of fish before cooking	16.728(S)	7	.019
8.	Use of preservative	31.077(S)	21	.072
9.	Use of marinate	39.071(S)	21	.010
10.	Method of cooking -1 (Boiling)	9.479(S)	7	.220
11.	Method of cooking -2 (Open pan dry roasting)	9.154(S)	7	.242
12.	Method of cooking -3 (Shallow frying)	9.985(S)	7	.189
13.	Method of cooking - 4 (Deep frying)	6.237(S)	7	.512
14.	Consumption of *Rohu*	4.007(S)	7	.779
15.	Consumption of *katla*	8.013(S)	7	.331
16.	Consumption of *Hilsa*	3.094(S)	7	.876
17.	Consumption of Pomfret	8.340(S)	7	.304
18.	Consumption of prawn	8.335(S)	7	.304
19.	Consumption of lobster	.762(NS)*	7	.998
20.	Consumption of other fish	12.412(S)	7	.088

*S= Significant *NS= Non-Significant*

This table shows that the observed chi square value is greater than the table value, which means all the values are statistically significant. It indicates that dependent variables have an association with the occupation of the surveyed population except the consumption of lobster is statistically non-significant that means there is no relation present between the occupation and the consumption of lobster. The data reveals that there is no occupational difference present regarding consumption pattern of lobster.

Overall analysis indicates that most of the dependent variables such as consumption pattern, preservation pattern and the use of conventional cooking methods have a relation with age, zone, economic status and occupation. But there is no such age group variation present regarding the use of open pan method for cooking and the consumption of *rohu* and prawn, and also no occupational difference present regarding consumption pattern of lobster. Moreover the data reveals that there is no zonal difference present regarding the method of preservation, the use of deep frying method for cooking and the consumption of *rohu* and prawn.

Chapter-6

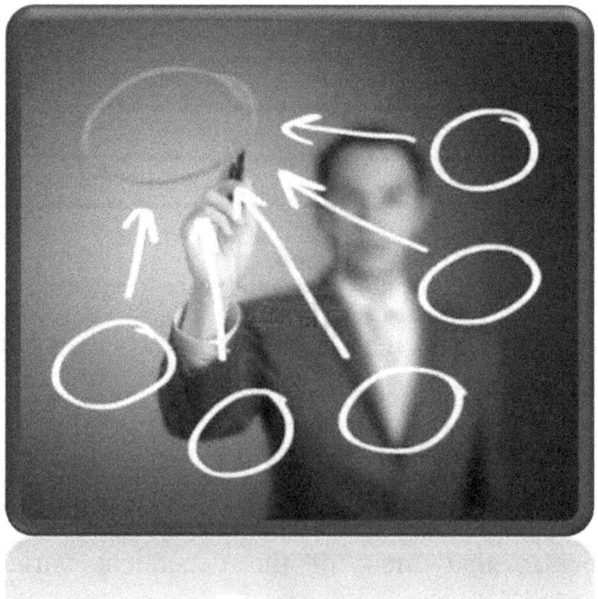

Conclusion

As a rich source of protein and enriched with other macro and micro nutrients, fish are commonly consumed in the state of West Bengal, where the present study has been carried out. Generally, conventional cooking methods are used, such as boiling, open pan dry roasting, shallow frying, deep frying, steaming and grilling to cook fish. But due to cooking, some nutrients are lost. The present study is based on the comparison of nutrient contents (carbohydrate, protein, fat, moisture, ash, calcium, iron and energy) among six most popular and available fish and other edible aquatic species in West Bengal, namely ***rohu*** *(Labeo rohita),* ***katla*** *(Catla catla),* **prawn** *(Fenneropenaeus indicus)* , **lobster** (*Macrobrachium rosenbergii*), **pomfret** (*Pampus argenteus*) and ***hilsa*** *(Tenualosa ilisha)*, after these are subjected to conventional cooking methods (boiling, open pan dry roasting, shallow frying and deep frying). Fish are perishable commodity and get easily spoilt, so these are generally preserved in the refrigerator for some days to prevent spoilage. This study also focuses on the preservation of fish and other edible aquatic species by the help of different preservation methods with preservatives (salt-turmeric and potassium metabisulphite) and without preservative at -20^{0}C up to 15 days. These samples are categorised into three groups such as sweet water or river water fish or carp, crustaceans and salt water fish. The comparisons of nutritive values are made among these three groups.

The present study is aimed to fulfill the following objectives which include-

- Estimation of the nutritive values of selected samples in the raw state and cooked conditions.
- Estimation of the nutritive values of the raw state samples after preservation on days 1, 2 and 14, 15.
- Estimation of the nutritive values of the above samples after cooking on days 1, 2 and 14, 15.
- Estimation of the nutritive values of the preserved raw state samples on days 1, 2 and 14, 15 in the raw condition (samples preserved with preservatives such as a combination of salt and turmeric and potassium metabisulphite).
- Estimation of the nutritive values of the raw state samples preserved with selected preservatives on days 1, 2 and 14, 15 after cooking.
    - After having estimated all the nutritive values the following comparisons are made between:
    - ➢ Raw state and cooked samples
    - ➢ samples with and without preservatives
    - ➢ Preservatives containing the raw state samples cooked on days 1, 2 and 14, 15
    - ➢ Salt water samples, sweet water samples and crustaceans
- Ascertaining the best cooking method for nutritive value restoration.
- Effect of preservatives on the nutritive value of the samples and identification of the best one among the selected preservatives.
- Determination of the best preservation day.

- Determination of the best fish from nutritional aspect.

Experimental results show that carbohydrate, protein, fat, moisture, ash, calcium, iron and energy contents of the raw state of the selected fish and other edible aquatic species under different cooking conditions vary from each other. Most of the nutrient contents are higher in the cooked samples compared to the raw state for all the selected samples. *Katla* contains the highest amount of carbohydrate, *hilsa* contains the highest amount of protein, iron, fat and energy, while pomfret contains the highest amount of moisture. Prawn contains the highest amount of ash and lobster contains the highest amount of calcium in the raw state in fresh condition. Most of the nutrient is present in fresh ***hilsa*** in the raw state. But when these fresh samples are subjected to cooking, the nutrient content changes. Boiling shows the restoration of carbohydrate and iron contents in *rohu*, whereas protein, moisture and ash contents in lobster, fat and energy contents in *hilsa,* and calcium content in prawn are restored. Open pan dry roasting shows the restoration of carbohydrate content in *katla*, protein, fat and calcium contents in *hilsa*, moisture content in lobster, ash content in *rohu*, iron content in *katla*, and energy content in *hilsa.* Shallow frying shows the restoration of carbohydrate, protein, fat, moisture, iron and energy content in *katla*, and ash and calcium contents in *rohu*. Deep frying shows the restoration of carbohydrate content in *hilsa,* protein, moisture, ash and energy contents in lobster, fat content in *katla*, and calcium and iron contents in *rohu*. Most of the nutrient restoration occurs by **boiling and shallow frying in *katla*, open pan dry roasting in *hilsa* and deep frying in lobster**. The probable reason for this may be due to the higher fat content of katla, which creates a barrier to eliminate the nutrient contents from the fish in boiling and shallow frying. *Hilsa* is a sea fish and it also contains a higher percentage of fatty layers, which may be the protective covering to prevent the leaching out of nutrients in open pan dry roasting. The flesh of lobster becomes hard after subjected to deep frying, which may create a layer of protection for the elimination of nutrients.

When the fresh raw fish and crustaceans are subjected to preservation in refrigerator at -20^{0}C without preservative, the nutrient contents again change. The changes of nutrient contents are observed at the interval of 24 hours, 48 hours, 14 days and 15 days. Experimental results reveal that there is a wide variation of nutrient contents among the preserved fish and crustaceans in the raw state. The carbohydrate content restores in 24 hours, 48 hours and 15 days in *rohu,* 14 days in *katla,* whereas protein content restores in 24 hours and 48 hours in *hilsa,* 14 days in prawn and 15 days in lobster, and fat content restores in 24 hours, 48 hours, 14 days and15 days in *hilsa*. The moisture content restores in 24 hours, 48 hours and 15 days in lobster, 14 days in prawn, whereas ash content restores in 24 hours in prawn and 48 hours, 14 days and 15 days in *katla,* and calcium content restores in 24 hours and 48 hours in pomfret, 14 days in lobster and 15 days in *rohu*. The iron content restores in 24 hours and 48 hours in pomfret and 14 days and 15 days in prawn, whereas energy content restores in 24 hours, 48 hours, 14 days and 15 days in *hilsa.* **In all of the observed preservation days, the raw state nutrient content analysis shows that carbohydrate content restoration occurs in *rohu* in 15 days, whereas protein as well as fat and energy restoration occurs in *hilsa* in 24 hours and 48 hours respectively, moisture content restoration occurs in lobster in 48 hours, ash content restoration occurs in *katla* in 15 days, and calcium and iron content restoration occurs in pomfret in 24 hours.** The probable reason for this may be due to the preservation for some days which can reduce the moisture content from the samples, leading to increased content of nutrients in most of the fish and crustaceans.

The preserved fish and crustaceans are also subjected to different cooking methods leading to changes in the nutrient contents among the samples. The changes of nutrient contents are observed at the interval of 24 hours, 48 hours, 14 days and 15 days. Experimental results indicate that there is a wide difference of nutrient contents among the preserved fish and crustaceans after cooking. Boiling shows the restoration of carbohydrate content in 24 hours, 48 hours and 15 days in *rohu* and 14 days in *hilsa*, whereas open pan dry roasting shows the restoration of carbohydrate content in 24 hours, 48 hours in *katla* and 14 days in pomfret and 15 days in *rohu*. Shallow frying shows the restoration of carbohydrate content in 24 hours, 48 hours in *rohu* and 14 days in pomfret and 15 days in *rohu*, whereas deep frying shows the restoration of carbohydrate content in 24 hours in *katla*, 48 hours in *rohu*, 14 days and 15 days in pomfret.

Boiling shows the restoration of protein content in 24 hours, 48 hours and 15 days in lobster and 14 days in pomfret, whereas open pan dry roasting shows the restoration of protein content in 24 hours, 48 hours in *katla* and 14 days in prawn and 15 days in pomfret. Shallow frying shows the restoration of protein content in 24 hours in *hilsa*, 48 hours in lobster and 14 days and 15 days in pomfret, whereas deep frying shows the restoration of protein content in 24 hours in lobster, 48 hours in *hilsa*, 14 days and 15 days in prawn.

Boiling shows the restoration of fat content in 24 hours, 14 days and 15 days in *hilsa* and 48 hours in pomfret, whereas open pan dry roasting shows the restoration of fat content in 24 hours in *katla*, 48 hours, 14 days and 15 days in *hilsa*. Shallow frying shows the restoration of fat content in 24 hours in *katla*, 48 hours in pomfret and 14 days and 15 days in *hilsa*, while deep frying shows the restoration of fat content in 24 hours in prawn, 48 hours, 14 days and 15 days in *hilsa*.

Boiling shows the restoration of moisture content in 24 hours in *rohu*, 48 hours and 15 days in lobster, 14 days in prawn, whereas open pan dry roasting shows the restoration of moisture content in 24 hours in lobster, 48 hours in pomfret, 14 days in lobster and 15 days in prawn. Shallow frying shows the restoration of moisture content in 24 hours in *katla*, 48 hours in pomfret and 14 days and 15 days in lobster, while deep frying shows the restoration of fat content in 24 hours and 48 hours in lobster, and 14 days and 15 days in prawn.

Boiling shows the restoration of ash content in 24 hours, 14 days and 15 days in *katla* and 48 hours in *hilsa*, while both open pan dry roasting and shallow frying show the restoration of ash content in 24 hours in prawn, 48 hours, 14 days and 15 days in *katla*. Deep frying shows the restoration of ash content in 24 hours, 48 hours, 14 days and 15 days in *hilsa*.

Boiling shows the restoration of calcium content in 24 hours in pomfret, 48 hours and 14 days in *katla*, and 15 days in prawn, while open pan dry roasting shows the restoration of calcium content in 24 hours in pomfret, 48 hours in *katla*, 14 days and 15 days in *hilsa*. Shallow frying shows the restoration of calcium content in 24 hours in pomfret, 48 hours in prawn and 14 days in *hilsa* and 15 days in *katla*, whereas deep frying shows the restoration of calcium content in 24 hours in *hilsa* and 48 hours, 14 days and 15 days in *katla*.

Boiling shows the restoration of iron content in 24 hours and 48 hours in pomfret and 14 days and 15 days in prawn, while open pan dry roasting shows the restoration of iron content in 24 hours and 48 hours in pomfret, 14 days in prawn and 15 days in lobster. Shallow frying shows the restoration of iron content in 24 hours and 48 hours in pomfret, 14 days in *rohu* and 15 days in *katla*, whereas deep frying shows the restoration of iron content in 24 hours and 48 hours in pomfret and 14 days in *katla* and 15 days in prawn.

Boiling shows the restoration of energy content in 24 hours, 14 days and 15 days in *hilsa* and 48 hours in pomfret, while open pan dry roasting shows the restoration of energy content in 24 hours in *katla*, 48 hours and 14 days in *hilsa*, 15 days in pomfret. Shallow frying shows the restoration of energy content in 24 hours in *katla*, in 48 hours and 15 days in pomfret and in 14 days in *hilsa*, whereas deep frying shows the restoration of energy content in 24 hours in *rohu* and in 48 hours, 14 days in *hilsa* and 15 days in pomfret.

After preservation of samples in the refrigerator at -20^0 C without preservative for some days and subjected to different cooking methods at the definite intervals, nutrient content analysis reveals that most of the **carbohydrate content retention occurs in *rohu* in 14 days and 15 days, protein content in lobster in 24 hours and pomfret in 14 days and 15 days, fat content in *hilsa* in 14 days and 15 days, moisture content in lobster in 48 hours and 14 days, ash content in *katla* in 14 days and 15 days, calcium content in *katla* in 48 hours, iron content in pomfret in 24 hours and 48 hours and energy content in *hilsa* in 14 days of preservation.** Most of the nutrient retention occurs in 14 days and 15 days, probably due to the elimination of moisture from the fish and crustaceans, concentrating the nutrient content. Moreover, cooking again helps to eliminate moisture due to direct heat.

In contrast, the fresh raw fish and crustaceans are subjected to preservation in the refrigerator at -20^{0}C with two preservatives, i.e. combination of salt-turmeric mixture and potassium metabisulphite, when the nutrient contents again change. The nutritive values of the preserved raw state samples are estimated on days 1, 2 and 14, 15 in the raw state. Experimental results reveal that there are differences present in the nutrient contents among the preserved fish and crustaceans with both the preservatives in the raw state. The effect of salt-turmeric preservation shows that carbohydrate content restores in 24 hours and 14 days in pomfret, 48 hours in *katla* and 14 days in *rohu,* whereas protein content restores in 24 hours in *katla,* 48 hours, 14 days and 15 days in lobster, and fat content restores in 24 hours, 48 hours, 14 days and 15 days in *hilsa*. The moisture content restores in 24 hours and 15 days in prawn, 48 hours and 14 days in lobster, whereas ash content restores in 24 hours in *rohu* and 48 hours and 15 days in lobster, 14 days in pomfret, and calcium content restores in 24 hours, 48 hours and 15 days in *hilsa*, 14 days in pomfret. The iron content restores in 24 hours and 48 hours in prawn and 14 days and 15 days in pomfret, whereas energy content restores in 24 hours, 48 hours, 14 days and 15 days in *hilsa.* **In all of the observed preservation days, the raw state nutrient content analysis shows that carbohydrate content restoration occurs in pomfret, protein and ash content restoration occurs in lobster, fat, calcium and energy content restoration occurs in *hilsa,* moisture content restoration occurs in lobster and prawn, and iron content restoration occurs in pomfret and prawn.** The probable reason for this may be due to the effectiveness of salt-turmeric preservation to restore nutrient and prevention of microbial growth on pomfret, lobster, *hilsa* and prawn.

The effect of potassium metabisulphite preservation shows that carbohydrate content restores in 24 hours and 15 days in lobster, 48 hours in *katla* and 14 days in pomfret, whereas protein content restores in 24 hours, 48 hours and 15 days in lobster, 14 days in prawn, and fat content restores in 24 hours, 48 hours, 14 days and 15 days in *hilsa*. The moisture content restores in 24 hours and 15 days in prawn, 48 hours and 14 days in lobster, whereas ash content restores in 24 hours in *rohu*, 48 hours, 14 days in lobster,15 days in prawn and calcium content restores in 24 hours in *hilsa*, 48 hours in *katla*, 14 days in *rohu* and 15 days in pomfret. The iron content restores in 24 hours in *katla*, 48 hours in pomfret, 14 days in *hilsa* and 15 days in prawn, whereas energy content restores in 24 hours, 48 hours, 14 days and 15 days in *hilsa.* **In all of the observed preservation days, the raw state nutrient content analysis shows that carbohydrate, protein and ash content restoration occurs in lobster; fat, calcium and energy content restoration occurs in *hilsa*; moisture content restoration occurs in lobster and prawn; and iron content restoration occurs in *katla*.** The probable reason for this may be due to the effectiveness of potassium metabisulphite preservation to restore nutrient and prevention of microbial growth on lobster, *hilsa, katla* and prawn.

The preserved fish and crustaceans with salt-turmeric and potassium metabisulphite are also subjected to different cooking methods leading to changes in the nutrient contents among the samples. The changes of nutrient contents are observed at the interval of 24 hours, 48 hours, 14 days and 15 days. Experimental results show that the nutrient contents vary among the preserved fish and crustaceans after cooking. The effect of salt-turmeric preservation indicates that boiling restores carbohydrate content in 24 hours and 14 days in pomfret and 48 hours and 15 days in *katla*, whereas open pan dry roasting shows the restoration of carbohydrate content in 24 hours in *katla*, 48 hours and 15 days in prawn and 14 days in *rohu* and 15 days in *rohu*. Shallow frying shows the restoration of carbohydrate content in 24 hours and 14 days in *rohu* and 48 hours in pomfret and 15 days in prawn, whereas deep frying shows the restoration of carbohydrate content in 24 hours and 15 days in prawn, 48 hours in pomfret, 14 days in *rohu*.

Boiling shows the restoration of protein content in 24 hours in prawn, 48 hours in *rohu*, 14 days and 15 days in lobster, whereas open pan dry roasting shows the restoration of protein content in 24 hours in *rohu*, 48 hours and 14 days in lobster and 15 days in prawn. Shallow frying shows the restoration of protein content in 24 hours in *rohu*, 48 hours and 14 days in prawn and 15 days in lobster, whereas deep frying shows the restoration of protein content in 24 hours in *rohu*, 48 hours and 14 days in prawn and 15 days in lobster.

Boiling shows the restoration of fat content in 24 hours, 48 hours, 14 days and 15 days in *hilsa*, whereas open pan dry roasting shows the restoration of fat content in 24 hours, 48 hours in pomfret, 14 days and 15 days in *hilsa*. Shallow frying shows the restoration of fat content in 24 hours, 14 days and 15 days in *hilsa* and 48 hours in pomfret, while deep frying shows the restoration of fat content in 24 hours, 48 hours and 14 days in pomfret and 15 days in *hilsa*.

Boiling shows the restoration of moisture content in 24 hours, 14 days and 15 days in lobster, 48 hours in prawn, whereas open pan dry roasting shows the restoration of moisture content in 24 hours in *rohu*, 48 hours and 15 days in lobster and 14 days in prawn. Both shallow frying and deep frying show the restoration of moisture content in 24 hours, 48 hours, 14 days and 15 days in lobster.

Boiling shows the restoration of ash content in 24 hours in *rohu*, 48 hours and 14 days in prawn and 15 days in lobster, while open pan dry roasting shows restoration of ash content in 24 hours and 14 days in *rohu,* 48 hours in prawn and 15 days in lobster. Deep frying shows the restoration of ash content in 24 hours in *rohu*, 48 hours and 14 days in *katla* and 15 days in lobster.

Boiling shows the restoration of calcium content in 24 hours, 48 hours, 14 days and 15 days in *hilsa*, while open pan dry roasting shows the restoration of calcium content in 24 hours in pomfret, 48 hours, 14 days and 15 days in *hilsa*. Shallow frying shows the restoration of calcium content in 24 hours, 48 hours and 15 days in *hilsa* and 14 days in *katla*, whereas deep frying shows the restoration of calcium content in 24 hours, 14 days and 15 days in *hilsa* and 48 hours in katla.

Boiling shows the restoration of iron content in 24 hours in *hilsa*, 48 hours and 14 days in *rohu*, 15 days in pomfret, while open pan dry roasting shows the restoration of iron content in 24 hours in lobster, 48 hours and 15 days in *rohu*, 14 days in *hilsa*. Shallow frying shows the restoration of iron content in 24 hours in lobster, 48 hours, 14 days and 15 days in *rohu*, whereas deep frying shows the restoration of iron content in 24 hours in *hilsa*, 48 hours and 14 days in *rohu*, 15 days in *katla*.

Boiling shows the restoration of energy content in 24 hours, 48 hours, 14 days and 15 days in *hilsa*, while open pan dry roasting shows the restoration of energy content in 24 hours, 48 hours, 14 days and 15 days in pomfret. Shallow frying shows the restoration of energy content in 24 hours, 48 hours and 15 days in pomfret, 14 days in *rohu*, whereas deep frying shows the restoration of energy content in 24 hours, 48 hours and 14 days in pomfret and 15 days in *katla*.

After preservation of samples in refrigerator at -20^0 C with salt and turmeric for some days and subjected to different cooking methods at definite intervals, nutrient content analysis reveals that most of the **carbohydrate retention occurs in *rohu* in 14 days, protein in lobster in 15 days, fat in *hilsa* in 15 days, moisture in lobster in 48 hours, 14 days and 15 days, ash in prawn in 48 hours, calcium in *hilsa* in 15 days, iron in *rohu* in 48 hours, and energy in pomfret in 24 hours.** Most of the nutrient retention occurs in 14 days and 15 days, probably due to the effectiveness of salt-turmeric preservation to reduce the microbial growth as well as the elimination of moisture from the fish and crustaceans, concentrating the nutrient content. Moreover, cooking again helps to eliminate moisture due to direct heat. **Salt-turmeric preservation is mostly effective for the preservation of *rohu*, lobster and *hilsa*.**

The effect of potassium metabisulphite preservation shows that boiling restores the carbohydrate content in 24 hours and 15 days in *katla,* 48 hours and 14 days in pomfret, whereas open pan dry roasting shows the restoration of carbohydrate content in 24 hours in prawn, 48 hours in *katla*, 14 days in *rohu*, 15 days in lobster. Shallow frying shows the restoration of carbohydrate content in 24 hours in prawn, 48 hours in *hilsa,* 14 days and 15 days in *rohu*, whereas deep frying shows the restoration of carbohydrate content in 24 hours and 48 hours in *hilsa*, 14 days in *katla* and 15 days in lobster.

Boiling shows the restoration of protein content in 24 hours and 48 hours in prawn, 14 days and 15 days in lobster, whereas open pan dry roasting shows the restoration of protein content in 24 hours in prawn, 48 hours, 14 days and 15 days in lobster. Shallow frying shows the restoration of protein content in 24 hours, 48 hours, 14 days and 15 days in lobster, whereas deep frying shows the restoration of protein content in 24 hours and 14 days in prawn, 48 hours in *hilsa* and 15 days in lobster.

Boiling shows the restoration of fat content in 24 hours, 48 hours, 14 days and 15 days in *hilsa*, whereas open pan dry roasting shows the restoration of fat content in 24 hours, 48 hours in pomfret, 14 days and 15 days in *hilsa*. Shallow frying shows the restoration of fat content in 24 hours, 48 hours and 15 days in pomfret and 14 days in *hilsa*, while deep frying shows the restoration of fat content in 24 hours, 48 hours and 14 days in pomfret and 15 days in *hilsa*.

Boiling shows the restoration of moisture content in 24 hours, 14 days and 15 days in lobster, 48 hours in *katla*, whereas open pan dry roasting and shallow frying show the restoration of moisture content in 24 hours and 15 days in *katla*, 48 hours and 15 days in lobster. Deep frying shows the restoration of moisture content in 24 hours, 48 hours and 14 days in lobster and 15 days in *katla*.

Boiling and open pan dry roasting show the restoration of ash content in 24 hours and 48 hours in *rohu*, 14 days and 15 days in prawn, while shallow frying shows the restoration of ash content in 24 hours in *rohu*, 48 hours, 14 days and 15 days in prawn. Deep frying shows the restoration of ash content in 24 hours in *hilsa*, 48 hours and 15 days in *katla*, and 14 days in prawn.

Boiling shows the restoration of calcium content in 24 hours and 14 days in *hilsa*, 48 hours in katla and 15 days in pomfret, while open pan dry roasting shows the restoration of calcium content in 24 hours in *hilsa*, 48 hours in prawn and 14 days and 15 days in pomfret. Shallow frying shows the restoration of calcium content in 24 hours in *hilsa*, 48 hours, 14 days and 15 days in pomfret, whereas deep frying shows the restoration of calcium content in 24 hours in *rohu*, 48 hours in *katla*, 14 days in pomfret and 15 days in lobster.

Boiling shows the restoration of iron content in 24 hours and 15 days in prawn, 48 hours in *hilsa* 14 days in pomfret and 15 days in prawn, while open pan dry roasting shows the restoration of iron content in 24 hours and 15 days in prawn, 48 hours in *hilsa*, 14 days in *rohu*. Shallow frying shows the restoration of iron content in 24 hours in *rohu*, 48 hours and 14 days in lobster, 15 days in prawn, whereas deep frying shows the restoration of iron content in 24 hours in *rohu*, 48 hours in pomfret and 14 days in lobster and 15 days in prawn.

Boiling shows the restoration of energy content in 24 hours, 48 hours, 14 days and 15 days in *hilsa*, while open pan dry roasting shows the restoration of energy content in 24 hours and 48 hours in pomfret, 14 days and 15 days in *hilsa*. Shallow frying shows the restoration of energy content in 24 hours, 48 hours and 15 days in pomfret and 14 days in *hilsa*, whereas deep frying shows the restoration of energy content in 24 hours and 14 days in pomfret and 48 hours and 15 days in *hilsa*.

After preservation of samples in the refrigerator at -20^0 C with potassium metabisulphite for some days and subjected to different cooking methods at definite intervals, nutrient content analysis reveals that most of the **carbohydrate retention occurs in *katla* in 48 hours, protein in lobster in 15 days, fat in *hilsa* in 14 days and 15 days, moisture in lobster in 14 days, ash in prawn in 14 days and 15 days, calcium in *hilsa* in 24 hours, iron in prawn in 15 days and energy in *hilsa* in 15 days.** Most of the nutrient retention occurs in 15 days, probably due to the addition of potassium metabisulphite which prevents the growth of microorganisms as well as the elimination of moisture from the fish and crustaceans, increasing the nutrient content. Moreover, cooking again helps to eliminate moisture due to direct heat. **Potassium metabisulphite preservation is mostly effective for the preservation of lobster, prawn and *hilsa*.**

After estimating all these above values, comparison is made between the raw and the cooked samples under different cooking methods and different preservation conditions. Overall analysis indicates that there is statistically **significant difference present between the raw and cooked values for all the fish and other edible aquatic species with respect to the carbohydrate, protein, fat, moisture, ash, iron, calcium and energy content**, which means that the carbohydrate, protein, fat, moisture, ash, iron, calcium and energy contents vary from the raw condition in different cooking methods. The probable reason for this is due to the application of heat, oil, water to the samples, leading to the loss of nutrients that makes the difference between the raw and cooked values for all the samples.

Another comparison is made between the samples preserved with salt-turmeric and potassium metabisulphite (KMS) and samples preserved without preservative. Overall experimental analysis reveals that salt and turmeric preservation is more effective to restore carbohydrate, protein, fat, moisture, ash, calcium, iron and energy content as compared to the preservation of samples without preservative for all the fish and crustaceans. Potassium metabisulphite preservation is more effective to restore fat, ash, calcium, iron and energy content as compared to preservation of samples without preservative for all the fish and crustaceans. **In most of the samples both the preservatives are effective as compared to the preservation without preservative.**

Yet another comparison is made between the raw state and the cooked samples preserved with salt-turmeric and potassium metabisulphite. Experimental analysis show that salt-turmeric is more effective than KMS preservation for *rohu* in 24 hours, 14 days and 15 days, prawn in 48 hours and 15 days, lobster in 48 hours and 14 days and pomfret in 14 days and 15 days, whereas KMS preservation is effective as compared to the salt and turmeric preservation for *katla* in 14 days, *hilsa* in 24 hours, 48 hours and 14 days to restore carbohydrate content.

KMS is effective than salt and turmeric preservation for *rohu* in 48 hours, *katla* in 48 hours, prawn in 24 hours, pomfret in 15 days and *hilsa* in 48 hours, 14 days and 15 days, whereas salt and turmeric is more effective than KMS for lobster in 24 hours to restore protein content.

Salt-turmeric is also effective than KMS preservation for *rohu* in 24 hours, 48 hours and 14 days, *katla* in 24 hours, pomfret in 15 days and *hilsa* in 15 days, whereas both the preservatives are similarly effective for prawn in 24 hours and 48 hours, lobster in 48 hours preservation to restore fat content.

Salt-turmeric is effective than KMS preservation for *rohu* in 24 hours and *katla* in 24 hours, prawn in 24 hours, 14 days and 15 days, lobster in 48 hours and 14 days, pomfret in 24 hours and 14 days and *hilsa* in 48 hours to restore moisture content.

Salt-turmeric is also effective than KMS preservation for *rohu* in 24 hours and 14 days, *katla* in 24 hours, 48 hours and 14 days, prawn in 48 hours, lobster in 15 days, pomfret in 48 hours and 14 days, and *hilsa* in 14 days to restore ash content.

Salt-turmeric is effective than KMS preservation for *rohu* in 24 hours, *hilsa* in 48 hours and 14 days, whereas KMS preservation is more effective than salt and turmeric for *katla* in 24 hours, prawn in 24 hours, 48 hours, 15 days, lobster and pomfret in 15 days to restore calcium content.

Salt-turmeric is effective than KMS preservation for *rohu* in 48 hours and 14 days, lobster in 24 hours and 48 hours, *hilsa* in 24 hours, whereas KMS preservation is more effective than salt and turmeric for prawn in 15 days, pomfret in 48 hours and both the preservatives are similarly effective for *katla* in 24 hours and 15 days to restore iron content.

Salt-turmeric is also effective than KMS preservation for *rohu* in 24 hours and 48 hours, *katla* in 48 hours, lobster in 24 hours, whereas KMS preservation is more effective than salt and turmeric for prawn in 24 hours, pomfret in 15 days, *hilsa* in 14 days and 15 days to restore energy content. There is significant difference present between the raw and cooked values and most of the nutrients are restored by using these preservatives. **Overall experimental analysis reveals that salt and turmeric preservation is effective for *rohu*, *katla*, *hilsa*, lobster, whereas potassium metabisulphite is effective for prawn and pomfret and both the preservatives are effective for *katla*, lobster and prawn to restore carbohydrate, protein, fat, moisture, ash, calcium, iron and energy content as compared to the preservation of samples without preservative for all the fish and crustaceans.**

A comparison is made among the salt water samples, sweet water samples and crustaceans regarding the restoration of nutrient contents after subjecting to different cooking methods under different preservation conditions. The statistical analysis indicates that there is significant difference present among the three groups i.e. carp, crustaceans and salt water fish with respect to the raw and cooked values regarding the carbohydrate, protein, fat, moisture, ash, calcium, iron and energy content, which means the nutrient contents vary among the three groups of samples. **Overall analysis reveals that carbohydrate, ash,**

iron contents are restored by carp, while protein and moisture contents are restored by crustaceans and fat, calcium and energy contents are restored by the sea fish.

This study focuses on the basic four objectives which include- the best cooking methods among the four different conventional cooking methods. The statistical analysis reveals that deep frying can mostly restore nutrient contents among the studied methods for most of the samples. Cooking methods can be graded in terms of nutrient restoration in the following manner- deep frying> shallow frying> boiling> open pan dry roasting. The probable reason may be that frying with oil provides a layer of protection to the cooked samples, thus nutrients cannot be eliminated, whereas most of the nutrients are water soluble so boiling can reduce the nutrient content as the nutrients are leached out in the boiling water. Open pan dry roasting provides the direct heat to the samples and the latter become charred and the elimination of protective fatty layers leads to the reduction of the nutrient contents.

The next objective is the determination of the best preservation day among the four observed preservation intervals. The statistical analysis exhibits that the 15th day is the best preservation day to preserve the crustaceans and 14th day is the best preservation day to preserve other studied fish, but *katla* cannot be preserved for prolonged period as the nutritional quality deteriorates. Preservation days can be graded in the following manner- 15 days>14 days>24 hours>48 hours. The probable reason maybe the elimination of moisture from the samples, concentrating the nutrient contents when preserved for prolonged period.

Another objective is the determination of the best preservation method among the three different preservation methods i.e. preservation without preservative, salt-turmeric preservation and potassium metabisulphite preservation. The statistical analysis indicates that the combination of salt and turmeric shows the highest value to preserve pomfret from the nutritional aspect. Thus it can be concluded that the combination of salt and turmeric preservation is the most effective among the other preservation methods. Probably salt-turmeric inhibits the growth of microorganisms in the samples when preserved for prolonged period, leading to restoration of the nutrient contents.

The last important objective is the best fish among the studied samples. The statistical analysis shows the overall comparison of nutrient contents among different samples and results indicate that prawn is rich in carbohydrate, protein and iron, pomfret contains the highest amount of fat, energy and moisture, while *katla* is rich in ash and calcium. Hence the study reveals that pomfret is highly nutritious amongst all the samples. The gradation of fish and other edible aquatic species according to the nutrient content analysis shows Pomfret>Prawn>*Katla*>*Hilsa*>*Rohu*>Lobster. Pomfret is a sea fish and it contains high amount of fatty tissues that create a barrier to eliminate the nutrient content after subjecting to different conventional cooking methods under different preservation conditions, hence restoring the nutrient contents[50] as compared to the other fish and crustaceans.

Survey results show that most people preserved fish for 48 hours whereas some preserved for 2 weeks. The nutrients losses also occur due to the preservation for a long time. But these losses can be reduced by the use of preservatives. In the present study, two types of preservatives such as a combination of salt and turmeric (natural preservative) and potassium metabisulphite (KMS, a synthetic preservative) are used in the fish for preservation for up to 2 weeks. Experimental analyses show that the nutritive value can be retained by the use of a preservative in comparison to the raw fish preservation without preservative. The combination of salt and turmeric is more effective than KMS. Survey results show that most of the people preserve fish without preservative in the raw condition, but they marinate fish with salt and turmeric before cooking. This indicates that nutritional awareness is poor in the surveyed population.

Among the four fish and two other aquatic edible species, pomfret is the most nutritious. It can be preserved for almost two weeks with the use of salt and turmeric with minimal loss of nutrients. Post cooking, nutrient loss is also minimal for this fish. Salt water fish are most nutritious among the three groups of study *viz.*, sweet water fish (Carp), salt water fish and crustacean. The surveyed population consumes mainly sweet water fish such as *rohu* and *katla*.

Finally, it can be concluded that Pomfret is the best fish among all the samples, the best cooking method is deep frying and fish can be preserved for 2 weeks but with the help of a combination of salt and turmeric. In the order of preference of the fish in all categories, this can be expressed in the following manner--Pomfret>Prawn>*Katla*>*Hilsa*>*Rohu*>Lobster.

Chapter-7

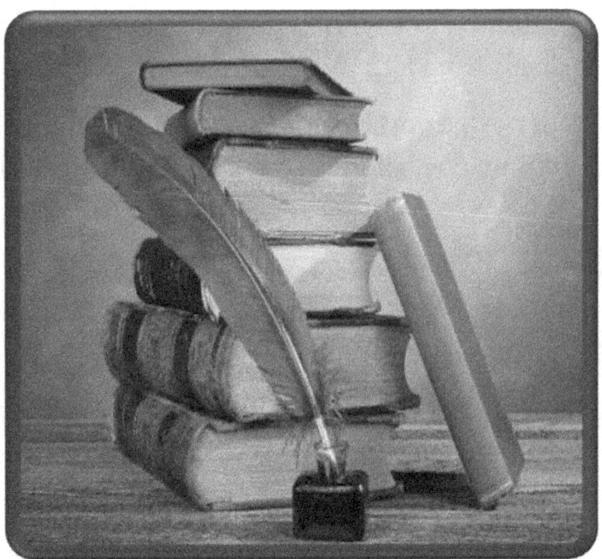

Bibliography

1. Uauy, R., Hoffman, D. R., Mena, P., Llanos, A., & Birch, E. E. (2003). Term infant studies of DHA and ARA supplementation on neurodevelopment: results of randomized controlled trials. *The Journal of pediatrics*, *143*(4), 17-25.

2. Water, I. I. I. (1990). The nutritive composition of the major groups of marine food organisms. *Seafood: Resources, nutritional composition, and preservation*, 29.

3. Erkan, N., & Özden, Ö. (2007). Proximate composition and mineral contents in aqua cultured sea bass (*Dicentrarchus labrax*), sea bream (*Sparus aurata*) analyzed by ICP-MS. *Food Chemistry*, *102*(3), 721-725.

4. Ersoy, B., Yanar, Y., Küçükgülmez, A., & Çelik, M. (2006). Effects of four cooking methods on the heavy metal concentrations of sea bass fillets (Dicentrarchus labrax Linne, 1785). *Food Chemistry*, *99*(4), 748-751.

5. Ghaly, A. E., Dave, D., Budge, S., & Brooks, M. S. (2010). Fish spoilage mechanisms and preservation techniques: review. *American Journal of Applied Sciences*, *7*(7), 859.

6. Yohanna, J. K., Fulani, A. U., & Aka'ama, W. (2011). Prospects for adaptable technological innovations in fresh fish processing and storage in rural areas of Doma LGA of Nasarawa State. *Journal of Agricultural Science*, *3*(3), 282.

7. Gandotra, R., Gupta, S., Koul, M., Gupta, V & Sharma, S. (2013). Nutritional and microbial quality changes in raw and brined frozen muscle of *Cyprinus carpio* (Linn.). *Asian Journal of Science and Technology*, *4*(06), 012-015.

8. Guide, R. (2017). Rohu Fish Farming Information Guide | Agrifarming.in. Agrifarming.in. Retrieved 15 June 2017, from http://www.agrifarming.in/rohu-fish-farming/.

9. Home Garden. (2017). Amazing Health Benefits of Rohu Fish. www.boldsky.com: retrieve on 14 June 2017, from http://www.boldsky.com/health/nutrition/2014/health-benefits-of-rohu-fish-carp-fish-049909.html.

10. ACHARI, A., Kumar, M., Dhanasekar, G., Kumar, p., Faizal, A., & Hassan, R. et al. (2017). Katla Fish | Modern Farming Methods. Modern Farming Methods. Retrieved 15 June 2017, from http://www.roysfarm.com/katla-fish/.

11. 15 Health Benefits of Eating Fish You Must Know | Find Home Remedy & Supplements. (2017).Findhomeremedy.com. Retrieved 15 June 2017, from http://www.findhomeremedy.com/15-health-benefits-of-eating-fish-you-must-know/.

12. FAO Fisheries & Aquaculture Penaeus indicus. (2017). Fao.org. Retrieved 15 June 2017, from http://www.fao.org/fishery/culturedspecies/Penaeus_indicus/en.

13. Fenneropenaeus indicus (Indian white shrimp). (2017). Cabi.org. Retrieved 15 June 2017, from http://www.cabi.org/isc/datasheet/71091.

14. Fenneropenaeus indicus, Indian white prawn: fisheries. (2017). Sealifebase.org. Retrieved 15 June 2017, from http://www.sealifebase.org/summary/Fenneropenaeus-indicus.html.

15. Stein, N. (2017). Can I Lose Weight If I Eat Shrimp?. LIVESTRONG.COM. Retrieved 15 June 2017, from http://www.livestrong.com/article/454942-can-i-lose-weight-if-i-eat-shrimp/.

16. Nutrition Facts for Prawns. (2017). LIVESTRONG.COM. Retrieved 15 June 2017, from http://www.livestrong.com/article/527990-nutrition-facts-for-prawns/.

17. Field guide for the edible crustacean of the Philippines. (2017). Aquaculture Department, Southeast Asian Fisheries Development Centre. Retrieved 16 June 2017 from https://repository.seafdec.org.ph/handle/10862/152.

18. Farming freshwater prawns. A manual for the culture of the giant river prawn (Macrobrachium rosenbergii). (2017). Fao.org. Retrieved 16 June 2017, from http://www.fao.org/docrep/y4100 e03. htm.

19. Food and Agriculture Organization of the United Nations. (2017). Farming freshwater prawns: A manual for the culture of the giant river prawn (Macrobrachium rosenbergii) Retrieved 16 June 2017 from http://www.fao.org/3/a-y4100.

20. 5 Surprising Benefits of Lobster | Organic Facts. (2017). Organic Facts. Retrieved 20 June 2017, from https://www.organicfacts.net/lobster.html.

21. Pomfret *pampus argenteus*: Topics by Science.gov. (2017). Science.gov. Retrieved 21 June 2017, from https://www.science.gov/topicpages/p/pomfret+pampus+argenteus.html.

22. FAO Fisheries & Aquaculture - Aquatic species. (2017). Fao.org. Retrieved 21 June 2017, from http://www.fao.org/fishery/species/3127/en.

23. Naser, S., & Naser, S. (2017). Silver pomfret, Pampus argenteus (Euphrasen, 1788) | BdFISH Feature. En.bdfish.org. Retrieved 21 June 2017, from http://en.bdfish.org/2011/08/silver-pomfret-pampus-argenteus/.

24. WHITE POMFRET FISH HEALTH BENEFITS AND NUTRITITON FACTS. (2017). Sun Samayal. Retrieved 21 June 2017, from http://sunsamayal.com/samayal/index.php/en/%E0%AE%AE%E0%AF%88%E0%AE%AF%E0%AE%B2%E0%AF%8D/health benefits-and-minerals/2054-white-pomfret-fish-health-benefits-and-nutrititon-facts.html.

25. Sunder, T., Debnath, S., Pradhan, b., & Hussain, m. (2017). Hilsa Fish | Modern Farming Methods. Modern Farming Methods. Retrieved 23 June 2017, from http://www.roysfarm.com/hilsa-fish/.

26. Mohanty, B. P., Das, S., Bhaumik, U., & Sharma, A. P. (2011). Tenualosa ilisha-A Rich Source of Omega-3 Fatty Acids (CIFRI Bulletin no. 171).

27. Oluwaniyi, O. O., & Dosumu, O. O. (2009). Preliminary Studies on the effect of processing methods on the quality of three commonly consumed marine fishes in Nigeria. *Biokemistri*, *21*(1), 1-7.

28. Erkan, N., Özden, Ö., & Selçuk, A. (2010). Effect of frying, grilling, and steaming on amino acid composition of marine fishes. *Journal of medicinal food*, *13*(6), 1524-1531.

29. Zhang, J. J., Ji, R., Hu, Y. Q., Chen, J. C., & Ye, X. Q. (2011). Effect of three cooking methods on nutrient components and antioxidant capacities of bamboo shoot. *Journal of Zhejiang University-Science B*, *12*(9), 752-759.

30. Mkandawire, K. T., & Masamba, K. G. (2014). Effect of lemon juice treatment and sun drying on vitamin C retention in three steam and water blanched indigenous vegetables over six weeks storage period. *African Journal of Food Science*, *8*(6), 316-321.

31. Yuan, G. F., Sun, B., Yuan, J., & Wang, Q. M. (2009). Effects of different cooking methods on health-promoting compounds of broccoli. *Journal of Zhejiang University Science*, *10*(8), 580-588.

32. Marimuthu, K., Thilaga, M., Kathiresan, S., Xavier, R., & Mas, R. H. M. H. (2012). Effect of different cooking methods on proximate and mineral composition of striped snakehead fish (Channa striatus, Bloch). *Journal of food science and technology*, *49*(3), 373-377.

33. Erkan, N., & Özden, Ö. (2010). Determination of mineral composition in three commercial fish species (Solea solea, Mullus surmuletus, and Merlangius merlangus). *International Journal of Environmental monitoring and assessment*, *170*(1), 353-363.

34. Ghada A. E., Y. B. Abu Gideiri, M. E. Ali & I. M. Abu Zied. (2012). Quality Preservation in Salted Fermented Labeo sp. during storage period. *New York Science Journal*, *5*(2), 32-38.

35. Angela.O, Onoabhagbe, Cynthia.A. (2013). Effect of brine and vinegar on nutrient composition and shelf life of dried cat fish. *Global journal of biology, agriculture & Health sciences*, *2*(3), 185-188.

36. Rickman, J. C., Barrett, D. M., & Bruhn, C. M. (2007). Nutritional comparison of fresh, frozen and canned fruits and vegetables. Part 1. Vitamins C and B and phenolic compounds. *Journal of the Science of Food and Agriculture*, *87*(6), 930-944.

37. Rahman, M. M., Zamri, M., & Fadilla, N. (2012). Effects of Deep Frying on Proximate Composition and Micronutrient of Indian Mackerel (*Rastrelliger kanagurta*), Eel (*Monopterus albus*) and Cockle (*Anadara granosa*). *Pakistan Journal of Biological Sciences*, *15*(12), 589.

38. Aberoumand, A., & Ziaei-Nejad, S. (2015). Effect of Cooking on Quality Commonly Consumed Marine Fish Platycephalidae (Platycephalus indicus) in Iran. *Turkish Journal of Agriculture-Food Science and Technology*, *3*(11), 891-893.

39. Ghaly, A. E., Dave, D., Budge, S., & Brooks, M. S. (2010). Fish spoilage mechanisms and preservation techniques: review. *American Journal of Applied Sciences*, *7*(7), 859.

40. Lomolino, G., Crapisi, A., & Cagnin, M. (2016). Study of elements concentrations of European seabass (*Dicentrarchus labrax*) fillets after cooking on steel, cast iron, teflon, aluminum and ceramic pots. *International Journal of Gastronomy and Food Science*, *5*, 1-9.

41. Tirtha, B., Tanushri, G., Dora, K. C., Sreekanta, S., & Chowdhury, S. (2016). Influence of chemical preservatives on the quality and shelf-life of dried Bombay duck (Harpodon nehereus). *Asian Journal of Animal Science*, *11*(1), 1-8.

42. Noordin, W. N. M., Shunmugam, N., & Huda, N. (2014). Application of salt solution and vacuum packaging in extending the shelf life of cooked fish balls for home and retail uses. *Journal of Food Quality*, *37*(6), 444-452.

43. Premarathna, A. D., Rajapakse, R. P. V. J., Pathirana, E., Senaratne, V. P., Karunarathna, S. C., & Jayasooriya, A. P. (2015). Nutritional analysis of some selected fish and crab meats and fatty acid

analysis of oil extracted from Portunus pelagicus. *International Journal of Technology Enhancements and Emerging Engineering Research*, *4*(7), 197-201.

44. Larsen, D., Quek, S. Y., & Eyres, L. (2010). Effect of cooking method on the fatty acid profile of New Zealand King Salmon (Oncorhynchus tshawytscha). *Food Chemistry*, *119*(2), 785-790.

45. Ersoy, B., & Özeren, A. (2009). The effect of cooking methods on mineral and vitamin contents of African catfish. *Food Chemistry*, *115*(2), 419-422.

46. Garcıa-Arias, M. T., Pontes, E. Á., Garcıa-Linares, M. C., Garcıa-Fernandez, M. C., & Sanchez-Muniz, F. J. (2003). Cooking–freezing–reheating (CFR) of sardine (Sardina pilchardus) fillets. Effect of different cooking and reheating procedures on the proximate and fatty acid compositions. *Food chemistry*, *83*(3), 349-356.

47. Steiner-Asiedu, M., Julshamn, K., & Lie, Ø. (1991). Effect of local processing methods (cooking, frying and smoking) on three fish species from Ghana: Part I. Proximate composition, fatty acids, minerals, trace elements and vitamins. *Food Chemistry*, *40*(3), 309-321.

48. Ågren, J. J., & Hänninen, O. (1993). Effects of cooking on the fatty acids of three freshwater fish species. *Food Chemistry*, *46*(4), 377-382.

49. Opstvedt, J., Miller, R., Hardy, R. W., & Spinelli, J. (1984). Heat-induced changes in sulfhydryl groups and disulfide bonds in fish protein and their effect on protein and amino acid digestibility in rainbow trout (Salmo gairdneri). *Journal of Agricultural and Food Chemistry*, *32*(4), 929-935.

50. Gall, K. L., Otwell, W. S., Koburgier, J. A., & Appledorf, H. (1983). Effects of four cooking methods on the proximate, mineral and fatty acid composition of fish fillets. *Journal of Food Science*, *48*(4), 1068-1074.

51. Omojowo, F. S., Idris, G. L., & Ihuahi, J. A. (2009). Comparative assessment of potassium sorbate and sodium metabisulphite on the safety and shelf life of smoked catfish. *Nature and Science*, *7*(10), 10-17.

52. Pezeshk, S., Rezaei, M., & Hosseini, H. (2011). Effects of Turmeric, Shallot Extracts, and Their Combination on Quality Characteristics of Vacuum-Packaged Rainbow Trout Stored at 4±1° C. *Journal of food science*, *76*(6), M387–M391.

53. Goulas, A. E., & Kontominas, M. G. (2005). Effect of salting and smoking-method on the keeping quality of chub mackerel (Scomber japonicus): biochemical and sensory attributes. *Food Chemistry*, *93*(3), 511-520.

54. Fagbenro, O., & Jauncey, K. (1993). Chemical and nutritional quality of raw, cooked and salted fish silages. Food Chemistry, *48*(4), 331-335.

55. Akter, T., Ahmed, A. T. A., Khaleque, M. A., & Begum, M. (2013). Effect of drying on quality of tengra (*Mystus vittatus*) treated with turmeric and salt. *Unique Research Journal of Biological Science*, *1*, 1-5.

56. Oluwaniyi, O. O., Dosumu, O. O., & Awolola, G. V. (2010). Effect of local processing methods (boiling, frying and roasting) on the amino acid composition of four marine fishes commonly consumed in Nigeria. *Food Chemistry*, *123*(4), 1000-1006.

57. Ampola, V. G., & Keller, C. L. (1985). Shelf life extension of drawn whole Atlantic cod, Gadus morhua, and cod fillets by treatment with potassium sorbate. *Marine Fisheries Review*, *47*, 26-29.

58. Kocatepe, D., Turan, H., Kaya, Y., Taşkaya, G., Erdoğdu, F., & Erden, R. (2014). Effect of potassium metabisulphite, glaze and vacuum on shelf life of frozen blacksea anchovy (*Engraulis encrasicolus*, Linnaeus1758), *9*(3)79-87.

59. Rotllant, G., Arnau, F., Garcia, J. A., García, N., Rodríguez, M., & Sardà, F. (2002). Note. Effect of Metabisulphite Treatments and Freezing on Melanosis Inhibition in Rose Shrimp Aristeus antennatus (Risso, 1816). *Revista de Agaroquimica y Tecnologia de Alimentos*, *8*(4), 243-247.

60. Pardio, V. T., Waliszewski, K. N., & Zuñiga, P. (2011). Biochemical, microbiological and sensory changes in shrimp (Panaeus aztecus) dipped in different solutions using face centred central composite design. *International journal of food science & technology*, 46(2), 305-314.

61. Candela, M., Astiasaran, I., & Bello, J. (1998). Deep-fat frying modifies high-fat fish lipid fraction. *Journal of Agricultural and Food Chemistry*, 46(7), 2793-2796.

62. Espe, M., & Lied, E. (1999). Fish silage prepared from different cooked and uncooked raw materials: chemical changes during storage at different temperatures. *Journal of the Science of Food and Agriculture*, 79(2), 327-332.

63. Devi, D. P., Hareesh, K., & Reddy, M. S. (2015). Studies on the Proximate Composition of Tropical Freshwater Prawn Macrobrachium rosenbergii. *International Journal of Fisheries and Aquatic Studies*, 3(1), 329-336

64. Begum, M., Bhowmik, S., Juliana, F. M., & Hossain, M. S. (2016). Nutritional Profile of *Hilsa* Fish [*Tenualosa ilisha* (Hamilton, 1822)] in Six Selected Regions of Bangladesh. *J Nutr Food Sci*, 6(567), 2.

65. Sankar, T. V., & Nair, P. V. (1988). Effect of pre-processing iced storage on deteriorative changes in lipids of silver pomfrets stored at-18° C. *Fishery Technology*, 25(2), 100-104.

66. Ersoy, B. (2011). Effects of cooking methods on the proximate, mineral and fatty acid composition of European eel (*Anguilla anguilla*). *International journal of food science & technology*, 46(3), 522-527.

67. Torres Filho, R., Cazedey, H., Fontes, P., Ramos, A., & Ramos, E. (2017). Drip Loss Assessment by Different Analytical Methods and Their Relationships with Pork Quality Classification. *Journal Of Food Quality*, 2017, 1-8.

68. Mu. G. (2014). Changes in the quality and yield of fish fillets due to temperature fluctuations during processing. *United Nations University Fisheries Training Programme*, Iceland [final project]. http://www.unuftp.is/static/fellows/document/mugang13prf.pdf

69. https://fedup.com.au/factsheets/additive-and-natural-chemical-factsheets/220-228-sulphite preservatives

70. Ludwig, T. G., & Goldberg, H. J. (1956). The anthrone method for the determination of carbohydrates in foods and in oral rinsing. *Journal of dental research*, *35*(1), 90-94.

71. Lowry. O. H., Rosebrough, N. J., Farr, A. L., & Randall, R. J. (1951). Protein measurement with the Folin phenol reagent. *Journal of biochemtry*, *193*(1), 265-275.

72. Manirakiza, P., Covaci, A., & Schepens, P. (2001). Comparative study on total lipid determination using Soxhlet, Roese-Gottlieb, Bligh & Dyer, and modified Bligh & Dyer extraction methods. *Journal of food composition and analysis*, *14*(1), 93-100.

73. Baker, A. S., & Smith, R. L. (1974). Preparation of solutions for atomic absorption analyses of iron, manganese, zinc, and copper in plant tissue. *Journal of agricultural and food chemistry*, *22*(1), 103-107.

74. Aberoumand, A. (2014). Nutrient composition analysis of gish fish fillets affected by different cooking methods. *International Food Research Journal*, *21*(5), 1989-1991.

75. Buskirk, E. R., & Mendez, J. (1980). Energy: caloric requirements, In Nutrition and the Adult (pp. 49-95). Springer US.

76. Yemm, E. W., & Willis, A. J. (1954). The estimation of carbohydrates in plant extracts by anthrone. *Biochemical journal*, 57(3), 508.

77. Waterborg, J. H. (2009). The Lowry method for protein quantitation. The protein protocols handbook, 7-10

78. Harwood, L. M., Moody, C. J., & Harwood, L. M. (1989). *Experimental organic chemistry: principles and practice*. Oxford, United Kingdom: Blackwell Scientific.

79. Pomeranz, Y. (Ed.). (2013). *Food analysis: theory and practice*. Springer Science & Business Media.

80. Jindal, V. K., & Siebenmorgen, T. J. (1987). Effects of oven drying temperature and drying time on rough rice moisture content determination. *Transactions of the ASABE (American Society of Agricultural and Biological Engineers)*, *30*(4), 1185-1192.

81. James, C. S. (Ed.). (2013). *Analytical chemistry of foods.* Springer Science & Business Media.

82. Southgate, D. A. T., & Durnin, J. V. G. A. (1970). Calorie conversion factors. An experimental reassessment of the factors used in the calculation of the energy value of human diets. *British Journal of Nutrition*, *24*(02), 517-535.

83. Adelakun, K.M., Mustapha, M.K, Amali, R.P. & Mohammed. N. (2017). Seasonal Variation in Nutritional Quality of Catfish (*Clarias gariepinus*) from Upper Jebba Basin, Nigeria. *Journal of Nutrition & Food Science*, 7(5), 1-4.

84. Gopalan, C., Rama Sastri, B.V. & Balashubramaniam, S.C., (1989). Nutritive value of Indian Foods, *Indian Council of Medical Research (ICMR)*, 54-56.

85. Longvah, T., Ananthan, R., Bhaskarachary, K. & Venkalah, K., (2017) Indian Food Composition Tables, *Indian Council of Medical Research (ICMR)*, 25-168.

86. Mukundan, A.K, Radhakrishnan et.al. (1986). Nutritional evaluation of some fresh water fishes, *Central Institute of Fisheries Technology,* 23, 189-195.

References for Figures

1.1 Labeo rohita (Rohu). (2017). Iucnredlist.org. Retrieved 12 October 2017, from http://www.iucnredlist.org/details/166619/0

1.1.1 *Rohu* overview. (2017). Icar.org.in. Retrieved 15 June 2017, from http://www.icar.org.in/rohudatabase/.

1.2 FAO Fisheries & Aquaculture *Labeo rohita* (2017). Fao.org Retrieved 15 June 2017, from http://www.fao.org/fishery/culturedspecies/Labeo_rohita/en.

1.3 Home Garden. (2017). amazing Health Benefits of Rohu Fish. www.boldsky.com: retrieve on 14.06.2017 from http://www.boldsky.com/health/nutrition/2014/health-benefits-of-rohu-fish-carp-fish-049909.html.

1.4 Gibelion catla (*Catla catla*). (2017). Iucnredlist.org. Retrieved 12 October 2017, from http://www.iucnredlist.org/details/166425/0.

1.4.1 *Catla* Fish Farming Information Guide | Agrifarming.in. Agrifarming.in. Retrieved 14 June 2017, from http://www.agrifarming.in/catla-fish-farming/.

1.5 FAO Fisheries & Aquaculture *Catla catla*. (2017). Fao.org. Retrieved 15 June 2017, from http://www.fao.org/fishery/culturedspecies/Catla_catla/en.

1.6 Katla Fish Curry | Krishna Dish. (2017). Krishna Dish. Retrieved 15 June 2017, from http://www.krishnadish.com/product/katla-fish-curry/.

1.7.1 Fenneropenaeus indicus (Indian white prawn) (Penaeus indicus). (2017).Uniprot.org. Retrieved 12October 2017, from http://www.uniprot.org/taxonomy/29960.

1.7 Indian Banana Prawn (Fenneropenaeus indicus). (2017). Noeyeddeer.com. Retrieved 15 June 2017, from http://noeyeddeer.com/fish/species/fenneropenaeus-indicus.html.

1.8 FAO Fisheries & Aquaculture Penaeus indicus. (2017). Fao.org. Retrieved 15 June 2017, from http://www.fao.org/fishery/culturedspecies/Penaeus_indicus/en.

1.9 Food, 1., Recipes, 1., Desk, N., Videos, R., Twist, V., & Kitchen, V. et al. (2017). 10 Best Prawn Recipes. food.ndtv.com. Retrieved 15 June 2017, from http://food.ndtv.com/lists/10-best-prawn-recipes-738477.

1.10 Macrobrachium rosenbergii (Giant Freshwater Prawn, Giant River Prawn). (2017). Iucnredlist.org. Retrieved 12 October 2017, from http://www.iucnredlist.org/details/197873/0

1.10.1 Beverage, F., & Dist., G. (2017). Giant Freshwater Prawn (Macrobrachium Rosenbergii) in Dist., Valsad | Penaeus Aquaculture. Tradeindia.com. Retrieved 16 June 2017, from https://www.tradeindia.com/fp2622583/Giant-Freshwater-Prawn-Macrobrachium-Rosenbergii-.html.

1.11 FAO Fisheries & Aquaculture Macrobrachium rosenbergii. (2017). Fao.org. Retrieved 16 June 2017 from http://www.fao.org/fishery/culturedspecies/Macrobrachium_rosenbergii/en.

1.12 Malaysian Giant Freshwater River Prawn | Photos & Videos | Texas Fishing Forum. (2017).Texasfishingforum.com. Retrieved 20 June 2017, from. http://texasfishingforum.com/forums/ubbthreadsphp/topics/4574634/all/Malaysian_Giant_Freshwater_Riv.

1.13 Pomadasys argenteus (Silver Javelin). (2017). Iucnredlist.org. Retrieved 12 October 2017, from http://www.iucnredlist.org/details/full/172404/0.

1.13.1 White Pomfret. (2017). Clovegarden.com. Retrieved 20 June 2017, from http://www.clovegarden.com/ingred/sf_pomfcsz.html.

1.14 *Pampus argenteus* summary page. (2017). FishBase. Retrieved 21 June 2017, from http://www.fishbase.org/summary/SpeciesSummary.php?ID=491&AT=silver+pomfret.

1.15 Seafood Recipes. (2017). Pinterest. Retrieved 21 June 2017, from https://www.pinterest.com/pin/446419381791084677/.

1.16 Tenualosa ilisha (Hilsa). (2017). Iucnredlist.org. Retrieved 12 October 2017, from http://www.iucnredlist.org/details/166442/0.

1.16.1 Tenualosa ilisha - ZipcodeZoo. (2017). Zipcodezoo.com. Retrieved 22 June 2017, from http://zipcodezoo.com/index.php/Tenualosa_ilisha.

1.17 Tenualosa ilisha summary page. (2017). FishBase. Retrieved 23 June 2017, from http://www.fishbase.org/summary/SpeciesSummary.php?ID=1596&AT=ilisha.

1.18 Fooooood. (2017). Pinterest. Retrieved 23 June 2017, from https://www.pinterest.com/pin/517914644344442929/.

4.1 Anthrone test for Carbohydrates quantitative analysis. (2017). All Medical Stuff. Retrieved 27 June 2017, from https://allmedicalstuff.com/anthrone-test-carbohydrates/.

4.2 Optimization of long-term storage procedures for the prebiotic cyanobacterium Arthrospira sp. S. platensis to milk (6 mg/ml) stimulated growth of Lactococcus. - ppt download. (2017). Slideplayer.com. Retrieved 27 June 2017, from http://slideplayer.com/slide/10804871/.

4.4 Physico-Chemical Analysis of Some Commercial Honey Samples from Telangana. (2017). Opensciencepublications.com. Retrieve 27 June 2017, from http://opensciencepublications.com/full textarticles/IJN-2395-2326-4-153.html.

4.5 Practical 2: Protein Experiment. (2017). Shinaebiochem.blogspot.in. Retrieved 3 July 2017, from http://shinaebiochem.blogspot.in/2013/04/practical-2-protein-experiment.html.

4.6 Protein and Proteomic Studies. (2017). G-Biosciences. Retrieved 30 June 2017, from https://www.gbiosciences.com/Educational-Products/Protein-and-Proteomic-Studies?page=1.

4.8 Folin–Ciocalteu reagent. (2017). En.wikipedia.org. Retrieved 27 June 2017, from https://en.wikipedia.org/wiki/Folin%E2%80%93Ciocalteu_reagent.

4.9 Principle of Soxhlet extraction and Experimental Setup of Soxhlet Extractor - Oleoresins. (2017). Oleoresins.melbia.com. Retrieved 3 July 2017, from http://oleoresins.melbia.com/principle-of-soxhlet-extraction-and-experimental-setup.html.

4.11 USA, M. (2017). Cold Vapor atomic absorption technology. Mercury-instrumentsusa.com. Retrieved 3 July 2017, from http://www.mercury-instrumentsusa.com/Technology.html.

ANNEXURE

QUESTIONNAIRE ON CONSUMPTION PATTERN AND PRESERVATION OF DIFFERENT TYPES OF FISH AND OTHER EDIBLE AQUATIC ANIMAL SPECIES

1. GENERAL INFORMATION

a. Name : ____________________

b. Age : ____________________

c. Residence : ____________________

d. Occupation : Govt. employee ☐ Private sector/ Corporate ☐ Teacher ☐ Doctor ☐ Self-employed ☐ Business☐ Home-maker ☐ Others (please specify) ____________________

e. Monthly income of family : Less than 20,000/-☐ 20,000 – 29,999/- ☐ 30,000 – 79,999/-☐ 80,000 – 1, 50,000/- ☐ More than 1,50,000/- ☐

2. CONSUMPTION PATTERN

a. How many days in a week do you consume fish (es)? 0-1 ☐ 2-4 ☐ 5 or more ☐

b. What are the kinds of fishes that you generally eat? *Rohu* ☐ *Katla* ☐ *Ilish* ☐ Pomfret ☐ Prawn ☐ Lobster ☐ others (please specify) ____________

c. The quantity of fish you eat per meal? 1 piece (50-60 gms) ☐ 2 pieces (100-120 gms) ☐

3. METHOD OF PREPARATION

a. What are the methods that you use for cooking fish?
Boiling ☐ Open pan dry roasting ☐ Shallow frying ☐ Deep frying ☐

b. Which method do you mostly use for cooking fish? (please tick only one)
Boiling ☐ Open pan dry roasting ☐ Shallow frying ☐ Deep frying ☐

c. What do you think is the most nutritious method for cooking fish? (please tick only one)
Boiling ☐ Open pan dry roasting ☐ Shallow frying ☐ Deep frying ☐

4. PRESERVATION

a. Do you preserve the fish before eating? Yes ☐ No ☐

b. If yes, for how long do you preserve? 24 hrs ☐ 48 hrs ☐ 14 days ☐ 15 days ☐

c. If no, then do you marinate the fish before cooking? Yes ☐ No ☐

d. What do you preserve your fish with? Only salt ☐ Only turmeric ☐ Salt and turmeric ☐ KMS (synthetic preservative) ☐ Others (please specify) ____________

e. If you only marinate, then with what do you marinate your fish before cooking?
Only salt ☐ only turmeric ☐ Salt and turmeric ☐ others (please specify) ________

Signature ------------------------

List of Publications

Research article

1. Jana, U. & Chakrabarti, S. (2015) Comparative analysis of macro nutrients between river fish *Rohu* (Labio rohita) and sea fish Pomfret (Pampus argenteus), treated under different cooking conditions, *International Journal of Current Research,7(8),*19306-19310.

2. Jana, U. & Chakrabarti, S. (2016), comparison of restoration of major mineral contents among different fish and other edible aquatic species treated under different preserving and cooking conditions, *International Journal of Agricultural Science and Research,6(4),*139-148.

3. Jana, U. & Chakrabarti, S. (2016), comparison of restoration of protein contents of preserved *Rohu* (Labio rohita), treated under different cooking conditions, *International Journal of Science and Research,* 5(3), 1374-1377.

4. Jana, U. & Chakrabarti, S. (2016), comparison of restoration of carbohydrate and protein contents among different fish and other edible aquatic species treated under different cooking conditions, *International Journal of Scientific and Engineering Research,7(1),*638-642.

5. Jana, U. & Chakrabarti, S. (2016), comparison of macro nutrients of preserved carp, treated under different cooking conditions, *International Research Journal of engineering and technology, 3(6),* 1174-1179.

6. Jana, U. & Chakrabarti, S. (2017), Comparative analysis of nutrient content between Prawn (*Fenneropenaeus indicus*) and Lobster (*Portunus sanguinolentus*), preserved and cooked under different conditions, *International Journal of Food science & Nutrition*, *2*(1), 90-96.

7. Jana, U. & Chakrabarti S. (2017), comparative analysis of nutritional quality Pomfret (Pampus *argenteus*) and Hilsa (*Hilsa ilisha*),preserved and cooked under different conditions of preserved carp, treated under different cooking conditions, *International Journal of fisheries & aquatic studies*, *5*(2), 258-263.

Conference proceedings

1. Food Value of a variety of Sea Fish: A Comparative Study. Sarmistha Chakrabarti & Uttiya Jana. Institute of Science & Technology (IST)-Journal on Business & Technology: Special Issue on ICWSET-2012 (Held on February 2-4, 2012) organised by Bangladesh Women Scientist Association and OWSD, Bangladesh Chapter: Volume 5 Number 1 December 2012.pp.67-71.

2. Nutritional Importance of three most popular Sea Fish. Sarmistha Chakrabarti and Uttiya Jana. UGC sponsored National Seminar on Bench Marking Environmental Initiatives held on 26th of March 2013 organised by the Department of Business Management, University of Calcutta.

3. Effect of cooking in fish and other aquatic species: An analysis of nutrients. Sarmistha Chakrabarti and Uttiya Jana. OWSD (formerly TWOWS) Fifth General Assembly and International Conference: Women Scientists in a Quest for Sustainability and Development. 17-20 September 2014, Cuernavaca, Mexico.pp.97-98.

COLLECTION OF PUBLICATIONS

ISSN: 0975-833X
INTERNATIONAL JOURNAL OF CURRENT RESEARCH
RESEARCH ARTICLE

COMPARATIVE ANALYSIS OF MACRONUTRIENTS BETWEEN RIVER FISH ROHU (LABIO ROHITA) AND SEA FISH POMFRET (PAMPUS ARGENTEUS), TREATED UNDER DIFFERENT COOKING CONDITIONS

Uttiya Jana and *Sarmistha Chakrabarti
Department of Home Science (Food & Nutrition), University of Calcutta, Kolkata 700 027, India

International Journal of Science and Research (IJSR)
ISSN (Online): 2319-7064
Index Copernicus Value (2013): 6.14 | Impact Factor (2014): 5.611

Comparison of Restoration of Protein Contents of Preserved *Rohu (Labio rohita)*, Treated under Different Cooking Conditions

Uttiya Jana, Sarmistha Chakrabarti

International Journal of Agricultural Science and Research (IJASR)
TRANS STELLAR

COMPARISON OF RESTORATION OF MAJOR MINERAL CONTENTS AMONG DIFFERENT FISH AND OTHER EDIBLE AQUATIC SPECIES, TREATED UNDER DIFFERENT PRESERVING AND COOKING CONDITIONS

UTTIYA JANA & SARMISTHA CHAKRABORTI

Comparison of restoration of carbohydrate and protein contents among different fish and other edible aquatic species, treated under different cooking conditions

Uttiya Jana & Sarmistha Chakrabarti

International Research Journal of Engineering and Technology (IRJET) e-ISSN: 2395-0056
www.irjet.net p-ISSN: 2395-0072

Comparison of macro nutrients of preserved carp, treated under different cooking conditions

Uttiya Jana & Sarmistha Chakrabarti *
Department of Home Science (Food & Nutrition), University of Calcutta, Kolkata 700 027, India

Abstract *Fish are rich sources of protein and are commonly consumed. This study is based on the comparison of contents of macro nutrients of carp, preserved with the combination of salt and turmeric and without preservative both up to 15 days. These preserved fishes were subjected to conventional cooking methods like open pan dry roasting, boiling, shallow frying and deep frying and macro nutrient contents were analysed after immediate (24hours) and long term (15 days) preservation. The nutrient contents of cooked fishes were significantly lower than those in the raw condition, changes occurring due to cooking. Loss of nutrients mainly occurred in boiling whereas it is better restored in deep frying method. The study significantly showed that the loss of nutrients occurred due to preservation but these losses can be reduced by using the combination of salt and turmeric. It was also found that among carp, restoration was greater for rohu.*

Keywords – **carp, macro nutrients, cooking methods, preservatives, deep fat frying**

International Journal of Fisheries and Aquatic Studies

Comparative analysis of nutritional quality between Pomfret (*Pampus argenteus*) and Hilsa (*Hilsa ilisha*), preserved and cooked under different conditions

Uttiya Jana and Sarmistha Chakrabarti

International Journal of Food Science and Nutrition
ISSN: 2455-4898, Impact Factor: RJIF 5.14
www.foodsciencejournal.com
Volume 2; Issue 1; January 2017; Page No. 90-96

Comparative analysis of nutrient content between Prawn (*Fenneropenaeus indicus*) and Lobster (*Portunus sanguinolentus*), preserved and cooked under different conditions

Uttiya Jana, Sarmistha Chakrabarti
Department of Home Science (Food & Nutrition), University of Calcutta, Kolkata, West Bengal, India

Abstract
Crustaceans are rich sources of protein and have lower cholesterol content compared to other animal food and thus commonly consumed. The content of this study was the comparison of nutrients between prawn and lobster. The nutrient contents of prawn were higher than lobster in the raw condition. These species were both subjected to conventional cooking methods like open pan dry roasting, boiling, shallow frying and deep frying. They were also preserved up to 15 days. The nutrient contents had changed due to preservation and the application of cooking methods. Losses of nutrients had taken place in both species. Most of the nutrient retention occurred in prawn than in lobster after preservation and cooking. The study significantly revealed that cooked prawn was beneficial due to adequate protein, fat and mineral restorations and it could be preserved up to 15 days with minimal loss as compared to lobster. Most of the nutrient retention occurred in shallow frying method.

Keywords: macronutrients, mineral contents, prawn, lobster, cooking methods, preservation

Available online at http://www.journalcra.com

International Journal of Current Research
Vol. 7, Issue, 08, pp.19306-19310, August, 2015

INTERNATIONAL JOURNAL OF CURRENT RESEARCH

ISSN: 0975-833X

RESEARCH ARTICLE

COMPARATIVE ANALYSIS OF MACRONUTRIENTS BETWEEN RIVER FISH *ROHU* (*LABIO ROHITA*) AND SEA FISH *POMFRET (PAMPUS ARGENTEUS)*, TREATED UNDER DIFFERENT COOKING CONDITIONS

Uttiya Jana and *Sarmistha Chakrabarti

Department of Home Science (Food & Nutrition), University of Calcutta, Kolkata 700 027, India

ARTICLE INFO

Article History:
Received 28th May, 2015
Received in revised form
15th June, 2015
Accepted 03rd July, 2015
Published online 31st August, 2015

Key words:
Macronutrients,
Rohu, Pomfret,
Cooking methods

ABSTRACT

Fish can be of two types according to habitat, i.e. river and sea fish. The content of this study was the comparison of macronutrients between *rohu* and *pomfret*. The carbohydrate and protein contents of *rohu* were higher than *pomfret* but the fat content was more in *pomfret* as compared to *rohu* in the raw condition. These fish were both subjected to conventional cooking methods like open pan dry roasting, boiling, shallow frying and deep frying. The nutrient contents had changed due to the application of cooking methods. Losses of nutrients had taken place in both fish. The carbohydrate and protein contents became higher in *pomfret* than in *rohu* after cooking whereas the fat content was higher in cooked *rohu* rather than in cooked *pomfret*. The study significantly showed that cooked *pomfret* was beneficial due to adequate protein and carbohydrate restoration whereas *rohu* was useful for fat restoration.

Citation: Uttiya Jana and *Sarmistha Chakrabarti, 2015. "Comparative analysis of macronutrients between river fish *Rohu (Labio rohita)* and sea fish *Pomfret (Pampus argenteus)*, treated under different cooking conditions", *International Journal of Current Research*, 7, (8), 19306-19310.

INTRODUCTION

Fish is a rich source of protein commonly consumed as an alternative source due to higher cost of other animal proteins. But the nutrient contents change when fish is cooked as shown in some studies previously carried out. In one study, three commonly available species of marine fish in Nigeria were subjected to boiling, frying and roasting and the effects of these cooking methods on the fish were observed. The results showed reduced protein content for all the fish types (Goldman *et al*., 1997). In yet another research, amino acid and proximate compositions were determined in six commonly consumed raw and cooked marine fish in Turkey. The changes in amino acid and proximate contents were found to be significant for all cooking methods in all fish species (Erkan *et al*., 2010). Another research showed that cooking methods were also applied for vegetable samples which could also be a reference for this present study. Three cooking methods, namely boiling, steaming and stir-frying were used to evaluate the effect on nutrient components of bamboo shoots, resulting in decreased contents of protein, soluble sugar and ash. Results indicated an appreciable loss in the total free amino acids in boiling method. All procedures were carried out for 10 minutes (Mkandawire *et al*., 2014). The effects of five domestic cooking methods, including steaming, microwaving, boiling, stir-frying and stir-frying followed by boiling on the nutrients and health-promoting compounds of broccoli were investigated. The results showed that all cooking treatments, except steaming, caused significant losses of total soluble proteins and soluble sugars (Yuan *et al*., 2009). The effects of different cooking methods (boiling, baking, frying and grilling) on proximate and mineral composition of snakehead fish were investigated. The changes in the amount of protein and fat were found to be significantly higher in frying and grilling fish (Marimuthu *et al*., 2012). The present study is significant due to the comparison of macronutrient contents between river fish and sea fish after being subjected to cooking. Cooking methods can cause loss of nutrients and the fish that can restore more nutrients after cooking is investigated in this study.

- This study aims to compare the nutritive values of river fish and sea fish in both raw and cooked conditions.
- This study aims at finding the nutritive values restored after cooking.

****Corresponding author: Sarmistha Chakrabarti,***
Department of Home Science (Food & Nutrition), University of Calcutta, Kolkata 700 027, India.

- To find the fish that is beneficial in the perspective of nutrition is the most important concern of this study.

MATERIALS AND METHODS

1.Sample preparation and cooking

Rohu (*Labio rohita*) with a length of 25 – 30 cm and weight of 1 kg and *pomfret* (*Pampus argenteus*) with a length of 12cm and weight of 250–300 g were obtained from the local fish market in Kolkata. They were kept in a plastic container, transported to the laboratory and washed with tap water several times to remove adhering blood and excessive mucous. Subsequently the fish samples were filleted and divided into five groups. The first group was left uncooked while the other four were boiled, dry roasted in open pan, shallow fried and deep fried. Boiling was performed at 99–101 °C (water temperature) for 10 minutes. Open pan dry roasting of fillets was performed in a pan at 180 °C for 10 minutes. The frying of fillets was performed in a domestic frying pan of 2 L capacity at a temperature of approximately 180 °C for 10 minutes. Mustard oil was used as the medium for frying. For shallow frying and deep frying 10 ml and 20 ml oil were used respectively. The fresh raw and cooked samples were then subjected to analysis.

2. Proximate composition analysis

Proximate composition analyses for homogenized samples of cooked and raw fish fillets were done in triplicate for carbohydrate, protein and lipid contents. The carbohydrate content was determined by Anthrone method (Clegg *et al.*, 1956) whereas the crude protein content was determined by the Lowry method (Lowry *et al.*, 1951). Total lipid was extracted from the muscle tissues by soxhlet (De Castro *et al.*, 1998).

a.Estimation of carbohydrate by Anthrone Method (Thomas *et al.*, 1956)

100mg of the sample was taken in a boiling tube and hydrolysed by immersing in boiling water for three hours with 5mL of 2.5 N HCl and cooled to room temperature. Then it was neutralized with solid sodium carbonate until the effervescence ceased. On dilution to 100 ml, the solution was centrifuged at 3000 RPM for 15 minutes. The supernatant was collected and 1 ml of it was used for analysis. 4 ml of Anthrone reagent was added to the solution after which it was heated for eight minutes in a boiling water bath and cooled rapidly. A green to dark green colour was appeared. Then the reading was taken at 630 nm by spectrophotometer (Perkin Elmer Lambda 25).

b.Estimation of protein by Lowry Method (Lowry *et al.* 1951)

200 mg of sample was taken and 20 ml of buffer containing sodium dihydrogen phosphate and disodium hydrogen phosphate was added and homogenized finely. Then it was kept overnight. After that it was cold centrifuged at 5000 RPM for 20 minutes. The supernatant was collected and 1 ml of it was used for analysis. Then 5 ml of Lowry reagent was added to the supernatant and allowed to incubate for 10 minutes. After that 0.5 ml of Folinciocaltue reagent was added and incubated for 30 minutes until a dark blue colour appeared. The reading was taken at 660 nm in a spectrophotometer (Perkin Elmer Lambda 25).

c.Estimation of fat by Soxhlet extraction method (de Castro *et al.* 1998)

The dried sample (5gms) was placed inside the thimble of the apparatus which was extracted with petroleum ether of 60 ^{0}c-80 ^{0}c boiling range which was placed in a distillation flask. On refluxing, the solvent vapour travelled up a distillation arm and flooded into the chamber housing the thimble of solid. The condenser ensured that any solvent vapour that cooled, dripped back down into the chamber housing the solid material. The chamber containing the solid material slowly filled with warm solvent. The fat present in the sample was dissolved in the solvent which was returned to the distillation flask. This cycle may be allowed to repeat for 12 hours. After complete extraction of fat, the solution, poured into a weighed petri dish was evaporated and the final weight of the petri dish containing the fat was taken. From this the amount of the fat was calculated.

3.Statistical analysis

The effect of different cooking methods on the proximate compositions of river fish and sea fish were analyzed using Mean and Standard Deviation. Paired sample t - test was done for comparing the nutritive values between the two fish. Differences were considered to be significant when p value is < 0.05. Data were analyzed by using SPSS package (Version 17).

RESULTS AND DISCUSSION

Table 1 showed the proximate compositions like carbohydrate, protein and fat contents of *rohu.* The raw and cooked values were displayed here. The proximate compositions were reduced due to application of different cooking methods. While the carbohydrate content was highest in shallow frying, the protein content was found to be highest in deep frying, whereas the fat content was restored best in shallow frying. The data showed that carbohydrate loss took place mainly in deep frying method. Protein loss occurred in boiling, whereas fat content was reduced in open pan dry roasting.

Table 2 showed the proximate compositions of *pomfret.* Here also the changes occur between the raw values and the cooked values. Deep frying could restore both carbohydrate and protein whereas shallow frying had increased the amount of fat content in the fish. Boiling could reduce both carbohydrate and protein contents whereas open pan dry roasting helped to reduce fat content of the fish.

Table 3 showed the difference of the proximate nutrient contents between *rohu* and *pomfret* in terms of raw and cooked value. Data showed that there was no significant difference present for carbohydrate content in raw, boiling and open pan

A.Nutrient content of Rohu

Nutrients	Raw	Boiling	Open Pan Dry roasting	Shallow fry	Deep fry
carbohydrate	4.40±0.10	2.83± 0.06	2.87± 0.06	3.17± 0.15	2.73± 0.15
protein	17.50± 0.50	3.03± 0.23	5.70± 0.10	5.03± 0.15	7.33± 0.15
fat	4.33± 0.12	3.47± 0.06	1.83± 0.06	10.77± 0.06	5.60±0.00

B.Nutrient content of Pomfret

Nutrients	Raw	Boiling	Open Pan Dry roasting	Shallow fry	Deep fry
carbohydrate	2.13 ±0.15	1.40± 0.10	1.70± 0.10	1.90± 0.10	2.07± 0.12
protein	16.33± 0.29	4.20± 0.20	6.20± 0.00	6.80± 0.00	7.90± 0.10
fat	5.07± 0.06	3.00± 0.00	2.33± 0.06	8.40± 0.00	5.10± 0.10

C.Comparison of Rohu and Pomfret

Nutrients	Raw	Boiling	Open Pan Dry roasting	Shallow fry	Deep fry
Carbohydrate	2.7661 (NS)	2.7679 (NS)	6.2604 (NS)	0.0002 (S)	0.0038 (S)
protein	0.0248 (S)	0.0027(S)	0.0009 (S)	3.6649 (NS)	0.0057 (S)
Fat	0.0005 (S)	0.0001 (S)	0.0004 (S)	2.3580 (S)	0.00094.4 (S)

(P value = <0.05 = significantly different) (S= significant, NS= Non significant)

D.Percentage of loss between Rohu & Pomfret

Nutrients Loss (%)	Boiling		Open pan Dry roasting		Shallow fry		Deep fry	
	Rohu	Pomfret	Rohu	Pomfret	Rohu	Pomfret	Rohu	Pomfret
Carbohydrate	35.68	34.27	34.77	20.18	27.95	10.79	37.95	2.81
protein	82.68	74.28	67.42	62.03	71.25	58.35	58.11	51.62
Fat	19.86	40.82	57.73	54.04	-59.79	-39.64	-22.67	-0.58

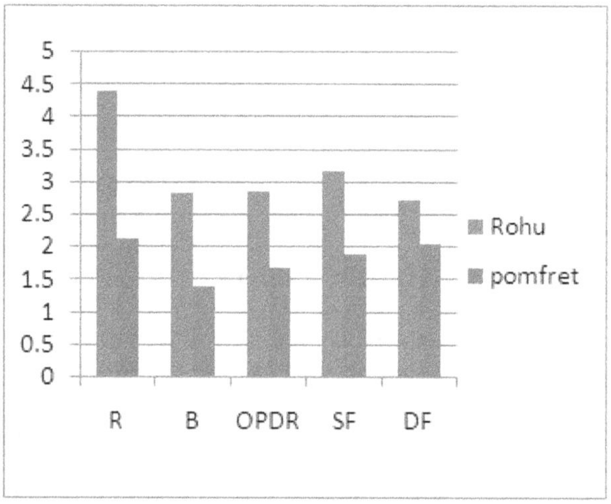

Fig. a. Comparison of carbohydrate content

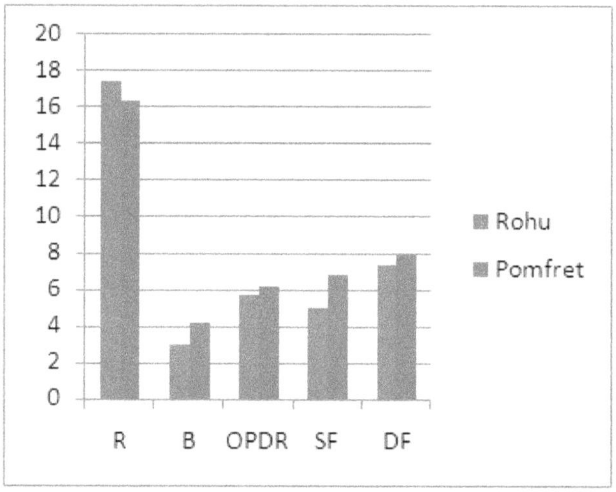

Fig. b. Comparison of protein content

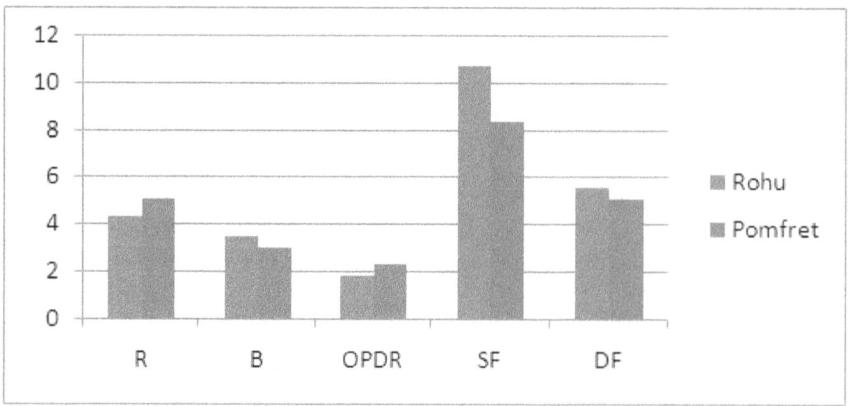

Fig. c. Comparison of fat content

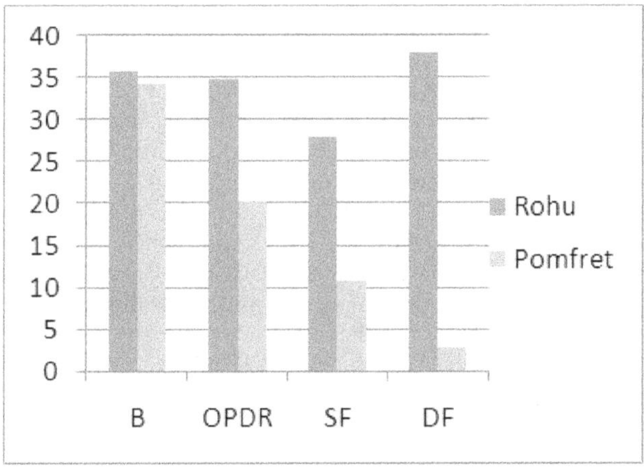

Fig. d. Percentage loss of carbohydrate

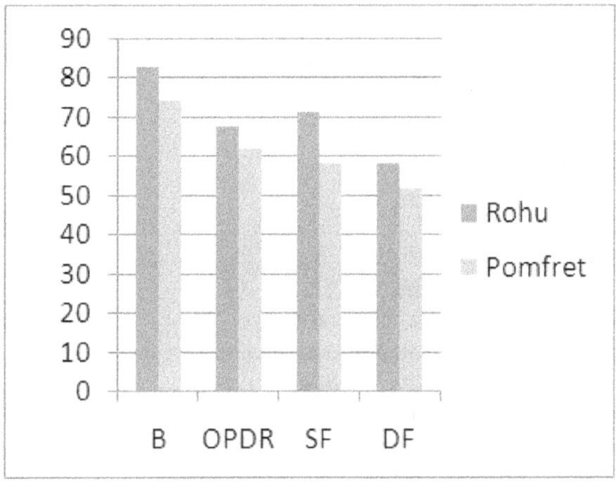

Fig. e. Percentage loss of protein

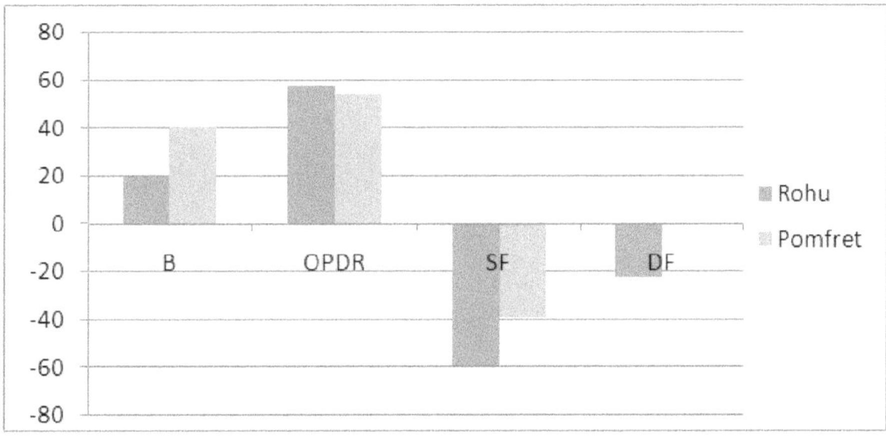

Fig. f. Percentage loss of fat

dry roasting but shallow and deep frying significantly differ in both the fish. Protein contents significantly differ in raw, boiling, open pan dry roasting and deep frying. Shallow frying had the non-significant difference. Fat content significantly differed in raw condition and also for all the four cooking methods. Protein and fat contents significantly differed in raw condition so that it was obvious that significant differences were also present for the cooked values.

Table 4 exhibited the percentage of losses due to cooking. Most of the carbohydrate and protein loss occurred in *rohu* rather than in *pomfret* after cooking. On the other hand, the loss of fat was higher in *pomfret* post cooking. But open pan dry roasting reduced the fat content of *rohu* more than that of *pomfret.* The fat contents increased for both the fish in shallow frying and deep frying methods in comparison to raw conditions due to the addition of mustard oil for frying.

Fig. a, b, c showed the difference among the carbohydrate, protein and fat contents of *rohu* and *pomfret*. These figures had suggested that in raw condition both carbohydrate and protein contents were higher in *rohu* and fat content was higher in *pomfret*. But after the application of cooking methods, carbohydrate contents were higher in *rohu* and protein contents were higher in *pomfret*.

The fat content was higher in *pomfret* in raw condition whereas it was found to be higher in *rohu* after cooking.

Fig c, d, e showed that the loss percentage of carbohydrate and protein contents was more in *rohu* after cooking, but fat loss was more in *pomfret*.

Conclusion

The maximum losses occurred in river fish after cooking rather than in sea fish. Losses occurred in both the fish but loss percentage for both carbohydrate and protein were higher in *rohu* rather than in *pomfret*. The loss of fat was more in *pomfret*. This might be due to the presence of extra fatty tissue in the sea fish which could give protection when it was subjected to cooking.

The fat loss was more for *pomfret* due to application of heat like open pan dry roasting which could eliminate oil from the fatty tissues. *Rohu* did not contain excessive fat so the loss also occurred in smaller amounts. In case of shallow and deep frying, oil was used, which increased the amount of fat contents. After considering all advantages and disadvantages, it can be said that sea fish is better than river fish in terms of nutrient restoration after cooking.

Acknowledgement

The University Grants Commission (UGC) is thanked for awarding a Junior Research Fellowship to Uttiya Jana.

REFERENCES

Clegg, K. M. 1956. The application of the anthrone reagent to the estimation of starch in cereals. *Journal of the Science of Food and Agriculture,* 7(1), 40-44.

De Castro, M. L., & Garcıa-Ayuso, L. E. 1998. Soxhlet extraction of solid materials: an outdated technique with a promising innovative future. *Analytica Chimica Acta.,* 369(1), 1-10.

Erkan, N., Özden, Ö., & Selçuk, A. 2010. Effect of frying, grilling, and steaming on amino acid composition of marine fishes. *Journal of Medicinal Food*, 13(6), 1524-1531.

Goldman, K. J. 1997. Regulation of body temperature in the white shark, Carcharodon carcharias. *Journal of Comparative Physiology B*, 167(6), 423-429.

Lowry, O. H., Rosebrough, N. J., Farr, A. L., & Randall, R. J. 1951. Protein measurement with the Folin phenol reagent. *J. Biol. Chem*, 193(1), 265-275.

Manirakiza, P., Covaci, A., & Schepens, P. 2001. Comparative study on total lipid determination using Soxhlet, Roese-Gottlieb, Bligh & Dyer, and modified Bligh & Dyer extraction methods. *Journal of Food Composition and Analysis*, 14(1), 93-100.

Marimuthu, K., Thilaga, M., Kathiresan, S., Xavier, R., & Mas, R. H. M. H. 2012. Effect of different cooking methods on proximate and mineral composition of striped snakehead fish (Channa striatus, Bloch). *Journal of Food Science and Technology*, 49(3), 373-377.

Mkandawire, K. T., & Masamba, K. G. 2014. Effect of lemon juice treatment and sun drying on vitamin C retention in three steam and water blanched indigenous vegetables over six weeks storage period. *African Journal of Food Science*, 8(6), 316-321.

Yuan, G. F., Sun, B., Yuan, J., & Wang, Q. M. 2009. Effects of different cooking methods on health-promoting compounds of broccoli. *Journal of Zhejiang University Science B*, 10(8), 580-588.

****

Comparison of Restoration of Protein Contents of Preserved *Rohu (Labio rohita)*, Treated under Different Cooking Conditions

Uttiya Jana[1], Sarmistha Chakrabarti[2]

Department of Home Science (Food & Nutrition), University of Calcutta, Kolkata 700 027, India

Abstract: ***Fish are rich sources of protein commonly consumed as an alternative source of protein due to higher cost of other animal proteins. This study was based on the comparison of protein contents of rohu preserved with the combination of salt and turmeric and without preservative for 24 hours, 48 hours, 14 days and 15 days. This preserved fish was subjected to conventional cooking methods like open pan dry roasting, boiling, shallow frying and deep frying. The protein contents of cooked fish were significantly lower than those in the raw condition. The nutrient contents change due to cooking. Loss of nutrients mainly occurs in boiling whereas it is better restored in deep fat frying method. The study significantly showed that the protein loss occurs due to preservation but this loss can be reduced by using the combination of salt and turmeric.***

Keywords: *Rohu*, protein, cooking methods, preservatives, deep fat frying

1. Introduction

Fish is consumed mainly as a rich source of protein. But the nutrient contents change when it is preserved and cooked as shown in some studies previously carried out. In one study, three commonly available species of marine fish in Nigeria were subjected to boiling, frying and roasting and the effects of these cooking methods on the fish were observed. The results showed reduced protein content for all the fish types [(1)]. In yet another research, amino acid and proximate compositions were determined in six commonly consumed raw and cooked marine fish in Turkey. The changes in amino acid and proximate contents were found to be significant for all cooking methods in all fish species [(2)]. Another research showed that cooking methods were also applied for vegetable samples which could also be a reference for this present study. Three cooking methods, namely boiling, steaming and stir-frying were used to evaluate the effect on nutrient components of bamboo shoots, resulting in decreased contents of protein, soluble sugar and ash. Results indicated an appreciable loss in the total free amino acids in boiling method. All procedures were carried out for 10 minutes [(3)]. The effects of five domestic cooking methods, including steaming, microwaving, boiling, stir-frying and stir-frying followed by boiling on the nutrients and health-promoting compounds of broccoli were investigated. The results showed that all cooking treatments, except steaming, caused significant losses of total soluble proteins and soluble sugars [(4)]. The effects of different cooking methods (boiling, baking, frying and grilling) on proximate and mineral composition of snakehead fish were investigated. The changes in the amount of protein and fat were found to be significantly higher in frying and grilling fish [(5)]. Another study was designed to observe the performance of turmeric and salt on *tengra* (Mystus vittatus) for several days, stored with preservatives of 2% of the sample weight, resulting in nutrient restoration.[(6)] The present study is significant due to the comparison of protein contents of *rohu* after being preserved for several days and then subjected to cooking. Preservation can cause loss of protein; however, the amount of protein that can be restored using a combination of salt and turmeric for 15 days, is investigated in this study.

- This study aims to estimate the protein contents of *rohu* in both raw and cooked conditions after being preserved for 24 hours, 48 hours, 14 days and 15 days with and without preservative.
- This study also aims at finding comparison of protein contents of preserved and cooked fish with and without preservative.
- To find the deterioration level of preserved fish in the perspective of protein content is the most important concern of this study.

2. Materials and Methods

1) Sample Preparation and Cooking

Rohu (*Labio rohita*), with a length of 25 – 30 cm and weight of 1 kg was obtained from the local fish market in Kolkata. It was kept in a plastic container, transported to the laboratory and washed with tap water several times to remove adhering blood and excessive mucous. Subsequently the fish sample was filleted into three sections and each section was divided into five groups. In the first section one group was left uncooked while the other four were boiled, dry roasted in open pan, shallow fried and deep fried. Boiling was performed at 99–101 °C (water temperature) for 10 minutes. Open pan dry roasting of fillets was performed in a pan at 180 °C for 10 minutes. The frying of fillets was performed in a domestic frying pan of 2 L capacity at a temperature of approximately 180 °C for 10 minutes. Mustard oil was used as the medium for frying. In case of shallow frying, 10 ml oil was used and for deep frying 20 ml. The other two sections were allowed to preserve up to15 days. Among these two sections, one was preserved in the refrigerator at -20^{0}C without preservative and the other section was preserved with the combination of salt and turmeric. The amount of combination of salt and turmeric was used as 2% of the weight of the fish sample preserved in 1:1 ratio. The raw, fresh and preserved samples were then subjected to analysis post cooking on the day of preservation of 1st, 2nd, 14th and 15th.

2) Proximate Composition Analysis

Proximate composition analyses for homogenized samples of fresh and preserved fish fillets, both raw and cooked, were done in triplicate for protein contents. The crude protein content was determined by the Lowry method (7).

Estimation of Protein by Lowry Method (7)

200 mg of sample was taken and 20 ml of buffer, containing sodium dihydrogen phosphate and disodium hydrogen phosphate, was added and homogenized finely. Then it was kept overnight. After that it was cold centrifuged at 5000 RPM for 20 minutes. The supernatant was collected and 1 ml of it was used for analysis. Then 5 ml of Lowry reagent was added to the supernatant and allowed to incubate for 10 minutes. After that 0.5 ml of Folinciocaltue reagent was added and incubated for 30 minutes until a dark blue colour appeared. The reading was taken at 660 nm by spectrophotometer (Perkin Elmer Lambda 25).

3) Statistical analysis

The effect of different cooking methods on protein content of fresh and preserved *rohu* was analyzed using Mean and Standard Deviations. Paired sample t - test was done for comparing the protein contents between preserved fish with and without preservative. Differences were considered to be significant when p value is < 0.05. Data were analyzed by using SPSS package (Version 17).

3. Result

Table 1: Protein content of fresh *rohu*

Raw	*Boiling*	*Dry roasting*	*Shallow frying*	*Deep frying*
17.50± 0.50	3.03± 0.23	5.70± 0.10	5.03± 0.15	7.33± 0.15

Table 2: Protein content of preserved *rohu* without preservative

Duration	*Raw*	*Boiling*	*Dry roasting*	*Shallow frying*	*Deep frying*
24 hours	16.50± 0.50	4.40±0.00	5.60± 0.20	4.46± 0.05	7.40± 0.17
48 hours	13.06±0.51	3.40±0.10	5.60±0.20	4.06±0.11	5.10±0.10
14 days	7.23±0.25	5.0±0.10	5.66±0.28	5.83±0.05	8.76±0.05
15 days	6.26±0.05	4.10±0.10	5.26±0.25	5.76±0.05	7.53±0.05

Table 3: Protein content of preserved *rohu* with the combination of salt and turmeric

Duration	*Raw*	*Boiling*	*Dry roasting*	*Shallow frying*	*Deep frying*
24 hours	16.83 ±0.15	6.20± 0.20	13.10± 0.17	13.26± 0.25	15.86± 0.1
48 hours	15.60± 0.17	7.03± 0.57	9.93± 0.11	5.80± 0.00	8.8± 0.10
14 days	14.06±0.05	5.26±0.05	8.6±0.10	6.8±0.20	11.8±0.05
15 days	12.03±0.05	4.93±0.11	6.10±0.10	6.26±0.17	8.6±0.05

Table 4: Comparison of protein content of preserved *rohu* with and without preservative

Duration	*Raw*	*Boiling*	*Dry roasting*	*Shallow frying*	*Deep frying*
24 hours	0.242(S)	0.004(S)	0.000(S)	0.000(S)	0.00(S)
48 hours	0.013(S)	0.000 (S)	0.000(S)	0.001(S)	0.000(S)
14 days	0.038(S)	0.057(NS)	0.003(S)	0.015(S)	0.000(S)
15 days	0.000(S)	0.002(S)	0.011(S)	0.023(S)	0.003(S)

(P value = <0.05 = significantly different) (S= significant, NS= Non significant

Table 5: Percentage of loss of protein in cooked *rohu* preserved without preservative

Duration	*Boiling*	*Dry roasting*	*Shallow frying*	*Deep frying*
24 hours	73.3	66.06	72.96	55.15
48 hours	74.01	57.12	68.86	60.94
14 days	30.84	21.71	19.36	- 21.16
15 days	34.50	15.97	7.98	- 20.28

Table 6: Percentage of loss of protein in cooked *rohu* preserved with salt and turmeric

Duration	*Raw*	*Boiling*	*Dry Roasting*	*Shallow Frying*	*Deep Frying*
24 hours	63.16	22.16	21.21	5.76	63.16
48 hours	54.93	36.34	62.82	43.58	54.93
14 days	62.58	38.83	51.63	16.07	62.58
15 days	59.01	49.29	48.46	28.01	59.01

Table 7: Percentage of loss of protein in preserved *rohu* without preservative in comparison to fresh

Duration	*Raw*	*Boiling*	*Dry Roasting*	*Shallow Frying*	*Deep Frying*
24 hours	5.71	- 45.21	1.75	11.33	- 1.36
48 hours	25.37	- 12.21	1.75	19.28	30.13
14 days	58.68	- 65.01	0.70	- 15.90	- 20.0
15 days	64.22	- 35.31	7.71	- 14.51	- 3.15

Table 8: Percentage of loss of protein in preserved *rohu* with preservative in comparison to fresh

Duration	*Raw*	*Boiling*	*Dry Roasting*	*Shallow Frying*	*Deep Frying*
24 hours	3.82	-104.62	-129.82	- 163.61	- 117.26
48 hours	10.85	- 132.01	- 74.21	- 15.30	- 20.54
14 days	19.65	- 73.59	- 50.87	- 35.18	-61.6
15 days	31.25	- 62.70	- 7.01	- 24.45	- 18.63

International Journal of Science and Research (IJSR)
ISSN (Online): 2319-7064
Index Copernicus Value (2013): 6.14 | Impact Factor (2014): 5.611

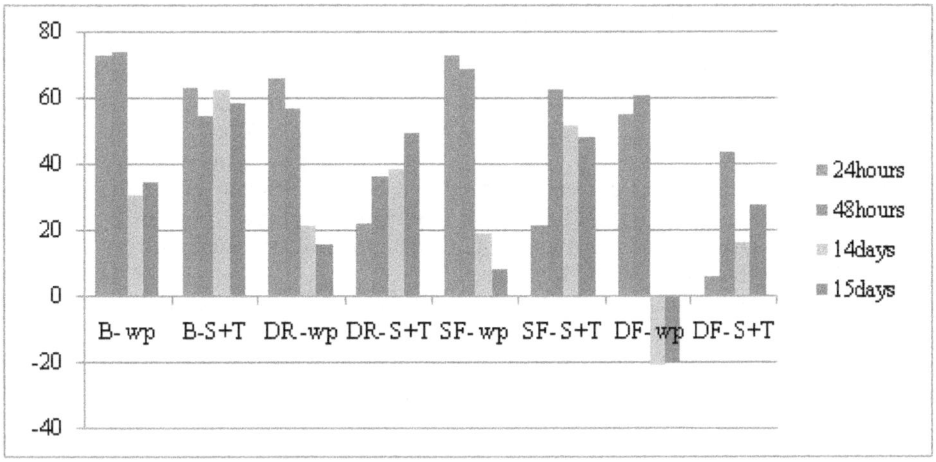

Figure (a): Percentage loss of preserved *rohu* in different cooking methods

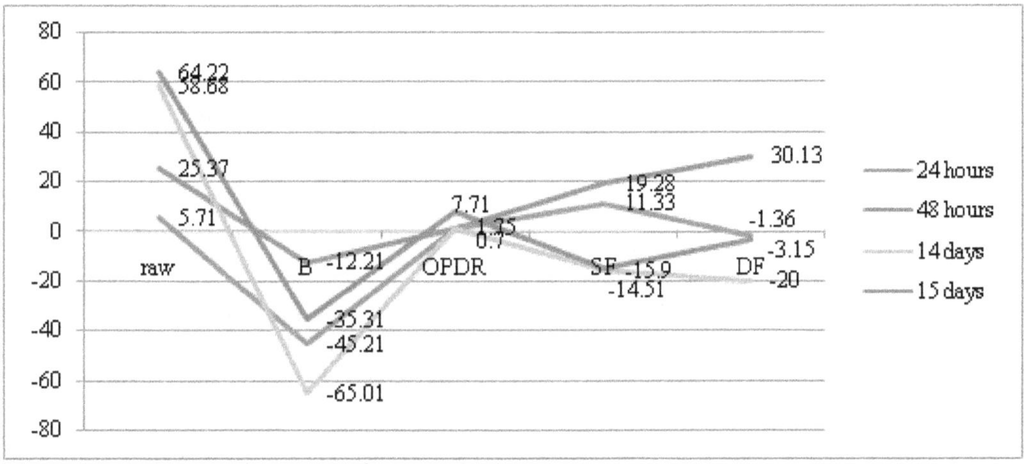

Figure (b): Percentage loss of preserved *rohu* without preservative in different cooking methods

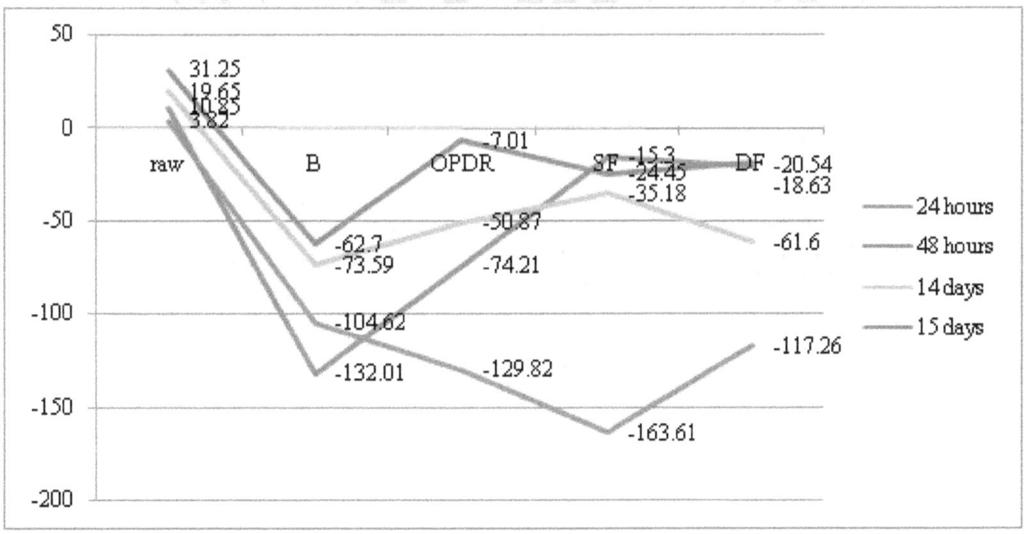

Figure (c): Percentage loss of preserved *rohu* with salt and turmeric in different cooking methods

4. Discussion

Table 1 showed the protein content of *rohu* after subjecting it to different cooking methods. The raw and cooked values were displayed here. The protein content was reduced due to application of different cooking methods. The highest loss occurs in boiling and it was found to be restored in deep frying method.

Table 2 showed the protein contents of preserved *rohu* without preservative for 24 hours, 48 hours, 14 days and 15 days respectively. Here also the changes occurred between the raw and the cooked values. Cooking methods significantly differed from the raw values. It also indicated that the highest loss was in boiling method whereas the lowest was in deep frying; rather the protein content was increased in this method after preservation for 14 and 15 days.

Table 3 showed the difference of the protein contents of the fish preserved with the combination of salt and turmeric in terms of raw and cooked value. Data showed that significant difference was present between both the values. Here also the loss occurred in the boiling method as compared to other cooking methods.

Table 4 exhibited the comparison of the protein contents of the fish preserved with and without preservative for short and long time durations. Data showed that the significant difference was present among the protein contents in terms of raw and cooked values.

Table 5 exhibited the percentage of protein losses post cooking of the preserved fish without preservative in respect of raw for each preservation day. Most of the loss occurred in boiling and the nutrient restoration occurred in deep frying.

Table 6 exhibited the percentage of protein losses following cooking of the preserved fish with the combination of salt and turmeric in respect of raw for each preservation day. Boiling causes the significant loss while deep frying causes protein restoration.

Table 7 exhibited the percentage of protein deterioration after cooking of the preserved fish without preservative in respect of fresh fish for each preservation day. Data indicated that protein loss occurred mostly in 48 hours.

Table 8 showed the percentage of protein reduction post cooking of the preserved fish with salt and turmeric in respect of fresh for each preservation day. Data indicated that loss of protein occurred gradually day by day preservation and the highest loss was found in the 15th day of preservation.

Fig. a showed the comparison of the loss percentage of protein contents post cooking of the fish preserved with and without preservative. It was found that losses were more in boiling whereas less in deep frying.

Fig. b showed the loss percentage in preserved fish without preservative and the line trend indicated the highest loss in 48 hours

Fig. c exhibited the percentage of losses in fish preserved upto 15 days by using preservative. The line indicated that there was gradual loss but maximum loss occurred in 15th day of preservation.

5. Conclusion

All cooking methods can reduce the protein content of the fish. The maximum restoration was found to be mostly in deep frying method while the loss occurred in boiling method. After preservation of this fish up to 15th day, the deterioration of protein occurred in 48 hours but this deterioration can be reduced to some extent with the use of natural preservative that is combination of salt and turmeric, which help to restore protein content up to 15th day of preservation. After considering all advantages and disadvantages, it can be said that deep frying is the best method for protein restoration among the other cooking methods and use of salt and turmeric can delay this deterioration post cooking.

6. Acknowledgement

The University Grants Commission (UGC) is thanked for awarding a Junior Research Fellowship to Uttiya Jana.

References

[1] Goldman, K. J. (1997). *Regulation of body temperature in the white shark, Carcharodon carcharias*. Journal of Comparative Physiology B, 167(6), 423-429.

[2] Erkan, N., Özden, Ö., & Selçuk, A. (2010). *Effect of frying, grilling, and steaming on amino acid composition of marine fishes*. Journal of medicinal food, 13(6), 1524-1531.

[3] Mkandawire, K. T., & Masamba, K. G. (2014). *Effect of lemon juice treatment and sun drying on vitamin C retention in three steam and water blanched indigenous vegetables over six weeks storage period*. African Journal of Food Science, 8(6), 316-321.

[4] Yuan, G. F., Sun, B., Yuan, J., & Wang, Q. M. (2009). *Effects of different cooking methods on health-promoting compounds of broccoli*. Journal of Zhejiang University Science B, 10(8), 580-588.

[5] Marimuthu, K., Thilaga, M., Kathiresan, S., Xavier, R., & Mas, R. H. M. H. (2012). *Effect of different cooking methods on proximate and mineral composition of striped snakehead fish (Channa striatus, Bloch)*. Journal of food science and technology, 49(3), 373-377.

[6] T. Akter 1 , A. T. A. Ahmed 1 , M. A. khaleque and M. Begum (2013), *Effect of drying on quality of tengra (Mystus vittatus)* treated with turmeric and salt. Unique Research Journal of Biological Science,1(1),001-005.

[7] Lowry, O. H., Rosebrough, N. J., Farr, A. L., & Randall, R. J. (1951). *Protein measurement with the Folin phenol reagent*. J Biol Chem, 193(1), 265-275.

International Journal of Scientific & Engineering Research, Volume 7, Issue 1, January-2016 638
ISSN 2229-5518

Comparison of restoration of carbohydrate and protein contents among different fish and other edible aquatic species, treated under different cooking conditions

Uttiya Jana & Sarmistha Chakrabarti

Abstract- Fish are rich sources of protein commonly consumed as an alternative source of protein due to higher cost of other animal proteins. This study was based on the comparison of carbohydrate and protein contents among different fish and other edible aquatic species namely *rohu, katla,* prawn, lobster, *pomfret* and *hilsa* after being subjected to conventional cooking methods. The carbohydrate and protein contents of cooked fish are significantly lower than those in the raw condition. These fish were subjected to conventional cooking methods like open pan dry roasting, boiling, shallow frying and deep frying, which altered their nutrient contents. Loss of nutrients mainly occurs in boiling, whereas it is better restored in deep fat frying method. The study significantly showed that cooked lobster was beneficial due to adequate protein and carbohydrate restoration compared to all other fish and edible aquatic species.

Keywords – carbohydrate, cooking methods, edible aquatics species, protein, sea fish, sweet water fish

Introduction

Fish is consumed mainly as a rich source of protein. But the nutrient contents change when it is cooked as shown in some studies previously carried out. In one study, three commonly available species of marine fish in Nigeria were subjected to boiling, frying and roasting and the effects of these cooking methods on the fish were observed. The results showed reduced protein content for all the fish types [(1)]. In yet another research, amino acid and proximate compositions were determined in six commonly consumed raw and cooked marine fish in Turkey. The changes in amino acid and proximate contents were found to be significant for all cooking methods in all fish species [(2)]. Another research showed that cooking methods were also applied for vegetable samples which could be a reference for this present study. Three cooking methods, namely boiling, steaming and stir-frying were used to evaluate the effect on nutrient components of bamboo shoots, resulting in decreased contents of protein, soluble sugar and ash. Results indicated an appreciable loss in the total free amino acids in boiling method. All procedures were carried out for 10 minutes [(3)]. Elsewhere, the effects of five domestic cooking methods, including steaming, microwaving, boiling, stir-frying and stir-frying followed by boiling, on the nutrients and health-promoting compounds of broccoli were investigated. The results showed that all cooking treatments, except steaming, caused significant losses of total soluble proteins and soluble sugars [(4)]. The effects of different cooking methods (boiling, baking, frying and grilling) on proximate and mineral composition of snakehead fish were investigated. The changes in the amount of protein and fat were found to be significantly higher in frying and grilling fish [(5)]. The present study is significant due to the comparison of carbohydrate and protein contents among river fish, sea fish and other edible aquatic species (crustaceans) after being subjected to cooking. Cooking methods can cause loss of nutrients and the fish that can restore more nutrients after cooking are investigated in this study.

This study aims to

- Estimate the nutritive values of different fish and other edible aquatic species in both raw and cooked conditions
- Find the nutritive values restored after cooking
- Find the fish that is beneficial in the perspective of nutrition

Materials and Methods

1. Sample preparation and cooking

Rohu (*Labio rohita*), *katla* (*Catla catla*), *hilsa* (*Hilsa ilisa*) with a length of 25 – 30 cm and weight of 1 kg, *pomfret* (*Pampus argenteus*) with a length of 12cm and weight of 250–300 g and prawn and lobster with a length of 10 cm and 15cm, and weight of 50 gm and 90 gm respectively were obtained from the local fish market in Kolkata. They were kept in a plastic containers, transported to the laboratory and washed with tap water several times to remove adhering blood and excessive mucous. Subsequently the fish samples were filleted and divided into five groups. The first group was left uncooked while the other four were boiled, dry roasted in open pan, shallow fried and deep fried. Boiling was performed at 99–101 °C (water temperature) for 10 minutes. Open pan dry roasting of fillets was performed in a pan at 180 °C for 10 minutes. The frying of fillets was performed in a domestic frying pan of 2 L capacity at a temperature of approximately 180 °C for 10 minutes.

Mustard oil was used as the medium for frying. In case of shallow frying 10 ml oil was used and for deep frying 20 ml oil. The fresh raw and cooked samples were then subjected to analysis.

2. Proximate composition analysis

Proximate composition analyses for homogenized samples of cooked and raw fish fillets were done in triplicate for carbohydrate and protein contents. The carbohydrate content was determined by Anthrone method [6] whereas the crude protein content was determined by the Lowry method [7].

a. Estimation of carbohydrate by Anthrone Method [6]

100mg of the sample was taken in a boiling tube. Hydrolysis was carried out by keeping it in a boiling water bath for three hours with 5mL of 2.5 N HCl followed by cooling to room temperature and neutralizing with solid sodium carbonate until the effervescence ceased. The volume was made up to 100 ml and centrifugation was done at 3000 RPM for 15 minutes. The supernatant was collected and 1 ml of it was used for analysis. Then 4 ml Anthrone was added to the solution. After that it was heated for eight minutes in a boiling water bath and was cooled rapidly. Green to dark green colour appeared. Then the reading was taken at 630 nm by a spectrophotometer (Perkin Elmer Lambda 25).

b. Estimation of Protein by Lowry Method [7]

200 mg of sample was taken and 20 ml of buffer, containing sodium dihydrogen phosphate and disodium hydrogen phosphate, was added and homogenized finely. Then it was kept overnight. After that it was cold - centrifuged at 5000 RPM for 20 minutes. The supernatant was collected and 1 ml was used for analysis. Then 5 ml of Lowry reagent was added to the supernatant and allowed to incubate for 10 minutes. After that 0.5 ml of Folinciocaltue reagent was added and incubated for 30 minutes until a dark blue colour appeared. The reading was taken at 660 nm with a spectrophotometer (Perkin Elmer Lambda 25).

3. Statistical analysis

The effect of different cooking methods on the proximate compositions of river fish, sea fish and crustaceans was analyzed using Mean and Standard Deviation. Paired sample t- test was done for comparing the nutritive values between the raw and cooked samples. Differences were considered to be significant when p value is < 0.05 and by the use of standard t- table. Data were analyzed by using SPSS package (Version 17).

Result

Table – 1

a. Nutrient contents of *rohu*

Nutrients	Raw	Boiling	Dry roasting	Shallow frying	Deep frying
carbohydrate	4.40± 0.10	2.83± 0.06	2.87± 0.06	3.17± 0.15	2.73± 0.15
protein	17.50 ± 0.50	3.03± 0.23	5.70± 0.10	5.03± 0.15	7.33± 0.15

b. Nutrient contents of *katla*

Nutrients	Raw	Boiling	Dry roasting	Shallow frying	Deep frying
carbohydrate	3.73± 0.15	2.70 ±0.10	2.93± 0.12	3.33± 0.15	3.17± 0.15
protein	21.17± 0.29	2.70± 0.00	6.20±0.00	10.90±0.00	5.00± 0.00

c. Nutrient contents of *pomfret*

Nutrients	Raw	Boiling	Dry roasting	Shallow frying	Deep frying
carbohydrate	2.13 ±0.15	1.40± 0.10	1.70± 0.10	1.90± 0.10	2.07± 0.12
protein	16.33± 0.29	4.20± 0.20	6.20± 0.00	6.80± 0.00	7.90± 0.10

d. Nutrient contents of *hilsa*

Nutrients	Raw	Boiling	Dry roasting	Shallow frying	Deep frying
carbohydrate	3.57± 0.12	2.37± 0.15	1.67± 0.12	2.13± 0.12	3.17± 0.06
protein	24.07± 0.12	6.53± 0.23	9.60± 0.17	10.70± 0.17	11.87 ± 0.12

e. Nutrient contents of prawn

Nutrients	Raw	Boiling	Dry roasting	Shallow frying	De fry
carbohydrate	1.03± 0.21	0.67± 0.12	0.97± 0.15	0.83± 0.06	0.5 0.1
protein	17.33±0.29	2.57± 0.12	6.47± 0.06	6.47± 0.06	11 0.(

f. Nutrient contents of lobster

Nutrients	Raw	Boiling	Dry roasting	Shallow frying	Deep frying

ISSN 2229-5518

carbohydrate	2.63± 0.12	2.13± 0.12	1.47± 0.12	2.43± 0.15	1.50± 0.10
protein	19.20 ±0.20	8.67± 0.15	7.93± 0.06	9.50±0.00	13.57±0 .12

Table – 2 : Comparison of carbohydrate contents of raw and cooked fish

Nutrients	Boiling	Dry roasting	Shallow frying	Deep frying
Rohu	1.94382(NS)	2.11732(NS)	0.000305(S)	9.34927(NS)
Katla	0.000607 (S)	0.001935(S)	0.032678(S)	0.01047(S)
Pomfret	0.006074 (S)	0.000245(S)	0.144704(NS)	0.000211(S)
Hilsa	0.006074 (S)	0.000245(S)	0.144704(S)	0.000211(S)
Prawn	0.055929 (S)	0.677869(NS)	0.184074(NS)	0.01613(S)
Lobster	0.006074 (S)	0.000245(S)	0.144704(NS)	0.000211(S)

(P value = <0.05 = significantly different)

(S= significant, NS= Non significant)

Table -3: Comparison of protein contents of raw and cooked fish and other edible aquatic species

Nutrients	Boiling	Dry roasting	Shallow frying	Deep frying
Rohu	1.39(S)	2.31(S)	2.05(S)	4.63(NS)
Katla	3.98(S)	9.22(NS)	4.16(S)	6.77(NS)
Pomfret	4.67(NS)	4.38(NS)	5.59(NS)	1.14(S)
Hilsa	3.13(S)	2.86(S)	3.92(S)	2.14(S)
Prawn	1.31(S)	3.59(S)	3.59(S)	3.05(S)
Lobster	2.17(S)	7.76(NS)	1.2(S)	1.88(S)

(P value is calculated by using the standard t-Table at the level of 5%.)

(S= significant, NS= Non significant)

Table - 4

Percentage of losses of carbohydrate among different fish and other edible aquatic species

Name of fish	Boiling	Dry Roasting	Shallow Frying	Deep Frying
Rohu	35.68	34.77	27.95	37.95
katla	27.6	21.4	10.7	15.0
Pomfret	34.27	20.18	10.79	2.81
Hilsa	33.61	53.22	40.3	11.2
Prawn	34.9	5.82	19.4	51.4
Lobster	19.0	44.10	7.60	42.9

Table - 5

Percentage of losses of protein among different fish and other edible aquatic species

Name of fish	Boiling	Dry Roasting	Shallow Frying	Deep Frying
Rohu	82.68	67.42	71.25	58.11
Katla	87.24	70.7	48.5	76.3
Pomfret	74.28	62.03	58.35	51.62
Hilsa	72.8	60.11	55.5	50.6
Prawn	85.17	62.6	62.6	35.94
Lobster	54.84	58.6	50.5	29.3

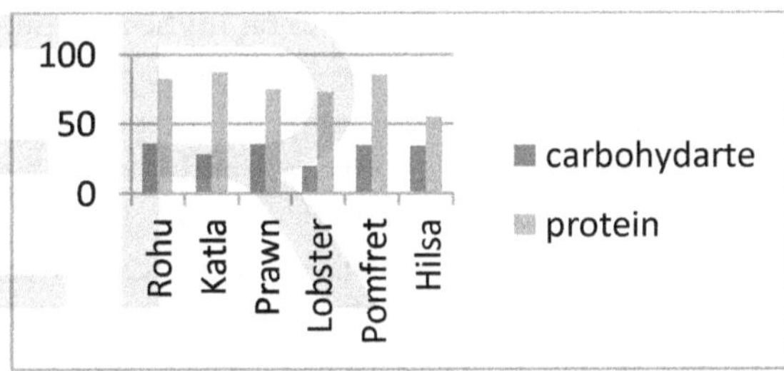

Fig a. Percentage loss in boiling

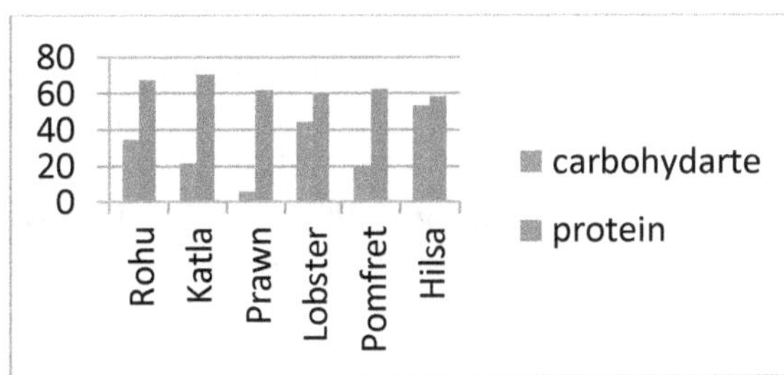

Fig b. Percentage loss in open pan dry roasting

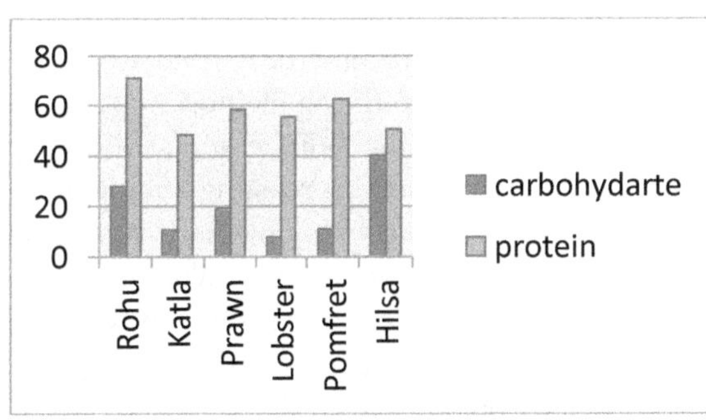

ISSN 2229-5518

Fig c. Percentage loss in shallow frying

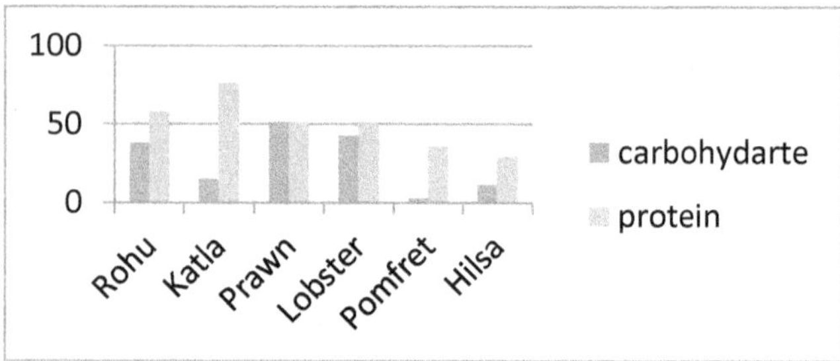

Fig d. Percentage loss in deep frying

Discussion

Table 1-a, b, c, d, e and f showed the proximate compositions like carbohydrate and protein contents of *rohu, katla, pomfret, hilsa,* prawn and lobster. The raw and cooked values were displayed here. The proximate compositions were reduced due to application of different cooking methods. While the carbohydrate content was highest in shallow frying for *rohu, katla,* prawn and lobster, the protein content was found to be highest in deep frying for all the fish. For the sea fish *pomfret* and *hilsa* the carbohydrate contents were better restored in deep frying. The data showed that carbohydrate and protein losses took place mainly in boiling method for *rohu, katla* and prawn whereas dry roasting was responsible for carbohydrate loss for *pomfret, hilsa* and lobster. Protein loss occurred in boiling for the sea fish.

Table 2 showed the comparison of carbohydrate contents of different fish. Here also the changes occurred between the raw and the cooked values. Boiling, open pan dry roasting and deep frying methods significantly differed from the raw values of *katla, pomfret, hilsa* and lobster whereas shallow frying significantly differed from the raw content of *rohu*. Boiling and deep frying could differ from the raw value of prawn.

Table 3 showed the difference of the protein contents of the fish in terms of raw and cooked value. Data showed that there was a significant difference present for protein content in raw, boiling and open pan dry roasting and shallow frying but deep frying method was non- significant for *rohu*, whereas in *katla*, boiling and shallow frying were significant, but open pan dry roasting and deep frying were non-significant. All the cooking methods significantly differ from the raw protein contents of prawn, lobster and *hilsa*. In case of *pomfret*, protein content significantly differs in deep frying whereas boiling, open pan dry roasting and shallow frying had the non-significant difference.

Table 4 exhibited the percentage of carbohydrate losses due to cooking. Most of the carbohydrate loss occurred in *rohu* after boiling. On the other hand, the loss was higher in *hilsa* post open pan dry roasting and shallow frying. But deep frying reduced the carbohydrate content in prawn the most. Losses mainly occurred in boiling while the nutrient restoration in deep frying.

Table 5 exhibited the percentage of protein losses post cooking. Most of the loss occurred in *katla* after boiling, open pan dry roasting and deep frying whereas shallow frying reduced the protein content the most in *rohu*. Protein losses mainly occurred in boiling and the nutrient restoration occurred in deep frying.

Fig. a. showed that the loss percentage of carbohydrate and protein contents of aquatic species occurred post boiling. It was found that losses were more in *rohu* and *katla* whereas it was low in lobster.

Fig. b. showed that the loss percentage of nutrient contents was more in *hilsa* and *katla* respectively whereas it was lower in prawn and lobster after open pan dry roasting.

Fig. c. showed that the losses were more in *hilsa* and *rohu* but less in lobster and *katla* after shallow frying.

Fig. d. showed that the loss percentage of carbohydrate and protein contents was more in prawn and *katla* but less in *pomfret* and lobster for deep frying method.

Conclusion

The maximum carbohydrate and protein contents were found to be highest in rohu and hilsa respectively in raw condition but prone to loss after cooking, although losses occurred after cooking for all the fish. The carbohydrate content was mostly restored in shallow frying for *rohu, katla* and lobster whereas deep frying helped to restore more in case of *pomfret* and *hilsa* but open pan dry roasting could reserve carbohydrate in prawn. Protein contents were retained mainly in deep frying for all the fish except *katla* whose protein restoration occurred in shallow frying. Most of the carbohydrate restoration occurred in prawn, lobster and *pomfret* post cooking whereas protein reservation occurred mostly in lobster. After considering all advantages and disadvantages, it can be said that boiling could reduce both carbohydrate and protein contents and deep frying can restore nutrients among the other cooking methods and lobster is the best among the other fish, regarding the restoration of nutrients post cooking.

Acknowledgement

ISSN 2229-5518
The University Grants Commission (UGC) is thanked for awarding a Junior Research Fellowship to Uttiya Jana.

Billiography

1. Goldman, K. J. (1997). *Regulation of body temperature in the white shark, Carcharodon carcharias*. Journal of Comparative Physiology B, 167(6), 423-429.

2. Erkan, N., Özden, Ö., & Selçuk, A. (2010). *Effect of frying, grilling, and steaming on amino acid composition of marine fishes*. Journal of Medicinal Food, 13(6), 1524-1531.

3. Mkandawire, K. T., & Masamba, K. G. (2014). *Effect of lemon juice treatment and sun drying on vitamin C retention in three steam and water blanched indigenous vegetables over six weeks storage period*. African Journal of Food Science, 8(6), 316-321.

4. Yuan, G. F., Sun, B., Yuan, J., & Wang, Q. M. (2009). *Effects of different cooking methods on health-promoting compounds of broccoli*. Journal of Zhejiang University Science B, 10(8), 580-588.

5. Marimuthu, K., Thilaga, M., Kathiresan, S., Xavier, R., & Mas, R. H. M. H. (2012). *Effect of different cooking methods on proximate and mineral composition of striped snakehead fish (Channa striatus, Bloch)*. Journal of Food Science and Technology, 49(3), 373-377.

6. Clegg et al. (1956). *The anthrone method for the determination of carbohydrates in foods and in oral rinsing*. Journal of Dental Research, 35(1), 90-94.

7. Lowry, O. H., Rosebrough, N. J., Farr, A. L., & Randall, R. J. (1951). *Protein measurement with the Folin phenol reagent*. J Biol Chem, 193(1), 265-275.

- Uttiya jana is currently pursuing Ph.D degree program in Food &Nutrition in University of Calcutta, India, PH- +919433659943. E-mail: Uttiya.2010@gmail.com
- Dr. Sarmistha Chakrabarti, Assistant Professor in Chemistry, University of Calcutta, India, PH- +919830356430E-mail: sarmisthac9@gmail.com

Comparison of macro nutrients of preserved carp, treated under different cooking conditions

Uttiya Jana & Sarmistha Chakrabarti #

Department of Home Science (Food & Nutrition), University of Calcutta, Kolkata 700 027, India

Phone no. +919830356430 / E-mail: sarmisthac9@gmail.com

Abstract :*Fish are rich sources of protein and are commonly consumed. This study is based on the comparison of contents of macro nutrients of carp, preserved with the combination of salt and turmeric and without preservative both up to 15 days. These preserved fishes were subjected to conventional cooking methods like open pan dry roasting, boiling, shallow frying and deep frying and macro nutrient contents were analysed after immediate (24hours) and long term (15 days) preservation. The nutrient contents of cooked fishes were significantly lower than those in the raw condition, changes occurring due to cooking. Loss of nutrients mainly occurred in boiling whereas it is better restored in deep frying method. The study significantly showed that the loss of nutrients occurred due to preservation but these losses can be reduced by using the combination of salt and turmeric. It was also found that among carp, restoration was greater for rohu.*

Keywords – **carp, macro nutrients, cooking methods, preservatives, deep fat frying**

Introduction

Fish is consumed mainly as a rich source of protein. But the nutrient contents change when it is preserved and cooked as shown in some studies previously carried out. In one study form Nigeria, three commonly available species of marine fish were subjected to boiling, frying and roasting and the effects of these cooking methods on the fish were observed. The results showed reduced protein content for all the fish types [(1)]. In yet another research, amino acid and proximate compositions were determined in six commonly consumed raw and cooked marine fish in Turkey. The changes in amino acid and proximate contents were found to be significant for all cooking methods in all fish species [(2)]. Another research showed that cooking methods were also applied for vegetable samples which could also be a reference for this present study. Three cooking methods, namely boiling, steaming and stir-frying were used to evaluate the effect on nutrient components of bamboo shoots, resulting in decreased contents of protein, soluble sugar and ash. Results indicated an appreciable loss in the total free amino acids in boiling method. All procedures were carried out for 10 minutes [(3)]. The effects of five domestic cooking methods, including steaming, microwaving, boiling, stir-frying and stir-frying followed by boiling, on the nutrients and health-promoting compounds of broccoli were investigated. The results showed that all cooking treatments, except steaming, caused significant losses of total soluble proteins and soluble sugars [(4)]. The effects of different cooking methods (boiling, baking, frying and grilling) on proximate and mineral composition of snakehead fish were investigated. The changes in the amount of protein and fat were found to be significantly higher in frying and grilling fish [(5)]. Another study was designed to observe the performance of turmeric and salt on *tengra* (Mystus vittatus) for several days, stored with preservatives of 2% of the sample weight, resulting in nutrient restoration.[(6)] The present study is significant due to the comparison of macro nutrient contents of carp after being preserved for several days and then subjected to cooking. Preservation can cause loss of nutrients; however, the amount of macro nutrients that can be restored using a combination of salt and turmeric for 15 days, is investigated in this study.

- This study aims to estimate the macro nutrient contents of preserved carp in both raw and cooked conditions after being preserved for 24 hours and 15 days with and without preservative.
- This study also aims at finding comparison of nutrient contents of preserved and cooked fish with and without preservative.
- To find out the deterioration level of preserved fishes in the perspective of the nutrient contents.
- To identify the best fish and the best cooking method in respect of nutrient restoration is the most important concern of this study.

Materials and Methods

1. **Sample preparation and cooking**

   Rohu (*Labio rohita*) and *katla* (Katla katla) with a length of 25 – 30 cm and weight of 1 kg was obtained from the local fish market in Kolkata. It was kept in a plastic container, transported to the laboratory and washed with tap water several times to remove adhering blood and excessive mucous. Subsequently the fish sample was filleted into three sections and each section was divided into five groups. In the first section one group was left uncooked while the other four were boiled, dry roasted in open pan, shallow fried and deep fried. Boiling was performed at 99–101 °C (water temperature) for 10 minutes. Open pan dry roasting of fillets was performed in a pan at 180 °C for 10 minutes. The frying of fillets was performed in a domestic frying pan of 2 L capacity at a temperature of approximately 180 °C for 10 minutes. Mustard oil was used as the medium for frying. In case of shallow frying, 10 ml oil was used and for deep frying 20 ml. The other two sections were allowed to preserve up to15 days. Among these two sections, one was preserved in the refrigerator at -20°C without preservative and the other section was preserved with the combination of salt and turmeric. The amount of combination of salt and turmeric was used as 2% of the weight of the fish sample preserved in 1:1 ratio. The raw, fresh and preserved samples were then subjected to analysis post cooking on the 1st and 15thdays of preservation.

2. Proximate composition analysis

Proximate composition analyses for homogenized samples of fresh and preserved fish fillets, both raw and cooked, were done in triplicate for carbohydrate, protein and fat contents.

a. **Estimation of carbohydrate by Anthrone Method** [7]

100mg of the sample was taken into a boiling tube. Hydrolysis was done by keeping it in a boiling water bath for three hours with 5mL of 2.5 N HCl and cooled to room temperature. Then it was neutralized with solid sodium carbonate until the effervescence ceased. The volume was made up to 100 ml and centrifugation was done at 3000 RPM for 15 minutes. The supernatant was collected and 1 ml was used for analysis, 4 ml anthrone was added to this solution after which it was heated for eight minutes in a boiling water bath and then cooled rapidly when a green to dark green colour appeared. The reading was then taken at 630 nm in a spectrophotometer (Perkin Elmer Lambda 25).

b. **Estimation of Protein by Lowry Method** [8]

200 mg of sample was taken and 20 ml of buffer, containing sodium dihydrogen phosphate and disodium hydrogen phosphate, was added and homogenized finely, kept overnight, after which it was cold centrifuged at 5000 RPM for 20 minutes. The supernatant was collected and 1 ml was used for analysis. Then 5 ml of the Lowry reagent was added to the supernatant and allowed to incubate for 10 minutes. After that 0.5 ml of Folinciocaltue reagent was added and incubated for 30 minutes until a dark blue colour appeared. The reading was taken at 660 nm in a spectrophotometer (Perkin Elmer Lambda 25).

c. **Estimation of fat by Soxhlet Extraction Method** [9]

5gm of dried sample was placed inside the thimble of the apparatus. Then the extraction solvent petroleum ether of 60- 80 boiling range was placed in a distillation flask and placed on the heating mantel. The solvent was heated to reflux when the solvent vapour travelled up a distillation arm and flooded into the chamber housing the thimble of solid. The condenser ensured that any solvent vapour cooled and dripped back down into the chamber housing the solid material. The chamber containing the solid material slowly filled with warm solvent. The fat present in the sample was dissolved in the solvent which returned to the distillation flask. This cycle may be allowed to repeat for 12 hours. After complete extraction of fat the solvent, poured into a weighed petridish, was evaporated and the final weight of the petridish containing fat was taken. From this the amount of the fat was calculated.

3.Statistical analysis

The effect of different cooking methods on macro-nutrient contents of fresh and preserved fishes was analyzed using Mean and Standard Deviations. One way ANOVA was done for comparing the nutrient contents in respect to cooking methods among preserved fishes with and without preservative. Differences were considered to be significant when F value was < 0.05. Data were analyzed by using SPSS package (Version 17).

Result

Table 1 - Carbohydrate content of fresh and preserved *rohu* with and without preservative

Duration	Raw	Boiling	Dry roasting	Shallow frying	Deep frying
Fresh	4.40± 0.10	2.80± 0.10	2.90± 0.10	3.20± 0.10	2.73± 0.15
24 hours	3.83± 0.15	2.50± 0.10	1.90± 0.10	3.16± 0.11	2.40±0.10
15 days	5.08± 0.06	4.16± 0.06	3.66± 0.16	3.64± 0.33	3.94±0.06
24hours(S+T)	4.78± 0.09	2.52± 0.07	1.68± 0.03	3.88± 0.03	4.50±0.05
15 days(S+T)	4.52± 0.05	3.84± 0.08	2.82± 0.02	3.66± 0.07	4.07±0.04

Table 2 - Protein content of fresh and preserved *rohu* with and without preservative

Duration	Raw	Boiling	Dry roasting	Shallow frying	Deep frying
fresh	17.5± 0.05	3.03±0.23	5.7±0.10	5.03±0.15	7.3±0.15
24 hours	16.50 ± 0.50	4.40± 0.00	5.60± 0.20	4.46± 0.05	7.40± 0.17
15 days	6.26± 0.05	4.10±0.10	5.26±0.25	5.76±0.05	7.53±0.05
24hours (S+T)	16.83 ±0.15	6.20± 0.20	13.10± 0.17	13.26± 0.25	15.86± 0.11
15 days(S+T)	12.03 ±0.05	4.93±0.11	6.10±0.10	6.20±0.17	8.66±0.05

Table 3 - Fat content of fresh and preserved rohu with and without preservative

Duration	Raw	Boiling	Dry roasting	Shallow frying	Deep frying
fresh	4.30 ±0.10	3.50± 0.10	1.89± 0.05	10.70± 0.10	5.65± 0.05
24 hours	1.30± 0.10	5.76± 0.15	6.10±0.1 0	9.7± 0.10	8.7± 0.10
15 days	2.38± 0.07	4.95±0 .05	9.80±0.1 0	8.70±0.1 0	5.06±0 .20
24hours (S+T)	5.66± 0.15	4.09±0 .08	5.30±0.1 0	10.50±0. 10	9.16±0 .15
15 days(S+T)	8.16± 0.15	3.05±0 .05	3.90±0.1 0	9.50±0.1 0	5.46±0 .15

Table 4 – Carbohydrate content of fresh and preserved katla with and without preservative

Duration	Raw	Boiling	Dry roasting	Shallow frying	Deep frying
fresh	3.73± 0.15	2.70± 0.10	2.93± 0.11	3.33± 0.15	3.17± 0.15
24 hours	3.30± 0.10	2.10± 0.10	2.20± 0.10	3.10± 0.10	2.63± 0.15
15 days	3.80± 0.14	1.15±0 .08	3.19±0.1 0	2.15±0.0 7	2.33±0 .08
24hours (S+T)	8.45± 0.07	2.18±0 .12	2.51±0.1 0	3.19±0.1 0	3.94±0 .07
15 days(S+T)	3.33± 0.07	1.93±0 .11	1.26±0.1 4	1.99±0.1 4	2.41±0 .20

Table 5 - Protein content of fresh and preserved katla with and without preservative

Duration	Raw	Boiling	Dry roasting	Shallow frying	Deep frying
fresh	21.16 ±0.14	2.70± 0.10	6.33± 0.15	10.80± 0.10	4.00± 0.10
24 hours	16.40 ± 0.53	5.40± 0.10	7.10± 0.10	7.30± 0.10	5.05± 0.05
15 days	12.20 ±0.16	5.67±0 .18	4.92±0.0 9	4.84±0.0 8	4.35±0.0 7
24hours(S+T)	17.30 ±0.36	6.20±0 .10	5.90±0.1 0	8.10±0.1 0	10.77±0. 15
15 days(S+T)	9.53± 0.15	3.50±0 .20	6.70±0.1 0	7.13±0.1 5	7.97±0.1 5

Table 6 - Fat content of fresh and preserved katla with and without preservative

Duration	Raw	Boiling	Dry roasting	Shallow frying	Deep frying
fresh	9.10± 0.10	8.0± 0.10	3.20± 0.20	9.03± 0.05	8.70± 0.10
24 hours	7.43± 0.06	8.10± 0.10	9.0± 0.10	11.50± 0.10	7.63± 0.15
15 days	10.10 ±0.10	6.27±0 .06	8.20±0.2 0	8.50±0 .10	5.43±0.0 6
24hours (S+T)	9.26± 0.23	10.16± 0.05	6.50±0.1 0	9.16±0 .15	6.10±0.1 0
15 days(S+T)	9.60± 0.10	5.36±0 .05	9.36±0.1 5	11.10 ±0.10	10.80±0. 10

Table 7- Comparison of carbohydrate content of preserved rohu and katla with and without preservative

Duration	Raw	Boiling	Dry roasting	Shallow frying	Deep frying
24 hours	0.007 (S)	0.008(S)	0.021(S)	0.492(NS)	0.091(NS)
15 days	0.000 (S)	0.000 (S)	0.014(S)	0.002(S)	0.000(S)
24hours(S+T)	0.000 (S)	0.014(S)	0.000(S)	0.000(S)	0.000(S)
15 days(S+T)	0.000 (S)	0.000(S)	0.000(S)	0.000(S)	0.000(S)

(P value = <0.05 = significantly different) (S= significant, NS= Non significant

Table 8 - Comparison of protein content of preserved rohu and katla with and without preservative

Duration	Raw	Boiling	Dry roasting	Shallow frying	Deep frying
24 hours	0.686(NS)	0.000(S)	0.000 (S)	0.000 (S)	0.000 (S)
15 days	0.000(S)	0.000 (S)	0.086 (S)	0.000 (S)	0.000 (S)
24hours(S+T)	0.108(NS)	1.000(NS)	0.000 (S)	0.000 (S)	0.000 (S)
15 days(S+T)	0.000(S)	0.010(S)	0.002 (S)	0.000 (S)	0.002 (S)

(P value = <0.05 = significantly different) (S= significant, NS= Non significant

Table 9 - Comparison of fat content of preserved rohu and katla with and without preservative

Duration	Raw	Boiling	Dry roasting	Shallow frying	Deep frying
24 hours	0.000 (S)	0.000 (S)	0.000 (S)	0.000(S)	0.001 (S)

15 days	0.000 (S)	0.000 (S)	0.000 (S)	0.070(NS)	0.042 (S)
24hours(S +T)	0.000 (S)	0.000 (S)	0.000 (S)	0.000(S)	0.000 (S)
15 days(S+T)	0.000 (S)	0.000 (S)	0.000 (S)	0.000(S)	0.000 (S)

(P value = <0.05 = significantly different) (S= significant, NS= Non significant)

Table 10 - Percentage of loss of carbohydrate in preserved rohu without preservative in comparison to fresh

Duration	Raw	Boiling	Dry Roasting	Shallow Frying	Deep Frying
24 hours	12.95	10.71	34.48	1.25	12.08
15 days	- 15.45	- 48.57	- 26.20	- 13.75	- 44.32
24hours(S+T)	- 8.63	10	42.06	- 21.25	- 64.83
15 days(S+T)	- 2.72	- 37.14	2.75	- 14.37	- 49.08

Table 11 - Percentage of loss of protein in preserved rohu with preservative in comparison to fresh

Duration	Raw	Boiling	Dry Roasting	Shallow Frying	Deep Frying
24 hours	5.71	-45.21	1.75	11.33	- 1.36
15 days	64.2 2	- 35.31	7.71	- 14.51	- 3.15
24hours(S +T)	3.82	- 104.62	- 129.8 2	- 163.6 1	-117.26
15 days(S+T)	31.2 5	- 62.70	- 7.01	- 24.45	- 18.63

Table 12 - Percentage of loss of fat in preserved rohu with preservative in comparison to fresh

Duration	Raw	Boiling	Dry Roasting	Shallow Frying	Deep Frying
24 hours	69.7 6	- 64.57	- 222.75	9.43	- 53.98
15 days	44.6 5	- 41.42	- 418.51	18.69	10.44
24 hours(S+ T)	- 31.6 2	- 16.85	- 180.42	1.86	- 62.12
15 days(S+T	- 89.7	12.85	- 106.34	11.21	3.36

)	6				

Table 13 - Percentage of loss of Carbohydrate in preserved katla with preservative in comparison to fresh

Duration	Raw	Boiling	Dry Roasting	Shallow Frying	Deep Frying
24 hours	11.52	22.22	24.91	6.90	17.03
15 days	-1.87	57.40	- 8.87	35.43	26.49
24 hours(S+ T)	- 127.3 4	19.25	14.33	4.20	- 24.29
15 days(S+T)	10.72	28.51	56.99	40.24	23.97

Table 14 - Percentage of loss of protein in preserved katla with preservative in comparison to fresh

Duration	Raw	Boiling	Dry Roasting	Shallow Frying	Deep Frying
24 hours	22.4 9	- 100.0 0	-12.16	32.40	- 26.25
15 days	42.3 4	- 110	22.27	55.18	- 8.75
24hours(S+ T)	18.2 4	- 129.6 2	6.79	25.0	- 169.2 5
15 days(S+T)	54.9 6	- 29.62	- 5.84	33.98	- 99.25

Table 15 - Percentage of loss of fat in preserved katla with preservative in comparison to fresh

Duration	Raw	Boiling	Dry Roasting	Shallow Frying	Deep Frying
24 hours	18.3 5	-1.25	-181.25	- 27.35	12.29
48 hours	- 10.9 8	21.62	- 156.25	5.86	37.58
14 days	- 1.78	- 27.0	- 103.12	- 1.43	29.88
15 days	5.49	33	- 192.50	- 22.92	- 24.13

Fig. a - Percentage of loss of carbohydrate in cooked rohu and katla preserved with and without preservative

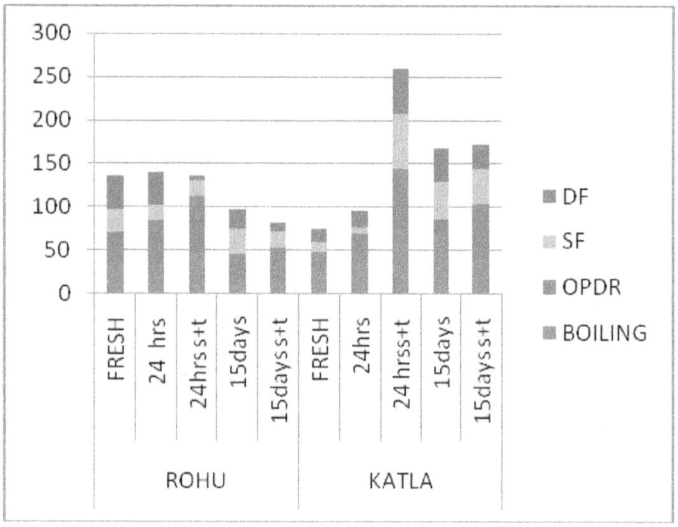

Fig. b - Percentage of loss of protein in cooked *rohu and katla* preserved with and without preservative

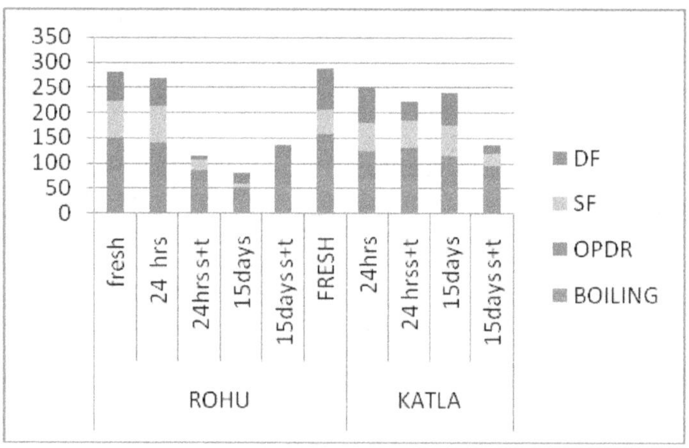

Fig. c - Percentage of loss of fat in cooked rohu and katla preserved with and without preservative

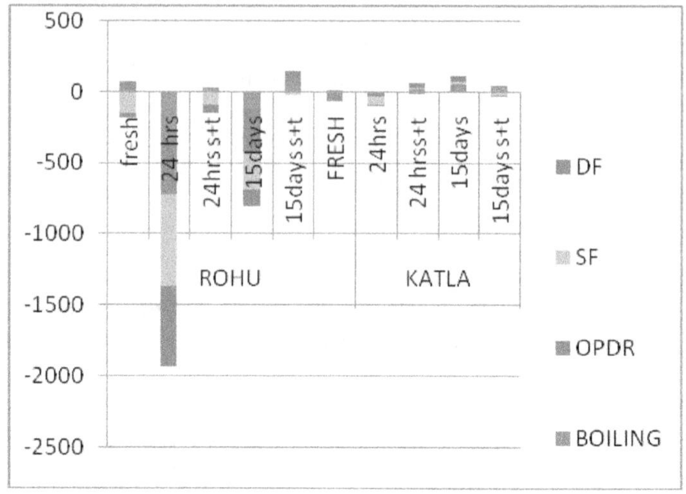

Discussion

Table 1, 2, 3 showed the carbohydrate, protein and fat contents of fresh and preserved *rohu* with and without preservative up to 15 days after subjecting it to different cooking methods. The raw and cooked values were displayed here. The nutrient contents were reduced due to application of different cooking methods. The highest loss occurred in boiling and it was found to be restored in deep frying method.

Table 4, 5, 6 exhibited the carbohydrate, protein and fat contents of the *katla* preserved with and without preservative for short and long time durations. Data showed that the significant difference was present in terms of raw and cooked values. Most of the loss occurred in boiling and the nutrient restoration occurred in deep frying.

Table 7, 8, 9 exhibited the comparison of carbohydrate, protein and fat contents of *rohu* and *katla*, preserved with and without preservative. Data indicated that there was a significant difference present between two fish in respect of different cooking methods and both short and long term preservation.

Table 10, 11, 12 showed the percentage of loss of carbohydrate, protein and fat contents post cooking of the preserved *rohu* with and without preservative in respect to the fresh values. Data indicated that deterioration occurred mainly in 24 hours of preservation but it can be restored with the combination of salt and turmeric up to 15th day of preservation.

Table 13, 14, 15 showed the deterioration value of carbohydrate, protein and fat contents post cooking of the preserved *katla* with and without preservative in respect to fresh values. Data indicated that losses occurred in both short and long term preservation but the use of preservative was not significantly effective for the restoration of nutrient contents of preserved *katla*.

Fig. a showed the loss percentage of carbohydrate contents of the cooked carp in respect of the raw values, preserved with and without preservative. It was found that losses were more in boiling whereas less in deep frying. Loss was more in *katla* rather than *rohu*. In case of rohu loss was restored by the use of combination of salt and turmeric but this is not effective for *katla*.

Fig. b showed the loss percentage of protein contents following cooking of the carp preserved with and without preservative. Data indicated that losses occurred mostly in boiling. Here also comparison showed that losses were more in *katla* than in *rohu* but losses were restored by the use of combination of salt and turmeric for both the carps.

Fig. c exhibited the loss percentage of fat contents after cooking of the carp preserved with and without preservative. Result showed that loss of fat was very low, rather fat content increased due to addition of cooking oil and loss of water from the fish due to temperature of cooking. The fat gain mainly occurred in *rohu* fish rather than in *katla*.

Conclusion

All cooking methods can reduce the nutrient contents of the carp. The maximum restoration was found to be mostly in deep frying method while the loss occurred in boiling method. After preservation of the fishes up to 15th day, the deterioration of nutrient occurred in 15th day but this deterioration could be reduced to some extent with the use of natural preservative that is combination of salt and turmeric, which help to restore nutrient contents up to 15th day of preservation. Maximum restoration occurred in 24 hours of preservation after using preservative. After considering all advantages and disadvantages, it can be said that deep frying is the best method for protein restoration among the other cooking methods and use of salt and turmeric can delay this deterioration post cooking and among the two fish, *rohu* is better than *katla* in respect of nutrient restoration.

Acknowledgement

The University Grants Commission (UGC) is thanked for awarding a Junior Research Fellowship to Uttiya Jana.

Bibliography

1. Goldman, K. J. "*Regulation of body temperature in the white shark, Carcharodon carcharias"*. Journal of Comparative Physiology B, 167(6), 423-429,1997.

2. Erkan, N., Özden, Ö., & Selçuk, A. *Effect of frying, grilling, and steaming on amino acid composition of marine fishes.* Journal of medicinal food, 13(6), 1524-15312010,.

3. Mkandawire, K. T., & Masamba, K. G. *Effect of lemon juice treatment and sun drying on vitamin C retention in three steam and water blanched indigenous vegetables over six weeks storage period.* African Journal of Food Science, 8(6), 316-321,2014.

4. Yuan, G. F., Sun, B., Yuan, J., & Wang, Q. M. *Effects of different cooking methods on health-promoting compounds of broccoli.* Journal of Zhejiang University Science B, 10(8), 580-588, 2009.

5. Marimuthu, K., Thilaga, M., Kathiresan, S., Xavier, R., & Mas, R. H. M. H. *Effect of different cooking methods on proximate and mineral composition of striped snakehead fish (Channa striatus, Bloch).* Journal of food science and technology, 49(3), 373-377, 2012.

6. T. Akter 1 , A. T. A. Ahmed 1 , M. A. khaleque and M. Begum, *Effect of drying on quality of tengra (Mystus vittatus)* treated with turmeric and salt. Unique Research Journal of Biological Science,1(1),001-005,2013.

7. Ludwig, T. G., & Goldberg, H. J, *The anthrone method for the determination of carbohydrates in foods and in oral rinsing.* Journal of dental research, 35(1), 90-94. 1956.

8. Lowry, O. H., Rosebrough, N. J., Farr, A. L., & Randall, R. J. *Protein measurement with the Folin phenol reagent.* J Biol Chem, 193(1), 265-275, 1951.

9. Manirakiza P, Covaci A, Schepens P(), *Comparative study on total lipid determination using Soxhlet*, Roese Gottlieb, Bligh and Dyer, and modified Bligh and Dyer extraction methods. J Food Comp Anal, 27(1), p 93-100,.

International Journal of Agricultural Science and Research (IJASR)
ISSN(P): 2250-0057; ISSN(E): 2321-0087
Vol. 6, Issue 4, Aug 2016, 139-148

COMPARISON OF RESTORATION OF MAJOR MINERAL CONTENTS AMONG DIFFERENT FISH AND OTHER EDIBLE AQUATIC SPECIES, TREATED UNDER DIFFERENT PRESERVING AND COOKING CONDITIONS

UTTIYA JANA & SARMISTHA CHAKRABORTI

Department of Home Science (Food & Nutrition), University of Calcutta, Kolkata, West Bengal, India

ABSTRACT

Fish are good sources of some important minerals. This study was based on the comparison of mineral contents among different fish and other edible aquatic species namely rohu, katla, prawn, lobster, pomfret and hilsa after preservation up to 15th day in refrigerator followed by subjecting to conventional cooking methods. The mineral contents of cooked fish were significantly lower than in the raw condition. These fish were subjected to conventional cooking methods like open pan dry roasting, boiling, shallow frying and deep frying. The mineral contents had changed from the raw value due to the application of cooking methods. Mineral restoration mainly occurred in both open-pan dry roasting and deep frying method whereas loss occurred in boiling. The study significantly showed that preserved pomfret followed by cooking was beneficial due to adequate iron and calcium restoration up to 14th day among all other fish and edible aquatic species.

***KEYWORDS:** Calcium, Iron, Edible Aquatics Species, Cooking Methods, Open Pan Dry Roasting, Deep Frying*

Received: Jun 21, 2016; **Accepted:** Jul 15, 2016; **Published:** Jul 20, 2016; **Paper Id.:** IJASRAUG201619

Original Article

INTRODUCTION

Fish is consumed mainly as a rich source of protein and minerals. But the nutrient contents change when it is cooked as shown in some studies previously carried out. In one study, three commonly available species of marine fish in Nigeria were subjected to boiling, frying and roasting and the effects of these cooking methods on the fish were observed. The results showed reduced protein and mineral contents for all the fish types [(1)]. In yet another research, amino acid and proximate compositions were determined in six commonly consumed raw and cooked marine fish in Turkey. The changes in amino acid and proximate contents, vitamins and mineral contents were found to be significant for all cooking methods in all fish species [(2)]. Another research showed that cooking methods were also applied for vegetable samples which could be a reference for this present study. Three cooking methods, namely boiling, steaming and stir-frying were used to evaluate the effect on nutrient components of bamboo shoots, resulting in decreased contents of protein, soluble sugar, and ash. Results indicated an appreciable loss in the total free amino acids in boiling method. All procedures were carried out for 10 minutes [(3)]. The effects of five domestic cooking methods, including steaming, microwaving, boiling, stir-frying and stir-frying followed by boiling on the nutrients and health-promoting compounds of broccoli were investigated. The results showed that all cooking treatments, except steaming, caused significant losses of total soluble proteins and soluble sugars and minerals [(4)]. The effects of different cooking methods (boiling, baking, frying and grilling) on proximate and mineral composition of snakehead fish were investigated. The changes in the amount of protein and fat were found to be significantly higher in frying and grilling fish [(5)]. Another study was carried out to determine the changes in the micro-mineral and macro-mineral composition of common sole (*Solea solea*), striped red mullet (*Mullus surmuletus*) and whiting (*Merlangius merlangus*) throughout the year. The researcher concluded that macro-mineral concentrations in edible parts of fish species were 444–1,559 mg/kg for Na, 1,975–5,130 mg/kg for K, 228–658 mg/kg for Mg, 187–1,105 mg/kg for Ca, and 2,341–7,341 for P respectively [(6)]. The present study is significant due to the comparison of calcium and iron contents among preserved river fish, sea fish and other edible aquatic species (crustaceans) after being subjected to conventional cooking. Cooking methods can cause loss of minerals and the fish that can restore more minerals post cooking is investigated in this study.

- This study aims to estimate the iron and calcium contents of different fish and other edible aquatic species in both raw and cooked conditions.
- This study also aims at finding the restoration of mineral contents after preservation up to 15 days followed by cooking.
- To find the fish and the cooking method that is beneficial in the perspective of mineral restoration is the most important concern of this study.

MATERIALS AND METHODS

- **Sample Preparation and Cooking**

Rohu (*Labio rohita*), *katla* (*Catla catla*) and *hilsa* (*Hilsa ilisa*), each with a length of 25 – 30 cm and weight of 1 kg and pomfret (*Pampus argenteus*) with a length of 12cm and weight of 250–300 g and prawn and lobster with a length of 10 cm, 15cm and weight of 50 gm and 90 gm respectively were obtained from the local fish market in Kolkata. They were kept in a plastic container, transported to the laboratory and washed with tap water several times to remove adhering blood and excessive mucous. Subsequently the fish sample was filleted into two sections and each section was divided into five groups. In the first section one group was left uncooked while the other four were boiled, dry roasted in open pan, shallow fried and deep fried. Boiling was performed at 99–101 °C (water temperature) for 10 minutes. Open pan dry roasting of fillets was performed in a pan at 180 °C for 10 minutes. The frying of fillets was performed in a domestic frying pan of 2 L capacity at a temperature of approximately 180 °C for 10 minutes. Mustard oil was used as the medium for frying. In case of shallow frying, 10 ml oil was used and for deep frying 20 ml. The other section was allowed to preserve up to15 days in the refrigerator at -20^{0}C. The raw, fresh and preserved samples were then subjected to analysis post cooking on the day of preservation of 1st, 2nd, 14th and 15th.

- **Mineral Contents Analysis**

Mineral contents analyses for homogenized samples of cooked and raw fish fillets were done in triplicate for the estimation of iron and calcium contents, determined by AOAC method. [(7)]

Estimation of Mineral by AOAC Method after Wet Digestion [(7)]

Dried sample (500 mg) was taken in a 25 ml volumetric flask and 10 ml of concentrated nitric acid was added in it and kept overnight. After that the volumetric flask was placed on the hot plate and allowed to boil for 8 hours. Then 4 ml of perchloric acid was added in it and boiled until brown fumes from the digestion stopped. After that volume was made up to the mark by double distilled water. Then the solution was used for the analysis of iron and calcium by atomic absorption spectrophotometer (Perkin Elmer)

- **Statistical analysis**

The effect of different cooking methods on the mineral contents of river fish, sea fish and crustaceans was analyzed using Mean and Standard Deviation. One way ANOVA was done for comparing the mineral contents between the raw and cooked samples along with the preservation days up to 15th. Differences were considered to be significant when p value is < 0.05. Data were analyzed by using SPSS package (Version 17).

RESULTS

Table 1: Iron Contents

Name of fish	Duration	Raw	Boiling	Dry roasting	Shallow fry	Deep fry
Rohu	fresh	2.7±0.02	3.16± 0.06	1.67± 0.02	1.49± 0.03	7.06± 0.04
	24 hours	0.38± 0.03	1.08± 0.03	2.05± 0.04	2.43± 0.08	1.07± 0.04
	48 hours	1.38±0.05	0.94±0.03	0.61±0.05	3.95±0.03	4.81±0.03
	14 days	1.51±0.03	2.03±0.05	1.86±0.05	4.55±0.03	1.56±0.03
	15 days	2.82±0.03	1.76±0.07	1.77±0.06	1.62±0.04	1.75±0.04
Katla	fresh	2.83±0.04	1.35±0.06	5.70±0.02	2.41±0.11	4.18±0.05
	24 hours	0.88±0.10	1.08±0.03	1.14±0.02	2.44±0.07	2.55±0.03
	48 hours	0.81±0.08	2.07±0.04	2.14±0.07	3.08±0.03	2.43±0.51
	14 days	1.36±0.06	3.04±0.03	1.02±0.09	1.44±0.03	4.64±0.12
	15 days	*1.19±0.06*	*1.44±0.02*	*1.82±0.09*	*4.98±0.07*	*1.68±0.05*
Prawn	fresh	1.40±0.02	1.45±0.03	1.51±0.01	0.93±0.02	0.68±0.06
	24 hours	2.51±0.01	1.81±0.08	1.77±0.04	3.36±0.06	2.46±0.04
	48 hours	1.58±0.06	1.36±0.05	2.06±0.02	2.31±0.03	2.29±0.08
	14 days	4.05±0.04	3.45±0.04	4.45±0.09	1.54±0.02	1.56±0.02
	15 day	3.15±0.06	2.15±0.13	1.42±0.02	2.65±0.03	2.83±0.04
Lobster	fresh	2.55±0.01	1.65±0.04	4.60±0.02	1.72±0.04	0.90±0.05
	24 hours	0.56±0.02	1.45±0.04	0.95±0.05	1.18±0.03	1.40±0.05
	48 hours	0.90±0.02	0.56±0.02	1.52±0.03	1.02±0.02	1.47±0.04
	14 days	0.62±0.07	1.63±0.05	0.57±0.04	0.70±0.05	1.08±0.03
	15 days	1.18±0.03	1.78±0.03	3.98±0.02	1.52±0.02	1.66±0.02
Pomfret	fresh	2.84±0.00	1.57±0.02	2.09±0.07	1.07±0.05	4.54±0.04
	24 hours	4.93±0.07	4.29±0.04	5.05±0.04	4.54±0.05	4.15±0.04
	48 hours	2.48±0.03	3.25±0.05	3.66±0.04	4.54±0.05	4.66±0.04
	14 days	3.56±0.02	3.05±0.04	1.85±0.03	2.92±0.08	2.92±0.07
	15 days	1.00±0.01	0.75±0.03	1.43±0.03	0.48±0.03	0.32±0.03
Hilsa	Fresh	3.28±0.01	1.28±0.03	2.38±0.26	1.66±0.04	1.82±0.05
	24 hour	3.25±0.05	1.74±0.05	3.22±0.03	2.98±0.04	3.48±0.03
	48 hours	1.87±0.02	1.72±0.03	0.87±0.02	1.78±0.03	1.95±0.04
	14 day	1.56±0.04	2.55±0.03	2.06±0.05	2.12±0.03	1.53±0.04
	15 days	1.56±0.03	2.55±0.03	3.52±0.03	2.56±0.04	2.54±0.05

Table 2: Calcium Contents

Name of fish	Duration	Raw	Boiling	Dry roasting	Shallow fry	Deep fry
Rohu	fresh	161±1.00	272± 2.51	271± 1.06	202± 2.64	434± 4.04
	24 hours	17.50±0.50	3.03± 0.23	5.70± 0.10	5.03± 0.15	7.33± 0.15
	48 hours	223±2.08	106±1.52	121±1.00	352±2.64	437±2.08
	14 days	121±1.00	231±1.00	216±1.52	181±1.52	232±2.00
	15 days	402±2.64	296±2.64	242±3.05	305±4.00	401±1.41
Katla	fresh	152±2.51	62.33±2.51	452±2.64	143±4.16	152±2.00
	24 hours	96±1.52	127±2.08	122±2.51	72±2.51	136±1.52
	48 hours	3.22±2.51	278±2.64	288±2.64	272±2.51	362±2.51
	14 days	52±2.51	301±1.00	66±1.52	203±3.21	531±1.00
	15 days	171±1.00	136±1.52	203±3.21	602±2.51	402±2.64
Prawn	fresh	177±2.08	302±2.00	251±1.00	50±1.00	39±0.25
	24 hours	216±1.52	248±2.64	131±1.00	201±2.08	126±1.52
	48 hours	176±1.52	206±1.52	336±1.00	501±2.08	201±1.52
	14 days	197±2.08	162±2.00	251±1.00	251±1.00	151±1.00
	15 day	151±1.52	502±1.00	152±1.00	291±1.52	185±0.70
Lobster	fresh	241±1.52	271±1.52	241±1.00	201±1.52	151±1.52
	24 hours	201±1.52	262±2.00	161±1.52	123±1.52	151±1.52
	48 hours	169±1.00	262±2.64	166±1.52	125±2.08	152±2.08
	14 days	351±1.00	501±1.00	281±1.00	1.65±2.08	151±1.52
	15 days	133±1.52	153±1.52	252±2.08	141±1.52	236±2.08
Pomfret	fresh	151±1.52	151±1.52	156±1.52	86±1.52	246±1.52
	24 hours	642±2.51	302±2.00	302±0.57	402±2.00	182±2.00
	48 hours	382±2.51	202±2.51	127±2.08	136±1.52	175±3.00
	14 days	195±3.00	297±2.08	417±2.51	185±3.00	243±3.60
	15 days	166±1.52	362±2.51	282±2.00	213±3.21	208±3.21
Hilsa	Fresh	201±1.52	277±2.08	301±1.00	352±2.00	151±1.52
	24 hour	221±1.52	196±1.52	161±1.52	292±2.00	501±2.08
	48 hours	222±2.00	201±1.53	219±1.53	402±2.00	192±2.00
	14 day	232±2.00	302±2.09	332±2.00	352±2.00	202±2.09
	15 days	202±2.00	228±2.08	501±1.53	242±2.52	752±1.53

Table 3: Comparisons of Iron Contents among Different Fish and Other Edible Aquatic Species

Name of fish	fresh	24 hours	48 hours	14 days	15 days
Rohu	0.00(S)	0.00(S)	0.00(S)	0.00(S)	0.00(S)
Katla	0.00(S)	0.00(S)	0.00(S)	0.00(S)	0.00(S)
Pomfret	0.00(S)	0.00(S)	0.00(S)	0.00(S)	0.00(S)
Hilsa	0.00(S)	0.00(S)	0.00(S)	0.00(S)	0.00(S)
Prawn	0.00(S)	0.00(S)	0.00(S)	0.00(S)	0.00(S)
Lobster	0.00(S)	0.00(S)	0.00(S)	0.00(S)	0.00(S)

(P value = <0.05 = significantly different) (S= significant, NS= Non significant)

Table 4: Comparisons of Calcium Contents among Different Fish and Other Edible Aquatic Species

Name of Fish	Fresh	24 Hours	48 Hours	14 Days	15 Days
Rohu	0.00(S)	0.00(S)	0.00(S)	0.00(S)	0.00(S)
Katla	0.00(S)	0.00(S)	0.00(S)	0.00(S)	0.00(S)
Pomfret	0.00(S)	0.00(S)	0.00(S)	0.00(S)	0.00(S)
Hilsa	0.00(S)	0.00(S)	0.00(S)	0.00(S)	0.00(S)
Prawn	0.00(S)	0.00(S)	0.00(S)	0.00(S)	0.00(S)
Lobster	0.00(S)	0.00(S)	0.00(S)	0.00(S)	0.00(S)

(P value = <0.05 = significantly different) (S= significant, NS= Non significant)

Table 5: Percentage of Loss of Iron of Different Preserved Fish and Other Edible Aquatic Species

Name of fish	Duration	Raw	Boiling	Dry roasting	Shallow fry	Deep fry
Rohu	24 hours	85.92	65.82	- 22.75	- 63.08	84.84
	48 hours	48.88	70.25	63.47	- 165.1	31.86
	14 days	43.7	35.75	- 11.37	- 205.36	85.69
	15 days	- 4.44	44.30	- 5.98	- 8.72	75.21
Katla	24 hours	68.90	20.00	80.00	- 1.24	38.99
	48 hours	71.37	- 53.33	62.45	- 27.80	41.86
	14 days	51.94	- 125.18	82.10	40.24	- 11.00
	15 days	57.95	- 6.66	68.07	- 106.63	59.80
Prawn	24 hours	79.28	- 24.82	- 17.21	- 261.29	- 261.76
	48 hours	- 12.85	6.20	- 36.42	- 148.38	- 236.76
	14 days	- 189.29	- 137.93	- 194.70	- 65.59	- 129.41
	15 day	- 89.28	- 48.27	5.96	- 184.94	- 316.17
Lobster	24 hours	78.03	12.12	79.34	31.39	- 55.55
	48 hours	64.70	66.06	66.95	40.69	- 63.33
	14 days	75.68	1.21	87.60	59.30	- 20.00
	15 days	53.72	- 7.87	13.47	11.62	- 84.44
Pomfret	24 hours	- 73.59	- 173.24	- 141.62	- 324.29	8.59
	48 hours	12.67	- 119.74	- 75.11	- 324.29	- 2.64
	14 days	- 25.35	- 94.26	11.48	- 172.89	35.68
	15 days	64.78	52.22	31.57	55.14	92.95
Hilsa	24 hour	- 73.59	- 35.93	- 35.29	-79.51	- 91.20
	48 hours	42.98	- 34.37	63.44	- 7.22	-7.14
	14 day	52.43	- 99.21	13.44	- 27.71	15.93
	15 days	52.43	- 99.21	- 47.89	- 54.21	- 39.56

Table 6: Percentage of Loss of Calcium of Different Preserved Fish and Other Edible Aquatic Species

Name of fish	Duration	Raw	Boiling	Dry roasting	Shallow fry	Deep fry
Rohu	24 hours	-15.52	51.83	43.91	26.23	- 53.45
	48 hours	- 38.50	61.02	55.35	-74.25	-0.69
	14 days	24.84	15.07	20.29	10.39	46.54
	15 days	- 149.68	- 8.82	10.70	- 50.99	7.60
Katla	24 hours	36.40	- 104.83	19.73	49.65	10.52
	48 hours	- 111.84	- 348.38	- 89.47	- 90.20	- 138.15
	14 days	65.78	- 385.48	56.57	- 41.95	- 249.34
	15 days	- 12.50	- 119.35	- 33.55	- 320.97	- 164.47
Prawn	24 hours	- 22.03	17.88	47.80	49.65	10.52
	48 hours	0.56	31.78	- 33.86	- 90.20	- 138.15
	14 days	- 11.29	46.35	0.00	- 41.95	- 249.34
	15 day	14.68	66.22	39.44	- 320.97	- 164.47
Lobster	24 hours	16.59	3.32	33.19	38.80	0.00
	48 hours	29.87	3.32	31.12	37.81	- 0.66
	14 days	- 45.64	- 84.87	- 16.59	17.91	0.00
	15 days	44.81	43.54	- 4.56	29.85	- 56.29
Pomfret	24 hours	- 325.16	-100.00	- 93.58	-367.44	26.01
	48 hours	- 152.98	- 33.77	18.58	- 58.13	28.86
	14 days	- 29.13	- 97.35	- 167.30	- 115.11	1.21
	15 days	- 9.93	- 139.73	- 80.76	- 147.67	15.44
Hilsa	24 hour	- 9.95	29.24	46.51	17.04	- 231.78
	48 hours	- 10.44	27.43	27.24	- 14.20	- 27.15
	14 day	-15.42	-9.02	- 10.29	0.00	-33.77
	15 days	- 0.49	17.68	- 66.44	31.25	-398.01

Table 7: Percentage of Loss of Iron of Different Cooked Fish and Other Edible Aquatic Species

Name of Fish	Duration	Boiling	Dry Roasting	Shallow Fry	Deep Fry
Rohu	Fresh	-17.03	38.14	44.81	- 161.48
	24 hours	- 184.21	- 439.47	- 539.40	-181.57
	48 hours	31.88	55.79	- 186.23	- 248.55
	14 days	-33.55	-22.36	- 199.34	- 2.63
	15 days	37.58	37.23	42.55	37.94
Katla	Fresh	52.29	- 101.41	14.84	-47.70
	24 hours	- 22.72	- 29.54	- 177.27	- 189.77
	48 hours	-155.55	-107.73	-280.24	-200.00
	14 days	-123.52	25.00	-5.88	-241.17
	15 days	-21.00	-52.94	-318.48	-41.17
Prawn	Fresh	-3.57	-7.85	33.57	57.42
	24 hours	27.88	29.48	- 33.86	1.99
	48 hours	13.92	-30.37	- 46.20	-44.93
	14 days	14.81	- 9.87	61.97	61.48
	15 day	31.74	54.92	15.87	10.15
Lobster	Fresh	35.29	- 80.39	32.54	64.70
	24 hours	-158.29	-69.64	-110.71	-150.00
	48 hours	37.77	-68.88	-13.33	-63.33
	14 days	-162.90	8.06	-12.90	- 74.11
	15 days	-50.84	- 237.29	- 28.8	-40.67
Pomfret	Fresh	44.71	26.40	62.32	-59.85
	24 hours	12.98	- 2.43	7.91	15.82
	48 hours	- 39.11	- 47.58	-83.06	-87.90
	14 days	14.32	48.03	17.97	17.97
	15 days	25.0	43.0	52.0	68.0
Hilsa	Fresh	60.97	27.43	49.39	44.51
	24 hour	46.46	0.92	8.30	7.07
	48 hours	8.02	53.47	4.81	- 4.27
	14 day	- 63.46	- 32.05	-35.89	1.92
	15 days	-63.46	-125.64	-64.10	-62.82

Table 8: Percentage of Loss of Calcium of Different Cooked Fish and Other Edible Aquatic Species

Name of fish	Duration	Boiling	Dry roasting	Shallow fry	Deep fry
Rohu	fresh	-68.94	-68.32	- 25.46	-169.56
	24 hours	29.56	80.27	19.89	- 8.60
	48 hours	52.46	45.73	-57.84	-95.96
	14 days	- 19.90	78.51	49.58	- 91.73
	15 days	26.36	39.80	24.12	0.24
Katla	fresh	59.21	0.00	5.92	0.00
	24 hours	-32.29	-27.08	25.0	-41.66
	48 hours	13.66	10.55	15.52	-12.42
	14 days	-478.84	-26.92	-290.38	-921.15
	15 days	20.46	-18.71	-252.04	-135.08
Prawn	fresh	-70.62	-41.80	71.75	77.96
	24 hours	-14.81	39.35	6.9	41.66
	48 hours	- 17.04	-90.90	-184.65	-14.20
	14 days	17.76	-27.41	-27.41	23.35
	15 day	232.45	-0.66	-92.71	-22.51
Lobster	fresh	-12.44	0.00	19.90	37.34
	24 hours	-30.34	19.90	38.84	24.87
	48 hours	-55.02	1.77	26.03	10.05

Table 8: Contd.,					
	14 days	-42.73	19.94	52.29	56.98
	15 days	-15.03	-98.47	-6.01	-77.44
Pomfret	Fresh	-70.62	-41.80	-71.75	77.96
	24 hours	-14.81	39.35	6.9	41.66
	48 hours	-17.04	-90.90	-184.65	-14.20
	14 days	17.76	-27.41	-27.41	23.35
	15 days	-232.45	-0.66	-92.71	-22.51
Hilsa	fresh	-37.81	-49.75	-75.12	-24.87
	24 hour	11.31	27.14	-32.12	-126.69
	48 hours	9.4	1.35	-81.08	13.51
	14 day	-30.17	-43.10	-51.72	12.93
	15 days	-12.87	-148.01	-19.80	-272.27

DISCUSSIONS

Table 1 showed the iron contents of *rohu, katla*, prawn, lobster, pomfret and *hilsa.* The raw and cooked values according to the days of preservation were displayed here. The iron contents were reduced due to application of different cooking methods. Iron contents were highest in deep frying for *rohu, katla,* prawn, pomfret and *hilsa* but it was better restored in open pan dry roasting for lobster. Restoration mainly occurred on 14th and 15th day. Fresh deep fried *rohu* contains most of the iron among all the other fish.

Table 2 showed the calcium contents of *rohu, katla,* prawn, lobster, pomfret and *hilsa.* Here also the raw and cooked values were displayed according to the days of preservation. The calcium contents were reduced due to application of heat, water and oil in different cooking methods. Calcium content was highest in deep frying for *rohu, katla* and *hilsa,* boiling for prawn and lobster, open pan dry roasting for pomfret but it was better restored in deep frying for *hilsa*. Restoration mainly occurred on 15th day for *rohu, katla,* pomfret and *hilsa* but in 48 hours for prawn and 14th day for lobster.

Tables 3 and 4 showed the comparison of the iron and calcium contents respectively of the fish and other edible aquatic species in terms of raw and cooked values according to the days of preservation along with fresh conditions. Data showed that there was a significant difference present in raw, boiling, open pan dry roasting, shallow frying and deep frying methods.

Table 5 exhibited the percentage of loss of iron contents of different preserved fish and other edible aquatic species due to preservation up to 15th day. Most of the iron loss occurred in 24hours for *katla* and prawn, in 48 hours for *rohu*, on 14th day for lobster and *hilsa* but on 15th day for pomfret. On the other hand, maximum restoration of iron occurred in 24 hours for *hilsa,* 48 hours for pomfret, 14th day for prawn and *katla* and 15th day for *rohu* and lobster. Maximum restoration occurred in prawn, *hilsa* and pomfret respectively after preservation up to 15th day.

Table 6 exhibited the percentage of loss of calcium contents of different preserved fish and other edible aquatic species due to preservation up to 15th day. Most of the calcium loss occurred in 24hours for *katla*, prawn, lobster and *hilsa,* in 48 hours for pomfret whereas on 14th day for *rohu*. On the other hand, maximum restoration of calcium occurred in 48 hours for *katla,* 14th days for prawn, lobster, *hilsa* and pomfret and on 15th day for *rohu*. Maximum restoration occurred in *katla*, pomfret and *hilsa* respectively after preservation up to 14th day.

Table 7 exhibited the percentage of iron losses post cooking. Most of the loss occurred in *katla,* lobster, pomfret and *hilsa* after boiling, in *rohu* after open pan dry roasting and in prawn after deep frying whereas open pan dry roasting restored the iron contents mostly in prawn, lobster, pomfret and *hilsa*. Deep frying can also lower the losses in *rohu* and *katla*. Data indicated that open pan dry roasting is useful for iron content restoration whereas boiling can cause losses of iron.

Table 8 exhibited the percentage of losses of calcium content following cooking. Most of the loss occurred in *rohu* and *katla* after boiling, in prawn and lobster after deep frying, in *hilsa* after open pan dry roasting whereas in pomfret after shallow frying. On the other hand boiling can restore the calcium contents mostly in prawn, lobster and *pomfret*. Deep frying can also lower the losses in *rohu* and *katla*. Shallow frying can reduce the loss in *hilsa*. Data showed that boiling is useful for calcium content restoration.

CONCLUSIONS

The maximum iron and calcium contents were found to be highest in *hilsa* and lobsters respectively in raw conditions as well as these were also prone to more loss after cooking, although losses occurred after cooking for all the fish. The iron content was mostly restored in open pan dry roasting for prawn, lobster, pomfret and *hilsa* whereas deep frying helped to restore more iron in case of *rohu* and *katla*. Calcium contents were retained mainly in boiling for prawn, lobster and pomfret where as in deep frying for *rohu* and *katla* and in shallow frying for pomfret. In short, both open-pan dry roasting and deep frying can restore iron and calcium contents in all the fish and other edible aquatic species. Pomfret and *hilsa* restore adequate amount of iron and calcium whereas prawn contains iron and *katla* contains calcium. Most of the fish can be preserved up to 14th day but *rohu, katla* and lobster can be preserved up to 15th days. After considering all advantages and disadvantages, it can be said that boiling can reduce the mineral contents and both deep frying and open pan dry roasting can restore iron and calcium almost for all the fish and pomfret is the best among the other fish, regarding the restoration of minerals post cooking. The fish can be preserved up to 14th day.

ACKNOWLEDGEMENTS

The University Grants Commission (UGC) is thanked for awarding a Junior Research Fellowship to Uttiya Jana.

REFERENCES

1. *Goldman, K. J. (1997). Regulation of body temperature in the white shark, Carcharodon carcharias. Journal of Comparative Physiology B, 167(6), 423-429.*
2. *Erkan, N., Özden, Ö., & Selçuk, A. (2010). Effect of frying, grilling, and steaming on amino acid composition of marine fishes. Journal of medicinal food, 13(6), 1524-1531.*
3. *Mkandawire, K. T., & Masamba, K. G. (2014). Effect of lemon juice treatment and sun drying on vitamin C retention in three steam and water blanched indigenous vegetables over six weeks storage period. African Journal of Food Science, 8(6), 316-321.*
4. *Yuan, G. F., Sun, B., Yuan, J., & Wang, Q. M. (2009). Effects of different cooking methods on health-promoting compounds of broccoli. Journal of Zhejiang University Science B, 10(8), 580-588.*
5. *Marimuthu, K., Thilaga, M., Kathiresan, S., Xavier, R., & Mas, R. H. M. H. (2012). Effect of different cooking methods on proximate and mineral composition of striped snakehead fish (Channa striatus, Bloch). Journal of food science and technology, 49(3), 373-377.*

6. *J. M. Hungerford & P. Cunniff (1998). Official method 938.08. Ash of seafood. Fish and other marine products. Official methods of analysis of AOAC International, 35(1),6.*

7. *A. S. Baker and R. L. Smith, J. Agric(1974). Preparation of Solutions for Atomic Absorption Analysis of Fe, Mn, Zn, and Cu in Plant Tissue Food Chem. 22, 103.*

International Journal of Food Science and Nutrition
ISSN: 2455-4898, Impact Factor: RJIF 5.14
www.foodsciencejournal.com
Volume 2; Issue 1; January 2017; Page No. 90-96

Comparative analysis of nutrient content between Prawn *(Fenneropenaeus indicus)* and Lobster *(Portunus sanguinolentus)*, preserved and cooked under different conditions

Uttiya Jana, Sarmistha Chakrabarti

Department of Home Science (Food & Nutrition), University of Calcutta, Kolkata, West Bengal, India

Abstract

Crustaceans are rich sources of protein and have lower cholesterol content compared to other animal food and thus commonly consumed. The content of this study was the comparison of nutrients between prawn and lobster. The nutrient contents of prawn were higher than lobster in the raw condition. These species were both subjected to conventional cooking methods like open pan dry roasting, boiling, shallow frying and deep frying. They were also preserved up to 15 days. The nutrient contents had changed due to preservation and the application of cooking methods. Losses of nutrients had taken place in both species. Most of the nutrient retention occurred in prawn than in lobster after preservation and cooking. The study significantly revealed that cooked prawn was beneficial due to adequate protein, fat and mineral restoration and it could be preserved up to 15 days with minimal loss as compared to lobster. Most of the nutrient retention occurred in shallow frying method.

Keywords: macronutrients, mineral contents, prawn, lobster, cooking methods, preservation

1. Introduction

Fish and other aquatic species are rich sources of protein commonly consumed in many parts of the world. But the nutrient contents change when they are cooked as shown in some studies previously carried out. In one study, three commonly available species of marine fish in Nigeria were subjected to boiling, frying and roasting and the effects of these cooking methods on the fish were observed. The results showed reduced protein content for all the fish types [1]. In yet another research, amino acid and proximate compositions were determined in six commonly consumed raw and cooked marine fish in Turkey. The changes in amino acid and proximate contents were found to be significant for all cooking methods in all fish species [2]. Another research showed that cooking methods were also applied for vegetable samples which could also be a reference for this present study. Three cooking methods, namely boiling, steaming and stir-frying were used to evaluate the effect on nutrient components of bamboo shoots, resulting in decreased contents of protein, soluble sugar, and ash. Results indicated an appreciable loss in the total free amino acids in boiling method. All procedures were carried out for 10 minutes [3]. The effects of five domestic cooking methods, including steaming, microwaving, boiling, stir-frying and stir-frying followed by boiling on the nutrients and health-promoting compounds of broccoli were investigated. The results showed that all cooking treatments, except steaming, caused significant losses of total soluble proteins and soluble sugars [4]. The effects of different cooking methods (boiling, baking, frying and grilling) on proximate and mineral composition of snakehead fish were investigated. The changes in the amount of protein and fat were found to be significantly higher in frying and grilling fish [5]. The present study is significant due to the comparison of macronutrient and micronutrient contents between prawn and lobster after being subjected to cooking and preservation up to 15 days. Cooking methods can cause loss of nutrients and the species that can restore more nutrients after preservation and cooking is investigated in this study.

- This study aims to compare the nutritive values of the two crustaceans under both raw and cooked conditions.
- It aims at finding the nutritive values restored after cooking and preservation.
- To find out the species that is beneficial in the perspective of nutrition is the most important concern of this study.

2. Materials and Methods

2.1 Sample preparation and cooking

Prawn *(Fenneropenaeus indicus)* and lobster *(Portunus sanguinolentus)* with a length of 10 cm, 15cm and weight of 50 gm, 90 gm respectively were obtained from the local fish market in Kolkata. They were kept in a plastic container, transported to the laboratory and washed with tap water several times to remove adhering dirt. Subsequently the samples were filleted and divided into two sections. The first section was sub-divided into five groups, one group was left uncooked while the other four were boiled, dry roasted in open pan, shallow fried and deep fried. Another section was preserved in the refrigerator at -20°C up to 15 days. Boiling was performed at 99–101 °C (water temperature) for 10 minutes. Open pan dry roasting of fillets was performed in a pan at 180 °C for 10 minutes. The frying of fillets was performed in a domestic frying pan of 2 L capacity at a temperature of approximately 180 °C for 10 minutes. Mustard oil was used as the medium for frying. In case of shallow frying 10 ml oil was used and 20 ml for deep frying. The fresh, preserved raw and cooked samples were then subjected to analysis.

2.2 Proximate composition analysis

Proximate composition analyses for homogenized samples of cooked and raw fish fillets were done in triplicate for carbohydrate, protein and lipid contents. The carbohydrate content was determined by Anthrone method [6] whereas the protein content was determined by the Lowry method [7]. Total lipid was extracted from the muscle tissues by soxhlet [8]. Mineral content was estimated by AOAC method [9] and energy content by energy conversion factor [10].

2.2.1 Estimation of carbohydrate by Anthrone Method [6]

100mg of the sample was taken into a boiling tube. Hydrolysis was carried out by keeping it in boiling water bath for three hours with 5mL of 2.5 N HCl and cooled to room temperature. Then it was neutralized with solid sodium carbonate until the effervescence ceased. Volume was made up to 100 ml and centrifuged at 3000 RPM for 15 minutes. The supernatant was collected and from it 1 ml was used for analysis. Then 4 ml Anthrone reagent was added to the solution. After that it was heated for eight minutes in a boiling water bath, cooled rapidly when green to dark green colour appeared. Then the reading was taken at 630 nm by spectrophotometer (Perkin Elmer Lambda 25).

2.2.2 Estimation of Protein by Lowry Method [7]

200 mg of sample was taken and 20 ml of buffer, containing sodium dihydrogen phosphate and disodium hydrogen phosphate, was added and homogenized finely. Then it was kept overnight. After that it was cold centrifuged at 5000 RPM for 20 minutes. The supernatant was collected and 1 ml of it was used for analysis. Then 5 ml of Lowry reagent was added to the supernatant and allowed to incubate for 10 minutes. After that 0.5 ml of Folinciocaltue reagent was added and incubated for 30 minutes until a dark blue colour appeared. The reading was taken at 660 nm by spectrophotometer (Perkin Elmer Lambda 25).

2.2.3 Estimation of fat by Soxhlet Extraction Method [8]

5gm of dried sample was placed inside the thimble of the apparatus, the extraction solvent petroleum ether of 60- 80^{0}C boiling range placed in a distillation flask and then on the heating mantel. The solvent was heated to reflux. The solvent vapour travelled up a distillation arm and flooded into the chamber housing the thimble. The condenser ensures that any solvent vapour that cooled, dripped back down into the chamber housing the solid material. The chamber containing the solid material slowly filled with warm solvent. The fat present in the sample was dissolved in the solvent which was returned to the distillation flask. This cycle was allowed to repeat for 12hours. After complete extraction of fat, the solvent was poured into a weighed petri dish, evaporated and the final weight of the petri dish containing the fat was taken. From this, the amount of the fat was calculated.

2.2.4 Estimation of mineral by AOAC method after wet digestion [9]

Dried sample (500 mg) was taken in a 25 ml volumetric flask and 10 ml of concentrated nitric acid was added to it and kept overnight. After that the volumetric flask was placed on the hot plate and allowed to boil for 8 hours. Then 4 ml of perchloric acid was added and boiled until brown fumes from the digestion stopped. After that the volume was made up to the mark by double distilled water and this solution was used for the analysis of iron and calcium by atomic absorption spectrophotometer (Perkin Elmer).

2.2.5 Determination of energy content by energy conversion factor [10]

The energy content of the sample was determined by the summation of the amount of energy from carbohydrate, protein and fat. The carbohydrate and protein contents were multiplied by the conversion factor 4.1 and 4 respectively and the fat content was multiplied by 9.3 and the total calorie content was represented in Kcal per 100 gm of a sample.

2.3 Statistical analysis

The effects of preservation and different cooking methods on the nutrient content of crustaceans were analyzed using Mean and Standard Deviation. One way ANOVA was applied for comparing the nutritive values between the two species. Differences were considered to be significant when p value is < 0.05. Data were analyzed by using SPSS package (Version 17).

3. Results

3.1 Nutrient content

Table 1: Carbohydrate content of samples (gm/100gm)

Sample	Duration	Raw	Boiling	Dry roasting	Shallow frying	Deep frying
Prawn	Fresh	1.06±0.20	0.71±0.07	0.98±0.12	0.85±0.06	0.50±0.09
	24 hours	0.88±0.10	0.41±0.09	0.55±0.13	0.88±0.10	0.51±0.17
	48 hours	1.03±0.20	0.52±0.02	1.01±0.0	0.71±0.0	0.95±0.04
	14 days	2.31±0.25	1.26±0.19	1.83±0.11	1.85±0.13	1.71±0.36
	15 day	2.25±0.05	0.63±0.079	0.62±0.06	1.61±0.07	1.87±0.19
Lobster	Fresh	2.65±0.13	2.15±0.13	1.51±0.14	2.47±0.13	1.51±0.10
	24 hours	1.65±0.13	1.51±0.09	1.11±0.10	1.63±0.11	1.29±0.06
	48 hours	1.15±0.13	0.95±0.15	0.78±0.11	1.16±0.08	0.19±0.05
	14 days	3.49±0.16	0.59±0.10	2.02±0.11	2.44±0.36	2.91±0.10
	15 days	3.22±0.20	0.54±0.10	1.17±0.21	2.19±0.17	2.21±0.19

Table 2: Protein content of samples (gm/100gm)

Sample	Duration	Raw	Boiling	Dry roasting	Shallow frying	Deep frying
Prawn	Fresh	17.36±0.27	2.59±0.14	6.50±0.02	6.48±0.07	11.12±0.02
	24 hours	14.20±0.28	4.60±0.02	6.99±0.09	6.51±0.08	7.17±0.15
	48 hours	12.69±0.27	3.60±0.09	5.06±0.05	5.08±0.08	6.57±0.13
	14 days	17.00±0.25	6.40±0.08	12.35±0.22	10.20±0.20	14.95±0.31
	15 day	14.75±0.25	10.00±0.39	7.51±0.08	9.99±0.41	16.93±0.41

Lobster	Fresh	19.20±0.20	8.69±0.11	7.96±0.04	9.53±0.04	13.60±0.11
	24 hours	16.06±0.05	6.70±0.16	7.06±0.05	7.63±0.14	9.03±0.11
	48 hours	11.72±0.56	5.63±0.17	5.85±0.05	5.90±0.05	6.25±0.04
	14 days	15.36±0.31	6.11±0.51	10.27±0.61	8.33±0.59	10.00±0.48
	15 days	15.25±0.25	12.89±0.51	8.40±0.40	7.43±0.59	12.37±0.48

Table 3: Fat content of samples (gm/100gm)

Sample	Duration	Raw	Boiling	Dry roasting	Shallow frying	Deep frying
Prawn	Fresh	2.46±0.04	3.02±0.04	3.04±0.05	6.46±0.04	4.35±0.07
	24 hours	1.85±0.03	1.59±0.03	1.94±0.05	9.78±0.03	9.29±0.01
	48 hours	0.86±0.04	0.76±0.04	1.56±0.06	2.57±0.04	3.62±0.03
	14 days	0.90±0.05	0.80±0.02	1.04±0.04	4.42±0.03	2.04±0.04
	15 day	0.78±0.06	0.63±0.02	0.97±0.06	6.40±0.02	2.04±0.04
Lobster	Fresh	2.09±0.07	2.58±0.05	2.02±0.02	6.75±0.06	6.14±0.06
	24 hours	0.88±0.02	0.58±0.03	0.63±0.01	4.20±0.05	4.07±0.04
	48 hours	1.09±0.07	1.339±0.04	0.56±0.04	5.78±0.05	7.76±0.03
	14 days	1.20±0.05	1.59±0.04	0.59±0.01	4.90±0.03	4.69±0.07
	15 days	1.01±0.04	1.14±0.04	0.98±0.09	7.72±0.07	4.68±0.03

Table 4: Iron content of samples (mg/100gm)

Sample	Duration	Raw	Boiling	Dry roasting	Shallow frying	Deep frying
Prawn	Fresh	1.40±0.01	1.45±0.02	1.51±0.01	0.93±0.01	0.67±0.05
	24 hours	2.52±0.02	1.80±0.08	1.74±0.05	3.45±0.03	2.50±0.02
	48 hours	1.58±0.05	1.32±0.02	2.03±0.04	2.32±0.02	2.23±0.04
	14 days	4.03±0.04	3.44±0.06	4.52±0.02	1.53±0.04	1.52±0.02
	15 day	3.12±0.02	2.16±0.05	1.41±0.01	2.65±0.03	2.84±0.04
Lobster	Fresh	2.55±0.01	1.65±0.03	4.60±0.02	1.72±0.04	0.89±0.05
	24 hours	0.56±0.02	1.45±0.03	0.94 ±0.04	1.17±0.02	1.40±0.05
	48 hours	0.90±0.02	0.55±0.02	1.52±0.02	1.05±0.04	1.46±0.04
	14 days	0.61±0.06	1.63±0.05	0.56±0.04	0.70±0.05	1.07±0.02
	15 days	1.17±0.02	1.77±0.02	3.97±0.02	1.51±0.01	1.66±0.01

Table 5: Calcium content of samples (mg/100gm)

Sample	Duration	Raw	Boiling	Dry roasting	Shallow frying	Deep frying
Prawn	Fresh	177.23±2.08	302.10±2.00	251.12±2.00	50.04±1.00	40.18±1.52
	24 hours	216.13±1.52	248.22±2.64	131.10±1.00	201.14±208	126.27±1.52
	48 hours	176.04±1.52	106.28±1.52	336.08±1.00	501.10±2.08	201.11±1.52
	14 days	136.10±1.52	136.34±1.52	227.33±2.51	202.65±2.64	162.39±2.00
	15 day	185.10±3.00	180.45±2.00	152.37±2.51	142.44±2.51	201.60±2.08
Lobster	Fresh	241.34±1.52	271.35±1.52	241.44±1.00	201.37±1.52	151.44±1.52
	24 hours	201.25±1.52	260.24±2.00	161.33±1.52	123.33±2.52	151.36±1.52
	48 hours	167.37±3.78	212.94±2.64	166.23±2.52	125.27±2.08	125.06±2.08
	14 days	351.95±1.00	501.65±1.00	281.88±1.00	265.32±2.08	151.36±1.52
	15 days	133.47±1.52	153.37±1.52	152.25±2.08	141.10±1.52	136.56±2.08

Table 6: Energy content of samples (kcal/100gm)

Sample	Duration	Raw	Boiling	Dry roasting	Shallow frying	Deep frying
Prawn	Fresh	96.61±1.74	41.26±0.61	58.36±0.29	89.55±0.24	87.01±0.72
	24 hours	77.54±1.30	34.86±0.56	48.22±1.24	124.48±0.25	171.13±0.85
	48 hours	62.88±0.11	23.53±0.61	38.70±0.58	47.04±0.33	63.79±0.56
	14 days	86.02±1.92	39.65±1.79	66.46±0.28	89.42±1.14	85.04±1.19
	15 day	75.25±0.50	48.41±1.80	41.59±3.07	105.95±2.00	93.19±0.74
Lobster	Fresh	106.87±0.53	67.37±0.35	56.71±0.94	110.87±0.91	117.54±1.28
	24 hours	78.82±0.31	38.25±0.49	38.60±0.40	76.16±0.41	79.04±0.34
	48 hours	61.91±2.19	39.35±0.62	30.66±2.13	82.03±0.27	97.90±0.54
	14 days	87.22±0.47	41.59±2.18	54.76±2.65	85.06±2.98	97.70±1.78
	15 days	83.30±1.98	64.31±2.61	47.24±2.36	110.28±2.21	101.96±2.44

3.2 Comparison between Prawn and Lobster

Table 7: One way anova for comparison of crustaceans

Nutrient	Duration	Raw	Boiling	Dry roasting	Shallow frying	Deep frying
Carbohydrate	Fresh	0.000(S)	0.000(S)	0.008(S)	0.000(S)	0.000(S)
	24 hours	0.002(S)	0.000(S)	0.004(S)	0.001(S)	0.002(S)
	48 hours	0.459(NS)	0.008(S)	0.045(S)	0.004(S)	0.000(S)
	14 days	0.003(S)	0.006(S)	0.111(NS)	0.058(NS)	0.005(S)

	15 day	0.001(S)	0.272(NS)	0.015(S)	0.006(S)	0.104(NS)
Protein	Fresh	0.001(S)	0.000(S)	0.000(S)	0.000(S)	0.000(S)
	24 hours	0.000(S)	0.000(S)	0.331(NS)	0.000(S)	0.000(S)
	48 hours	0.055(NS)	0.000(S)	0.000(S)	0.000(S)	0.017(S)
	14 days	0.002(S)	0.617(NS)	0.005(S)	0.006(S)	0.000(S)
	15 days	0.070(NS)	0.001(S)	0.120(NS)	0.000(S)	0.003(S)
Fat	Fresh	0.001(S)	0.000(S)	0.000(S)	0.002(S)	0.000(S)
	24 hours	0.010(S)	0.000(S)	0.000(S)	0.000(S)	0.000(S)
	48 hours	0.000(S)	0.000(S)	0.000(S)	0.000(S)	0.000(S)
	14 days	0.002(S)	0.000(S)	0.000(S)	0.000(S)	0.000(S)
	15 day	0.005(S)	0.000(S)	0.879(NS)	0.000(S)	0.000(S)
Iron	Fresh	0.000(S)	0.001(S)	0.000(S)	0.000(S)	0.008(S)
	24 hours	0.000(S)	0.002(S)	0.000(S)	0.000(S)	0.000(S)
	48 hours	0.000(S)	0.000(S)	0.000(S)	0.000(S)	0.000(S)
	14 days	0.000(S)	0.000(S)	0.000(S)	0.000(S)	0.000(S)
	15 days	0.000(S)	0.000(S)	0.000(S)	0.000(S)	0.000(S)
Calcium	Fresh	0.000(S)	0.000(S)	0.000(S)	0.000(S)	0.000(S)
	24 hours	0.000(S)	0.002(S)	0.000(S)	0.000(S)	0.000(S)
	48 hours	0.017(S)	0.033(S)	0.000(S)	0.000(S)	0.000(S)
	14 days	0.000(S)	0.000(S)	0.000(S)	0.000(S)	0.561(NS)
	15 day	0.000(S)	0.000(S)	0.000(S)	0.000(S)	0.000(S)
Energy	Fresh	0.001(S)	0.000(S)	0.044(S)	0.000(S)	0.000(S)
	24 hours	0.173(S)	0.001(S)	0.000(S)	0.000(S)	0.000(S)
	48 hours	0.489(NS)	0.000(S)	0.003(S)	0.000(S)	0.000(S)
	14 days	0.354(NS)	0.300(NS)	0.002(S)	0.077(NS)	0.001(S)
	15 days	0.002(S)	0.001(S)	0.065(NS)	0.066(NS)	0.004(S)

(P value = <0.05 = significantly different) (S= significant, NS= Non significant)

Table 8: Percentage of loss of preserved Prawn & Lobster up to 24 hours

Nutrients Loss (%)	Raw		Boiling		Open pan Dry roasting		Shallow fry		Deep fry	
	Prawn	**Lobster**	**Prawn**	**Lobster**	**Prawn**	**Lobster**	**Prawn**	**Lobster**	**Prawn**	**Lobster**
Carbohydrate	16.98	37.73	42.25	29.76	43.87	26.49	-3.53	34.00	-2.00	14.56
protein	18.20	16.35	77.60	22.89	-7.53	11.30	-0.46	19.93	35.52	33.60
Fat	24.79	57.89	24.79	77.51	47.35	68.81	-51.39	37.77	-113.56	33.71
Iron	-80.00	78.03	-24.13	12.12	-15.23	79.56	-270.96	31.97	-273.13	-57.30
Calcium	-22.03	16.59	17.88	4.05	47.80	33.19	-302.00	38.80	-215.00	0.00
Energy	19.73	26.24	15.51	43.22	17.37	31.93	-34.53	31.30	-96.67	32.78

Table 9: Percentage of loss of preserved Prawn & Lobster up to 48 hours

Nutrients Loss (%)	Raw		Boiling		Open pan Dry roasting		Shallow fry		Deep fry	
	Prawn	**Lobster**	**Prawn**	**Lobster**	**Prawn**	**Lobster**	**Prawn**	**Lobster**	**Prawn**	**Lobster**
Carbohydrate	2.83	56.60	26.76	55.81	-3.06	48.34	16.47	53.03	-90.00	87.41
protein	26.90	38.95	-38.99	35.21	22.15	26.50	21.60	38.09	40.91	54.04
Fat	65.04	47.84	74.83	46.12	48.68	72.27	60.21	14.37	16.78	-26.38
Iron	-12.85	64.70	8.96	66.66	-34.43	66.95	-149.46	38.95	-232.83	-64.04
Calcium	0.56	30.70	64.90	21.77	-33.86	31.12	-902.00	37.81	-402.50	17.21
Energy	34.91	42.06	42.97	41.59	33.56	45.93	47.47	26.01	26.74	16.74

Table 10: Percentage of loss of preserved Prawn & Lobster up to 14days

Nutrients Loss (%)	Raw		Boiling		Open pan Dry roasting		Shallow fry		Deep fry	
	Prawn	Lobster	Prawn	Lobster	Prawn	Lobster	Prawn	Lobster	Prawn	Lobster
Carbohydrate	-117.92	-31.69	-77.46	72.55	-86.73	-33.77	-11.76	1.21	-242	-92.71
Protein	2.07	20	-147.10	29.68	-90	-29.02	-57.40	12.59	-34.44	26.47
Fat	63.41	42.58	73.50	38.37	65.78	70.79	31.57	27.40	53.10	23.61
Iron	-187.85	76.07	-37.24	-7.27	-99.33	87.82	-64.51	59.30	-128.35	-20.22
Calcium	-11.29	-45.64	46.35	-84.87	0.00	-16.59	-402	-31.84	-277.50	0.00
Energy	10.96	18.38	3.90	38.26	-13.87	3.43	0.14	23.27	2.26	16.91

Table 11: Percentage of loss of preserved Prawn & Lobster up to 15days

Nutrients Loss (%)	Raw		Boiling		Open pan Dry roasting		Shallow fry		Deep fry	
	Prawn	Lobster	Prawn	Lobster	Prawn	Lobster	Prawn	Lobster	Prawn	Lobster
Carbohydrate	-112.26	-21.50	11.26	74.88	36.73	22.51	-89.41	11.33	2.74	-46.35
Protein	15.03	20.57	-286.10	-48.33	-15.53	-5.52	-54.16	22.03	-52.24	9.64
Fat	68.29	51.67	79.13	55.81	68.09	51.48	0.92	-14.37	53.10	23.77
Iron	-122.85	54.11	-48.96	-7.27	6.62	13.69	-184.94	12.20	-184.94	-86.51
Calcium	14.68	44.81	-66.22	43.54	39.44	36.92	-482	29.85	-365	9.93
Energy	22.10	22.05	-17.32	4.54	28.73	16.69	-18.31	0.53	-7.10	13.29

3.3 Comparison of percentage of nutrient loss due to cooking

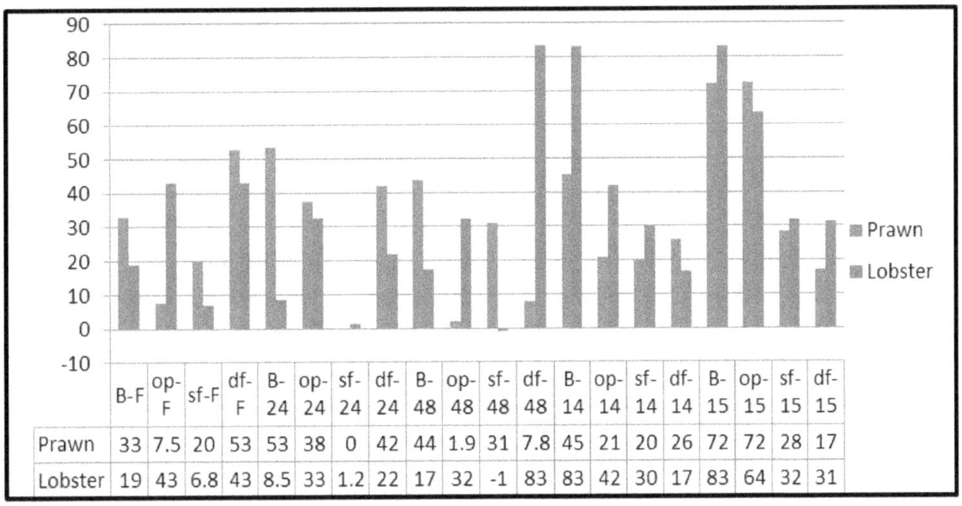

	B-F	op-F	sf-F	df-F	B-24	op-24	sf-24	df-24	B-48	op-48	sf-48	df-48	B-14	op-14	sf-14	df-14	B-15	op-15	sf-15	df-15
Prawn	33	7.5	20	53	53	38	0	42	44	1.9	31	7.8	45	21	20	26	72	72	28	17
Lobster	19	43	6.8	43	8.5	33	1.2	22	17	32	-1	83	83	42	30	17	83	64	32	31

Fig 1: Carbohydrate content

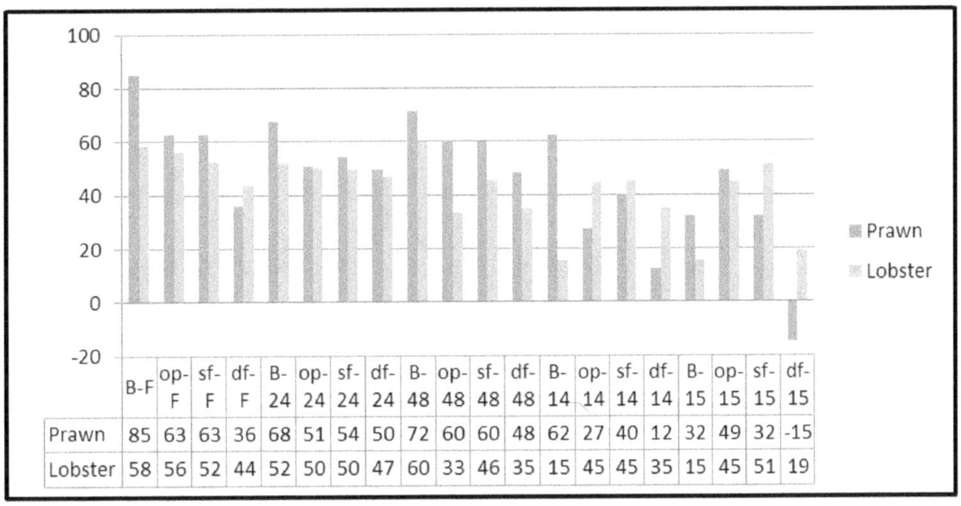

	B-F	op-F	sf-F	df-F	B-24	op-24	sf-24	df-24	B-48	op-48	sf-48	df-48	B-14	op-14	sf-14	df-14	B-15	op-15	sf-15	df-15
Prawn	85	63	63	36	68	51	54	50	72	60	60	48	62	27	40	12	32	49	32	-15
Lobster	58	56	52	44	52	50	50	47	60	33	46	35	15	45	45	35	15	45	51	19

Fig 2: Protein content

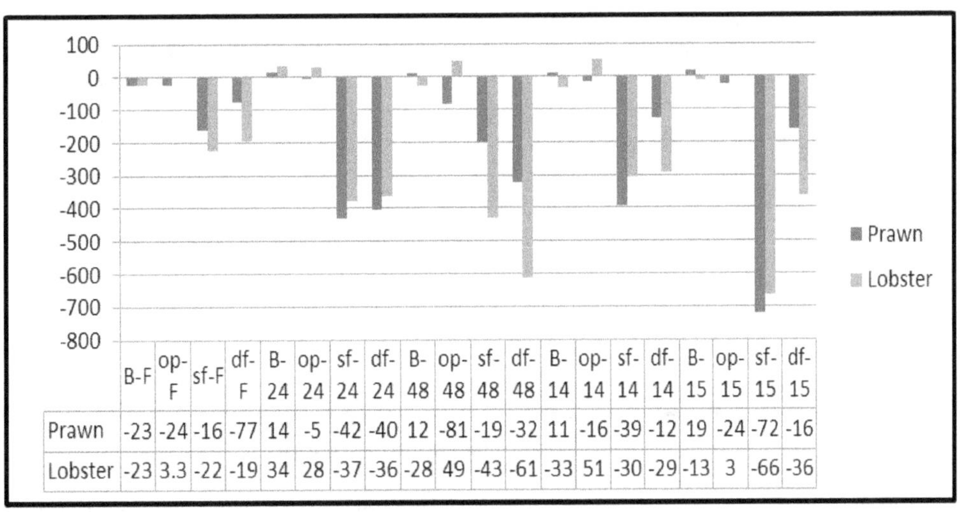

	B-F	op-F	sf-F	df-F	B-24	op-24	sf-24	df-24	B-48	op-48	sf-48	df-48	B-14	op-14	sf-14	df-14	B-15	op-15	sf-15	df-15
Prawn	-23	-24	-16	-77	14	-5	-42	-40	12	-81	-19	-32	11	-16	-39	-12	19	-24	-72	-16
Lobster	-23	3.3	-22	-19	34	28	-37	-36	-28	49	-43	-61	-33	51	-30	-29	-13	3	-66	-36

Fig 3: Fat content

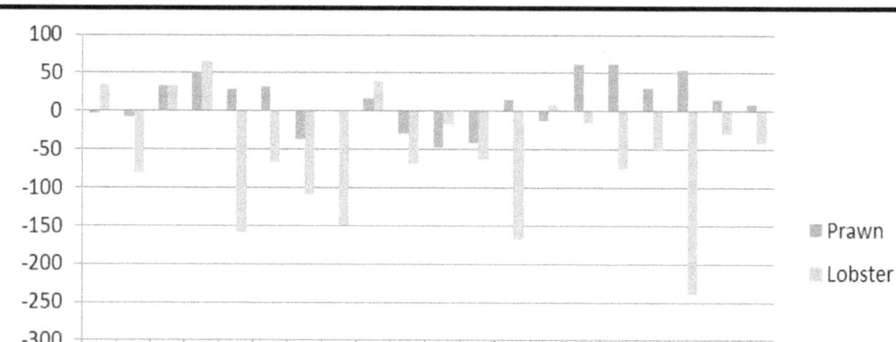

	B-F	op-F	sf-F	df-F	B-24	op-24	sf-24	df-24	B-48	op-48	sf-48	df-48	B-14	op-14	sf-14	df-14	B-15	op-15	sf-15	df-15
Prawn	-4	-8	34	52	29	31	-37	0.8	16	-28	-47	-41	15	-12	62	62	31	55	15	9
Lobster	35	-80	33	65	-15	-68	-10	-15	39	-69	-17	-62	-16	8.2	-15	-75	-51	-23	-29	-42

Fig 4: Iron content

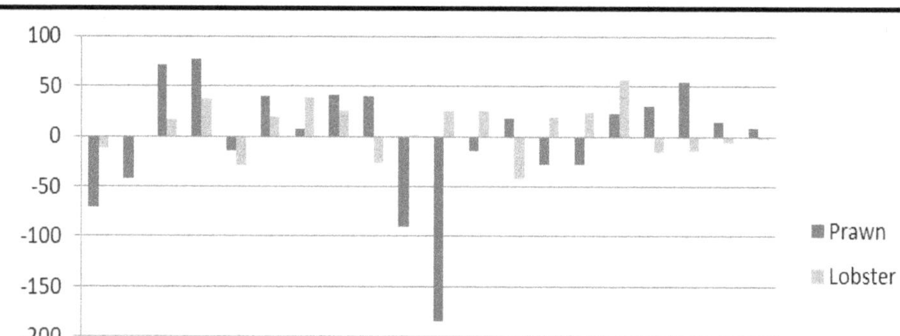

	B-F	op-F	sf-F	df-F	B-24	op-24	sf-24	df-24	B-48	op-48	sf-48	df-48	B-14	op-14	sf-14	df-14	B-15	op-15	sf-15	df-15
Prawn	-71	-42	72	77	-15	39	6.9	42	40	-91	-18	-14	18	-27	-27	23	31	55	15	9
Lobster	-12	0	17	37	-29	20	39	25	-27	0.6	25	25	-43	20	25	57	-15	-14	-6	-2

Fig 5: Calcium content

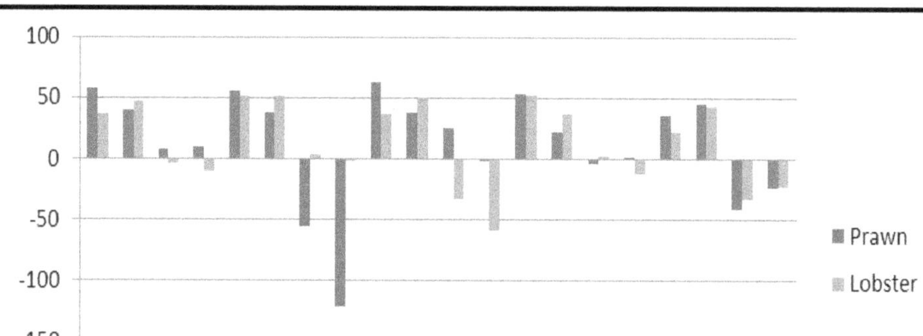

	B-F	op-F	sf-F	df-F	B-24	op-24	sf-24	df-24	B-48	op-48	sf-48	df-48	B-14	op-14	sf-14	df-14	B-15	op-15	sf-15	df-15
Prawn	57	40	7.3	9.9	55	38	-55	-12	63	38	25	-1	54	23	-4	1.1	36	45	-41	-24
Lobster	37	47	-4	-10	51	51	3.4	-0	36	50	-32	-58	52	37	2.5	-12	23	43	-32	-22

Fig 6: Energy content

4. Discussion

Table I, II, III, IV, V, VI showed the nutrient contents like carbohydrate, protein, fat, iron, calcium and energy contents of prawn and lobster. The raw and cooked values were displayed here along with the preservation days up to 15th. The proximate compositions and the mineral contents were reduced due to application of different cooking methods and preservation up to 15days.The table showed the changes between the raw values and the cooked values. Most of the nutrient content was highest in lobster rather than in prawn in fresh raw condition but due to cooking and preservation nutrient restoration occurred mainly in prawn.

Table VII showed the comparison between the two crustaceans. Most of the values are significant ($P<0.05$) which means there is significant difference present between the fresh and preserved raw and cooked samples.

Table VIII, IX, X, XI showed the percentage of loss due to preservation of prawn and lobster for 24 hours, 48hours, 14days and 15 days preservation. The values show that nutrient loss occurred in both 24 and 48 hours but most of the nutrient restoration occurred in 14th and 15th days of preservation. Due to prolonged preservation moisture loss occurred from the crustaceans so the nutrients become more concentrated and when these are subjected to cooking further some moisture loss occurred which could increase the amount of nutrients than in fresh condition. Prawn can restore most of the nutrients than lobster during preservation.

Fig. 1, 2, 3, 4, 5, 6 showed the percentage of loss of nutrients due to cooking of both fresh and preserved crustaceans. The carbohydrate and protein content reduced due to cooking. The percentage of loss was more for lobster than for prawn. Fat content is increased for both of the crustaceans due to moisture loss as a result of application of heat. Iron content also increased for both of them due to use of iron pan for cooking. Iron content mostly increased in lobster than in prawn whereas calcium content reduced mostly in lobster rather than in prawn. Energy content is increased in shallow frying and deep frying method mainly for oil absorption of the crustaceans.

5. Conclusion

The maximum losses occur in lobster after preservation and cooking rather than in prawn. Losses occur in both the crustaceans but loss percentage due to cooking and preservation for carbohydrate, protein, calcium and energy are higher in prawn rather than in lobster, both due to cooking and preservation, whereas fat and iron content are better restored in lobster. Boiling and open pan dry roasting can mostly reduce the nutrient content whereas shallow frying retains more nutrients. They can be preserved almost up to 2 weeks. After considering all pros and cons, it can be concluded that prawn is better than lobster in terms of nutrient restoration after cooking and preservation.

6. Acknowledgement

The University Grants Commission (UGC) is thanked for awarding a Junior Research Fellowship to Uttiya Jana.

7. References

1. Goldman KJ. *Regulation of body temperature in the white shark, Carcharodon carcharias*. Journal of Comparative Physiology B, 1997; 167(6):423-429.
2. Erkan N, Özden Ö, Selçuk A. *Effect of frying, grilling, and steaming on amino acid composition of marine fishes*. Journal of medicinal food. 2010; 13(6):1524-1531.
3. Mkandawire KT, Masamba KG. *Effect of lemon juice treatment and sun drying on vitamin C retention in three steam and water blanched indigenous vegetables over six weeks storage period.* African Journal of Food Science. 2014; 8(6):316-321.
4. Yuan GF, Sun B, Yuan J, Wang QM. *Effects of different cooking methods on health-promoting compounds of broccoli*. Journal of Zhejiang University Science B. 2009; 10(8):580-588.
5. Marimuthu K, Thilaga M, Kathiresan S, Xavier R, Mas RHMH. *Effect of different cooking methods on proximate and mineral composition of striped snakehead fish (Channa striatus, Bloch).* Journal of food science and technology, 2012; 49(3):373-377.
6. Ludwig TG, Goldberg HJ. The anthrone method for the determination of carbohydrates in foods and in oral rinsing. Journal of dental research. 1956; 35(1):90-94.
7. Lowry OH, Rosebrough NJ, Farr AL, Randall RJ. Protein measurement with the Folin phenol reagent. Journal of biochemtry, 1951; 193(1):265-275.
8. Manirakiza P, Covaci A, Schepens P. Comparative study on total lipid determination using Soxhlet, Roese-Gottlieb, Bligh & Dyer, and modified Bligh & Dyer extraction methods. Journal of food composition and analysis, 2001; 14(1):93-100.
9. Baker AS, Smith RL. Preparation of solutions for atomic absorption analyses of iron, manganese, zinc, and copper in plant tissue. Journal of agricultural and food chemistry, 1974; 22(1):103-107.
10. Buskirk ER, Mendez J. Energy: caloric requirements, In Nutrition and the Adult. Springer US, 1980, 49-95.

International Journal of Fisheries and Aquatic Studies

E-ISSN: 2347-5129
P-ISSN: 2394-0506
(ICV-Poland) Impact Value: 5.62
(GIF) Impact Factor: 0.549
IJFAS 2017; 5(2): 258-263

www.fisheriesjournal.com
Received: 05-01-2017
Accepted: 06-02-2017

Uttiya Jana
Department of Home Science (Food & Nutrition), University of Calcutta, West Bengal, India

Sarmistha Chakrabarti
Department of Home Science (Food & Nutrition), University of Calcutta, West Bengal, India

Correspondence
Uttiya Jana
Department of Home Science (Food & Nutrition), University of Calcutta, West Bengal, India

Comparative analysis of nutritional quality between Pomfret (*Pampus argenteus*) and Hilsa (*Hilsa ilisha*), preserved and cooked under different conditions

Uttiya Jana and Sarmistha Chakrabarti

Abstract
The present study was conducted to compare the nutrients between *Pampus argenteus* and *Hilsa ilisha*. The nutrient contents of *P. argenteus were* higher than *H. ilisha* in the raw condition. They were both subjected to conventional cooking methods like open pan dry roasting, boiling, shallow frying and deep frying. They were also preserved raw up to 15 days with the preservative *viz.* a combination of salt and turmeric. The nutrient contents had changed due to preservation and cooking but the losses could be retained by the use of preservative. Nutrient retention mostly occurred in pomfret than in *hilsa*. The present study significantly revealed that cooked pomfret was beneficial due to adequate nutrient restoration and it could be preserved with preservative up to 15 days with minimal loss as compared to *hilsa*. Nutrient retention occurred mostly in deep frying method.

Keywords: Macronutrients, mineral contents, pomfret, *hilsa,* cooking methods, preservative

1. Introduction

Fish and other aquatic species are rich sources of protein commonly consumed in many parts of the world. But the nutrient contents change when they are cooked as shown in some studies previously carried out, which include- three commonly available species of marine fish in Nigeria were subjected to boiling, frying and roasting and the effects of these cooking methods on the fish were observed. The results showed reduced protein content for all the fish types [1]. In yet another research, amino acid and proximate compositions were determined in six commonly consumed raw and cooked marine fish in Turkey. The changes in amino acid and proximate contents were found to be significant for all cooking methods in all fish species [2]. Another research showed that cooking methods were also applied for vegetable samples which could also be a reference for this present study. Three cooking methods, namely boiling, steaming and stir-frying were used to evaluate the effect on nutrient components of bamboo shoots, resulting in decreased contents of protein, soluble sugar, and ash. Results indicated an appreciable loss in the total free amino acids in boiling method. All procedures were carried out for 10 minutes [3]. The effects of five domestic cooking methods, including steaming, microwaving, boiling, stir-frying and stir-frying followed by boiling on the nutrients and health-promoting compounds of broccoli were investigated. The results showed that all cooking treatments, except steaming, caused significant losses of total soluble proteins and soluble sugars [4]. The effects of different cooking methods (boiling, baking, frying and grilling) on proximate and mineral composition of snakehead fish were investigated. The changes in the amount of protein and fat were found to be significantly higher in frying and grilling fish [5]. The present study is significant due to the comparison of macronutrient and micronutrient contents between prawn and lobster after being subjected to cooking and preservation up to 15 days. Cooking methods can cause loss of nutrients and the species that can restore more nutrients after preservation and cooking is investigated in this study. The present study had three objectives as follows:

- This study aims to compare the nutritive values of the two sea fish under both raw and cooked conditions.
- It aims at finding the nutritive values restored after cooking and preservation with preservative.

- To find the fish that is beneficial in the perspective of nutrition is the most important concern of this study.

2. Materials and Methods

2.1. Sample preparation and cooking

Pomfret (*Pampus argenteus*) with a length of 12cm and weight of 250–300 g and *hilsa (Hilsa ilisha)* with a length of 25–30 cm and weight of 1 kg were obtained from the local fish market in Kolkata. They were kept in a plastic container, transported to the laboratory (University of Calcutta, Laboratory of Food Science) and washed with tap water several times to remove adhering dirt. Subsequently the samples were filleted and divided into three sections. The first section was sub-divided into five groups, one group was left uncooked while the other four were boiled, dry roasted in open pan, shallow fried and deep fried. Another section was preserved in the refrigerator at -20 °C up to 15 days without preservative and the other section was preserved up to 15 days with the combination of salt and turmeric (2% of the weight of the fish). The preservatives were used in the ratio of 1:1. Boiling was performed at 99–101 °C (water temperature) for 10 minutes. Open pan dry roasting of fillets was performed in a pan at 180 °C for 10 minutes. The frying of fillets was performed in a domestic frying pan of 2 L capacity at a temperature of approximately 180 °C for 10 minutes. Mustard oil was used as the medium for frying. In case of shallow frying 10 ml oil was used and 20 ml for deep frying. The fresh, preserved raw and cooked samples were then subjected to analysis.

2.2. Nutrient analysis

Nutrient analyses for homogenized samples of cooked and raw fish fillets were done in triplicate for carbohydrate, protein and lipid contents. The carbohydrate content was determined by Anthrone method [6] whereas the protein content was determined by the Lowry method [7]. Total lipid was extracted from the muscle tissues by soxhlet [8], Moisture and ash were determined by weight difference method [9], mineral content was estimated by AOAC method [10] and energy content by energy conversion factor [11].

2.2.1. Estimation of carbohydrate by Anthrone Method

100mg of the sample was taken into a boiling tube. Hydrolysis was carried out by keeping it in boiling water bath for three hours with 5mL of 2.5 N HCl and cooled to room temperature. Then it was neutralized with solid sodium carbonate until the effervescence ceased. Volume was made up to 100 ml and centrifuged at 3000 RPM for 15 minutes. The supernatant was collected and from it 1 ml was used for analysis. Then 4 ml Anthrone reagent was added to the solution. After that it was heated for eight minutes in a boiling water bath, cooled rapidly when green to dark green colour appeared. Then the reading was taken at 630 nm by spectrophotometer (Perkin Elmer Lambda 25) [6].

2.2.2. Estimation of Protein by Lowry Method

200 mg of sample was taken and 20 ml of buffer, containing sodium dihydrogen phosphate and disodium hydrogen phosphate, was added and homogenized finely. Then it was kept overnight. After that it was cold centrifuged at 5000 RPM for 20 minutes. The supernatant was collected and 1 ml of it was used for analysis. Then 5 ml of Lowry reagent was added to the supernatant and allowed to incubate for 10 minutes. After that 0.5 ml of Folinciocaltue reagent was added and incubated for 30 minutes until a dark blue colour appeared. The reading was taken at 660 nm by spectrophotometer (Perkin Elmer Lambda 25) [7].

2.2.3. Estimation of fat by Soxhlet Extraction Method

5gm of dried sample was placed inside the thimble of the apparatus, the extraction solvent petroleum ether of 60- 80 ^{0}C boiling range placed in a distillation flask and then on the heating mantel. The solvent was heated to reflux. The solvent vapour travelled up a distillation arm and flooded into the chamber housing the thimble. The condenser ensures that any solvent vapour that cooled, dripped back down into the chamber housing the solid material. The chamber containing the solid material slowly filled with warm solvent. The fat present in the sample was dissolved in the solvent which was returned to the distillation flask. This cycle was allowed to repeat for 12hours. After complete extraction of fat, the solvent was poured into a weighed petri dish, evaporated and the final weight of the petri dish containing the fat was taken. From this, the amount of the fat was calculated [8].

2.2.4. Estimation of moisture by weight difference method

10 gm sample was taken in a previously weighed petri dish and placed in an oven, maintained at 60 ^{0}C. The sample was placed there for 7 consecutive days and the weight of the sample was checked at specific intervals until the weight became constant. The difference between the initial weight and the final weight of sample containing Petri dish was converted into a percentage of moisture present in the sample [9].

2.2.5. Estimation of ash by weight difference method

5 gm of dried sample was taken in a previously weighed crucible and placed in a muffle furnace at temperature 600 ^{0}C for 8 hours. The weight was checked after that and the crucible was again placed in the furnace for at least 4 hours. The weight was checked again and the process was repeated until the weight became constant. The difference between the initial and the final weights of the sample containing crucible was used for the calculation of ash content of the sample [9].

2.2.6. Estimation of mineral by AOAC method after wet digestion

Dried sample (500 mg) was taken in a 25 ml volumetric flask and 10 ml of concentrated nitric acid was added to it and kept overnight. After that the volumetric flask was placed on the hot plate and allowed to boil for 8 hours. Then 4 ml of perchloric acid was added and boiled until brown fumes from the digestion stopped. After that the volume was made up to the mark by double distilled water and this solution was used for the analysis of iron and calcium by atomic absorption spectrophotometer (Perkin Elmer) [10].

2.2.7. Determination of energy content by energy conversion factor

The energy content of the sample was determined by the summation of the amount of energy from carbohydrate, protein and fat. The carbohydrate and protein contents were multiplied by the conversion factor 4.1 and 4 respectively and the fat content was multiplied by 9.3 and the total calorie content was represented in Kcal per 100 gm of a sample [11].

3. Statistical analysis

The effects of preservative and different cooking methods on the nutrient content of sea fish were analyzed by using Mean and Standard Deviation. One way ANOVA was applied for comparing the nutritive values between the two fish. Differences were considered to be significant when p value is < 0.05. Data were analyzed by using SPSS package (Version 17).

4. Results

4.1. Nutrient content

Table 1, 2, 3, 4, 5, 6, 7, 8 showed the nutrient contents like carbohydrate, protein, fat, iron, calcium, moisture, ash, and energy contents of pomfret and hilsa. The raw and cooked values were displayed here along with the preservation days with and without preservative up to 15th. The proximate compositions and the mineral contents were reduced due to application of different cooking methods and preservation up to 15days. The table showed the changes between the raw and the cooked values.

Table 1: Carbohydrate content of samples (gm/100gm)

Sample	Duration	Raw	Boiling	Dry roasting	Shallow frying	Deep frying
Pomfret	Fresh	2.17±0.17	1.42±0.07	1.74±0.11	1.90±0.10	2.14±0.09
	15 days	2.63±0.11	1.33±0.12	2.59±0.09	2.60±0.07	4.33±0.10
	15 day (S+T)	4.19±0.11	2.08±0.08	2.08±0.07	2.76±0.04	3.20±0.05
Hilsa	Fresh	3.59±0.14	2.37±0.15	1.72±0.14	2.30±0.10	3.25±0.10
	15 days	1.72±0.08	2.40±0.10	1.27±0.08	2.05±0.05	2.50±0.08
	15 day (S+T)	3.25±0.05	0.65±0.05	1.65±0.05	1.75±0.05	2.62±0.13

Table 2: Protein content of samples (gm/100gm)

Sample	Duration	Raw	Boiling	Dry roasting	Shallow frying	Deep frying
Pomfret	Fresh	16.36±0.31	4.22±0.20	6.24±0.04	6.82±0.02	7.93±0.12
	15 days	7.50±0.25	6.66±0.33	11.04±0.52	10.43±0.43	10.00±0.55
	15 day (S+T)	7.50±0.25	3.33±0.33	8.40±0.55	6.95±0.43	7.75±0.25
Hilsa	Fresh	24.07±0.11	6.58±0.20	9.64±0.18	10.73±0.17	11.92±0.11
	15 days	11.42±0.87	4.84±0.41	4.09±0.19	2.96±0.37	3.85±0.30
	15 day (S+T)	5.25±0.25	2.80±0.40	2.98±0.44	3.36±0.40	3.50±0.50

Table 3: Fat content of samples (gm/100gm)

Sample	Duration	Raw	Boiling	Dry roasting	Shallow frying	Deep frying
Pomfret	Fresh	1.71±0.09	2.78±0.07	5.78±0.08	5.43±0.04	4.47±0.04
	15 days	13.07±0.03	8.83±0.04	11.76±0.07	12.59±0.03	7.38±0.04
	15 day (S+T)	21.95±0.04	9.69±0.07	13.88±0.08	15.65±0.05	9.06±0.05
Hilsa	Fresh	13.21±0.17	13.12±0.10	6.28±0.03	6.14±0.04	3.62±0.04
	15 days	29.10±0.10	20.52±0.03	14.89±0.09	13.18±0.03	9.64±0.06
	15 day (S+T)	21.98±0.04	20.37±0.06	14.62±0.10	16.10±0.10	10.81±0.10

Table 4: Iron content of samples (mg/100gm)

Sample	Duration	Raw	Boiling	Dry roasting	Shallow frying	Deep frying
Pomfret	Fresh	2.84±0.00	1.56±0.02	2.09±0.07	1.07±0.05	4.53±0.03
	15 days	0.03±0.01	0.75±0.03	1.43±0.02	0.47±0.02	0.32±0.02
	15 day (S+T)	3.52±0.02	2.21±0.01	1.12±0.02	1.02±0.02	1.72±0.02
Hilsa	Fresh	3.28±0.01	1.27±0.02	2.38±0.02	1.65±0.03	1.82±0.05
	15 days	1.56±0.03	2.55±0.03	3.52 ±0.02	2.56±0.03	2.54±0.04
	15 day (S+T)	1.62±0.02	1.51±0.01	1.92±0.02	1.92±0.02	2.42±0.02

Table 5: Calcium content of samples (mg/100gm)

Sample	Duration	Raw	Boiling	Dry roasting	Shallow frying	Deep frying
Pomfret	Fresh	151±1.52	151±1.52	156±1.52	86±1.52	246±1.52
	15 days	166±1.52	362±2.51	282±2.00	213±3.21	208±3.21
	15 day (S+T)	284±2.00	64±2.00	68±1.52	42±2.00	64±3.05
Hilsa	Fresh	201±1.52	277±2.08	301±1.00	351±2.00	151±1.52
	15 days	202±2.00	227±2.08	501±1.52	242±2.51	251±1.52
	15 day (S+T)	602±2.51	552±2.00	504±4.16	337±2.51	351±1.00

Table 6: Moisture content of samples (gm/100gm)

Sample	Duration	Raw	Boiling	Dry roasting	Shallow frying	Deep frying
Pomfret	Fresh	80.74±1.97	55.78±0.05	25.31±0.10	31.64±0.14	18.41±0.07
	15 days	76.03±0.04	51.02±0.62	42.93±0.52	45.21±0.50	30.77±0.24
	15 day (S+T)	75.36±0.47	39.90±0.26	46.98±0.58	45.53±0.31	29.60±0.36
Hilsa	Fresh	69.76±0.25	50.06±0.0.05	36.81±0.10	24.54±0.06	11.53±0.05
	15 days	66.60±3.32	59.47±0.50	27.30±0.77	32.94±0.48	23.81±1.80
	15 day (S+T)	57.36±0.47	54.67±0.22	35.57±0.49	41.24±0.66	24.57±0.50

Table 7: Ash content of samples (gm/100gm)

Sample	Duration	Raw	Boiling	Dry roasting	Shallow frying	Deep frying
Pomfret	Fresh	4.19±0.10	1.68±0.05	1.08±0.07	0.97±0.03	1.06±0.05
	15 days	3.05±0.05	1.03±0.04	1.27±0.04	2.65±0.05	3.35±0.03
	15 day (S+T)	2.30±0.05	1.59±0.08	1.40±0.05	1.82±0.03	3.24±0.04
Hilsa	Fresh	2.07±0.06	1.08±0.08	1.49±0.07	1.10±0.10	3.69±0.07
	15 days	1.25±0.08	0.60±0.10	0.34±0.03	0.34±0.02	0.93±0.04
	15 day (S+T)	3.36±0.06	2.75±0.03	1.78±0.08	2.43±0.04	2.66±0.06

Table 8: Energy content of samples (kcal/100gm)

Sample	Duration	Raw	Boiling	Dry roasting	Shallow frying	Deep frying
Pomfret	Fresh	89.22±0.23	48.45±0.17	85.72±0.95	85.38±0.76	81.85±0.49
	15 days	162.00±1.30	114.14±1.90	163.96±2.04	169.24±1.43	125.99±2.18
	15 day (S+T)	250.97±1.30	111.79±1.76	171.05±2.79	184.46±2.18	128.08±1.01
Hilsa	Fresh	233.90±0.14	161.15±5.41	103.83±0.60	109.28±0.50	94.63±0.38
	15 days	323.16±3.71	219.94±1.43	159.95±1.09	142.66±1.35	114.25±2.73
	15 day (S+T)	238.42±1.19	203.27±1.65	154.48±1.57	170.16±1.42	125.03±1.98

4.2. Comparison between Pomfret and Hilsa

Table 9 showed the comparison between the two sea fish. Most of the values are significant (*P*<0.05) which means there is significant difference present between the fresh and preserved with and without preservative raw and cooked samples.

Table 9: One way ANOVA for comparison of sea fish

Nutrient	Duration	Raw	Boiling	Dry roasting	Shallow frying	Deep frying
Carbohydrate	Fresh	0.000(S)	0.000(S)	0.797(NS)	0.009(S)	0.000(S)
	15days	0.000(S)	0.000(S)	0.000(S)	0.000(S)	0.000(S)
	15day (S+T)	0.000(S)	0.000(S)	0.001(S)	0.000(S)	0.002(S)
Protein	Fresh	0.000(S)	0.000(S)	0.000(S)	0.000(S)	0.000(S)
	15days	0.002(S)	0.004(S)	0.000(S)	0.000(S)	0.000(S)
	15day (S+T)	0.000(S)	0.151(NS)	0.000(S)	0.000(S)	0.000(S)
Fat	Fresh	0.000(S)	0.000(S)	0.000(S)	0.000(S)	0.000(S)
	15days	0.000(S)	0.000(S)	0.000(NS)	0.000(S)	0.000(S)
	15day (S+T)	0.054(NS)	0.000(S)	0.001(S)	0.002(S)	0.000(S)
Moisture	Fresh	0.001(S)	0.000(S)	0.000(S)	0.000(S)	0.000(S)
	15days	0.008(S)	0.000(S)	0.000(S)	0.000(S)	0.003(S)
	15day (S+T)	0.000(S)	0.000(S)	0.000(S)	0.001(S)	0.000(S)
Ash	Fresh	0.000(S)	0.000(S)	0.002(S)	0.107(NS)	0.000(S)
	15days	0.000(S)	0.002(S)	0.000(S)	0.000(S)	0.000(S)
	15day (S+T)	0.000(S)	0.000(S)	0.002(S)	0.000(S)	0.000(S)
Iron	Fresh	0.000(S)	0.000(S)	0.003(S)	0.000(S)	0.000(S)
	15days	0.000(S)	0.000(S)	0.000(S)	0.000(S)	0.000(S)
	15day (S+T)	0.000(S)	0.000(S)	0.006(S)	0.000(S)	0.000(S)
Calcium	Fresh	0.000(S)	0.000(S)	0.000(S)	0.000(S)	0.000(S)
	15days	0.000(S)	0.000(S)	0.000(S)	0.000(S)	0.000(S)
	15day (S+T)	0.017(S)	0.033(S)	0.000(S)	0.000(S)	0.000(S)
Energy	Fresh	0.000(S)	0.000(S)	0.000(S)	0.000(S)	0.000(S)
	15days	0.000(S)	0.000(S)	0.000(S)	0.000(S)	0.000(S)
	15day (S+T)	0.000(S)	0.000(S)	0.000(S)	0.000(S)	0.000(S)

(P value = <0.05 = significantly different) (S= significant, NS= Non- significant)

Table 10, 11 showed the percentage of loss due to preservation with and without preservative of pomfret and hilsa up to 15 days. The values showed that nutrient loss occurred due to preservation for long period but most of the nutrient restoration could be done by using salt and turmeric.

Table 10: Percentage of loss of preserved Pomfret and Hilsa up to 15days without preservative

Nutrients Loss (%)	Raw		Boiling		Open pan Dry roasting		Shallow fry		Deep fry	
	Pomfret	*hilsa*	Pomfret	*hilsa*	Pomfret	*hilsa*	Pomfret	*hilsa*	Pomfret	*hilsa*
Carbohydrate	-21.19	52.08	6.33	-1.26	-48.85	26.16	-43.68	10.86	-102.33	23.07
protein	54.15	52.55	-57.81	26.44	-76.92	57.57	-52.93	72.41	-26.10	67.70
Fat	-664.32	-120.2	-217.62	-56.40	-103.46	-137.10	-131.86	-114.6	-65.10	-166.29
Moisture	5.83	4.52	8.53	-18.79	-69.61	25.83	-42.88	-34.22	-67.13	-106.50
Ash	25.79	39.61	38.69	44.44	-17.59	77.18	-173.19	69.09	-216.03	74.79
Iron	98.94	52.43	51.92	-100.7	31.57	-47.89	56.07	-55.15	92.93	-39.56
Calcium	9.93	-0.49	-139.73	18.05	-66.44	-66.44	-31.05	31.25	-66.22	-66.22
Energy	-81.57	-38.16	-135.57	-36.48	-91.27	-54.04	-98.21	-30.54	-53.92	-20.73

Table 11: Percentage of loss of preserved Pomfret and Hilsa up to 15days with salt and turmeric

Nutrients Loss (%)	Raw		Boiling		Open pan Dry roasting		Shallow fry		Deep fry	
	Pomfret	*hilsa*	Pomfret	*hilsa*	Pomfret	*hilsa*	Pomfret	*hilsa*	Pomfret	*hilsa*
Carbohydrate	-93.08	9.47	-46.47	72.57	-48.85	4.06	-45.26	23.91	-96.72	19.38
protein	54.15	78.18	21.09	57.44	-34.61	69.08	-1.90	68.68	2.26	70.63
Fat	-1183.6	-66.38	-248.56	-55.25	-140.13	-132.80	-188.21	-162.21	-102.68	-226.2
Moisture	6.66	17.77	28.46	-9.20	-85.61	3.36	-43.90	-68.05	-60.78	-113.0
Ash	44.03	-62.31	5.35	-154.6	-29.62	-19.46	-87.62	-120.90	-205.66	27.91
Iron	-23.94	68.90	-41.66	0.00	46.41	57.14	4.67	-10.30	62.03	43.95
Calcium	-88.07	-199.5	-23.46	-23.46	-116.61	-116.61	-14.81	-14.48	-148.34	-148.3
Energy	-181.29	-1.93	-130.73	-26.13	-99.54	-48.78	-116.04	-55.71	-56.48	-32.12

4.3. Comparison of percentage of nutrient loss due to cooking

Fig. 1, 2, 3, 4, 5, 6, 7, 8 showed the percentage of loss of nutrients of pomfret and hilsa due to cooking of both fresh and preserved with and without preservative. The carbohydrate, protein, moisture, iron and energy content were reduced more in hilsa than in pomfret whereas ash and calcium content were reduced more in pomfret than in hilsa.

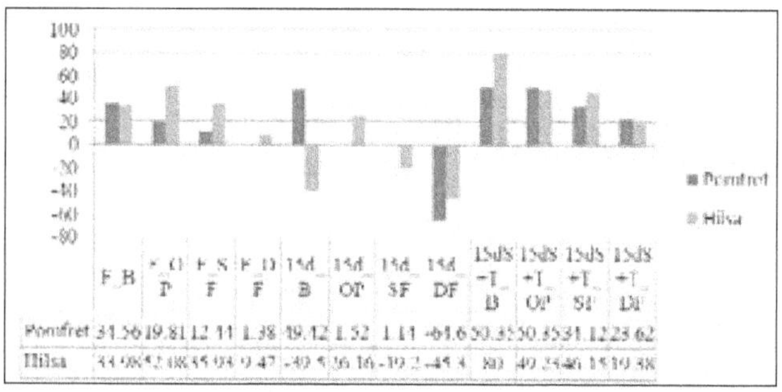

Fig 1: Carbohydrate content of Pomfret and Hilsa

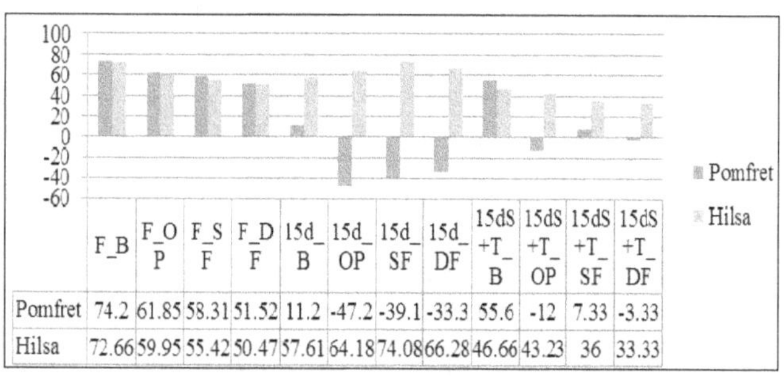

Fig 2: Protein content of Pomfret and Hilsa

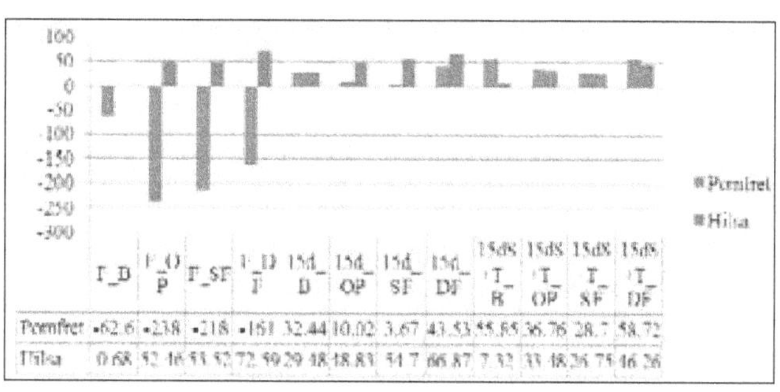

Fig 3: Fat content of Pomfret and Hilsa

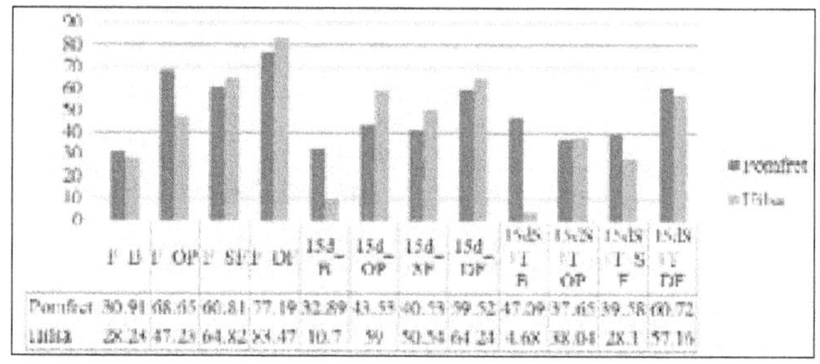

Fig 4: Moisture content of Pomfret and Hilsa

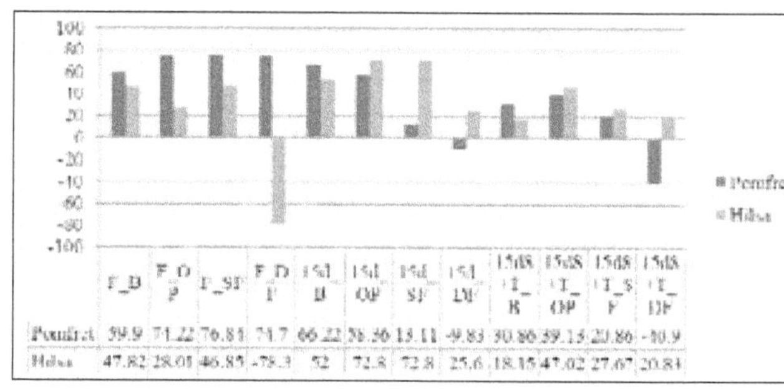

Fig 5: Ash content of Pomfret and Hilsa

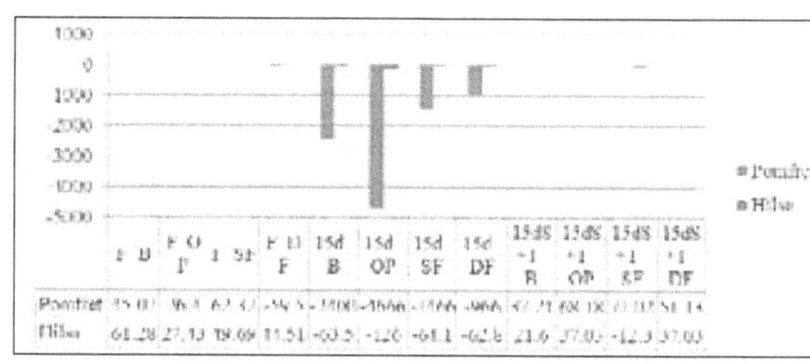

Fig 6: Iron content of Pomfret and Hilsa

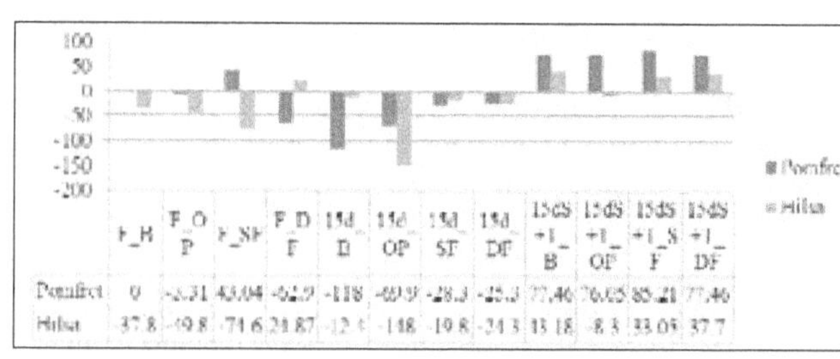

Fig 7: Calcium content of Pomfret and Hilsa

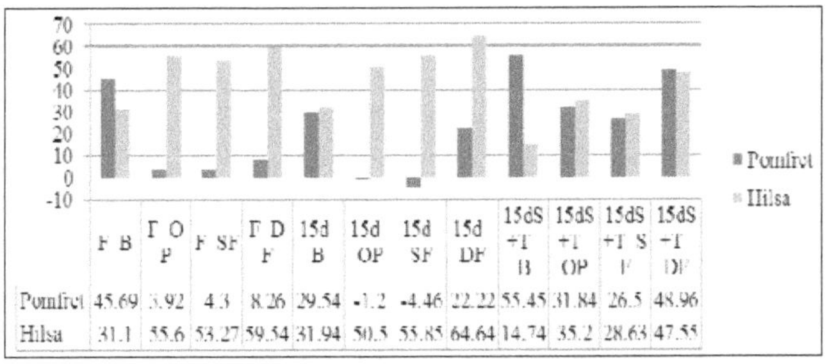

Fig 8: Energy content of Pomfret and Hilsa

5. Discussion

In fresh condition carbohydrate, protein, moisture, ash and energy contents were higher in hilsa but during cooking and preservation nutrient restoration occurred in pomfret. Fat, iron and calcium contents were higher in hilsa rather than in pomfret both in fresh, preserved and cooked conditions. The nutrient content reduced after cooking for both the fish due to application of heat, cooking oil, water [4]. Due to prolonged preservation moisture loss occurred from the sea fish so the nutrients become more concentrated and when these were subjected to cooking, further some moisture loss occurred which could increase the amount of some nutrients than in fresh condition. Pomfret could restore most of the nutrients than hilsa during preservation, mainly when preserved with salt and turmeric. Some nutrient contents were increased in some conditions for both of the fish due to moisture loss as a result of application of heat. Iron content also increased for both of them due to use of iron pan for cooking. Iron content mostly increased in pomfret than in hilsa whereas calcium content reduced mostly in pomfret rather than in hilsa. Energy and fat content is increased in shallow frying mainly due to excess oil consumption whereas other nutrient contents were increased in deep frying. In deep frying method the fish were exposed to excess oil which create a layer of fat surrounding the fish, intern a barrier was formed which reduced the elimination of nutrients from the fish [2]. Most of the losses occurred in boiling. The nutrients were dissolved in cooking water during boiling and throwing out this boiled water could reduce the nutrient contents of the fish [3]. The percentage of loss due to cooking could be reduced by using salt and turmeric. These are the natural preservative which can prevent the microbial growth as well as reduce the protein denaturation and reduce the moisture content of the fish during storage which help to increase the nutrient content of the fish but it is most effective for pomfret rather than hilsa.

6. Conclusion

The maximum losses occurred in hilsa after preservation and cooking rather than in pomfret. The loss percentage due to cooking and preservation for carbohydrate, protein, fat, moisture, iron and energy were higher in hilsa rather than in pomfret, whereas ash and calcium content were better restored in hilsa. Boiling mostly reduced the nutrient content whereas deep frying retained more nutrients. They could be preserved almost up to two weeks but the nutrient retention was better in both the sea fish when preserved with salt and turmeric. After considering all pros and cons, it can be concluded that pomfret is better than hilsa in terms of nutrient restoration after cooking and preservation and the use of combination of salt and turmeric as preservative is effective.

7. Acknowledgement

The University Grants Commission (UGC) is thanked for awarding a Junior Research Fellowship to Uttiya Jana.

8. References

1. Goldman KJ. Regulation of body temperature in the white shark, Carcharodon carcharias. Journal of Comparative Physiology B. 1997; 167(6):423-429.
2. Erkan N, Özden Ö, Selçuk A. Effect of frying, grilling, and steaming on amino acid composition of marine fishes. Journal of medicinal food. 2010; 13(6):1524-1531.
3. Mkandawire KT, Masamba KG. Effect of lemon juice treatment and sun drying on vitamin C retention in three steam and water blanched indigenous vegetables over six weeks storage period. African Journal of Food Science. 2014; 8(6):316-321.
4. Yuan GF, Sun B, Yuan J, Wang QM. Effects of different cooking methods on health-promoting compounds of broccoli. Journal of Zhejiang University Science B. 2009; 10(8):580-588.
5. Marimuthu K, Thilaga M, Kathiresan S, Xavier R, Mas RHMH. Effect of different cooking methods on proximate and mineral composition of striped snakehead fish (Channa striatus, Bloch). Journal of food science and technology. 2012; 49(3):373-377.
6. Ludwig TG, Goldberg HJ. The anthrone method for the determination of carbohydrates in foods and in oral rinsing. Journal of dental research. 1956; 35(1):90-94.
7. Lowry OH, Rosebrough NJ, Farr AL, Randall RJ. Protein measurement with the Folin phenol reagent. Journal of biochemtry. 1951; 193(1):265-275.
8. Manirakiza P, Covaci A, Schepens P. Comparative study on total lipid determination using Soxhlet, Roese-Gottlieb, Bligh & Dyer, and modified Bligh & Dyer extraction methods. Journal of food composition and analysis. 2001; 14(1):93-100.
9. Aberoumand A. Nutrient composition analysis of gish fish fillets affected by different cooking methods. International Food Research Journal. 2014; 21(5):1989-1991.
10. Baker AS, Smith RL. Preparation of solutions for atomic absorption analyses of iron, manganese, zinc, and copper in plant tissue. Journal of agricultural and food chemistry. 1974; 22(1):103-107.
11. Buskirk ER, Mendez J. Energy: caloric requirements, In Nutrition and the Adult, Springer US. 1980, 49-95.

www.ingramcontent.com/pod-product-compliance
Lightning Source LLC
LaVergne TN
LVHW082008200926
848481LV00010B/2821
* 9 7 9 8 2 3 3 6 6 3 8 1 9 *